Perioperative Medi
for Total Joint Arth

Andrea Baldini • Patrizio Caldora
Editors

Perioperative Medical Management for Total Joint Arthroplasty

How to Control Hemostasis, Pain and Infection

Foreword by Thomas P. Sculco

Springer

Editors
Andrea Baldini
Orthopaedics Unit
IFCA Clinic
Florence
Italy

Humanitas Clinical and Research Center
Milan
Italy

Patrizio Caldora
San Donato Hospital
Arezzo
Italy

ISBN 978-3-319-07202-9 ISBN 978-3-319-07203-6 (eBook)
DOI 10.1007/978-3-319-07203-6
Springer Cham Heidelberg New York Dordrecht London

Library of Congress Control Number: 2014950403

Printed on acid-free paper

Springer is part of Springer Science+Business Media (www.springer.com)

To my mentors Paolo Aglietti and Roberto Buzzi, who taught me the scientific methodology. To my mother and father Nicoletta and Renzo, who taught me that everything is possible with positive thinking. To my beloved wife Irene and to my children Alessandro and Ester, to whom I ask forgiveness for all the moments when I was writing, operating or seeing patients

Andrea Baldini

To my wife Cecilia and to my children Giacomo and Ginevra

Patrizio Caldora

Foreword

Total joint arthroplasty is truly one of the great surgical advances of the twentieth century. It has led to relief of pain and improved mobility in countless sufferers of arthritis throughout the world. The surgical techniques and advances in implant design have led to outstanding outcomes in the vast majority of patients undergoing these procedures. In many hospital centers, joint replacement surgery has become a common procedure, and protocols and clinical pathways continue to evolve in the management of these patients. Certainly, as important as surgical outcome is the perioperative management of patients undergoing joint replacement. Today, arthroplasty surgeons are performing replacement surgery on patients who are complex medically and require proficient perioperative management to mitigate serious complications. These include thromboembolic, wound and periprosthetic infection which can be life threatening and catastrophic. Pain management, particularly after total knee replacement, continues to be a problem in a subset of patients and can lead to a poor surgical result. Drs. Andrea Baldini and Patrizio Caldora have edited a magnificent and much needed text which provides crucial information on the perioperative management of the arthroplasty patient. To my knowledge, there is no other text that covers this material in a comprehensive way and brings a multidisciplinary approach to the topic.

The editors have provided current and evidence-based approaches to blood management, thromboembolic prophylaxis, pain management, infection, and wound problem prevention and treatment. Many of these areas remain heavily debated, but each author documents literature-based rationale for the treatment options recommended. The international perspective is another strength of this book in that authors represent a broad spectrum of arthroplasty expertise globally. Each chapter begins with the "open questions" which are still debated and then provides scientific data for the answers to these controversial questions. Do we need potent anticoagulant agents in patients undergoing joint replacement, how can we prevent allogeneic transfusion and when should we transfuse a patient, what is the best anesthetic technique for arthroplasty, how do you manage the recalcitrant pain after arthroplasty, how do you prevent this pain from occurring at all, and what should you do with a draining wound—these are but a few of the important and constantly debated questions in the arthroplasty patient, and answers are provided in this book.

Cost-effectiveness is a topic which is of global concern in heath care and particularly in joint replacement surgery. This is addressed thoroughly in Baldini and Caldora's book in many areas of recovery from joint replacement. Early mobilization of the patient is important to reduce thromboembolic problems, and accelerated clinical pathways have led to early discharge from the hospital. It is crucial, however, that quality and patient safety not be compromised in any measures which reduce cost to the arthroplasty intervention. Often, hospitals harbor virulent and resistant organisms, and the safest environment for the patient is home, and this is emphasized in this text.

I congratulate Drs. Baldini and Caldora on a superb accomplishment in providing a much needed and comprehensive book. It deals with issues of perioperative medicine which are present in a fragmented way in other arthroplasty texts. Here in one place physicians, anesthesiologists, pain management providers, infectious disease experts, and orthopedic surgeons will find the most useful and evidence-based information on significant topics that often determine surgical outcome. It should become a text that is on the desk not sitting on the book shelf of every physician and surgeon that cares for arthroplasty patients.

Thomas P. Sculco
Hospital for Special Surgery
New York, NY, USA

Preface

Scientific research on the medical management of patients undergoing arthroplasty has offered new and useful insights to clinical practice in the last decade. In the field of hip and knee arthroplasty surgery, the medical aspects that most affect the final outcome of the procedure are pain management, hemostasis balance, and infection control.

For this reason, we have asked leading national and international experts to participate in the preparation of this volume, which is divided into three sections: each of these parts include topics related to the management of pain, hemostasis, and infection. The authors – and we thank them deeply – represent all medical figures who work every day around the arthroplasty patient: orthopedic surgeons, anesthesiologists, cardiologists, physiatrists, rheumatologists, and infectious disease specialists.

Enhanced control of postoperative pain and bleeding is nowadays allowing faster recovery of patients compared to the past decades, without associated complication risks. This positively reflects on a multitude of health-related factors. We believe that the orthopedic surgeon should be sensitive to the improvements in the medical management of their patients with the same emphasis they have for the advancements in implant design, materials, and surgical technique.

Several medical aspects in the management of the arthroplasty patients are still controversial. For this reason, some chapters are composed by two authors who are presenting their different points of view around the same topic.

Each chapter is characterized by a specific format, which begins with a list of typical, open questions, the most common issues that the practitioner usually wants to clear in their daily practice; they are answered to throughout the chapter; and they are then outlined in the final list of key points.

We hope that readers of these chapters will find the contents full of hints for learning, practical, and most of all useful. The final beneficiaries of this book will be our patients, who will definitely benefit, during their journey through arthroplasty surgery, from the application of the knowledge and tips offered by our admirable authors.

Florence, Italy — Andrea Baldini
Arezzo, Italy — Patrizio Caldora

Contents

Contributors

Rosanna Abbate Department of Experimental and Clinical Medicine, AOU Careggi, University of Florence, Florence, Italy

Paolo Adravanti Department of Orthopaedics, "Città di Parma" Clinic, Parma, Italy

Jacques Albanese Department of Anaesthesiology, Hôpital de la Conception, Aix-Marseille University, Marseille, France

Pouya Alijanipour Rothman Institute of Orthopaedics at Thomas Jefferson University, Philadelphia, PA, USA

Aldo Ampollini Department of Orthopaedics, "Città di Parma" Clinic, Parma, Italy

Lorenzo Andreani Ortopedia e Traumatologia I, Azienda Ospedaliera Universitaria Pisana, Pisa, Italy

Jean-Noël Argenson Department of Orthopedic Surgery, Institute for Locomotion, Aix-Marseille University, Marseille, France

Tiziana Ascione Department of Infectious Diseases, "D. Cotugno" Hospital, AORN "Dei Colli", Naples, Italy

Giovanni Balato Department of Orthopaedic Surgery, University 'Federico II', Naples, Italy

Andrea Baldini Orthopaedics Unit, IFCA Clinic, Florence, Italy

Humanitas Clinical and Research Center, Milan, Italy

Leonardo Bolognese Cardiovascular and Neurological Department, Azienda Ospedaliera, Arezzo, Italy

Davide Edoardo Bonasia Azienda Ospedaliera Citta' della Salute e della Scienza, Centro Traumatologico Ortopedico Hospital, University of Torino, Torino, Italy

Matteo Bruzzone Mauriziano Umberto I Hospital, University of Torino, Torino, Italy

Giuseppe Calafiore Department of Orthopaedics, "Città di Parma" Clinic, Parma, Italy

Christian Carulli Orthopaedic Clinic, University of Florence, Florence, Italy

Priscilla K. Cavanaugh Rothman Institute of Orthopaedics at Thomas Jefferson University, Philadelphia, PA, USA

Jonathan Lorenzo Chiti Orthopaedic Unit, IFCA Clinic, Florence, Italy

Gabriele Cioni Department of Experimental and Clinical Medicine, AOU Careggi, University of Florence, Florence, Italy

Roberto Civinini Orthopaedic Clinic, University of Florence, Florence, Italy

Giorgio Danelli Department of Anesthesia, Analgesia and Perioperative Medicine, Istituti Ospitalieri di Cremona, Cremona, Italy

David Delahaye Department of Anaesthesiology, Hôpital Sainte-Marguerite, Aix-Marseille University, Marseille, France

Federico Dettoni Mauriziano Umberto I Hospital, University of Torino, Torino, Italy

Lorenzo Drago Clinical-Chemistry and Microbiology Lab, Istituto Ortopedico IRCCS Galeazzi, Milan, Italy

Alberto Farese Infectious and Tropical Diseases Unit, Azienda Ospedlaiero Universitaria Careggi, Florence, Italy

Matteo Carlo Ferrari Hip Orthopedics and Prosthesis, Humanitas Clinical and Research Center, Rozzano, Milan, Italy

Marco Gardini Department of Anesthesia, Intensive Care and Pain Therapy, Azienda Ospedaliero-Universitaria di Parma, Parma, Italy

Grazia Gentilini Immunohematology and Transfusion Service, Azienda Ospedaliero–Universitaria Careggi, Florence, Italy

Alejandro Gonzalez Della Valle Department of Orthopaedic Surgery, Hospital for Special Surgery, New York, NY, USA

Angelo Graceffa Department of Orthopaedic Surgery, Center of Excellence for Articular Replacement (Centro Eccellenza Sostituzioni Articolari Toscana, CESAT), University of Florence, Florence, Italy,

"In Cammino" Foundation, Fucecchio, Florence, Italy

Guido Grappiolo Hip Orthopedics and Prosthesis, Humanitas Clinical and Research Center, Rozzano, Milan, Italy

Irina Grosu Department of Anesthesiology, Cliniques Universitaires St Luc, Brussels, Belgium

Caterina Guarducci Orthopaedics Unit, IFCA Clinic, Florence, Italy

Antonino Gurgone Hip and Knee Arthroplasty and Arthroscopic Unit, Humanitas Clinical and Research Center, Rozzano, Milan, Italy

Snir Heller Rothman Institute of Orthopaedics at Thomas Jefferson University, Philadelphia, PA, USA

Henrik Husted Orthopedic Department, Hvidovre University, Hospital of Copenhagen, Hvidovre, Denmark

Pier Francesco Indelli Department of Orthopaedic Surgery, Center of Excellence for Articular Replacement (Centro Eccellenza Sostituzioni Articolari Toscana, CESAT), University of Florence, Florence, Italy

"In Cammino" Foundation, Fucecchio, Florence, Italy

The Breyer Center for Overseas Study, Stanford University in Florence, Florence, Italy

Massimo Innocenti Orthopaedic Clinic, University of Florence, Florence, Italy

Patricia Lavand'homme Department of Anesthesiology, Cliniques Universitaires St Luc, Brussels, Belgium

Michele Lisanti Ortopedia e Traumatologia I, Azienda Ospedaliera Universitaria Pisana, Pisa, Italy

Nicola Logoluso Center for Reconstructive Surgery and Osteoarticular Infections (Centro di Chirurgia Ricostruttiva e delle Infezioni Osteo-articolari – C.R.I.O.), Istituto Ortopedico IRCCS Galeazzi, Milan, Italy

James H. MacDonald Orthopaedic and Sports Medicine Center, Anne Arundel Medical Center, Annapolis, MD, USA

Massimiliano Marcucci Department of Orthopaedic Surgery, Center of Excellence for Articular Replacement (Centro Eccellenza Sostituzioni Articolari Toscana, CESAT), University of Florence, Florence, Italy

"In Cammino" Foundation, Fucecchio, Florence, Italy

Federica Martorelli Hip and Knee Arthroplasty and Arthroscopic Unit, Humanitas Clinical and Research Center, Rozzano, Milan, Italy

Fabrizio Matassi Orthopaedic Clinic, University of Florence, Florence, Italy

Lorenzo Mattei Mauriziano Umberto I Hospital, University of Torino, Torino, Italy

Francesco Menichetti U.O. Malattie Infettive, Azienda Ospedaliera Universitaria Pisana, Pisa, Italy

Irene Miniati Orthopaedics Unit, IFCA Clinic, Florence, Italy

Giuseppe Musumeci Cardiovascular Department, AO Papa Giovanni XXIII, Bergamo, Italy

Pasquale Pagliano Department of Infectious Diseases, "D. Cotugno" Hospital, AORN "Dei Colli", Naples, Italy

Paolo Parchi Ortopedia e Traumatologia I, Azienda Ospedaliera Universitaria Pisana, Pisa, Italy

Sébastien Parratte Department of Orthopedic Surgery, Institute for Locomotion, Aix-Marseille University, Marseille, France

Javad Parvizi Rothman Institute of Orthopaedics at Thomas Jefferson University, Philadelphia, PA, USA

Maddalena Pazzi Department of Experimental and Clinical Medicine, AOU Careggi, University of Florence, Florence, Italy

Xuan-Phien Pham The Breyer Center for Overseas Study, Stanford University in Florence, Florence, Italy

Nicola Piolanti Ortopedia e Traumatologia I, Azienda Ospedaliera Universitaria Pisana, Pisa, Italy

Giovanni Riccio Regional Center for Infectious Diseases and Septic Orthopedics (Centro Specialistico Regionale Malattie Infettive e Ortopedia Settica, MIOS), Local Healthcare Unit ASL 2 Savonese, Ospedale Santa Maria di Misericordia, Albenga, Italy

Alvaro Ringressi Immunohematology and Transfusion Service, Azienda Ospedaliero–Universitaria Careggi, Florence, Italy

Gabriele Ristori Orthopaedic Clinic, University of Florence, Florence, Italy

Carlo Luca Romanò Center for Reconstructive Surgery and Osteoarticular Infections (Centro di Chirurgia Ricostruttiva e delle Infezioni Osteo-articolari – C.R.I.O.), Istituto Ortopedico IRCCS Galeazzi, Milan, Italy

Lorenza Rossi Department of Experimental and Clinical Medicine, AOU Careggi, University of Florence, Florence, Italy

Roberto Rossi Mauriziano Umberto I Hospital, University of Torino, Torino, Italy

Lorenzo Castellani Reconstructive Articular Surgery Unit, IFCA – Villa Ulivella, Florence, Italy

Roberta Rossini Cardiovascular Department, AO Papa Giovanni XXIII, Bergamo, Italy

Federica Rosso Mauriziano Umberto I Hospital, University of Torino, Torino, Italy

Eduardo A. Salvati Department of Orthopaedic Surgery, Hospital for Special Surgery, New York, NY, USA

Marco Scardino Hip and Knee Arthroplasty and Arthroscopic Unit, Humanitas Clinical and Research Center, Rozzano, Milan, Italy

Erik Schnaser Department of Orthopaedic Surgery, Hospital for Special Surgery, New York, NY, USA

Nigel Sharrock Department of Orthopaedic Surgery, Hospital for Special Surgery, New York, NY, USA

Enrico Tagliaferri U.O. Malattie Infettive, Azienda Ospedaliera Universitaria Pisana, Pisa, Italy

Emmanuel Thienpont Department of Orthopaedics, University Hospital Saint Luc, Brussels, Belgium

Francesco Traverso Hip and Knee Arthroplasty and Arthroscopic Unit, Humanitas Clinical and Research Center, Rozzano, Milan, Italy

Sandrine Wiramus Department of Anaesthesiology, Hôpital de la Conception, Aix-Marseille University, Marseille, France

Part I

Hemostasis Control (Bleeding/ Thromboembolism)

Modern Patient Blood Management in Arthroplasty

1

Grazia Gentilini and Alvaro Ringressi

Open Questions

- Which are the modern transfusion risks and disadvantages?
- How feasible is a patient blood management program in the clinical daily practice?
- How should it be treated preoperative anemia?
- When is autologous blood donation advisable?

1.1 Introduction

One of the oldest and still commonest procedures in clinical practice, allogeneic blood transfusion (ABT), is not fully supported by available evidence. In the last few decades, increasing concerns about unfavorable outcomes associated with ABT, anticipation of future insufficient blood supply, and awareness of the cost (direct and indirect) of transfusion have led to the promotion of patient blood management (PBM) as a cost-effective strategy, beneficial for patients as well as for society (Shander et al. 2010). PBM programs utilize a series of measures with a proven ability to reduce ABT and to be cost-effective. Despite that the impact of PBM on patient clinical outcomes needs to be fully defined and future studies are needed, PBM should be adopted as a new standard of care.

G. Gentilini (✉) • A. Ringressi
Immunohematology and Transfusion Service, Azienda Ospedaliero–Universitaria Careggi, 3, L.go Brambilla, Florence 50134, Italy
e-mail: gentilinig@aou-careggi.toscana.it

1.2 Background

The complex of measures undertaken with a multiprofessional and multidisciplinary approach by medical and surgical staffs, in order to perform planned surgery without transfusion and to improve patient's clinical outcomes, has been termed patient blood management. This issue, regarded as one of the ten key advances in transfusion medicine over the past 50 years, has been fully developed in the last decade, in response to the different needs that emerged at the turn of the millennium. At that time the scenario shows that allogeneic blood transfusion (ABT) is universally considered part of the standard cure in major elective surgery, but relevant variations exist in the use of blood and blood products between countries and both between and within hospitals in the same country. Even limited to lower limb arthroplasty, heterogeneity in the likelihood of transfusion is very large: a 16–85 % and a 7.5–87 % rate of transfusion, for hip and

A. Baldini, P. Caldora (eds.), *Perioperative Medical Management for Total Joint Arthroplasty: How to Control Hemostasis, Pain and Infection*, DOI 10.1007/978-3-319-07203-6_1,

knee surgery, respectively, have been reported (Rosencher et al. 2003; Gombotz et al. 2007). These numbers suggest that standards of care for patients undergoing elective orthopedic surgery are poorly defined, since transfusion rate does not appear to be related to case mix, surgical technique, or anesthetic practices.

Drivers for a change in blood management are different in nature but have contributed to strongly motivate international and national authorities to approve resolutions addressed to national governments and scientific societies. In Rec (2002)11, the European Council recommends member states to arrange appropriate regulatory and advisory bodies both at the national and local levels in order to implement policies encompassing the use of alternatives to allogeneic blood transfusion and preventive strategies to reduce blood loss. In 2010, the World Health Assembly in "Resolution on availability, safety and quality of blood products" (WHA 63.12), "Bearing in mind that patient blood management means that before surgery every reasonable measure should be taken to optimize the patient's own blood volume, to minimize the patient's blood loss and to harness and optimize the patient-specific physiological tolerance of anemia following WHO's guide for optimal clinical use (three pillars of patient blood management)," urged all member states to "promote the availability of transfusion alternatives including, where appropriate, autologous transfusion and patient blood management." Thereafter, regulatory agencies and scientific societies worldwide have developed guidelines and recommendations aimed to reduce the use of allogeneic blood transfusion and also to implement PBM programs. Among others, worthy of mention, the Australian National Blood Authority is in the process of developing six comprehensive modules of a PBM guideline. In particular, Module 2 (available at http://www.blood.gov.au/pbm-module-2) regards PBM in the perioperative setting. In Italy, the national scientific society of transfusion medicine (SIMTI) has emanated a complex of comprehensive recommendations (Liumbruno et al. 2011a, b, c). Also, useful guidelines are found in Leal-Noval et al. (2013).

Historical drives for advances toward the development of PBM have been:

1. Known and unknown risks of transfusion
2. Preservation of national blood inventory
3. Constraints from escalating costs

1.2.1 Risks of Transfusion

Adverse effects to transfusion are traditionally distinguished in acute reactions, which occur in minutes to hours, and delayed, which occur within days to months. Acute reactions include acute hemolytic reactions, febrile nonhemolytic reactions, allergic reactions, transfusion-associated circulatory overload (TACO), transfusion-related acute lung injury (TRALI), and transfusion-related sepsis. Also, hyperkalemia, citrate toxicity, coagulopathy, and hypothermia may occur, especially in the case of massive transfusion. Delayed transfusion reactions include delayed hemolytic reactions, active immunization toward blood cell antigens, iron overload, transfusion-transmitted infections, autoimmunization and posttransfusion purpura, and transfusion-associated graft-versus-host disease.

All these adverse effects, among which some are mostly ascribable to human errors (acute hemolytic reactions, TACO, that are among the main causes of transfusion-associated deaths), are well known, thanks to the reports of nation-based hemovigilance systems. "Haemovigilance is required to identify and prevent occurrence or recurrence of transfusion related unwanted events, to increase the safety, efficacy and efficiency of blood transfusion, covering all activities of the transfusion chain from donor to recipient." The system should include monitoring, identification, reporting, investigation, and analysis of adverse events, near misses, and reactions related to transfusion and manufacturing (WHO, http://www.who.int/bloodsafety/haemovigilance/en). Hemovigilance carries extremely important conclusions and recommendations but entails intrinsic limits. It essentially uses an incident-reporting methodology, where underreporting is common, since adverse effects may be not recognized or not ascribed to transfusion, or due to the lack of a rigorous reporting system. More importantly, some relevant adverse outcomes are not comprehended by an even well-established hemovigilance system but require large clinical studies for coming into light. On the basis of several observational studies and some RCTs, a causative relationship with transfusion has been shown for unfavorable outcomes, including higher mortality, more thrombotic events, organ dysfunction, infections, delayed wound healing, and increased length of hospital stay; transfusion has also been associated with cancer recurrence and insurgence of non-Hodgkin lymphoma (for comprehensive reviews, see Vamvakas and Blajchman 2009; Shander et al. 2011). A dose relationship is present, but complications can be observed after administration of minimal amounts of RBC units (Rubinstein et al. 2013).

In high-income countries, because of the currently adopted diagnostic measures for HBV, HCV, and HIV, the relative transfusion-transmitted infections have been dramatically reduced. For HBV the rate is slightly higher (around 1:200,000), because of the prolonged window period before serologic conversion and because of occult HBV infection (OBI), but further reduction is possible after the introduction of the triplex HBV/HCV/HIV NAT test in some countries (among which Italy) on the basis of HBV infection prevalence. In the last decade, west nile virus (WNV) has constituted a growing challenge for the blood bank system, forcing national authorities in North America and Europe to implement plans for either testing or referring donations, adapted on the base of national and/or local epidemiology reports. Dynamics of migrating populations and tourism are also taken into account as a possible source of infections by epidemiology control bodies, which blood management national authorities refer to. In this respect, reports of transmission through transfusion of newly emerging and reemerging infections, due to protozoan parasites (malaria, babesiosis, Chagas disease, etc.), viruses (dengue, chikungunya, influence strains, coronavirus, etc.), and prions (vCJD), are a matter of concern. Implementation of specific tests for infrequent infections is not an option for unacceptable cost/benefit ratio, and selection of donors has to be guided by up-to-date protocols.

1.2.2 Concerns About Blood Inventory

In high-income countries, ongoing demographic dynamics are characterized by what is described as the "age dependency ratio," that is, the burden of the nonworking population sustained by the working population. Operating a translation in our field, the "total transfusion dependency ratio" (TTDR; Hofmann et al. 2009) has been proposed, that is, non-donating population (aged <17 or >65 years), divided by donating population, multiplied by 100. Such index is suggestive since aged patients account for a large part of all RBC transfused (45 % for patients aged >70 years). In the recently past years, the TTDR was well less than 50 %, but a rapid climb is expected in the next 20 years, escalating over 55 % in several high-income countries (Farmer et al. 2013). In this perspective, a blood supply fulfilling even a steady request can no longer be taken for granted.

1.2.3 Escalating Costs

According to the WHO Global Database on Blood Safety, in 2011, 92 million units of blood were donated, approximately half of which in high-income countries, where direct costs of blood components have progressively increased, due to ameliorated procedures of collection, testing, and processing. When considering real costs of transfusion, a long series of activities involving material resources, technologies, and personnel both in transfusion service laboratories and in the wards (indirect costs) are to be taken into account. Through activity-based costing methodology (Shander et al. 2010), it has been calculated that on average, to transfuse a single RBC unit costs $726–1,183 in the USA and $522–611 in Europe.

This initial approach, mainly aimed to reduce the use of ABT, has evolved toward a patient-centered perspective, where PBM is established in order to ultimately ameliorate patient's clinical outcomes and experience. Still, browsing papers for this discussion, we can realize that PBM continues to be interpreted as the plain concept of avoiding ABT. Even if reduction of ABT in the perioperative course rate remains one of the main end points and this kind of data is easily obtainable, clinical research should develop instruments in order to derive outcomes more relevant for the patient's pathway.

1.3 Focus on PBM

PBM is based on three "pillars":

1. Detection and treatment of perioperative anemia
2. Reduction of surgical blood loss and perioperative coagulopathy
3. Harnessing and optimizing physiological tolerance of anemia

1.3.1 Preoperative Anemia

In the general population, the prevalence of anemia increases with age, being reported as much as 11 and 10.2 % in men and women, respectively, aged more than 65 years (Guralnik et al. 2004). In particular, among candidates for elective orthopedic surgery, one out of three to five is expected to be anemic at preadmission (Bierbaum et al. 1999; Saleh et al. 2007; Spahn 2010). Therefore, till recently, the presence of low-grade anemia has been accepted as a matter of facts, eventually to be corrected through the liberal use of RBC concentrates. Blood components were considered safe, quickly effective, readily available, and relatively inexpensive. As a consequence, preoperative anemia is a predictive factor for perioperative transfusion and still drives a relevant consumption of blood units (Khanna et al. 2003; Shander et al. 2004; Myers et al. 2004; Gruson et al. 2009), as much as 8 % for major orthopedic hip and knee surgery, in a study conducted in north England (Wells et al. 2002).

Preoperative anemia has been independently associated with an increased risk of perioperative adverse outcomes in noncardiac surgery (Carson et al. 1996; Gruson et al. 2002; Dunne et al. 2002; Beattie et al. 2009; Wu et al. 2007; Musallam et al. 2011). Moreover, low preoperative hemoglobin concentration and high patient age are constantly associated with increased risk of transfusion; additional factors are represented by comorbidity, low body weight, complexity of surgery, and female sex (Boralessa et al. 2009; Barr et al. 2011).

1.3.2 Physiological Tolerance of Anemia

Oxygen supply is essential for aerobic metabolism, where it is employed in the process of extraction of energy from organic molecules. In multicellular, complex organisms, the atmospheric oxygen reaches the tissues by diffusing through specifically developed organs and vascular structures in a liquid system, that is, blood, from which it can diffuse in peripheral tissues. More complex organisms rely on a high-efficiency carrier for oxygen in the bloodstream, for at the atmospheric partial pressure of oxygen (21 %), the amount dissolved in the water solvent would not be sufficient for life. Therefore, in mammals, the presence of an adequate quota of oxygen in the inhaled air, anatomical and functional integrity of the lungs and its vascularization, and adequate blood flow and hemoglobin content are critical for the survival of cells. Even simple organisms have developed mechanisms for sensing reduction in oxygen delivery; in more complex organisms, oxygen sensors are multiple, existing in cells (hypoxia-inducible factor, HIF), organelle (aortic and carotid chemoreceptors), and organs (kidney). When hypoxia occurs, these mechanisms become activated, ultimately leading to the adaptive phenomena that we observe during blood loss and anemia. In acute anemia, partial pressure of oxygen in arterial blood (PaO_2) and hemoglobin-oxygen saturation (SaO_2) are maximized by means of an increased ventilation and a more efficient ventilation/perfusion matching, occurring through a NO-mediated mechanism. The cardiovascular system undergoes fundamental modifications in response to acute normovolemic anemia: through activation of the sympathetic nervous system, after stimulation of vascular chemoreceptors, both heart rate and stroke volume are increased, the resulting cardiac output (CO) augmented up to threefold in the presence of intact adaptive mechanisms. Moreover, vasodilation occurs, determining a reduction in systemic vascular resistance. Importantly, regional differences in CO are established, through differentiated degrees of vasodilation; thus, vital organs are initially preserved, the heart and the brain receiving a higher proportion of CO. Instead, the kidney appears to have a lower margin for compensation and becomes injured earlier, insomuch as hemoglobin concentration drops below 7 g/dl, during cardiac surgery (Habib et al. 2003; Karkouti et al. 2005). Increased CO is also related to reduced blood viscosity and increased venous return, associated with vasoconstriction in the splanchnic district. The relevance of adrenergic activation as a compensative mechanism is highlighted by what has been considered a paradoxical effect of β-blockade during blood loss, that is, an increased rate of perioperative myocardial infarction (van Klei et al. 2009) and stroke (Devereaux et al. 2008), following administration of adrenergic antagonists. Another compensative mechanism for tissue hypoxia is an increased peripheral oxygen extraction, consequent to lowered hemoglobin-oxygen affinity (for increased 2,3-DPG, reduced pH, and NO-mediated events) and overall enlarged capillary bed. On the other hand, some organs reduce their oxygen demand, in front of an increase in consumption by the myocardium.

In humans, tolerance of anemia has been addressed in observational studies, involving patients for whom transfusion is not an option, for unavailability or refuse; also, experimental investigations have been carried out in voluntaries. When normovolemia is maintained, Hb concentrations as low as 5 g/dl can be tolerated without adverse systemic effects (Weiskopf et al. 1998). After noncardiac surgery, Hb levels ≤ 7 g/dl are associated with some morbidity, but not mortality; risk of mortality increases by a factor of 1.5, for every 1 g/dl decrement below 7 g/dl (Carson et al. 2002).

In healthy subjects at steady conditions, oxygen delivery (DO_2) meets tissue oxygen demand (VO_2), exceeding fivefold the consumption at rest. However, there are relevant intraindividual differences in oxygen consumption depending on metabolic requirement. More importantly, wide interindividual differences in anemia tolerance exist, due to impairment in ill subjects of part of the compensatory mechanisms described above. In surgery settings, comorbidity, primarily cardiovascular disease, ultimately greatly increases the rate of death in postoperatively anemic patients (Carson et al. 1996, 2002).

Perioperatively, an acute blood loss is anticipated, and medical support is aimed to maintain normovolemia and to optimize the oxygen delivery/oxygen demand ratio, in order to prevent ischemic organ injury. Possible strategies therefore include measures aimed to increase DO_2 and possibly to reduce VO_2. Since $DO_2 = CaO_2 \times CO$ (where CaO_2 is the arterial oxygen content), a feasible approach to increase CaO_2 is hyperoxic ventilation, with the aim to maximize the amount of the gas physically dissolved in plasma that can become a relevant quota available for tissue oxygenation in the presence of low Hb concentrations. To support CO, inotropic drugs are used in acute normovolemic anemia. On the other hand, a reduced oxygen demand can be obtained with neuromuscular blockade, as well as induction of anesthesia. Depth of anesthesia also affects anemia tolerance, but handling this tool is not commonly practicable (see Meier and Gombotz 2013).

Current existing guidelines covering transfusion thresholds in acutely anemic patients rely on these and a number of other observational studies, as well as randomized clinical trials. This issue will be addressed in this volume by Husted and Gentilini and Ringressi. Overall, compliance with available guidelines, compiled by scientific societies and advisory bodies (see Carson et al. 2012; Retter et al. 2013; Shander et al. 2013), is a main cornerstone of PBM programs and must be highlighted when such programs are offered.

It must be stated that benefits, effectiveness, and cost-effectiveness of complete PBM programs have been not fully proven yet. It is difficult to argue against the overall beneficial outcomes of a program encompassing several measures, all aimed to reduce ABT, improve clinical outcomes, and reduce costs. Nevertheless, although the effects of single measures are mostly known, we cannot really anticipate the effect of a complex of measures, possibly being addictive, synergistic, or even paradoxically counteracting. Studies involving a large population are needed in order to address this question, in the form of CRTs, targeting clinically relevant outcomes, or in the form of registries collecting safety and effectiveness data on patients managed in a PBM program (Gross et al. 2013). So far, initiatives involving local institutions have demonstrated the feasibility of implementing PBM programs, achieving extremely relevant goals such as fewer transfusion administered, reduced mortality and complications, lenght of stay (LOS), readmissions, and costs (Kotzé et al. 2012; Leahy et al. 2012). A recently published study (So-Osman et al. 2014a), combining restrictive transfusion thresholds, erythropoietin administration, and/or autologous blood reinfusion, reports effectiveness (but not cost-effectiveness) of erythropoietin administration, but it shows lack of benefit for cell salvage/drain reinfusion in patients with Hb levels 10–13 g/dl.

PBM therefore is not simply a transfusion alternative, as PBM programs consider a complex of practical measures, also including alternatives to transfusion. A series of tools utilizable in PBM programs is listed in Table 1.1. Single programs do not encompass all the possible measures (indeed, some are necessarily alternative),

Table 1.1 Tools for PBM programs in elective orthopedic surgery

Preadmission	Evaluation	Detect anemia and diagnose
		Detect hemostasis defects and diagnose
		Anticipate intraoperative blood loss
		Type and screen
	Interval	Treat anemia (iron, ESAs, vitamin B12, folate)
		Optimize hemostasis (withdrawal of interfering drugs)
		PABD
Admission		
Surgery		Preoperative normovolemic hemodilution
		Physical tools (body position, tourniquet, etc.)
		Blood-saving surgical techniques
		Blood-saving anesthesiology measures, including regional anesthesia
		Normothermia
		Normotension (controlled hypotension)
		Tranexamic acid
		Pharmacological support to increase CO
		Hyperoxic ventilation
		Fibrin sealants and other topic treatments
		Transfusion guidelines
		Intraoperative cell salvage
		Limit blood drawing for tests
Postoperative period		Normothermia
		Iron ± ESA
		No drain
		Postoperative shed blood reinfusion
		Transfusion guidelines
		Pharmacological support to increase DO_2
		Hyperoxic ventilation
		Limit blood drawing for tests

but a combination of some, of which a priority has to be put on the treatment of preoperative anemia, blood-sparing surgery technique, adequate hemostasis, medical support for optimization of anemia tolerance, and adhesion to protocols concerning transfusion thresholds. The choice of the measures to be undertaken has to be done on the basis of the patient's characteristics, expected blood loss, and kind of surgery, but also it has to be driven by organizational features that can condition the patient's pathway. Even though a whole process of validation of PBM programs has not been carried out, PBM in elective surgery is to be regarded as a new standard of care, and there is no reason to delay further its implementation in our institutions.

1.4 Structure of PBM Programs

As mentioned above, PBM is a multiprofessional and multidisciplinary strategy; therefore, from a managerial standpoint, its implementation will require drawing a new pathway for patients candidate for elective orthopedic surgery, with involvement of different specialists, among which anesthetists are to play a major role. The draw should be robust, including detailed algorithms for the management of patients with different features and needs, going through the various steps (e.g., see Kotzé et al. 2012). Also, organization of continue education and controlled communication processes should be included.

1.4.1 Preoperative Management

1.4.1.1 Preoperative Assessment

In elective surgery, a preadmission assessment of patient's clinical conditions is generally performed some 30 days before surgery. Potential benefits include increased patient safety, reduced cancellation or delay of surgery, reduced LOS, and increased quality of patient experience. Pillars of preanesthesia evaluation are medical records, patient interview, and physical examination and tests, where indicated (NICE 2003; ASA 2012): major surgery schedule for adults includes a complete blood cell count and blood typing (T&S).

In a PBM program, such schedule is to be further integrated with the ultimate aim of optimizing patient's medical health prior to surgery, ultimately avoiding unnecessary transfusions. For the weight that anemia has as a prognostic factor of unfavorable outcome, its diagnosis is central to subsequent correction. Etiology is heterogeneous, and unexpected diseases such as chronic kidney failure or occult malignancy are to be considered. In these cases, referral to appropriate specialist is necessary, before planning any elective surgery. Overall, iron-restricted erythropoiesis as the most relevant abnormal condition in elderly and chronic inflammation are common in candidates for lower limb arthroplasty (Spahn 2010). Consequently, the "iron status" must be assessed, by measuring blood ferritin and TSAT, together with an inflammation index (CRP). These tests can be ordered contemporaneously to full blood cell count or later, only for anemic patients, depending on organizational constrains (Goodnough et al. 2011; Royal Cornwall Hospitals 2013).

All the collected data will lead to discriminate among three possible conditions:

- Absolute iron deficiency, due to blood loss, nutritional deficiency, or malabsorption
- Functional iron deficiency, for increased erythron iron requirements (treatment with ESAs, hemoglobinopathies, or hemolytic anemias)
- Iron sequestration, in the presence of inflammation, through a hepcidin-dependent mechanism (Weiss and Goodnough 2005)

In elderly population, also vitamin B12 and folate deficiency are relatively common (Bisbe et al. 2008; Saleh et al. 2007). We suggest to order their dosage (as a reflex test) when defects are suspected, i.e., when macrocytosis is present.

In order to minimize blood loss during surgery, the assessment of hemorrhagic risk constitutes a priority. Algorithms for scoring the risk are available (Tosetto et al. 2007; Nichols et al. 2008). Fundamental is the interview, where any personal and family history of bleeding disorders must be uncovered, as well as the use of medicaments, both prescribed or not. Besides anticoagulant or antiplatelet drugs, agents that are able to interfere with hemostasis include NSAIDs, serotonin reuptake inhibitor antidepressants, and herbal remedies such as garlic, ginkgo biloba, ginseng, and others (Ang-Lee et al. 2001).

Preoperative evaluation must also assess a transfusion strategy, beginning with the prediction of the need for ABT. Apposite algorithms have been elaborated (Mercuriali and Inghilleri 1996; Noticewala et al. 2012; Park et al. 2013), taking into account surgical technique, procedure duration, hemostatic measures, and patient's features. On the basis of that, alternatives to transfusion are to be planned, including the use of autologous blood and/or pharmacological treatments.

For major surgery, a preadmission ABO/Rh typing should be ordered. Instead, the usefulness of a red cell antibody screening depends on patient's history (previous transfusions) and on organizational peculiarities, i.e., it is advisable if pre-transfusion tests and cross-matched blood may be not available because of time constraints, when surgery occurs shortly after admission.

1.4.1.2 Preoperative Measures

Nutritional deficiencies should be treated by proper vitamin and/or mineral medicament, besides a correct diet. Treatment of iron-restricted erythropoiesis is particularly important for the prevalence of preoperative anemia and for its unfavorable consequences. It is based on the availability of two classes of agents: iron, in oral and IV formulations, and erythropoiesis-stimulating agents (ESAs).

1.4.1.3 Iron Therapy

In brief, oral iron therapy, when tolerated, will work appropriately in most iron-deficient patients, unless an absorption defect is present. When a diagnosis is made of functional iron deficiency, iron sequestration, or mixed anemia, IV iron therapy may be necessary, particularly in the presence of a systemic inflammatory response, because of inhibition of gastrointestinal absorption caused by increased hepcidin levels. At present, IV iron is included in guidelines as a recommended pharmacological measure aimed to reduce transfusion rate (Leal-Noval et al. 2013). Several formulations are available for IV use, currently for different anemic conditions. High-molecular-weight iron dextran (HMWD) should be abandoned in favor of low-molecular-weight iron dextran (LMWD), for a lower rate of adverse reactions. Ferric gluconate and iron sucrose are formulations widely used in chronic kidney disease, but adverse effects are not rare. The recently introduced ferumoxytol does not require dilution for slow IV use, in contrast to iron sucrose and sodium ferric gluconate. Ferric carboxymaltose and iron isomaltoside, still in the course of study for some applications, are proposed, as well as ferumoxytol, for total dose infusion, that is, a slow infusion of 1–1.5 g. The European Medicines Agency's Committee for Medicinal Products for Human Use (CHMP; 2013) has emanated new recommendations to manage risk of allergic reactions with intravenous iron-containing medicines indicating that IV iron medicines are used when iron supplements given by mouth cannot be used or do not work and staff trained to evaluate and manage anaphylactic and anaphylactoid reactions must be immediately available, as well as resuscitation facilities. Moreover, the utility of test dose is underscored, and a 30-min period of observation after infusion is prescribed.

1.4.1.4 Erythropoiesis-Stimulating Agents (ESAs)

In the late 1980s, ESAs were first approved for use in chronic kidney disease patients, who mostly continue to benefit of this therapy. Later on, ESAs have also been approved for oncology patients suffering from chemotherapy-induced anemia and for patients candidate for elective surgery, even though not universally. In particular, in many European countries, ESA preoperative use is not approved, unless preoperative autologous blood donation (PABD) is scheduled. More recently, following post-approval clinical trials, targeting risk of thrombotic adverse effects of ESAs, and overall increased rate of morbidity and mortality, limits for their use have been indicated, in respect to Hb levels and an appropriate antithrombotic prophylaxis, by regulatory agencies.

Used preoperatively, ESAs are able to increase Hb levels, being the equivalent of 1 RBC unit produced by day 7 of treatment. In the course of a PABD program, 5 units can be produced with a timing compatible with storage and use during surgery (Goodnough et al. 1992). Most effective dosage and timing of administration are debated, and diverse schedules are used. Low doses of erythropoietin (400 U/kg over a 2-week period) are sufficient to exert a significant stimulus on erythropoiesis (Sans et al. 1996). Even a single administration of erythropoietin plus iron, 1 day before surgery, has been found to be effective in reducing the need in ABT in cardiac surgery (Yoo et al. 2011). Aggressive schedules are employed in the course of a PABD program, when the RBC mass produced on a 3-week period, directly related to erythropoietin dosage, can be anticipated: RBC volume (ml per kg) = 6.34 + 0.0013*X*, where *X* equals the total units of erythropoietin administered, per kg body weight (Goodnough et al. 1994). Throughout the course of ESA treatment, iron supplementation is necessary to maximize the RBC production stimulated by ESAs.

1.4.1.5 Withdrawal of Drugs

In order to prevent severe blood loss, withdrawal of anticoagulant or antiplatelet drugs is recommended, unless critical for patient's safety. Under usual circumstances, warfarin and aspirin should be discontinued, 5 days before surgery, but at least 7 days of withdrawal are necessary for clopidogrel. Stopping aspirin and/or clopidogrel for secondary prevention should be carefully weighted case by case, after discussion with the prescribing cardiologist, but maintaining low-dose aspirin is mostly recommended (Korte et al. 2011; Royal Cornwall Hospitals 2013). Experiences of urgent orthopedic surgery in patients on antiplatelet drugs should relieve general concerns about excessive perioperative bleeding (Collinge et al. 2012; Feely et al. 2013). The BRIDGE trial, targeting bridging for anticoagulation, is still ongoing.

The use of other, nonprescribed drugs and herbal remedies possibly interfering with the hemostatic process is to be discouraged. Classical NSAIDs, because of their short half-life, usually do not raise concern of intraoperative bleeding; also, there is no indication for withdrawal of COX-2 inhibitors, provided adverse cardiac effects are taken into account. Serotonin reuptake inhibitor antidepressants have been imputed to enhance perioperative bleeding, but so far a clear evidence of increased risk of ABT is lacking; it is advisable to avoid coadministration with aspirin (Movig et al. 2003; van Haelst et al. 2010). For recommended behavior regarding perioperative use of drugs, see a list in Royal Cornwall Hospitals (2013).

1.4.1.6 Autologous Blood Donation

Preoperative autologous blood donation (PABD), consisting of collecting and storing the patient's own blood prior to surgery, has been widely practiced in different surgical settings, offered to patients as a main alternative to ABT. Indeed, PABD programs in major orthopedic surgery have caused a reduction in risk of ABT (Rosencher et al. 2003; Carless et al. 2004). Greater effectiveness is obtained when a PABD program is integrated with treatment with an ESA. Yet, the overall risk of transfusion is increased, entailing an increased risk of clerical errors as well as some kind of complication also presented by PABD (TACO, fever and chills, infections, possibly immunomodulation). These and other disadvantages (over-collection, outdating, wasting) are to be taken into account in order to evaluate PABD cost/benefit ratio. The British Committee for Standards in Hematology (2007) emanated internationally recognized guidelines that do not recommend PABD unless specific conditions are present. In particular, patients still considerable candidate for PABD are children with scoliosis, patients who refuse transfusion but would consent to PABD, bearers of rare blood groups, or who are poly-immunized. A PABD program, in combination with blood salvage, may be beneficial in bilateral TKA (Boettner et al. 2009).

1.4.2 Intraoperative Management

Normothermia should be maintained intra- and postoperatively, in order to sustain physiologic hemostasis and reduce blood loss and need for transfusion (Rajagopalan et al. 2008). For methods of fulfilling this requirement, refer to specific literature.

Acute normovolemic hemodilution, consisting of the collection of 2–4 units of whole blood exchanged with crystalloid/colloid solutions and performed in the operating theater, immediately preceding surgery, doesn't seem beneficial in the orthopedic setting (Carless et al. 2004). It is to be considered only in combination with other blood-sparing measures in selected patients undergoing spine surgery (Shander and Rijhwani 2004).

Intraoperative cell salvage is restricted to settings concerning high risk of intraoperative bleeding. In arthroplasty, it may be considered for hip surgery in a subpopulation of patients in which an expected substantial blood loss cannot be prevented by different means.

The use of antifibrinolytic drugs (i.e., tranexamic acid) has been found to be effective in minimizing blood loss in lower limb arthroplasty, more remarkably in TKA, also proving cost-effectiveness (see Henry et al. 2011; Ker et al. 2013; Irisson et al. 2012). Concerns about its safety are not completely relieved: they would be not justified for some authors (Henry et al. 2011; Sukeik et al. 2011), whereas Australian authors solicit a post-market surveillance program (Bruce et al. 2013). Different schedules are used for administering tranexamic acid, taking into account its short half-life. In TKA, when a tourniquet is used, administration must precede its release, given the activation of fibrinolysis occurring thereafter. Tranexamic acid has also been used topically in TKA and THA, obtaining a significant reduction of postoperative blood loss, without relevant complications (Wong et al. 2010; Ishida et al. 2011; Alshryda et al. 2013a, b).

In TKA, topically applied blood components, such as fibrin sealants, have been shown to be safe and effective in reducing total blood loss and ABT rate (Liu et al. 2013). In addition, some authors (Everts et al. 2006), but not others (Diiorio et al. 2012), have also found platelet gel to be effective. As a consequence, definitive recommendations on topically applied blood components cannot at present be drawn.

1.4.3 Postoperative Management

In TKA, some 50 % of the total blood loss occurs during the postoperative period (Sehat et al. 2004). Therefore, drainage is a common practice, aimed to reduce the occurrence of wound hematomas and compression of vital structures, meanwhile permitting the application of salvage/reinfusion systems. To date, two kinds of blood salvage systems are considered safe and effective, therefore widely used, including or not washing of blood cells. About the discussion on the features and safety profiles of the two systems, see Muñoz et al. (2011).

Recently, the real efficacy of closed suction drainage has been questioned, emerging that it causes an increased need for allogeneic blood transfusion (Parker et al. 2007). Instead, the use of low-vacuum drains with salvage/reinfusion systems is associated with a reduced rate of ABT and LOS (Markar et al. 2012; Haien et al. 2013). On the other hand, the use of antifibrinolytic drugs appears to be as effective as reinfusion drains in lowering the risk of ABT (Sasanuma et al. 2011) and significantly reduces the volume of shed blood, therefore rendering useless its collection (Iwai et al. 2013; Oremus et al. 2014).

To date, randomized trials comparing low-vacuum drain/blood salvage versus no drain in TKA are still insufficient. One recent study with such a design shows that the "drain" group of patients presents a higher Hb level during a 3-day postoperative period, together with lower net blood loss (Horstmann et al. 2013). This study was not powered enough to detect significant differences in either ABT or complication rate.

It seems reasonable to argue that if postoperative drains are to be used, especially on the basis of an expected high postoperative blood loss in diverse conditions, such as in hemophilic patients (Kang et al. 2014), application of a low-vacuum salvage/reinfusion system still represents the best option in order to prevent ABT need. Cost-effectiveness is debated, as Muñoz et al. (2013) found that in TKA, postoperative blood salvage would also be cost-effective in most cases, that is, in patients presenting at surgery with Hb ≤15 g/dl; instead, for patients presenting with Hb >13 g/dl, any form of blood salvage would be useless and would increase costs, according to So-Osman et al. (2014b). Indeed, it is to be considered that institutions in which postsurgery strategies generally do not include drainage would afford relevant costs in case of sporadic use of postoperative blood salvage, because of both cost of devices and skill maintenance.

The use of iron and ESAs has also been proposed as immediate postoperative treatment aimed to accelerate early recovery from postoperative anemia. More trials are needed to draw any conclusion, but the use of one of two different IV iron formulations on postoperative days of lower limb arthroplasty has been effective in reducing rate of transfusion, without incremental costs (Muñoz et al. 2014).

In conclusion, in this discussion we have focused on the philosophy of PBM and on the instruments that can be used when drawing PBM programs. Aware of difficulties that may hamper their implementation, we solicit managers of public and private institutions to actively promote projects for implementation of beneficial and cost-effective PBM pathways.

Key Points

- PBM strategy has been developed because of concerns about safety of blood transfusion, future blood supply shortage, and escalating costs.
- Presently, PBM strategy is "patient centered," aiming not only to avoid blood transfusion but also target patient clinical outcomes.
- PBM implementation requires a solid design, including algorithms for management of all kinds of patients and taking into account educational and communication issues.
- Priority must be given to the treatment of preoperative anemia, improving anemia tolerance, reduction of blood loss by means of blood-sparing surgical techniques and careful hemostasis, and adherence to protocols for administering ABT.
- Despite scarcity of evidence concerning the whole protocol of PBM, adequate rationale exists for promoting wide implementation of PBM programs. Further studies are needed in order to target relevant clinical outcomes.

References

Alshryda S, Mason J, Sarda P, Nargol A, Cooke N, Ahmad H, Tang S, Logishetty R, Vaghela M, McPartlin L, Hungin AP (2013a) Topical (intra-articular) tranexamic acid reduces blood loss and transfusion rates following total hip replacement: a randomized controlled trial (TRANX-H). J Bone Joint Surg Am 95(21):1969–1974

Alshryda S, Mason J, Vaghela M, Sarda P, Nargol A, Maheswaran S, Tulloch C, Anand S, Logishetty R, Stothart B, Hungin AP (2013b) Topical (intra-articular) tranexamic acid reduces blood loss and transfusion rates following total knee replacement: a randomized controlled trial (TRANX-K). J Bone Joint Surg Am 95(21):1961–1968

Ang-Lee MK, Moss J, Yuan CS (2001) Herbal medicines and perioperative care. JAMA 286(2):208–216

ASA (2012) Practice advisory for preanesthesia evaluation: an updated report by the American Society of Anesthesiologists Task Force on Pre Transfusion Anesthesiol 116(3):522–538

Barr PJ, Donnelly M, Cardwell C, Alam SS, Morris K, Parker M, Bailie KE (2011) Drivers of transfusion decision making and quality of the evidence in orthopedic surgery: a systematic review of the literature. Transfus Med Rev 25(4):304–316.e1–6

Beattie WS, Karkouti K, Wijeysundera DN, Tait G (2009) Risk associated with preoperative anemia in noncardiac surgery: a single-center cohort study. Anesthesiology 110(3):574–581

Bierbaum BE, Callaghan JJ, Galante JO, Rubash HE, Tooms RE, Welch RB (1999) An analysis of blood management in patients having a total hip or knee arthroplasty. J Bone Joint Surg Am 81(1):2–10

Bisbe E, Castillo J, Sáez M, Santiveri X, Ruiz A, Muñoz M (2008) Prevalence of preoperative anemia and hematinic deficiencies in patients scheduled for elective major orthopedic surgery. Transfus Alternat Transfus Med 10(4):166–73

Boettner F, Sculco P, Altneu E, Capar B, Sculco TP (2009) Efficiency of autologous blood donation in combination with a cell saver in bilateral total knee arthroplasty. HSS J 5(1):45–48

Boralessa H, Goldhill DR, Tucker K, Mortimer AJ, Grant-Casey J (2009) National comparative audit of blood use in elective primary unilateral total hip replacement surgery in the UK. Ann R Coll Surg Engl 91(7):599–605

British Committee for Standards in Haematology, Transfusion Task Force, Boulton FE, James V (2007) Guidelines for policies on alternatives to allogeneic blood transfusion. 1. Predeposit autologous blood donation and transfusion. Transfus Med 17(5):354–365

Bruce W, Campbell D, Daly D, Isbister J (2013) Practical recommendations for patient blood management and the reduction of perioperative transfusion in joint replacement surgery. ANZ J Surg 83(4):222–229

Carless P, Moxey A, O'Connell D, Henry D (2004) Autologous transfusion techniques: a systematic review of their efficacy. Transfus Med 14(2):123–144

Carson JL, Duff A, Poses RM, Berlin JA, Spence RK, Trout R, Noveck H, Strom BL (1996) Effect of anaemia and cardiovascular disease on surgical mortality and morbidity. Lancet 348(9034):1055–1060
Carson JL, Noveck H, Berlin JA, Gould SA (2002) Mortality and morbidity in patients with very low postoperative Hb levels who decline blood transfusion. Transfusion 42(7):812–818
Carson JL, Grossman BJ, Kleinman S, Tinmouth AT, Marques MB, Fung MK, Holcomb JB, Illoh O, Kaplan LJ, Katz LM, Rao SV, Roback JD, Shander A, Tobian AA, Weinstein R, Swinton McLaughlin LG, Djulbegovic B, Clinical Transfusion Medicine Committee of the AABB (2012) Red blood cell transfusion: a clinical practice guideline from the AABB*. Ann Intern Med 157(1):49–58
Collinge CA, Kelly KC, Little B, Weaver T, Schuster RD (2012) The effects of clopidogrel (Plavix) and other oral anticoagulants on early hip fracture surgery. J Orthop Trauma 26(10):568–573
Devereaux PJ, Yang H, Yusuf S, Guyatt G, Leslie K, Villar JC, Xavier D, Chrolavicius S, Greenspan L, Pogue J, Pais P, Liu L, Xu S, Málaga G, Avezum A, Chan M, Montori VM, Jacka M, Choi P (2008) Effects of extended-release metoprolol succinate in patients undergoing non-cardiac surgery (POISE trial): a randomised controlled trial. Lancet 371(9627): 1839–1847
Diiorio TM, Burkholder JD, Good RP, Parvizi J, Sharkey PF (2012) Platelet-rich plasma does not reduce blood loss or pain or improve range of motion after TKA. Clin Orthop Relat Res 470(1):138–143
Dunne JR, Malone D, Tracy JK, Gannon C, Napolitano LM (2002) Perioperative anemia: an independent risk factor for infection, mortality, and resource utilization in surgery. J Surg Res 102(2):237–244
European Medicines Agency's Committee for Medicinal Products for Human Use (CHMP) (2013) http://www.ema.europa.eu/docs/en_GB/document_library/Press_release/2013/06/WC500144874.pdf. Last accessed on 31 Jan 2013
Everts PA, Devilee RJ, Brown Mahoney C, Eeftinck-Schattenkerk M, Box HA, Knape JT, van Zundert A (2006) Platelet gel and fibrin sealant reduce allogeneic blood transfusions in total knee arthroplasty. Acta Anaesthesiol Scand 50(5):593–599
Farmer SL, Towler SC, Leahy MF, Hofmann A (2013) Drivers for change: Western Australia Patient Blood Management Program (WA PBMP), World Health Assembly (WHA) and Advisory Committee on Blood Safety and Availability (ACBSA). Best Pract Res Clin Anaesthesiol 27(1):43–58
Feely MA, Mabry TM, Lohse CM, Sems SA, Mauck KF (2013) Safety of clopidogrel in hip fracture surgery. Mayo Clin Proc 88(2):149–156
Gombotz H, Rehak PH, Shander A, Hofmann A (2007) Blood use in elective surgery: the Austrian benchmark study. Transfusion 47(8):1468–1480
Goodnough LT, Price TH, Rudnick S, Soegiarso RW (1992) Preoperative red cell production in patients undergoing aggressive autologous blood phlebotomy with and without erythropoietin therapy. Transfusion 32(5):441–445
Goodnough LT, Verbrugge D, Marcus RE, Goldberg V (1994) The effect of patient size and dose of recombinant human erythropoietin therapy on red blood cell volume expansion in autologous blood donors for elective orthopedic operation. J Am Coll Surg 179(2):171–176
Goodnough LT, Maniatis A, Earnshaw P, Benoni G, Beris P, Bisbe E, Fergusson DA, Gombotz H, Habler O, Monk TG, Ozier Y, Slappendel R, Szpalski M (2011) Detection, evaluation, and management of preoperative anaemia in the elective orthopaedic surgical patient: NATA guidelines. Br J Anaesth 106(1):13–22
Gross I, Shander A, Sweeney J (2013) Patient blood management and outcome, too early or not? Best Pract Res Clin Anaesthesiol 27(1):161–172
Gruson KI, Aharonoff GB, Egol KA, Zuckerman JD, Koval KJ (2002) The relationship between admission hemoglobin level and outcome after hip fracture. J Orthop Trauma 16(1):39–44
Gruson KI, Accousti KJ, Parsons BO, Pillai G, Flatow EL (2009) Transfusion after shoulder arthroplasty: an analysis of rates and risk factors. J Shoulder Elbow Surg 18(2):225–230
Guralnik JM, Eisenstaedt RS, Ferrucci L, Klein HG, Woodman RC (2004) Prevalence of anemia in persons 65 years and older in the United States: evidence for a high rate of unexplained anemia. Blood 104(8): 2263–2268
Habib RH, Zacharias A, Schwann TA, Riordan CJ, Durham SJ, Shah A (2003) Adverse effects of low hematocrit during cardiopulmonary bypass in the adult: should current practice be changed? J Thorac Cardiovasc Surg 125(6):1438–1450
Haien Z, Yong J, Baoan M, Mingjun G, Qingyu F (2013) Post-operative auto-transfusion in total hip or knee arthroplasty: a meta-analysis of randomized controlled trials. PLoS One 8(1):e55073
Henry DA, Carless PA, Moxey AJ, O'Connell D, Stokes BJ, Fergusson DA, Ker K (2011) Anti-fibrinolytic use for minimising perioperative allogeneic blood transfusion. Cochrane Database Syst Rev (3):CD001886
Hofmann A, Farmer S, Shander A (2009) Cost-effectiveness in haemotherapies and transfusion medicine. ISBT Sci Ser 4(2):423–435
Horstmann W, Kuipers B, Ohanis D, Slappendel R, Kollen B, Verheyen C (2013) Autologous re-transfusion drain compared with no drain in total knee arthroplasty: a randomised controlled trial. Blood Transfus 26:1–6
Irisson E, Hémon Y, Pauly V, Parratte S, Argenson JN, Kerbaul F (2012) Tranexamic acid reduces blood loss and financial cost in primary total hip and knee replacement surgery. Orthop Traumatol Surg Res 98(5):477–483
Ishida K, Tsumura N, Kitagawa A, Hamamura S, Fukuda K, Dogaki Y, Kubo S, Matsumoto T, Matsushita T, Chin T, Iguchi T, Kurosaka M, Kuroda R (2011) Intra-articular injection of tranexamic acid reduces not only blood loss but also knee joint swelling after total knee arthroplasty. Int Orthop 35(11):1639–1645

Iwai T, Tsuji S, Tomita T, Sugamoto K, Hideki Y, Hamada M (2013) Repeat-dose intravenous tranexamic acid further decreases blood loss in total knee arthroplasty. Int Orthop 37(3):441–445

Kang DG, Khurana S, Baek JH, Park YS, Lee SH, Kim KI (2014) Efficacy and safety using autotransfusion system with postoperative shed blood following total knee arthroplasty in haemophilia. Haemophilia 20(1): 129–132

Karkouti K, Beattie WS, Wijeysundera DN, Rao V, Chan C, Dattilo KM, Djaiani G, Ivanov J, Karski J, David TE (2005) Hemodilution during cardiopulmonary bypass is an independent risk factor for acute renal failure in adult cardiac surgery. J Thorac Cardiovasc Surg 129(2):391–400

Ker K, Prieto-Merino D, Roberts I (2013) Systematic review, meta-analysis and meta-regression of the effect of tranexamic acid on surgical blood loss. Br J Surg 100(10):1271–1279

Khanna MP, Hébert PC, Fergusson DA (2003) Review of the clinical practice literature on patient characteristics associated with perioperative allogeneic red blood cell transfusion. Transfus Med Rev 17(2):110–119

Korte W, Cattaneo M, Chassot PG, Eichinger S, von Heymann C, Hofmann N, Rickli H, Spannagl M, Ziegler B, Verheugt F, Huber K (2011) Peri-operative management of antiplatelet therapy in patients with coronary artery disease: joint position paper by members of the working group on Perioperative Haemostasis of the Society on Thrombosis and Haemostasis Research (GTH), the working group on Perioperative Coagulation of the Austrian Society for Anesthesiology, Resuscitation and Intensive Care (ÖGARI) and the Working Group Thrombosis of the European Society for Cardiology (ESC). Thromb Haemost 105(5):743–749

Kotzé A, Carter LA, Scally AJ (2012) Effect of a patient blood management programme on preoperative anaemia, transfusion rate, and outcome after primary hip or knee arthroplasty: a quality improvement cycle. Br J Anaesth 108(6):943–952

Leahy MF, Roberts H, Mukhtar SA, Farmer S, Tovey J, Jewlachow V, Dixon T, Lau P, Ward M, Vodanovich M, Trentino K, Kruger PC, Gallagher T, Koay A, Hofmann A, Semmens JB, Towler S (2012) Western Australian Patient Blood Management Program. anesthesia Evaluation. A pragmatic approach to embedding patient blood management in a tertiary hospital. Anesthesiology 116(3):522–538

Leal-Noval SR, Muñoz M, Asuero M, Contreras E, García-Erce JA, Llau JV, Moral V, Páramo JA, Quintana M (2013) Spanish Expert Panel on Alternatives to Allogeneic Blood Transfusion. Spanish Consensus Statement on alternatives to allogeneic blood transfusion: the 2013 update of the "Seville document". Blood Transfus 11(4):585–610

Liu J, Cao JG, Wang L, Ma XL (2013) Effect of fibrin sealant on blood loss following total knee arthroplasty: a systematic review and meta-analysis. Int J Surg 12(2):95–102, pii: S1743-9191(13)01111-4

Liumbruno GM, Bennardello F, Lattanzio A, Piccoli P, Rossetti G, Italian Society of Transfusion Medicine and Immunohaematology (SIMTI) Working Party (2011a) Recommendations for the transfusion management of patients in the peri-operative period. I. The pre-operative period. Blood Transfus 9(1):19–40

Liumbruno GM, Bennardello F, Lattanzio A, Piccoli P, Rossetti G, Italian Society of Transfusion Medicine and Immunohaematology (SIMTI) Working Party (2011b) Recommendations for the transfusion management of patients in the peri-operative period. II. The intra-operative period. Blood Transfus 9(2):189–217

Liumbruno GM, Bennardello F, Lattanzio A, Piccoli P, Rossetti G, Italian Society of Transfusion Medicine and Immunohaematology Working Party (2011c) Recommendations for the transfusion management of patients in the peri-operative period. III. The postoperative period. Blood Transfus 9(3):320–335

Markar SR, Jones GG, Karthikesalingam A, Segaren N, Patel RV (2012) Transfusion drains versus suction drains in total knee replacement: meta-analysis. Knee Surg Sports Traumatol Arthrosc 20(9):1766–1772

Meier J, Gombotz H (2013) Pillar III–optimisation of anaemia tolerance. Best Pract Res Clin Anaesthesiol 27(1):111–119

Mercuriali F, Inghilleri G (1996) Proposal of an algorithm to help the choice of the best transfusion strategy. Curr Med Res Opin 13(8):465–78

Movig KL, Janssen MW, de Waal Malefijt J, Kabel PJ, Leufkens HG, Egberts AC (2003) Relationship of serotonergic antidepressants and need for blood transfusion in orthopedic surgical patients. Arch Intern Med 163(19):2354–2358

Muñoz M, Slappendel R, Thomas D (2011) Laboratory characteristics and clinical utility of post-operative cell salvage: washed or unwashed blood transfusion? Blood Transfus 9(3):248–261

Muñoz M, Ariza D, Campos A, Martín-Montañez E, Pavía J (2013) The cost of post-operative shed blood salvage after total knee arthroplasty: an analysis of 1,093 consecutive procedures. Blood Transfus 11(2):260–271

Muñoz M, Gómez-Ramírez S, Cuenca J, García-Erce JA, Iglesias-Aparicio D, Haman-Alcober S, Ariza D, Naveira E (2014) Very-short-term perioperative intravenous iron administration and postoperative outcome in major orthopedic surgery: a pooled analysis of observational data from 2547 patients. Transfusion 54(2):289–299

Musallam KM, Tamim HM, Richards T, Spahn DR, Rosendaal FR, Habbal A, Khreiss M, Dahdaleh FS, Khavandi K, Sfeir PM, Soweid A, Hoballah JJ, Taher AT, Jamali FR (2011) Preoperative anaemia and postoperative outcomes in non-cardiac surgery: a retrospective cohort study. Lancet 378(9800):1396–1407

Myers E, O'Grady P, Dolan AM (2004) The influence of preclinical anaemia on outcome following total hip replacement. Arch Orthop Trauma Surg 124(10): 699–701

NICE (2003) http://www.nice.org.uk/nicemedia/pdf/CG3NICEguideline.pdf

Nichols WL, Hultin MB, James AH, Manco-Johnson MJ, Montgomery RR, Ortel TL, Rick ME, Sadler JE,

Weinstein M, Yawn BP (2008) von Willebrand disease (VWD): evidence-based diagnosis and management guidelines, the National Heart, Lung, and Blood Institute (NHLBI) Expert Panel report (USA). Haemophilia 14(2):171–232

Noticewala MS, Nyce JD, Wang W, Geller JA, Macaulay W (2012) Predicting need for allogeneic transfusion after total knee arthroplasty. J Arthroplasty 27(6):961–967

Oremus K, Sostaric S, Trkulja V, Haspl M (2014) Influence of tranexamic acid on postoperative autologous blood retransfusion in primary total hip and knee arthroplasty: a randomized controlled trial. Transfusion 54(1):31–41

Park JH, Rasouli MR, Mortazavi SM, Tokarski AT, Maltenfort MG, Parvizi J (2013) Predictors of perioperative blood loss in total joint arthroplasty. J Bone Joint Surg Am 95(19):1777–1783

Parker MJ, Livingstone V, Clifton R, McKee A (2007) Closed suction surgical wound drainage after orthopaedic surgery. Cochrane Database Syst Rev (3): CD001825

Rajagopalan S, Mascha E, Na J, Sessler DI (2008) The effects of mild perioperative hypothermia on blood loss and transfusion requirement. Anesthesiology 108(1): 71–77

Retter A, Wyncoll D, Pearse R, Carson D, McKechnie S, Stanworth S, Allard S, Thomas D, Walsh T, British Committee for Standards in Haematology (2013) Guidelines on the management of anaemia and red cell transfusion in adult critically ill patients. Br J Haematol 160(4):445–464

Rosencher N, Kerkkamp HE, Macheras G, Munuera LM, Menichella G, Barton DM, Cremers S, Abraham IL, OSTHEO Investigation (2003) Orthopedic Surgery Transfusion Hemoglobin European Overview (OSTHEO) study: blood management in elective knee and hip arthroplasty in Europe. Transfusion 43(4): 459–469

Royal Cornwall Hospitals (2013) http://www.rcht.nhs.uk/DocumentsLibrary/RoyalCornwallHospitalsTrust/Clinical/Anaesthetics/PreOperativeAssessmentGuidelines.pdf. Last accessed 31 Jan 2014

Rubinstein C, Davenport DL, Dunnagan R, Saha SP, Ferraris VA, Xenos ES (2013) Intraoperative blood transfusion of one or two units of packed red blood cells is associated with a fivefold risk of stroke in patients undergoing elective carotid endarterectomy. J Vasc Surg 57(2 Suppl):53S–57S

Saleh E, McClelland DB, Hay A, Semple D, Walsh TS (2007) Prevalence of anaemia before major joint arthroplasty and the potential impact of preoperative investigation and correction on perioperative blood transfusions. Br J Anaesth 99(6):801–808

Sans T, Bofil C, Joven J, Clivillé X, Simó JM, Llobet X, Peró A, Galbany J (1996) Effectiveness of very low doses of subcutaneous recombinant human erythropoietin in facilitating autologous blood donation before orthopedic surgery. Transfusion 36(9):822–826

Sasanuma H, Sekiya H, Takatoku K, Takada H, Sugimoto N, Hoshino Y (2011) Efficient strategy for controlling postoperative hemorrhage in total knee arthroplasty. Knee Surg Sports Traumatol Arthrosc 19(6):921–925

Sehat KR, Evans RL, Newman JH (2004) Hidden blood loss following hip and knee arthroplasty. Correct management of blood loss should take hidden loss into account. J Bone Joint Surg Br 86(4):561–565

Shander A, Rijhwani TS (2004) Acute normovolemic hemodilution. Transfusion 44(12 Suppl):26S–34S

Shander A, Knight K, Thurer R, Adamson J, Spence R (2004) Prevalence and outcomes of anemia in surgery: a systematic review of the literature. Am J Med 116(Suppl 7A):58S–69S

Shander A, Hofmann A, Ozawa S, Theusinger OM, Gombotz H, Spahn DR (2010) Activity-based costs of blood transfusions in surgical patients at four hospitals. Transfusion 50(4):753–765

Shander A, Fink A, Javidroozi M, Erhard J, Farmer SL, Corwin H, Goodnough LT, Hofmann A, Isbister J, Ozawa S, Spahn DR, International Consensus Conference on Transfusion Outcomes Group (2011) Appropriateness of allogeneic red blood cell transfusion: the international consensus conference on transfusion outcomes. Transfus Med Rev 25(3):232–246.e53

Shander A, Gross I, Hill S, Javidroozi M, Sledge S (2013) A new perspective on best transfusion practices. Blood Transfus 11(2):193–202

So-Osman C, Nelissen RG, Koopman-van Gemert AW, Kluyver E, Pöll RG, Onstenk R, Van Hilten JA, Jansen-Werkhoven TM, van den Hout WB, Brand R, Brand A (2014a) Patient blood management in elective total hip- and knee-replacement surgery (part 1): a randomized controlled trial on erythropoietin and blood salvage as transfusion alternatives using a restrictive transfusion policy in erythropoietin-eligible patients. Anesthesiology 120(4):839–851

So-Osman C, Nelissen RG, Koopman-van Gemert AW, Kluyver E, Pöll RG, Onstenk R, Van Hilten JA, Jansen-Werkhoven TM, van den Hout WB, Brand R, Brand A (2014b) Patient blood management in elective total hip- and knee-replacement surgery (part 2): a randomized controlled trial on blood salvage as transfusion alternative using a restrictive transfusion policy in patients with a preoperative hemoglobin above 13 g/dl. Anesthesiology 120(4):852–860

Spahn DR (2010) Anemia and patient blood management in hip and knee surgery: a systematic review of the literature. Anesthesiology 113(2):482–495

Sukeik M, Alshryda S, Haddad FS, Mason JM (2011) Systematic review and meta-analysis of the use of tranexamic acid in total hip replacement. J Bone Joint Surg Br 93(1):39–46

Tosetto A, Castaman G, Rodeghiero F (2007) Assessing bleeding in von Willebrand disease with bleeding score. Blood Rev 21(2):89–97

Vamvakas EC, Blajchman MA (2009) Transfusion-related mortality: the ongoing risks of allogeneic blood transfusion and the available strategies for their prevention. Blood 113(15):3406–3417

van Haelst IM, Egberts TC, Doodeman HJ, Traast HS, Burger BJ, Kalkman CJ, van Klei WA (2010) Use of

serotonergic antidepressants and bleeding risk in orthopedic patients. Anesthesiology 112(3):631–636
van Klei WA, Bryson GL, Yang H, Forster AJ (2009) Effect of beta-blocker prescription on the incidence of postoperative myocardial infarction after hip and knee arthroplasty. Anesthesiology 111(4):717–724
Weiskopf RB, Viele MK, Feiner J, Kelley S, Lieberman J, Noorani M, Leung JM, Fisher DM, Murray WR, Toy P, Moore MA (1998) Human cardiovascular and metabolic response to acute, severe isovolemic anemia. JAMA 279(3):217–221. Erratum in: JAMA 1998 Oct 28;280(16):1404
Weiss G, Goodnough LT (2005) Anemia of chronic disease. N Engl J Med 352(10):1011–1023
Wells AW, Mounter PJ, Chapman CE, Stainsby D, Wallis JP (2002) Where does blood go? Prospective observational study of red cell transfusion in north England. BMJ 325(7368):803
WHO Global Database on Blood Safety. http://www.who.int/bloodsafety/global_database/en. Last accessed 31 Jan 2014
Wong J, Abrishami A, El Beheiry H, Mahomed NN, Roderick Davey J, Gandhi R, Syed KA, Muhammad Ovais Hasan S, De Silva Y, Chung F (2010) Topical application of tranexamic acid reduces postoperative blood loss in total knee arthroplasty: a randomized, controlled trial. J Bone Joint Surg Am 92(15):2503–2513
Wu WC, Schifftner TL, Henderson WG, Eaton CB, Poses RM, Uttley G, Sharma SC, Vezeridis M, Khuri SF, Friedmann PD (2007) Preoperative hematocrit levels and postoperative outcomes in older patients undergoing noncardiac surgery. JAMA 297(22):2481–2488
Yoo YC, Shim JK, Kim JC, Jo YY, Lee JH, Kwak YL (2011) Effect of single recombinant human erythropoietin injection on transfusion requirements in preoperatively anemic patients undergoing valvular heart surgery. Anesthesiology 115(5):929–937

How to Reduce Blood Transfusion to a Minimum in Total Knee Arthroplasty

2

Irene Miniati, Caterina Guarducci, Andrea Baldini, and Emmanuel Thienpont

Open Questions

- How should tourniquet and drains be managed? Is their use still justified?
- How should surgeons stop bleeding from the bony surfaces?
- Which are the optimal dose and timing for tranexamic acid?
- Are hemostatic matrices and bipolar sealing devices cost-effective?
- What works and what does not in the immediate postoperative time to control bleeding?

I. Miniati • C. Guarducci
Orthopaedics Unit, IFCA Clinic, Florence, Italy

A. Baldini (✉)
Orthopaedics Unit, IFCA Clinic, Florence, Italy

Humanitas Clinical and Research Center, Milan, Italy
e-mail: drbaldiniandrea@yahoo.it

E. Thienpont
Department of Orthopaedics, University Hospital Saint Luc, Brussels, Belgium
e-mail: emmanuel.thienpont@uclouvain.be

2.1 Introduction

Primary total knee arthroplasty (TKA) and even more revision knee arthroplasty are surgical procedures which can lead to a significant amount of blood loss with the consequence of a high rate of blood transfusions if not properly addressed (Keating et al. 2002).

Total blood loss during arthroplasty consists of visible blood loss and hidden blood loss. Visible blood loss can be intraoperatively estimated measuring the volume of blood from suction device bottles and weighting the sponges, while postoperatively it can be assessed quantifying the drain output, although irrigation fluids and exudates may influence the accuracy of the data (Kluba et al. 2012). Hidden blood loss represents 40 % of total blood loss and can be identified with Hb and HTC changes (total blood loss (TBL) = blood volume × [HTC pre − HTC post]) (Sehat et al. 2004).

Exposed bony surfaces or drill holes, surgical trauma to tissues and blood vessels as well as fibrinolysis, anticoagulant medication, and coagulopathies or platelet dysfunction are all factors that contribute to intraoperative bleeding (Moonen et al. 2006). The average drop in hemoglobin (Hb) levels reported in the literature after TKA and total hip arthroplasty (THA) is approximately 4.0 ± 1.5 g/dL. While after revision TKA and THA the hemoglobin decrease is expected to be approximately 5–6 g/dL (Nuttall et al. 1996;

A. Baldini, P. Caldora (eds.), *Perioperative Medical Management for Total Joint Arthroplasty: How to Control Hemostasis, Pain and Infection*, DOI 10.1007/978-3-319-07203-6_2,

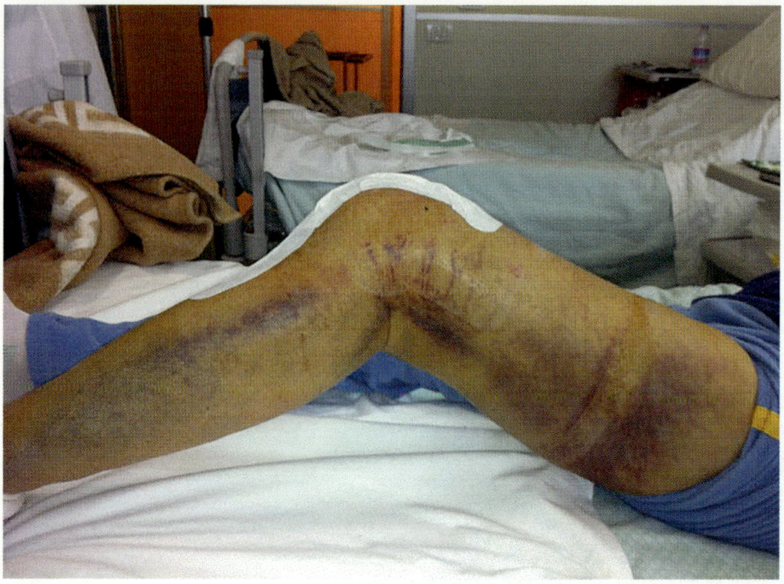

Fig. 2.1 Example of diffused hematoma after total knee arthroplasty

Keating et al. 1998, 1999; Keating and Meding 2002; Keating and Ritter 2002). Blood loss up to 1,500 mL and transfusion rates ranging from 7.5 to 13 % have been observed (Pietsch et al. 2013; Sehat et al. 2000, 2004; Vundelinckx et al. 2013; Thienpont et al. 2014).

Bleeding can lead to clinical complications such as pain, swelling, delayed rehabilitation, stiffness, arthrofibrosis, oozing wounds, and increased infection risk as well as a greater likelihood for blood transfusion along with its related complications (Fig. 2.1) (Everts et al. 2007). In general, the threshold for anemia leading to a transfusion trigger is set at 8 g/dL, but of course clinical symptoms like cardiac symptoms, dyspnea, palpitations, and fatigue should be considered.

Blood transfusion carries significant risks of immunological reactions, intravascular hemolysis, transmission of disease, renal failure, transfusion-induced coagulopathy, admission to intensive care, and even death (Cardone and Klein 2009; Kumar 2009; Lemaire 2008). A variety of blood-saving techniques including autologous blood transfusion, intraoperative blood-saving methods, hypotensive anesthesia, and the use of antifibrinolytic agents have been introduced to reduce allogenic blood transfusion in total knee arthroplasty (Cardone and Klein 2009; Sharrock and Salvati 1996; Flynn and Csenesitz 1979; Cowell 1937).

Autologous transfusion is not risk-free; autologous donors tend to be older and less healthy and as such have a greater likelihood to face complications (Mcvay and Toy 1996; Yomtovian 1996). Autologous donation may also lead to postoperative decreased hemoglobin levels, resulting in transfusion in patients who might not have needed it had they not predonated, thus lowering their preoperative hemoglobin level (Cohen and Brecher 1995).

Preoperative risk factors for transfusion are advanced age, low preoperative Hb or RBC volume (anemia or small patient), female gender, renal insufficiency, preoperative administration of antiplatelet or antithrombotic drugs, revision surgery, and cardiac comorbidity. Preoperative anemia is frequently present in a TKA population (Jans et al. 2014)

By analyzing 31 independent variables in 644 primary unilateral TKA, Noticewala et al. attempted to develop a predictive model (90 % sensitive and 52.5 % specific) to forecast the need for a postoperative allogenic blood transfusion. Their analysis showed especially that patient's age, comorbidity leading to anemia, preoperative

Hb levels, and surgical time are statistically significant predictors of postoperative blood transfusion (Noticewala et al. 2012).

Postoperative vigor is correlated to the hematocrit (HTC) level and plays an important role in rehabilitation and the quality of life after surgery (Keating 1999; Cleeland et al. 1999). Anemic patients who received an immediate postoperative transfusion showed better outcomes, less complications, and a better sense of well-being after TKA than those who received a delayed transfusion (Lotke et al. 1999).

Several studies reported a greater likelihood to receive blood transfusion in patients undergoing surgery for rheumatic arthritis (RA) than in those for osteoarthritis; however, these findings were supposedly related to lower preoperative hemoglobin in patients diagnosed with RA and moreover not statistically significant (Bong et al. 2004; Prasad et al. 2007).

The aim of modern total knee surgery should therefore be to try to reduce postoperative transfusion by a threefold strategy. Firstly, the patient condition should be optimized preoperatively to obtain the best possible Hb level before surgery; secondly, during the surgery, careful attention to potential bleeding by the surgeon should reduce the visible blood loss; and finally, an optimization strategy of the postoperative care should reduce hidden blood loss to a minimum.

2.2 Preoperative Optimization of Patients Undergoing Joint Arthroplasty

A baseline preoperative blood test should screen patients for their preoperative Hb and HTC levels and their iron and vitamin levels. According to a recent study by Jans et al., about 13 % of patients undergoing fast-track joint replacement present preoperative anemia according to WHO criteria (Jans et al. 2014). The possible causes of anemia should be investigated and if possible treated before the surgery. Patients with an Hb <12 g/dL for women and Hb <13 g/dL for men should go through the anemia clinic for further checkup.

In the presence of anemia and low iron levels, gastrointestinal complaints should be screened and treated to eliminate potential neoplastic syndromes.

Patients who present macrocytic anemia should be screened for a deficiency in vitamin B levels and possible comorbidity identified and treated.

Patients with microcytic anemia should be screened for iron deficiency. For those with moderate iron deficiency, chronic disease and inflammation should be ruled out. Patients with mild iron depletion should have their renal function checked, and chronic kidney disease should be ruled out by consulting a nephrologist. Anemia by iron depletion can be treated with an erythropoietin (EPO) program combined with iron supplementation.

The dose of EPO should be related to the level of Hb and the time of potential treatment before the surgery. Four EPO injections should be considered for an Hb <10 g/dL and reduced by one injection by g/dL of Hb with only one injection for Hb levels of 13 g/dL. Of course iron therapy should be added with 300 mg/day or 500 mg/week if IV (Rosencher et al. 2008).

2.3 Perioperative Reduction of Blood Loss by the Surgeon

2.3.1 Anesthetic Technique

The use of regional anesthesia in orthopedic surgery has shown measurable reduction in blood loss compared with general anesthesia (Flordal and Neander 1991; Sculco and Ranawat 1975; Sharrock et al. 1993). This has been linked to the potential influences of the anesthetic drugs on the postoperative platelet function. The addition of a hypotensive regimen to the epidural anesthesia (HEA) has led to further decrease in blood loss, simultaneously improving a bloodless field at the bony surfaces for better implant fixation and leading to shorter surgical time (Sharrock et al. 1993; Davis et al. 1974; An et al. 1991; Mallory 1973; Nelson and Bowen 1986). Hypotensive epidural anesthesia is one of the techniques used to reduce perioperative blood loss by achieving an epidural block at least as far as the T2 level and to establish a sufficiently extensive and dense block of the cardio-acceleratory fibers of the thoracic sympathetic chain (Moonen et al. 2006). Patients tolerate the use of HEA well without additional morbidity and with a decreased rate of postoperative deep venous thrombosis. An added benefit has been the improved analgesia produced by using a patient-controlled system of postoperative pain medication through the indwelling epidural catheter, avoiding bleeding by pain-induced hypertension.

In a prospective, randomized clinical study, Eroglu et al. (2005) compared hypotensive epidural anesthesia (HEA) with bupivacaine and hypotensive total intravenous anesthesia (HTIVA) with propofol and remifentanil on blood loss on 40 patients (ASA scores I–III) undergoing primary hip arthroplasty. The study resulted in less intraoperative blood loss and a minor percentage of patients receiving blood and total packed red blood cells transfusions as well as a lower intraoperative mean central venous pressure in patients receiving HEA.

A comparison between HEA and spinal anesthesia (SPA) by Niemi et al. (2000) on patients undergoing primary total hip arthroplasty documented a minor blood loss and a reduced number of transfused units of packed cells (UPC) in the HEA group, in which coagulation system was considered to be better preserved than in SPA group.

Sometimes it can be necessary to titrate epinephrine intravenously to keep the blood pressure at an acceptable level for tissue oxygenation. Epinephrine-augmented hypotensive epidural anesthesia is effective in avoiding the use of tourniquet in TKA without negative effects on perioperative hemoglobin values, as documented by Kiss et al. (2005).

Anesthesia and surgery itself may cause perioperative hypothermia. Mild perioperative hypothermia increases the incidence of myocardial morbidity, reduces the resistance to surgical wound infection, causes coagulopathy resulting from platelet inhibition, and prolongs both postanesthetic recovery and hospitalization. Postoperative blood loss has been shown to be significantly greater in hypothermic patients (Schmied et al. 1995). It is therefore recommended that patients be kept normothermic during orthopedic surgery using warmed fluids, heated blankets, and a warm airflow with inflatable devices on the body of the patient. New technologies like a double-heated blanket (HotDog® Augustine Temperature Management, Eden Prairie, MN, USA, or EasyWarm® Mölnlycke Health Care AB, Göteborg, Sweden) can keep patients normothermic without needing a general raise of the room temperature or forced airflows in the room which may disrupt the laminar airflow (Fig. 2.2).

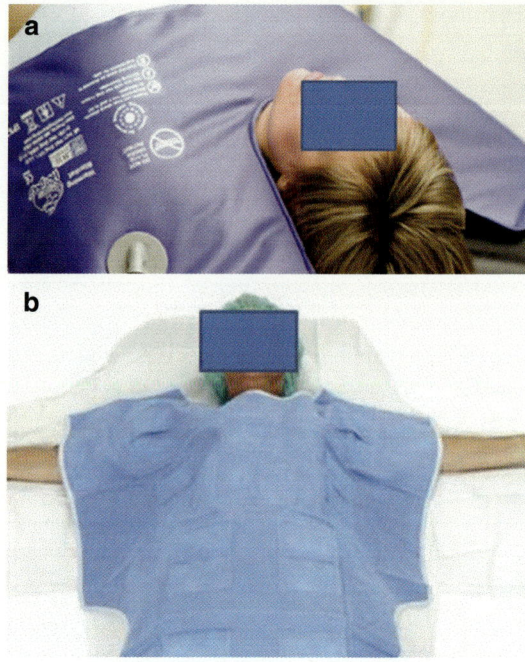

Fig. 2.2 Examples of new technologies for patients' normothermia are the double-heated blanket HotDog® (Augustine Temperature Management, Eden Prairie, MN, USA) (**a**) or EasyWarm® (Mölnlycke Health Care AB, Göteborg, Sweden) (**b**), which can keep patients normothermic without needing a general raise of the room temperature or forced air flows in the room which may disrupt the laminar air flow

Preoperative acute normovolemic hemodilution (ANH) can be considered appropriate for

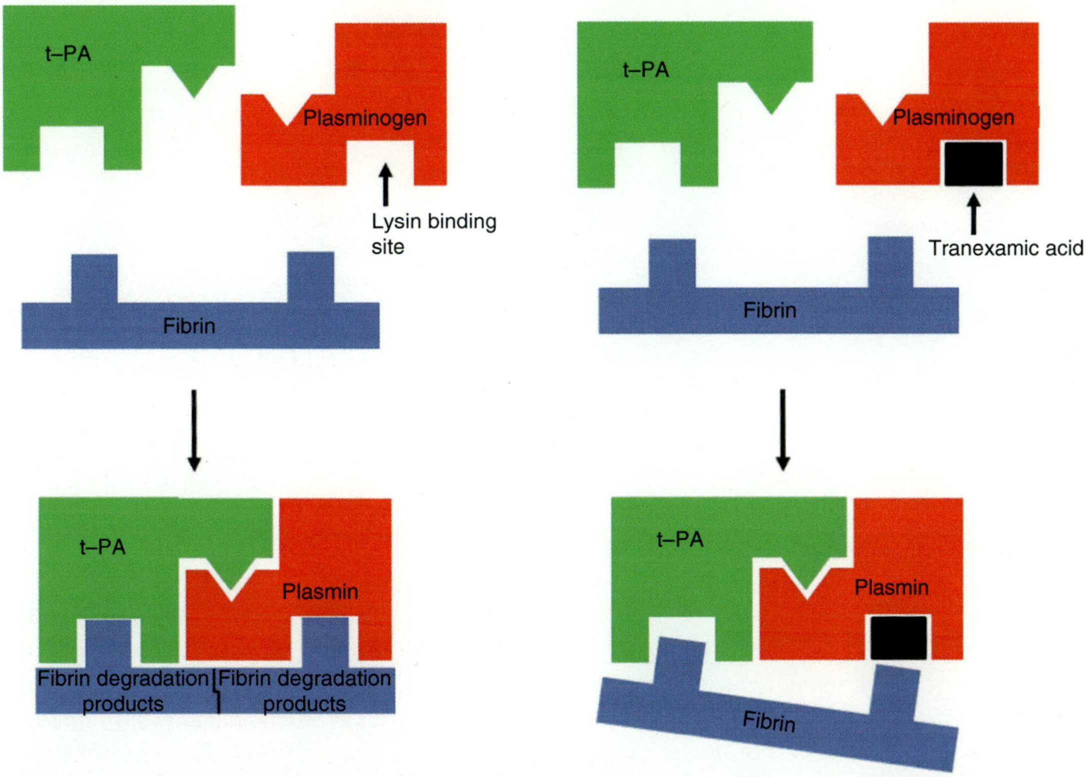

Fig. 2.3 Tranexamic acid (TXA) reduces surgery-induced fibrinolysis and blood loss thanks to antifibrinolytic properties. TXA has been shown to inhibit fibrinolysis by competitively blocking the lysine-binding sites of plasminogen

patients with high Hb levels undergoing potentially high bleeding surgery, like complicated revisions. The predonation of 20 % of their total blood volume will make a few UPC available for after the procedure, and because the hemoglobin concentration of the blood is lower, it will lead to less valuable blood loss. This technique is especially indicated for patients with high-viscosity diseases that present increased risks of DVT after surgery (Juelsgaard et al. 2002).

2.3.2 Pharmacologic Agents: Tranexamic Acid

To reduce tourniquet and surgery-induced fibrinolysis and blood loss, drugs with antifibrinolytic properties such as tranexamic acid (TXA) can be used. TXA has been shown to inhibit fibrinolysis by competitively blocking the lysine-binding sites of plasminogen (Fig. 2.3). Tranexamic acid has been diffusely tested in orthopedic surgery and particularly after TKA (Dunn and Goa 1999; Engel et al. 2001; Eubanks 2010). In a review study, Wind et al. (2013) observed a statistically significant decrease in blood transfusion in patients receiving TXA via IV infusion ($p=0.001$) and in topical application of TXA ($p=0.019$) compared to the control group. While both systematic and topical TXA reduced blood loss after TKA, the effect of either treatment is influenced by doses and timing of administration. Tanaka et al. (2001) compared two different single-dose regimens and a split-dose regimen (before and during surgery), finding the latter to be the more efficacious even though the total amount of TXA used was the same. Maniar et al. (2012) found a single-dose regimen to be least

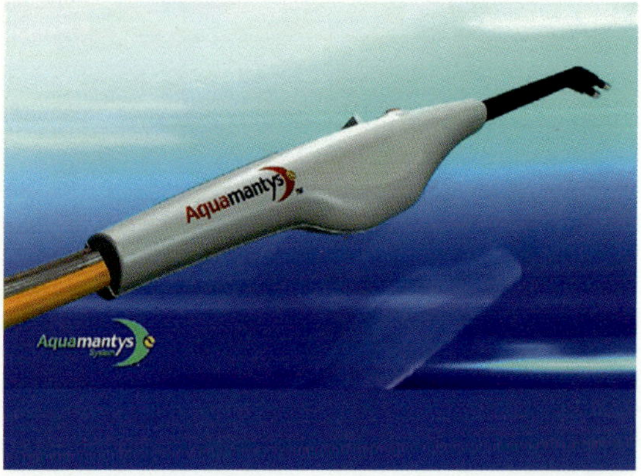

Fig. 2.4 The bipolar device Aquamantys (Medtronic, Minneapolis, MN, USA)

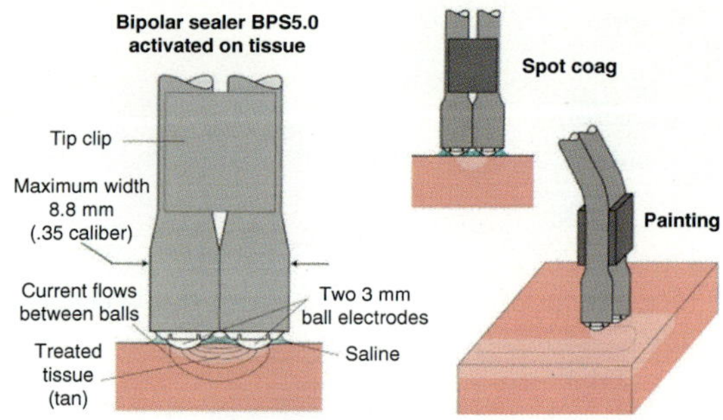

efficacious, while administering TXA before and during surgery was more efficacious than during and after surgery. As for topical TXA administration, Wong et al. (2010) found that only a high concentration reduces transfusion rate whereas low concentration does not. After TKA, a second phase of fibrinolysis can be observed after 6 h (Fedi et al. 1999; Aglietti et al. 2000). It can therefore be important to use a second dose of TXA before this new fibrinolytic episode starts (Maniar et al. 2012; Blanié et al. 2013). Regardless of the dose, timing, and route of administration, several studies reported no increase in the incidence of deep vein thrombosis (DVT) or pulmonary embolism (PE) (Wind et al. 2013; Kim et al. 2014).

2.3.3 Direct Hemostasis

2.3.3.1 Mechanical Hemostasis

If a mechanical blockade exists that is stronger than the local blood pressure of the blood vessel, the result will be local hemostasis. Direct pressure, clips, sutures, bandaging, and bone wax are all means of mechanical hemostasis. As for bone wax, hemostasis can be achieved using the classical Bone Wax® (Ethicon, Johnson & Johnson, Somerville, NJ, USA) or Ostene® (Baxter Healthcare Corporation, Fremont, CA, USA) which looks and feels like bone wax, is biocompatible, does not interfere with bone healing nor increases infection rates, and does not lead to inflammation due to beeswax (Wellisz et al. 2008). These types of mechanical devices can be used to fill the drill holes around the femur and tibia and unresurfaced areas around the implants if present.

2.3.3.2 Cauterization

Hemostasis can be achieved via thermal cautery like the classic bovey or monopolar/bipolar radiofrequency (RF) devices. Recently more advanced devices such as laser or vessel sealing devices have been used too. In a prospective, randomized study, Plymale et al. (2012) investigated whether unipolar or bipolar hemostasis is more effective in reducing blood loss in TKA. The study showed no significant difference in postoperative drain output, postoperative Hb levels, or hematocrit values nor transfusion requirements. A different result was found by Pfeiffer et al. who compared 20 TKAs treated with a bipolar device (Aquamantys, Medtronic, Minneapolis, MN, USA) versus 20 controls and found a significant reduction in total blood loss from 1,130 to 1,580 mL on average (Fig. 2.4) (Pfeiffer et al. 2005). Results in primary THA have been described by Zeh et al. (2010). In 105 cases, they were not able to find significant differences in total blood loss using a bipolar device. Cost-effectiveness has been judged by the paper of Falez et al. in 95 primary THAs randomly

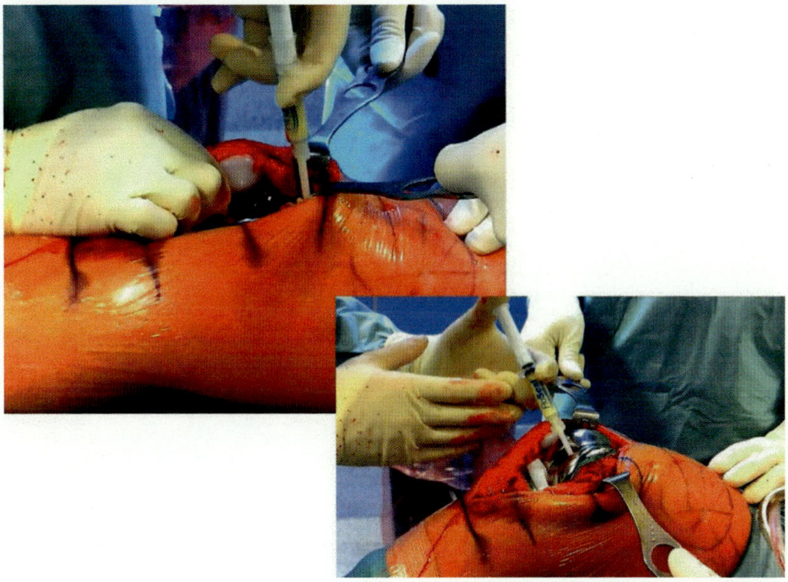

Fig. 2.5 FloSeal® (Baxter Healthcare Corporation, Fremont, CA, USA), a topical, absorbable, thrombin-based hemostat

assigned in 3 groups. A fibrin sealant outperformed the use of bipolar device and controls in term of blood loss savings (Falez et al. 2013). Authors calculated their costs of fibrin sealant ranging between 450 and 675 euros versus the bipolar device which costed 1,440 euros on average. Blood loss savings for the fibrin sealant group ranged from 235 to 642 mL and for the bipolar device group from 96 to 296 mL. Two studies from the same group on THA and TKA revisions in postinfected cases showed an effective reduction in blood loss using a bipolar device only for the hip cohort (Clement et al. 2012; Derman et al. 2013).

2.3.3.3 Chemical Hemostasis

Chemical hemostasis can be achieved with vasoconstrictors (local infiltration analgesia: ropivacaine + adrenaline + clonidine) or with topical absorbable hemostats that can be thrombin based such as FloSeal (FloSeal®, Baxter Healthcare Corporation, Fremont, CA, USA) (Fig. 2.5), (Kim et al. 2012; Heyse et al. 2014) or with fibrin sealants such as Quixil (Omrix Biopharmaceuticals, Brussels, Belgium) (Levy et al. 1999) or fibrinogen sealants such as Evicel (J&J, Somerville, NJ, USA) (Skovgaard et al. 2013) (Fig. 2.6).

The effect on blood loss for local infiltration analgesia (LIA) using vasoconstrictors has not been extensively described in the literature on this analgesic regimen. A study from Hospital for Special Surgery comparing the effect on blood loss of LIA with adrenaline versus a fibrin sealant did not show a significant difference on total blood loss between the two techniques thereby demonstrating a significant efficacy for LIA on bleeding control after TKA (Reinhardt et al. 2013).

Collagen-based products, such as gelatin sponges, gelatin matrices, and microfibrillar collagen, stimulate the intrinsic pathway of the coagulation cascade. Plant-based compounds use cellulose to activate the intrinsic pathway hence facilitate hemostasis.

Thrombin converts fibrinogen into fibrin and is often used in combination with other topical agents. Platelet-rich plasma (PRP) sprays and fibrin sealants are topically applied hemostatic agents that have demonstrated beneficial effects, including reducing blood loss (Thoms and Marwin 2009; Carless et al. 2003).

Diiorio et al. retrospectively reviewed 134 patients who received an intraoperative application of PRP during TKA and 139 patients who

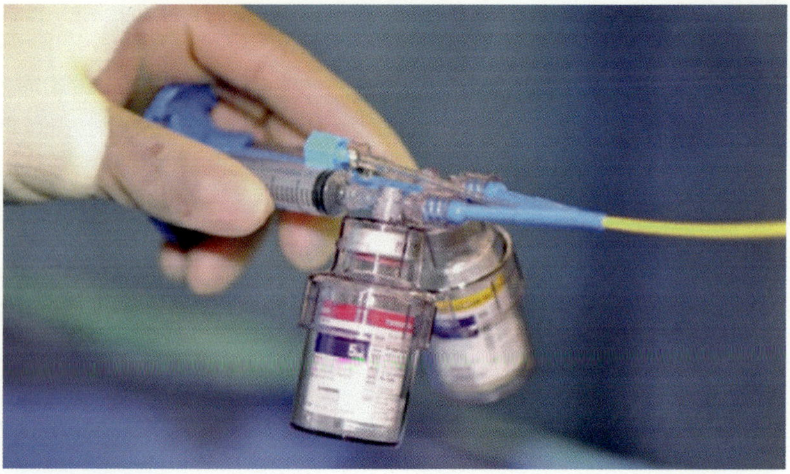

Fig. 2.6 Evicel (J&J, Somerville, NJ, USA), a fibrinogen sealant

did not receive PRP (Diiorio et al. 2012). The blood loss up to 1,500 mL and transfusion rates ranging from 7.5 to 13 % have been observed. Differences in passive ROM (88° versus 88°), narcotic requirement (27 vs. 32 morphine equivalent), and length of stay (2.4 vs. 2.6 days) were also similar.

Fibrin sealants achieve their local hemostatic effects by reproducing the last step of the coagulation cascade thereby facilitating the formation of a stable fibrin clot and subsequent hemostasis (Albala and Lawson 2006). Everts et al. (2006) evaluated the efficacy of autologous platelet gel and fibrin sealant in unilateral TKA. Study group patients presented a higher postoperative hemoglobin level, a decreased need for allogenic blood transfusions, a shorter hospital stay, and a significant less incidence in wound leakage and healing disturbances than control patients.

In a prospective, randomized study on patients undergoing TKA, Notarnicola et al. (2012) compared two groups of patients treated with different dosages of fibrin sealant (5 and 10 mL) and a control group. The two study groups achieved a lower decrease in the postoperative hemoglobin level as well as a lower need for blood transfusion than the control group. Both 5 and 10 mL dosages led to a comparable outcome hence the hypothesis to reserve the higher dosage to patients at higher risk of bleeding in order to reduce costs.

Several studies reported a better functional recovery, a superior ROM, and fewer cases of arthrofibrosis in patients treated with fibrin sealants during TKA (Everts et al. 2007; Notarnicola et al. 2012).

Kluba et al. (2012) found that the application of a low dose of fibrin sealant (2 mL) led to no statistically significant difference between treated and control patients in the means of postoperative hemoglobin loss, hospital length of stay, or amount of blood transfusion while showing a significant lower levels in postoperative fluid loss in the treated group ($p=0.026$). A recent prospective randomized study compared blood loss volume in 62 TKAs treated with Evicel® or not. They were not able to find any difference between the two groups in terms of total blood loss and transfusion rate (Randelli et al. 2014).

Two recent meta-analysis concluded that the use of fibrin sealant in total knee arthroplasty was effective and safe, reduced hemoglobin decline, postoperative drainage volume, incidence of hematomas and need for blood transfusion, and did not increase the risk of complications. Due to the limited quality of the evidence currently available, more high-quality RCTs are required (Li et al. 2014; Liu et al. 2014).

2.3.3.4 Good Surgical Practice

Good surgical practice is essential in order to reduce intraoperative bleeding. Surgical steps to keep in mind in order to reduce bleeding to a minimum in TKA are as follows: coagulate the medal genicular arteries during the approach, coagulate the femoral insertion of the PCL in cruciate resection, and coagulate the lateral genicular artery at meniscal resection. Several studies showed that plugging the defect made by the femoral intramedullary rod in TKA with autologous bone or cement significantly reduces total blood loss and transfusion rate (Ko et al. 2003; Kumar et al. 2000; Raut et al. 1993). The use of cement fixation also reduces bony bleeding in TKA (Christodoulou et al. 2004).

2.3.3.5 Synovectomy

Surgical removal of the synovial layer during TKA inevitably exposes a multitude of vessels. Bleeding from the resected layer should be addressed by intraoperative diathermic coagulation. A study by Zhaoning et al. randomized 187 TKA patients into two groups, one of which underwent synovectomy. Total bleeding was higher in the synovectomy group compared with the control group. There were no significant differences in blood transfusion rate ($p=0.882$), hospital stay ($p=0.805$), or range of movement of the knee ($p=0.413$) between the two groups. These authors concluded that synovectomy conferred no clinical advantages in TKA while subjecting patients to higher levels of bleeding. The same conclusions were found by Kilicarslan et al. in a cohort of 50 patients undergoing bilateral simultaneous TKA in which one side only received the synovectomy. Mean blood loss in the study group (with synovectomy) was significantly higher than the control, while pain relief and Knee Society Score did not differ between the two groups at follow-up (Kilicarslan et al. 2011).

2.3.3.6 Avoidance of Opening the Femoral Canal

Controversial data exists about the blood preservation potential of not opening the femoral canal. Several studies showed that less blood loss was observed if navigation or patient-specific instruments (PSI) were used (Pietsch et al. 2013; Vundelinckx et al. 2013; Thienpont et al. 2014). Other studies however could not confirm those findings (Ajwani et al. 2012; Mohanial et al. 2013; Baldini and Adravanti 2009; Thiengwittayaporn et al. 2009; Thienpont et al. 2014). The difference of these observations can probably be linked to differences in surgical technique. The use of a tourniquet and extramedullary tibial cutting guides or the efficient sealing with cortical bone of the drill hole makes a statistical difference for the reduction of both visible and hidden blood losses (Thienpont et al. 2014).

2.3.3.7 Tourniquet

Tourniquets are widely used in total knee arthroplasty in order to achieve a better visualization of the structures, reduced intraoperative bleeding, and a better cementation. However, there are complications associated with tourniquet use such as skin burns, soft tissue and muscle damage, injury of calcified vessels, increased swelling and stiffness of the joint, nerve injury, and paralysis, as well as an ongoing debate concerning tourniquet application and deep vein thrombosis (DVT) as TKA is followed by a hypercoagulative state (Aglietti et al. 2000; Irvine and Chan 1986; Abdel-Salam and Eyres 1995; Silver et al. 1986; Newman 1984; O'Leary et al. 1990; Din and Geddes 2004; Harvey et al. 1997).

A systematic review and meta-analysis of randomized controlled trials, carried out by Alcelik et al. (2012), reported that the use of tourniquet during TKA does not significantly reduce the duration of surgery nor reduces postoperative blood loss while reduces intraoperative bleeding, although there appears to be no correlation between blood loss and tourniquet time. Subsequentially total blood loss (intraoperative + postoperative) is statistically reduced by the use of tourniquet ($p<0.001$). Although it would appear that there is a better early flexion in patients without tourniquet, no difference was shown in the long term. Deep vein thrombosis (DVT) and pulmonary embolism had not a significantly different incidence in either non-tourniquet or tourniquet patients, although the latter group presented more minor complications (14.4 % vs. 5.6 %).

A recent meta-analysis evaluated the differences between tourniquet and non-tourniquet surgery on the following items: total measured blood loss, calculated blood loss, and intraoperative and postoperative blood loss. The total and intraoperative blood loss was higher when non-tourniquet surgery was used maybe due to a prolonged surgical time. On the other hand,

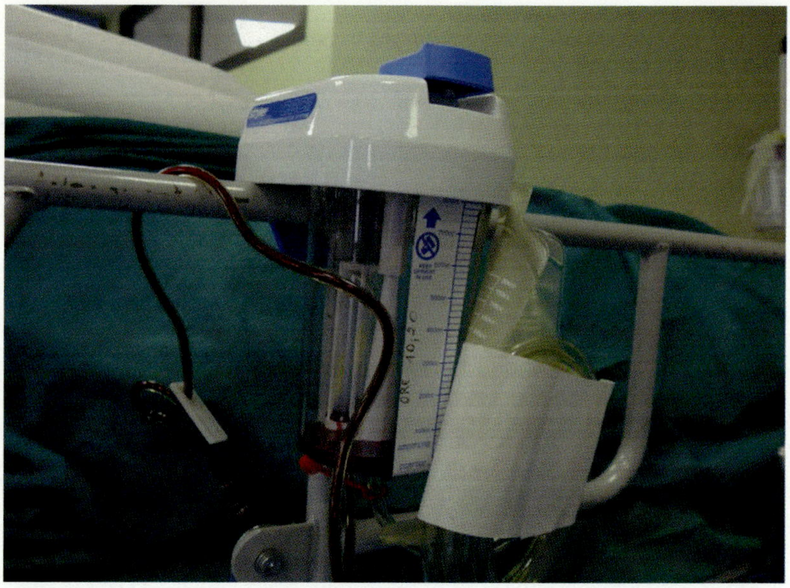

Fig. 2.7 Example of a reinfusion drain with very limited blood collection due to the application of multimodal strategies for bleeding control after TKA

calculated and postoperative blood loss data were in favor of non-tourniquet surgery. In conclusion the use of tourniquet does not seem to reduce the overall blood loss effectively (Tai et al. 2011). The limit of this analysis is that hidden blood loss was not considered.

The timing of tourniquet release is another controversial issue. According to some authors, the tourniquet release after the wound closure is associated with a lower blood loss (Ishii and Matsuda 2005).

A meta-analysis including 11 studies reports that early release of the tourniquet increased the total measured blood loss and blood loss as calculated on the basis of the maximum decrease in hemoglobin concentration. On the other hand, the rate of reoperations due to postoperative complications was higher when the tourniquet was released after wound closure.

According to the literature, it seems that there is no substantial advantage in using a tourniquet in TKA, but the common use may be justified since it increases visualization of the surgical field and reduces operation time (Smith and Hing 2010).

Christodoulou and associates (Christodoulou et al. 2004) estimated that intraoperative tourniquet release is related with a greater blood loss ($p<0.001$) and a longer operating time ($p<0.05$) and demands more blood transfusions than postoperative tourniquet release.

Rama et al. (2007) reported intraoperative tourniquet release to lead to a better hemostatic control of major bleeding events which may have closure can be associated with lower reoperation rate.

2.3.3.8 Surgical Drains

The use of drainage and the eventual postoperative blood collected reinfusion has been applied in TKA for the last decade (Fig. 2.7). Various methods of clamping have been reported in the literature, but no consensus has been achieved. It has been reported that drainage reduces postoperative hematoma formation (Martin et al. 2004), provides a better wound outcome in orthopedic surgery (Berman et al. 1990), and is associated with a lower postoperative pain, swelling, and incidence of infections (Kim et al. 1998). Some authors have estimated the volume of blood in the dressing by measuring the weight of the dressing, which was lower in the drainage group (Esler et al. 2003; Tao et al. 2006). It has been also shown that the use of drainage was associated with a smaller area of ecchymosis (Holt et al. 1997; Kim et al. 1998) and a smaller volume of hematoma measured through musculoskeletal ultrasound (Omonbude et al. 2010).

Concerning infection occurrence, a recent meta-analysis showed a lower incidence of infection in the drainage group (0.5 % versus 1.2 % in the non-drainage group), but pooled data demonstrated no significant difference (Zhang et al. 2011).

Since drainage use reduces postoperative knee swelling, it has been postulated that it may reduce the risk of thromboembolism, but several studies comparing the incidence of DVT between the drainage and non-drainage groups found no significant difference (Holt et al. 1997; Adalberth et al. 1998; Mengal et al. 2001)). According to more recent studies (Parker et al. 2004; Jones et al. 2007), using a drain seems not only to have no benefits but also to increase blood loss, resulting in a more severe drop of hemoglobin (Tai et al. 2010), a higher need of blood transfusion (Cao et al. 2009), with a consequent longer hospitalization both for a delayed rehabilitation program (due to the longer drainage permanence in the knee) and the bleeding complications. No consensus has been achieved to date on the use of temporary or no clamping drainage. Some authors assessed that temporarily clamping the drainage tube can create a tamponade effect (Shen et al. 2005), but a recent meta-analysis showed no differences between the 2 drainage strategies on wound-related complications and the occurrence of DVT. Despite this, a trend of a smaller number of patients requiring transfusions was observed when using the temporary clamping drainage (Huang et al. 2012). The authors concluded that an ideal drainage strategy would maintain the balance between a tamponade effect and wound complications.

As most of the blood loss occurs during the first postoperative hours (37 % in 2 h and 55 % in 4 h) (Jou and Yang 1993), the temporary clamping strategy should provide an initial tamponade effect after surgery reducing the amount of blood loss while delayed unclamping should limit hematoma formation. Some studies demonstrate that the use of clamping for 4 h or more is associated with a smaller need of transfusion per person (Stucinskas et al. 2009; Pornrattanamaneewong et al. 2012). These data are in contrast with another study in which no difference in total blood loss and range of motion (ROM) was observed between intermittent clamping with intra-articular epinephrine through the drain tube and no clamping drainage; however, intermittent clamping was associated with a higher rate of oozing wounds (Jung et al. 2013).

Table 2.1 Literature data on percentage per time of volume drained after TKA

Author	Volume drained	Time drain maintained
Leeman (2006)	78 % in 6 h	24 h
Senthil (2005)	84 % in 12 h	24 h
	94 % in 24 h	48 h
Zamora-Navas et al. (1999)	87 % in 12 h	24 h
	91 % in 12 h, 97 % in 24 h	48 h

Another issue that has been raised is the length of time that the drainage should be maintained (Table 2.1). In a retrospective study, three different population of patients have been examined: one undergoing conventional TKA, one minimally invasive technique, and another group unicompartmental knee arthroplasty. The persistence of bleeding was significantly longer in the first group where the mean was 16 h versus 14.2 h and 14.8 h, respectively. For that reason, the authors suggest that the ideal timing of drain removal is about 17 h after surgery. Besides this they found that a higher number of drains, especially when superficial, were related to a higher risk of continuous bleeding.

The blood salvage system and reinfusion does not prevent bleeding, but it acts when the damage has already been done. The blood is suctioned intraoperatively and can be transfused as whole blood or, once filtered, as a concentrate of red blood cells; only about 60 % of red blood cells can be collected and reinfused.

According to a survey analysis on 434 members of the American Association of Hip and Knee Surgeons, 62 % always used a postoperative drain in TKA, 24 % reported not draining the knee, 8 % rarely used, and 4 % occasionally used; about half of respondents used drains with reinfusion potential (Lee et al. 2005).

Data on the efficacy have been recently reported on a meta-analysis including 6 RCT: the number of patients requiring at least one unit of

ABT and the overall red cell units of ABT were lower when blood salvage was applied. Despite the fact that drain reinfusion is a reparative method, less blood loss was detected in reinfused patients as if blood loss can be reduced by preventing the use of banked blood. For that reason, the authors suggest to limit the use of ABT only when patients need and symptoms require it (Haien et al. 2013).

Although all these data encourage the use of drain reinfusion, the limit of this procedure in TKA is that it requires a significant blood loss to obtain enough product to reinfuse.

2.4 Optimization of the Reduction of Postoperative Blood Loss

2.4.1 Limb Positioning

Hip and knee flexion during surgery is an efficacious temporary method to reduce bleeding as it decreases venous bleeding due to the elevated limb position, and it increases the intra-articular pressure due to the knee flexion (Fig. 2.8).

In a study by Li et al., 110 patients undergoing TKA were randomized in 2 groups. Both groups had a 30° hip flexion for the first 72 h after surgery, but patients in the experimental group maintained also a 30° knee flexion and the control group maintained knee extension. The results showed that blood loss, swelling, and hematoma were significantly lower in the experimental group. Active ROM after 3 and 7 days and the number of patients who managed straight leg raises after 1 and 3 days were significantly higher in the experimental group. The authors concluded that postoperative knee flexion was associated with a lower blood loss and a better functional recovery without the risk of residual flexion contracture (Li et al. 2012).

Ong and Taylor found that knee flexion and knee elevation in extension reduced hemoglobin loss by 25 %. Compromise to tissue oxygenation has been reported with prolonged knee flexion. The author recommended elevation of the leg at 35° from the hip with the knee extended (Ong and Taylor 2003).

In a randomized controlled trial (RCT) of 420 TKAs, patients were randomized to one of three postoperative knee positions: flexion for 3 or 6 h postoperatively or knee extension. Positioning of the knee in flexion for 6 h immediately after surgery significantly reduced blood loss ($p=0.002$). These authors reported an incidence of 4.7 % of lower limb sensory neuropathy at their 3-month review when flexion was prolonged more than 6 h (Napier et al. 2014).

2.4.2 Compression Bandaging

The modified Robert Jones dressing (MRJD) is a splint bandage consisting of many layers of soft material wrapped around a joint or extremity covered by an elastic layer with more tension distally than proximally in an effort to promote venous drainage (Fig. 2.9). This dressing was proposed to limit edema of the extremity, effusions, and hemarthrosis. However, a recent randomized controlled trial (RCT) comparing MRJD and a conventional wound dressing did not show any differences in total mean drainage, hematocrit, and transfusion rates between the two groups (Pinsornsak and Chumchuen 2013). The limits of this study were first that the hidden blood loss was not evaluated, the pressure under the bandage in each patient with the

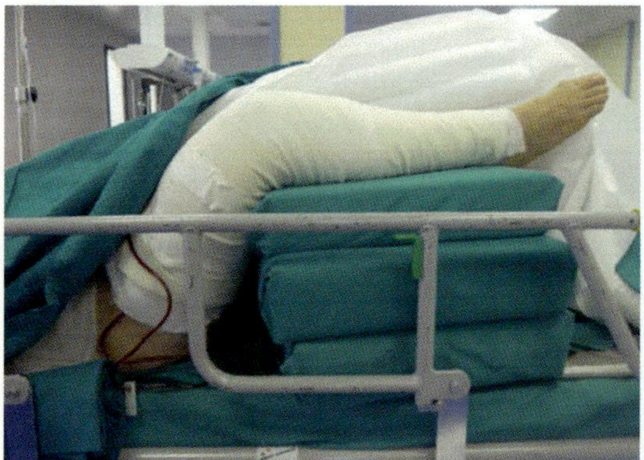

Fig. 2.8 The elevated limb decreases venous bleeding and knee flexion increases intra-articular pressure; for this reason, hip and knee flexion during surgery is an effective temporary method to reduce bleeding. This particular limb position should be maintained for a period of time inferior to 4–5 h

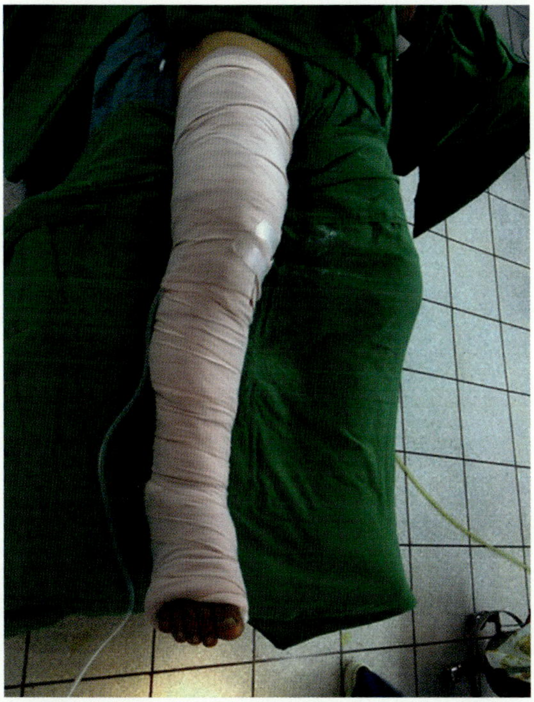

Fig. 2.9 The modified Robert-Jones dressing (MRJD) is a splint bandage consisting of many layers of soft material wrapped around a joint or extremity covered by an elastic layer with more tension distally than proximally in an effort to promote venous drainage. This dressing was proposed to limit edema of the extremity, effusions and hemarthroses

MRJB dressing was not measured, so the pressures underneath might have been different with each application. A previous study comparing the advantage of the MRJD with the elastic support bandage (Hughes et al. 1995) found no differences in pain (VAS), ROM, and analgesic need from the initial period to 3 weeks postoperative. However, the authors reported an elastic support bandage made the patients feel more comfortable than the MRJD during the first week in the early post injury period.

2.4.3 Adequate Pain Control

When postoperative pain is not properly controlled, the alert status of the patient may translate to higher blood pressure peaks. This cardiocirculatory postoperative status of the patient with a painful postoperative experience may elicit bleeding from vessels which are opened during the surgical procedure and not completely coagulated thereafter.

At this regard, Guay evaluated the effect of pain on perioperative blood loss in patients undergoing primary total knee replacement. Data from 60 patients undergoing TKA were prospectively collected (Guay 2006). They found a significant positive correlation between measured blood loss and morphine consumption from 12 to 18 h ($p=0.006$) and between calculated blood loss and preoperative mean arterial blood pressure ($p=0.01$) and preoperative hemoglobin value ($p=0.02$)

2.4.4 Cryotherapy

Cryotherapy has for centuries been considered to help in the reduction of pain, swelling, and blood loss after surgery, but despite some early gains, it yields no apparent lasting benefits. A recent systematic review and meta-analysis including 11 prospective RCT showed that cryotherapy has small benefits on blood loss and early ROM recovery; no benefits have been seen in transfusion requirements, pain, analgesia use, swelling, and length of stay. However, cryotherapy seems to be beneficial in pain control when regularly exchanged, and when added to a compressive dressing, it had additive range of motion benefits to compression alone (Adie et al. 2010). This leads to a recent randomized trial where ice packs were compared with continuous controlled temperature cryotherapy (Waegener, Beerse, Belgium). In this study, no benefits for advanced cryotherapy could be noted whilst a lower range of flexion was observed in the advanced cryotherapy group due to the many treatment hours spent lying down with the leg in extension during the treatment periods. The effect of cryotherapy is limited to the local anesthetic effect of the nerve endings in the skin which determines a subjective better feeling to patients, however, without any more important effect on the healing of postsurgical patients (Thienpont et al. 2014).

Cryopneumatic devices seem to offer additional benefit to cryotherapy alone. In a

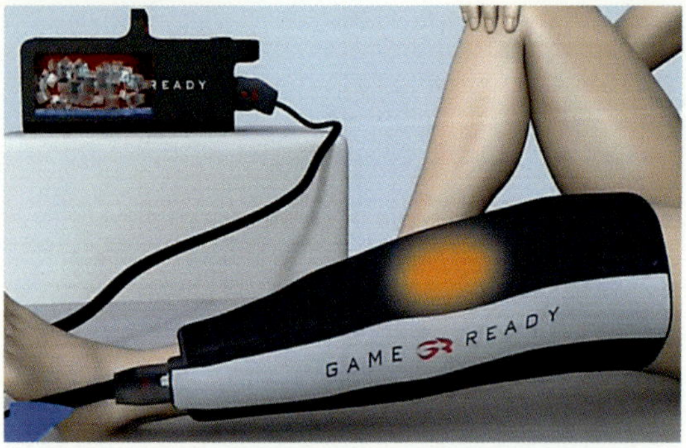

Fig. 2.10 A cryopneumatic device (Game Ready®, CoolSystems Inc., Concord, CA) provides joint compression while the cooling system is in action

multicenter study, 280 patients were randomized for a postoperative treatment either with a cryopneumatic device (Game Ready®, CoolSystems Inc., Concord, CA) or classic ice packings (Fig. 2.10). Both treatments were initiated within 3 h postoperation and used at least four times per day for 2 weeks. There was a significant difference in the satisfaction scores of patients with their cooling regimen, with greater satisfaction in the treatment group ($p<0.0001$). Narcotics consumption in the first 2 weeks was significantly lower in the study group (Su et al. 2012).

2.5 Prospective Randomized Study Performed at IFCA Clinic, Florence, Italy

2.5.1 Aim of the Study

This prospective randomized study was aimed to compare blood loss in three groups of patients. Ninety consecutive patients treated with TKA for osteoarthritis were randomized in the following groups:

1. Multimodal protocol (MM)
2. Multimodal protocol + hemostatic matrix (MM + HM)
3. Drain reinfusion only (controls)

The primary endpoints was the estimated blood loss volume.

Secondary endpoints were the drainage effusion (mL), blood transfusion rate, intraoperative bleeding, the need of synovectomy, ROM, and VAS at day 2 and discharge.

The following adverse events were collected: hematoma, hemarthrosis, the need for a lower dose of LMWH, and slow functional recovery.

2.6 Materials and Methods

From May 2013 to February 2014, all patients undergoing posterior stabilized cemented TKA in our institution for knee osteoarthritis were selected to take part in this prospective randomized study. Exclusion criteria were as follows: patients previously treated with LMWH (low-molecular-weight heparin) or oral anticoagulants and patients not tolerating LMWH or needing a different anticoagulant treatment for comorbidity, coagulopathies, all diagnosis other than primary osteoarthritis, and preoperative or intraoperative decision to perform the procedure without tourniquet. In our earlier patient treated with a standard protocol (drainage reinfusion only), the average postoperative blood loss over 5 days was approximately 2,000 ± 600 mL. We considered a reduction of this loss to approximately 1,500 ± 600 mL as clinically important. If any of the treatment groups caused such a reduction, the study should have a power of 80 % to detect it at a significance level of 5 %. Using these inputs, the STATA 10.0 software (StataCorp, College Station, TX, USA) found a sample size of 20 per group would be needed. In order to add statistical power, we decided to enroll 30 patients per group. Ninety consecutive patients were randomly assigned to three groups with a 1:1:1 ratio using closed envelopes.

In all patients, epidural anesthesia was used. Pneumatic tourniquet was inflated before incision (at a pressure ranging from 250 to 300 mmHg) and released just before wound closure. A less invasive surgical approach was used in every case with limited parapatellar incision without everting the patella.

The drainage was applied before wound closure and maintained for about 24 h. Robert Jones dressing and classic ice-packing cryotherapy were maintained for the first 24 h.

Table 2.2 Preoperative characteristics of the three groups of patients

	MM	MM+HM	Controls	*p* value
Age[a]	69±9.71	73.28±7.35	69.90±10.51	0.90
Sex				
Males	12	13	7	0.71
Females	18	17	13	
Basal Hb levels[a]	13.5±1.73	14.01±1.03	14.84±1.54	0.65
Basal HCT[a]	41.6±2.33	42.17±2.54	42.08±2.03	0.70

MM multimodal protocol, *MM+HM* multimodal protocol+hemostatic matrix, *Controls*. The three groups have been compared using chi-square test for sex and ANOVA for the others: no significant differences between the three groups were observed

[a]Age and basal levels of Hb and hct are expressed as mean±SD

The two experimental groups (group MM and MM+HM) have been treated with the same multimodal procedure including:

- IV *tranexamic acid* (*TA*: 10 mg/kg), 10 min before the tourniquet release and another identical dose 3 h after surgery.
- *Adrenaline* (*1/3 vial*) *and ropivacaine* (300 mg) intra-articular before wound closure
- *Postoperative 70° hip and knee flexion for 3 h*

Group 2 (MM+HM) had an additional treatment with a thrombin-based hemostatic matrix (FloSeal®, Baxter Healthcare Corporation, Fremont, CA, USA). After tourniquet deflation, 5 mL of FloSeal was applied in the suprapatellar area, in the medial and lateral patellofemoral gutters, and in every visible bleeding site. Group 2 received also a collagen topical hemostatic matrix (GentaFleece Baxter Healthcare Corporation, Fremont, CA, USA), which was inserted in the posterior recess between the implant and the posterior capsule.

The preoperative demographic data of the patients in the three groups are summarized in Table 2.2.

Drainage was removed about 24 h after surgery. On day 1, patients were helped by a physiotherapist to sit on the bedside; on day 2, they started passive motion and walked assisted. They were discharged 5–7 days after surgery. The blood hemoglobin concentration was determined preoperatively and on days 1, 2, 3, and 5 after surgery for all patients and on day 4 where indicated.

Blood transfusions were given to patients whose hemoglobin was less than 8.5 g/dL or less that 10 g/dL in case of symptomatic anemia. All patients consented to transfusion when required.

DVT prophylaxis protocol with LMWH was started the day before surgery (and maintained for 5 weeks after surgery); patients started ankle and foot movement exercises as soon as the anesthesia effect wore off; compressive stockings were prescribed to all patients from day 2 after surgery as soon as they were made to stand and started walking with crutches.

The total blood loss was evaluated through the following formula:

$$\text{Estimated blood loss}(\text{EBV}) = \text{weight}(\text{kg}) \times \text{average blood volume}$$

$$\text{Allowable blood loss}(\text{ABL}) = \frac{[\text{EBV} \times (\text{Hi} - \text{Hf})]}{\text{Hi}}$$

Intraoperative bleeding was quantified by the surgeon as follows:

- Grade I (+−−): below average, controllable by limited cauterization
- Grade II (++−): average bleeding, controllable by careful cauterization
- Grade III (+++): more than average, difficult to be completely controllable by cauterization

2.6.1 Statistical Analysis

Primary and secondary endpoints were analyzed using one-way ANOVA with STATA 10.0 software (StataCorp, College Station, TX, USA). If a significant difference among the groups was found, pairwise differences between groups were examined by Scheffe's test. The significance level

Table 2.3 Primary endpoints

Variable	Controls	MM	MM+HM	*p* value
EBV day 1 (in mL)	1,377.5±388.57	1,068±383.5	1,042.5±234	0.0027
MM	0.015			
MM+HM	0.007	0.96		
EBV day 2 (in mL)	1,812.5±915.3	1,238±739.2	1,254±323.5	0.0021
MM	0.043			
MM+HM	0.002	0.71		
EBV day 3 (in mL)	1,963.5±572	1,347±435.5	1,453.5±431	0.0026
MM	0.025			
MM+HM	0.006	0.86		
EBV day 5 (in mL)	1,876.5±612	1,567±864.3	1,441±368	0.024
MM	0.065			
MM+HM	0.056	0.97		

Blood loss (mL) at days 1, 2, 3, and 5 is reported as mean±SD; *p* value comparing the difference between the three groups and groups' subanalysis is also reported

used for all tests was $p<0.05$. Multiple regression was used to investigate a possible association between total blood loss and intraoperative data (synovectomy and intraoperative bleeding).

2.7 Results

Total blood loss was significantly lower in the experimental groups than in the control group. During the study, we found an unacceptable rate of bleedings in the controls (group 3) compared to the other groups. For this ethical reason, we decided to stop the control group when the number of 20 enrolled patients had been reached. The two experimental groups enrolled 30 patients each for a total of 80 patients in the entire study cohort.

Using Scheffe's test the total blood loss was comparable in the two experimental groups (Table 2.3). Similar results were found for the drainage effusion. ROM and VAS at day 2 and discharge were comparable in the three groups (Table 2.4).

Intraoperative data are reported in Table 2.5. The occurrence of synovectomy was higher in the DR and MM+HM groups. Only two patients in the control group had a severe intraoperative bleeding requiring protocol violation: in these two patients, a rescue with TA was given postoperatively.

No serious side effects were observed in the protocol. As previously reported, in two patients of the control group, TA was administered because of a severe intraoperative bleeding. No complications were observed in the follow-up of these two patients. LMWH dose reduction and compressive bandage were successfully applied in two patients of the control group for a mild-moderate hemarthrosis.

Transfusion rate was higher in the control group: four patients received ABT (20 %), one of them received 2 units of concentrated red blood cells (trigger Hb=7.4 g/dL), and two patients in MM group (6.6 %) and three patients in the MM+HM group (10 %) received 1 unit of red blood cells each. Using chi-square test, a trend toward a statistical significance was found between the three groups ($p=0.075$) but maybe because of the limited number of cases or because of the predominant male population starting with a higher Hb level, the proportion of patients requiring ABT did not significantly differ among the three groups. Fisher exact test was used to compare the proportion of patients requiring ABT between control and the two experimental groups which was significantly higher than the first one ($p=0.016$, OR 3.22) indicating that patients treated only with DR are at the higher risk of ATB.

Table 2.4 Secondary endpoints

Variable	Controls	MM	MM+HM	*p value*
Drainage (in mL)	749.5±221	260.5±91.5	175±110.5	0.0001
MM	0.0001			
MM+HM	0.0001	0.173		
VAS day 2 (0–10)	2.5±2	1.9±1	1±0.75	0.42
MM	0.81			
MM+HM	0.43	0.81		
VAS discharge (0–10)	2.5±2	0.8±0.6	0.7±0.3	0.58
MM	0.96			
MM+HM	0.61	0.75		
ROM day 2	65±14.5	77±16.5	86±12.2	0.61
MM	0.57			
MM+HM	0.53	0.64		
ROM discharge	67±14.1	93±15.4	89±12.3	0.64
MM	0.51			
MM+HM	0.43	0.69		

Drainage effusion is reported in mL
ROM only the maximum flexion has been considered for statistical analysis

Table 2.5 Intraoperative data concerning rate of synovectomy and classification of visual bleeding score by surgical team

	DR	MM	MM+HM
Synovectomy	8/20	11/30	12/30
Bleeding+−−/3	8/20	17/30	16/30
Bleeding ++−/3	10/20	13/30	14/30
Bleeding +++/3	2/20	0/30	0/30

Looking at the intraoperative data, a possible association between synovectomy, intraoperative bleeding, and blood loss has been investigated through multiple regression using a stepwise selection. The maximum blood loss for each patient was taken into consideration, independently from which postoperative day (nadir). No relation was detected between synovectomy and total blood loss ($R^2=0.046$, $p=0.24$).

The relation between functional ability and total blood loss was also evaluated through linear regression, taking in consideration the maximum knee flexion at day 2 and discharge. While at day 2, there is a positive, but limited, association between the two items ($R^2=0.081$, $p=0.023$), this positive trend is lost during hospitalization since at discharge no association has been found.

2.8 Discussion

According to our data, a multimodal protocol is effective in bleeding control independently from the association of a topic HM. As a matter of fact, no statistically significant differences have been detected between the two treatment groups in terms of total blood loss and drainage effusion. However, the limit of this study is still the small population due to the strict exclusion criteria that have more than halved the number of potentially enrollable patients. Despite the comparable results in the two experimental groups, a potential use of HM may be cost-effective in patients at high risk of bleeding, especially patients with coagulopathies or previously exposed to oral anticoagulants or LMWH, or in revision procedures in which this device may foster hemostasis locally.

The effect of synovectomy has been recently reported in an RCT on 50 patients undergoing bilateral TKA within the same procedure; synovectomy was done in one randomly assigned knee and was associated with higher blood loss and hemarthrosis occurrence; no association with pain and functional rehabilitation was observed (Kilicarslan et al. 2011). These data are in contrast with our results in which no relation between synovectomy and EBV has been detected. However, our data are influenced by the different treatments as TA and HM.

The effect of the different regimens of treatment was very limited on functional recovery evaluated through ROM: a mild effect during the follow-up at the hospital. At discharge all patients had a satisfactory functional recovery, and almost all of them reached a ROM 0–90; in only one patient of the control group, ROM was limited to 0–60, and she was successfully treated with femoral nerve block 1 day before discharge.

Looking at the safety, it is evident that patients treated only with reinfusion drains had a higher blood loss since surgery (two patients were rescued with TA for that reason). According to our analysis, the risk of requiring ATB is more than three times more than patients treated with multimodal protocol independently from the association of HM. For that reason, it should be strongly recommended not to use DR alone in TKA so far. MM protocol is a simple, cheap, safe, and efficacious method for bleeding control in primary TKA. The association with HM seems not to influence blood loss; for that reason, HM should not be used in the routine practice of TKA; further studies on patients at high risks of bleeding, both for comorbidities and concomitant medications and for type of surgery, are necessary to evaluate their role in bleeding control when more hemostasis is required.

Key Points

- There is a growing tendency toward avoidance of postoperative drains use, particularly when associated to a multimodal protocol which limits hemarthrosis.
- The use of tourniquet has known advantages and disadvantages. If properly utilized, it may represent a valid tool to control intraoperative bleeding.
- Occult bleeding is a major contributor to blood loss after arthroplasty. Intraoperative care should be taken to limit the potential sources which enhance it.
- Tranexamic acid usage for lower limb arthroplasty procedures has reached the level of standard of care for obvious benefits and no side effects.
- When a multimodal protocol for bleeding control in hip and knee arthroplasty is employed, the role of expensive tools such as hemostatic matrices and bipolar sealing devices may be justified for specific conditions at higher risk of bleeding.
- Patient positioning associated with new cryotherapy regimens have a key role in limiting intra- and periarticular bleeding and in improving the functional recovery.

References

Abdel-Salam A, Eyres KS (1995) Effects of tourniquet during total knee arthroplasty. A prospective randomised study. J Bone Joint Surg Br 77:250

Adalberth G, Bystrom S, Kolstad K et al (1998) Postoperative drainage of knee arthroplasty is not necessary: a randomized study of 90 patients. Acta Orthop Scand 69:475

Adie S, Naylor JM, Harris IA (2010) Cryotherapy after total knee arthroplasty a systematic review and meta-analysis of randomized controlled trials. J Arthroplasty 25(5):709–715

Aglietti P, Baldini A, Vena LM et al (2000) Effect of tourniquet use on activation of coagulation in total knee replacement. Clin Orthop 371:169–177

Ajwani SH, Jones M, Jarrat JW et al (2012) Computer assisted versus conventional total knee replacement: a comparison of tourniquet time, blood loss and length of stay. Knee 19:606–610

Albala DM, Lawson JH (2006) Recent clinical and investigational applications of fibrin sealant in selected surgical specialties. J Am Coll Surg 202:685–697

Alcelik I, Pollock RD, Sukeik M et al (2012) A comparison of outcomes with and without a tourniquet in total knee arthroplasty: a systematic review and meta-analysis of randomized controlled trials. J Arthroplasty 27(3):331–340

An HS, Mikhail WE, Jackson WT et al (1991) Effects of hypotensive anesthesia, nonsteroidal antiinflammatory drugs, and poly- methylmethacrylate on bleeding in total hip arthroplasty patients. J Arthroplasty 6:245–250

Baldini A, Adravanti P (2009) Less invasive TKA: extramedullary femoral reference without navigation. Clin Orthop Relat Res 466(11):2694–2700

Berman AT, Fabiano D, Bosacco SJ et al (1990) Comparison between intermittent (spring- loaded) and continuous closed suction drainage of orthopedic wounds: a controlled clinical trial. Orthopedics 13:309–314

Blanié A, Bellamy L, Rhayem Y et al (2013) Duration of postoperative fibrinolysis after total hip or knee replacement: a laboratory follow-up study. Thromb Res 131(1):e6–e11

Bong MR, Patel V, Chang E et al (2004) Risks associated with blood transfusion after total knee arthroplasty. J Arthroplasty 3:281–287

Cao L, Ablimit N, Mamtimin A et al (2009) Comparison of no drain or with a drain after unilateral total knee arthroplasty: a prospective randomized controlled trial. Zhonghua Wai Ke Za Zhi 47:1390–1393

Cardone D, Klein AA (2009) Perioperative blood conservation. Eur J Anesth 26:722–729

Carless PA, Henry DA, Anthony DM (2003) Fibrin sealant use for minimising peri- operative allogeneic blood transfusion. Cochrane Database Syst Rev 2:CD004171

Christodoulou AG, Ploumis AL, Terzedis IP et al (2004) The role of timing on tourniquet release and cementing on perioperative blood loss in total knee replacement. Knee 11:313–317

Cleeland CS, Demetri GD, Glaspy J et al (1999) Identifying hemoglobin level for optimal quality of life: results of an incremental analysis (Abstract). Proc Am Soc Clin Oncol 18:547a

Clement RC, Kamath AF, Derman PB et al (2012) Bipolar sealing in revision total hip arthroplasty for infection: efficacy and cost analysis. J Arthroplasty 27(7): 1376–1381

Cohen JA, Brecher ME (1995) Preoperative autologous blood donation: benefit or detriment; a mathematical analysis. Transfusion 35:640–644

Cowell HR (1937) Editorial. Prior deposit of autologous blood for transfusion. J Bone Joint Surg 69A:319

Davis NJ, Jennings JJ, Harris WH (1974) Induced hypotensive anesthesia for total hip replacement. Clin Orthop 101:93–98

Derman PB, Kamath AF, Lee GC (2013) Saline-coupled bipolar sealing in revision total knee arthroplasty for infection. Am J Orthop (Belle Mead NJ) 42(9): 407–411

Diiorio TM, Burkholder JD, Good RP et al (2012) Platelet-rich plasma does not reduce blood loss or pain or improve range of motion after TKA. Clin Orthop Relat Res 470(1):138–143

Din R, Geddes T (2004) Skin protection beneath the tourniquet. A prospective randomized trial. ANZ J Surg 74:721

Dunn CJ, Goa KL (1999) Tranexamic acid: a review of its use in surgery and other indications. Drugs 57:1005

Engel JM, Jojaus T, Ruwoldt R et al (2001) Regional hemostatic status and blood requirements after total knee arthroplasty with and without tranexamic acid or aprotinin. Anesth Analg 92:775

Eroglu A, Uzunlar H, Erciyes N (2005) Comparison of hypotensive epidural anesthesia and hypotensive total intravenous anesthesia on intraoperative blood loss during total hip replacement. J Clin Anesth 17:420–425

Esler CN, Blakeway C, Fiddian NJ (2003) The use of a closed- suction drain in total knee arthroplasty. A prospective, randomised study. J Bone Joint Surg Br 85:215

Eubanks JD (2010) Antifibrinolytics in major orthopaedic surgery. J Am Acad Orthop Surg 92:775

Everts PAM, Devilee RJJ, Brown MC et al (2006) Platelet gel and fibrin sealant reduce allogeneic blood transfusions in total knee arthroplasty. Acta Anaesthesiol Scand 50:593–599

Everts PAM, Devilee RJJ, Oosterbos CJM et al (2007) Autologous platelet gel and sealant enhance the efficacy of total knee arthroplasty: improved range of motion, decreased length of stay and a reduced incidence of arthrofibrosis. Knee Surg Sports Traumatol Arthrosc 15:888–894

Falez F, Meo A, Panegrossi G et al (2013) Blood loss reduction in cementless total hip replacement with fibrin spray or bipolar sealer: a randomised controlled trial on ninety five patients. Int Orthop 37(7):1213–1217

Fedi S, Gori AM, Falciani M et al (1999) Procedure-dependence and tissue factor-independence of hypercoagulability during orthopaedic surgery. Thromb Haemost 81(6):874–878

Flordal PA, Neander G (1991) Blood loss in total hip replacement: a retrospective study. Arch Orthop Trauma Surg 111:34–38

Flynn JC, Csenesitz TA (1979) Present status of intraoperative blood recovery during orthopaedics surgery. Jefferson Orthop J 8:22–25

Guay J (2006) Postoperative pain significantly influences postoperative blood loss in patients undergoing total knee replacement. Pain Med 7(6):476–482

Haien Z, Yong J, Baoan M et al (2013) Post-operative auto-transfusion in total hip or knee arthroplasty: a meta-analysis of randomized controlled trials. PLoS One 8(1):e55073. doi:10.1371/journal.pone.0055073

Harvey EJ, Leclerc J, Brooks CE et al (1997) Effect of tourniquet use on blood loss and incidence of deep vein thrombosis in total knee arthroplasty. J Arthroplasty 12(3):291–296

Heyse T, Haas SB, Drinkwater D et al (2014) Intraarticular fibrinogen does not reduce blood loss in TKA: a randomized clinical trial. Clin Orthop Relat Res 472: 272–276

Holt BT, Parks NL, Engh GA et al (1997) Comparison of closed-suction drainage and no drainage after primary total knee arthroplasty. Orthopedics 20:1121–1124

Huang Z, Shen B, Ma J et al (2012) Mini-midvastus versus medial parapatellar approach in TKA: muscle damage and inflammation markers. Orthopedics 35(7):e1038–e1045

Hughes DL, Crosby AC (1995) Treatment of knee sprains: modified Robert Jones or elastic support bandage?. J Accid Emerg Med 12(2):115–8

Irvine GB, Chan RN (1986) Arterial calcification and tourniquets. Lancet 2:1217

Ishii Y, Matsuda Y (2005) Effect of the timing of tourniquet release on perioperative blood loss associated with cementless total knee arthroplasty: a prospective randomized study. J Arthroplasty 20(8):977–983

Jans Ø, Jørgensen C, Kehlet H et al (2014) Role of preoperative anemia for risk of transfusion and postoperative morbidity in fast-track hip and knee arthroplasty. Transfusion 54(3):717–726

Jones AP, Harrison M, Hui A (2007) Comparison of autologous transfusion drains versus no drain in total knee arthroplasty. Acta Orthop Belg 73(3):377–385

Jou IM, Lai Ka, Yang CY (1993) Blood loss associated with total knee arthroplasty. J Orthop Surg (ROC) 10:213

Juelsgaard P, Møller M, Larsen U (2002) Preoperative Acute Normovolaemic Hemodilution (ANH) in combination with Hypotensive Epidural Anaesthesia (HEA) during knee arthroplasty surgery. No effect on transfusion rate. A randomized controlled trial [ISRCTN87597684]. BMC Anesthesiol 2(1):1

Jung WH, Chun CW, Lee JH et al (2013) No difference in total blood loss, haemoglobin and haematocrit between continues and intermittent wound drainage after total knee arthroplasty. Knee Surg Sports Traumatol Arthrosc 21(12):2831–2836

Keating EM (1999) Current options and approaches for blood management in orthopaedic surgery. Instr Course Lect 48:655–665

Keating EM, Meding JB (2002) Perioperative blood management practices in elective orthopaedic surgery. J Am Acad Orthop Surg 10:393–400

Keating EM, Ritter MA (2002) Transfusion options in total joint arthroplasty. J Arthroplasty 17(Suppl 1): 125–128

Keating EM, Meding JB, Faris PM et al (1998) Predictors of transfusion risk in elective knee surgery. Clin Orthop 357:50–59

Keating EM, Faris PM, Meding JB et al (1999) Comparison of the midvastus muscle-splitting approach with the median parapatellar approach in total knee arthroplasty. J Arthroplasty 14:29–32

Kilicarslan K, Yalcin N, Cicek H et al (2011) The effect of total synovectomy in total knee arthroplasty: a prospective randomized controlled study. Knee Surg Sports Traumatol Arthrosc 19(6):932–935

Kim YH, Cho SH, Kim RS (1998) Drainage versus nondrainage in simultaneous bilateral total knee arthroplasties. Clin Orthop Relat Res 347:188–193

Kim HJ, Fraser MR, Kahn B et al (2012) The efficacy of a thrombin-based hemostatic agent in unilateral total knee arthroplasty: a randomized controlled trial. J Bone Joint Surg Am 94:1160–1165

Kim TK, Chang CB, Koh IJ (2014) Practical issues for the use of tranexamic acid in total knee arthroplasty: a systematic review. Knee Surg Sports Traumatol Arthrosc 22(8):1849–1858

Kiss H, Raffl M, Neumann D et al (2005) Epinephrine-augmented hypotensive epidural anesthesia replace tourniquet use in total knee replacement. Clin Orthop Relat Res 436:184–189

Kluba T, Fiedler K, Kunze B et al (2012) Fibrin sealant in orthopaedic surgery: practical experiences derived from use of QUIXIL in total knee arthroplasty. Arch Orthop Trauma Surg 132:1147–1152

Ko PS, Tio MK, Tang YK et al (2003) Sealing the intramedullary femoral canal with autologous bone plug in total knee arthroplasty. J Arthroplasty 18:6–9

Kumar A (2009) Perioperative management of anemia: limits of blood transfusion and alternatives to it. Cleve Clin J Med 76:112–118

Kumar N, Saleh J, Gardiner E et al (2000) Plugging the intramedullary canal of the femur in total knee arthroplasty: reduction in postoperative blood loss. J Arthroplasty 15:947–949

Lee GC, Hawes T, Cushner FD et al (2005) Current trends in blood conservation in total knee arthroplasty. Clin Orthop Relat Res 440:170–174

Leeman MF, Costa ML, Costello E, Edwards D (2006) Timing of re-transfusion drain removal following total knee replacement. Ann R Coll Surg Engl 88(2): 134–5

Lemaire R (2008) Strategies for blood management in orthopaedic and trauma surgery. J Bone Joint Surg Br 90:1128–1136

Levy O, Martinowitz U, Oran A et al (1999) The use of fibrin tissue adhesive to reduce blood loss and the need for blood transfusion after total knee arthroplasty. A prospective, randomized, multicenter study. J Bone Joint Surg Am 81(11):1580–1588

Li B, Wen Y, Liu D et al (2012) The effect of knee position on blood loss and range of motion following total knee arthroplasty. Knee Surg Sports Traumatol Arthrosc 20(3):594–599

Li ZJ, Fu X, Tian P (2014) Fibrin sealant before wound closure in total knee arthroplasty reduced blood loss: a meta-analysis. Knee Surg Sports Traumatol Arthrosc Feb 12. [Epub ahead of print]

Liu J, Cao JG, Wang L et al (2014) Effect of fibrin sealant on blood loss following total knee arthroplasty: a systematic review and meta-analysis. Int J Surg 12(2):95–102. doi:10.1016/j.ijsu.2013.11.011. Epub 2013 Dec 4

Lotke PA, Barth P, Garino JP et al (1999) Predonated autologous blood transfusions after total knee arthroplasty: immediate versus delayed administration. J Arthroplasty 14:647–650

Mallory TH (1973) Hypotensive anesthesia in total hip replacement. JAMA 224:248

Maniar RN, Kumar G, Singhi T et al (2012) Most effective regimen of tranexamic acid in knee arthroplasty: a prospective randomized controlled study in 240 patients. Clin Orthop Relat Res 470(9):2605–2612

Martin A, Prenn M, Spiegel T et al (2004) Relevance of wound drainage in total knee arthroplasty–a prospective comparative study. Z Orthop Ihre Grenzgeb 142:46–50

Mcvay PA, Toy PT (1996) Very severe outcomes associated with autologous blood donation [letter]. Transfusion 36:761

Mengal B, Aebi J, Rodriguez A et al (2001) A prospective randomized study of wound drainage versus non-

drainage in primary total hip or knee arthroplasty. Rev Chir Orthop Reparatrice Appar Mot 87:29
Mohanial PK, Sandiford N, Skinner JA et al (2013) Comparison of blood loss between computer assisted and conventional total knee arthroplasty. Indian J Orthop 47:63–66
Moonen AF, Neal TD, Pilot P (2006) Peri-operative blood management in elective orthopaedic surgery. A critical review of the literature. Injury 37S:511–516
Napier RJ, Bennett D, McConway J et al (2014) The influence of immediate knee flexion on blood loss and other parameters following total knee replacement. Bone Joint J 96-B(2):201–209
Nelson CL, Bowen WS (1986) Total hip arthroplasty in Jehovah's Witnesses without blood transfusion. J Bone Joint Surg Am 68:350–353
Newman RJ (1984) Metabolic effects of tourniquet ischaemia studied by nuclear magnetic resonance spectroscopy. J Bone Joint Surg Br 66-B:434
Niemi TT, Syrijala M, Rosenbemrg PH (2000) Comparison of hypotensive epidural anaesthesia and spinal anaesthesia on blood loss and coagulation during and after total hip arthroplasty. Acta Anaesthesiol Scand 44:457–464
Notarnicola A, Moretti L, Martucci A et al (2012) Comparative efficacy of different doses of fibrin sealant to reduce bleeding after total knee arthroplasty. Blood Coagul Fibrinolysis 23(4):278–284
Noticewala MS, Nyce JD, Wang W et al (2012) Predicting need for allogenetic transfusion after total knee arthroplasty. J Arthoplasty 27(6):961–967
Nuttall GA, Santrach PJ, Oliver WC Jr et al (1996) The predictors of red cell transfusions in total hip arthroplasties. Transfusion 36:144–149
O'Leary AM, Veall G, Butler P et al (1990) Acute pulmonary oedema after tourniquet release. Can J Anaesth 37:826
Omonbude D, El MM, O'Connor PJ et al (2010) Measurement of joint effusion and haematoma formation by ultrasound in assessing the effectiveness of drains after total knee replacement: a prospective randomised study. J Bone Joint Surg Br 92:51
Ong SM, Taylor GJ (2003) Can knee position save blood following total knee replacement? Knee 10(1):81–85
Parker MJ, Roberts CP, Hay D (2004) Closed suction drainage for hip and knee arthroplasty. A meta-analysis. J Bone Joint Surg Am 86-A:1146
Pfeiffer M, Bräutigam H, Draws D, Sigg A (2005) A new bipolar blood sealing system embedded in perioperative strategies vs. a conventional regimen for total knee arthroplasty: results of a matched-pair study. Ger Med Sci 13;3:Doc10.
Pietsch M, Djahani O, Zweiger C et al (2013) Custom-fit minimally invasive total knee arthroplasty: effect on blood loss and early clinical outcomes. Knee Surg Sports Traumatol Arthrosc 21(10):2234–2240
Pinsornsak P, Chumchuen S (2013) Can a modified Robert Jones bandage after knee arthroplasty reduce blood loss? A prospective randomized controlled trial. Clin Orthop Relat Res 471:1677–1681
Plymale MF, Capogna BM, Lovy AJ et al (2012) Unipolar vs bipolar hemostasis in total knee arthoplasty: a prospective randomized trial. J Arthroplasty 27(6):1133–1137
Pornrattanamaneewong C, Narkbunnam R, Siriwattanasakul P et al (2012) Three-hour interval drain clamping reduces postoperative bleeding in total knee arthroplasty: a prospective randomized controlled trial. Arch Orthop Trauma Surg 132(7): 1059–1063
Prasad N, Padmanabhan V, Mullaji A (2007) Blood loss in total Knee arthroplasty: an analysis of risk factors. Int Orthop 31:31–44
Rama KR, Apsingi S, Poovali S et al (2007) Timing of tourniquet release in knee arthroplasty. Meta-analysis of randomized, controlled trials. J Bone Joint Surg Am 89:699–705
Randelli F, D'Anchise R, Ragone V et al (2014) Is the newest fibrin sealant an effective strategy to reduce blood loss after total knee arthroplasty? A randomized controlled study. J Arthroplasty. doi:10.1016/j.arth.2014.02.024, pii: S0883-5403(14)00116-8
Raut VV, Stone MH, Wroblewski BM (1993) Reduction of postoperative blood loss after press-fit condylar knee arthroplasty with use of a femoral intramedullary plug. J Bone Joint Surg Am 75:1356–1357
Reinhardt KR, Osoria H, Nam D et al (2013) Reducing blood loss after total knee replacement: a fibrin solution. Bone Joint J 95-B(11 Suppl A):135–139
Rosencher N, Bellamy L, Chabbouh T et al (2008) Blood conservation approaches in orthopedic surgery. Transfus Clin Biol 15(5):294–302
Schmied H, Kurz A, Sessler DI et al (1995) Mild hypothermia increases blood loss and transfusion requirements during total hip arthroplasty. Lancet 147:289–292
Sculco TP, Ranawat C (1975) The use of spinal anesthesia for total hip-replacement arthroplasty. J Bone Joint Surg Am 57:173–177
Sehat KR, Evans R, Newman JH (2000) How much blood is really lost in total knee arthroplasty? Correct blood loss management should take hidden loss into account. Knee 7:151–155
Sehat KR, Evans RL, Newman JH (2004) Hidden blood loss following hip and knee arthroplasty. Correct management of blood loss should take hidden loss into account. J Bone Joint Surg Br 86(4):561–565
Senthil KG, Von Arx OA, Pozo JL (2005) Rate of blood loss over 48 hours following total knee replacement. Knee 12(4):307–309
Sharrock NE, Salvati EA (1996) Hypotensive epidural anesthesia for total hip arthroplasty. Acta Orthop Scand 67:91–107
Sharrock NE, Mineo R, Urquhart B et al (1993) The effect of two levels of hypotension on intraoperative blood loss during total hip arthroplasty performed under lumbar epidural anesthesia. Anesth Analg 76:580–584
Shen PC, Jou IM, Lin YT et al (2005) Comparison between 4-hour clamping drainage and nonclamping drainage after total knee arthroplasty. J Arthroplasty 20:909–913

Silver R, De la Garza J, Rang M et al (1986) Limb swelling after release of a tourniquet. Clin Orthop Relat Res 206:86

Skovgaard C, Holm B, Troelsen A et al (2013) No effect of fibrin sealant on drain output or functional recovery following simultaneous bilateral total knee arthroplasty: a randomized, double-blind, placebo-controlled study. Acta Orthop 84(2):153–158

Smith TO, Hing CB (2010) Is a tourniquet beneficial in total knee replacement surgery? A meta-analysis and systematic review. Knee 17(2):141–147

Stucinskas J, Tarasevicius S, Cebatorius A et al (2009) Conventional drainage versus four hour clamping drainage after total knee arthroplasty in severe osteoarthritis: a prospective, randomised trial. Int Orthop 33(5):1275–1278

Su EP, Perna M, Boettner F et al (2012) A prospective, multi-center, randomised trial to evaluate the efficacy of a cryopneumatic device on total knee arthroplasty recovery. J Bone Joint Surg Br 94(11 Suppl A): 153–156

Tai TW, Jou IM, Chang CW et al (2010) Non-drainage is better than 4-hour clamping drainage in total knee arthroplasty. Orthopedics 33(3):156–160

Tai TW, Lin CJ, Jou IM et al (2011) Tourniquet use in total knee arthroplasty: a meta-analysis. Knee Surg Sports Traumatol Arthrosc 19(7):1121–1130

Tanaka N, Sakahashi H, Sato E et al (2001) Timing of the administration of tranexamic acid for maximum reduction in blood loss in arthroplasty of the knee. J Bone Joint Surg Br 83:702–705

Tao K, Wu HS, Li XH et al (2006) The use of a closed-suction drain in total knee arthroplasty: a prospective, randomized study. Zhonghua Wai Ke Za Zhi 44:1111–1114

Thiengwittayaporn S, Junsee D, Tanavalee A (2009) A comparison of blood loss in minimally invasive surgery with and without electromagnetic computer navigation in total knee arthroplasty. J Med Assoc Thai 92:S27–S32

Thienpont E, Grosu I, Paternostre F (2014) The use of patient-specific instruments does not reduce blood loss during minimally invasive total knee arthroplasty? Knee Surg Sports Traumatol Arthrosc Mar 27. [Epub ahead of print]

Thoms RJ, Marwin SE (2009) The role of fibrin sealants in orthopaedic surgery. J Am Acad Orthop Surg 17:727–736

Vundelinckx BJ, Bruckers L, De Mulder K et al (2013) Functional and radiographic short-term outcome evaluation of the Visionaire system, a patient-matched instrumentation system for total knee arthroplasty. J Arthroplasty 28:964–970

Wellisz T, An YH, Wen X et al (2008) Infection rates and healing using bone wax and soluble polymer material. Clin Orthop Relat Res 466:481–486

Wind TC, Bartfield WR, Moskal JT (2013) The effect of tranexamic acid on blood loss and transfusion rate in primary total knee arthroplasty. J Arthroplasty 28: 1080–1083

Wong J, Abrishami A, El Beheiry H et al (2010) Topical application of tranexamic acid reduces postoperative blood loss in total knee arthroplasty: a randomized, controlled trials. J Bone Joint Surg Am 92:2503–2513

Yomtovian R (1996) Autologous transfusion complications. In: Popovsky MA (ed) Transfusion reactions. American Association of Blood Banks Press, Bethesda, pp 237–280

Zamora-Navas P, Collado-Torres F, de la Torrie-Solis F (1999) Closed suction drainage after knee arthroplasty. A prospective study of the effectiveness of the operation and of bacterial contamination. Acta Orthop Belg 65(1):44–47

Zeh A, Messer J, Davis J et al (2010) The Aquamantys system – an alternative to reduce blood loss in primary total hip arthroplasty? J Arthroplasty 25(7):1072–1077

Zhang QD, Guo WS, Zhang Q et al (2011) Comparison between closed suction drainage and nondrainage in total knee arthroplasty: a meta-analysis. J Arthroplasty 26(8):1265–1272

Antiplatelet Therapy in Patients with Coronary Stent Undergoing Orthopedic Surgery: Is It Still No Man's Land?

3

Roberta Rossini, Giuseppe Musumeci, and Leonardo Bolognese

Open Questions

- When is it safe to undergo an arthroplasty procedure after cardiac stenting?
- How much is postoperative bleeding risk increased without discontinuation of antiplatelet therapy?
- Which is the optimal antiplatelet regimen in patients with stents undergoing an arthroplasty procedure?
- In case of perioperative suspension of antiplatelet therapy, which is the right "bridging" therapy to do?

3.1 Introduction

Percutaneous coronary intervention (PCI) in patients with coronary artery disease is increasing worldwide. Every year more than one million PCIs are performed in the United States and Europe (Roger et al. 2011; Moschovitis et al. 2010). In more than 85 % of cases, a coronary stent is implanted (Savonitto et al. 2011), and prolonged antiplatelet therapy is mandatory after stent implantation. International guidelines recommend dual antiplatelet therapy (DAPT) for at least 4 weeks after bare metal stent (BMS) and 6–12 weeks after drug-eluting stent (DES) implantation (Task Force on Myocardial Revascularization of the ESC 2010). Premature withdrawal of antiplatelet therapy is associated with a significantly higher risk of cardiac ischemic events, due to stent thrombosis (ST). This is a rare but life-threatening complication, which occurs most of the time as acute myocardial infarction with a mortality of 10–40 %. Stent thrombosis is up to 90 times higher after premature discontinuation of DAPT (Iakovou et al. 2005). The prevalence and causes of premature discontinuation of DAPT after DES implantation have been assessed in previous studies, showing that premature discontinuation was not a rare event (more than one patient out of ten). The most common causes of discontinuation were surgery and bleeding events and were often associated with a poor prognosis (Rossini et al. 2011; Ferreira-González et al. 2010).

Aspirin can significantly reduce the risk of cardio-cerebrovascular events in secondary prevention (Antithrombotic Trialists' Collaboration 2002). Its abrupt discontinuation can be associated with a rebound effect (Biondi-Zoccai et al. 2006). Of note, surgical interventions increase per se coagulation (Priebe 2004). Previous studies

R. Rossini • G. Musumeci
Cardiovascular Department, AO Papa Giovanni XXIII, Bergamo, Italy

L. Bolognese (✉)
Cardiovascular and Neurological Department, Azienda Ospedaliera, Arezzo, Italy
e-mail: leonardobolognese@hotmail.com

A. Baldini, P. Caldora (eds.), *Perioperative Medical Management for Total Joint Arthroplasty: How to Control Hemostasis, Pain and Infection*, DOI 10.1007/978-3-319-07203-6_3,

demonstrated that perioperative discontinuation of aspirin therapy is associated with a significant increase of major adverse cardiac events (MACEs) (Biondi-Zoccai et al. 2006; Oscarsson et al. 2010). Also in coronary artery by-pass grafting (CABG), the maintenance of aspirin in the perioperative phase is associated with a significant reduction of mortality (Mangano 2002; Topol 2002).

Data on the effect of the association of aspirin and clopidogrel is lacking and derives mostly from post hoc analyses of randomized trials and from registries (Yusuf et al. 2001; Firanescu et al. 2009).

The incidence of perioperative MACE is high especially if surgery is performed early after coronary stenting (Berger et al. 2010).

The increase of MACE might be, in part, due to the perioperative discontinuation of antiplatelet therapy (Albaladejo et al. 2011; Schouten et al. 2007; Artang and Dieter 2007). In Shouten's series, the overall population experienced 2.6 % of MACE, which rose up to 13.3 % in patients undergoing early surgery (Artang and Dieter 2007). However, data on the protective effect of perioperative antiplatelet therapy are not consistent in previous studies (Anwaruddin et al. 2009; van Kuijk et al. 2009). These (apparently) discordant data might be explained by a patients' selection bias: antiplatelet therapy maintenance might identify a population at high risk for MACE, which seems likely the results of complex unidentified interactions between clinical and surgical risk factors. Previous studies demonstrated that the risk of perioperative MACE is higher within the first months after stent implantation (Cruden et al. 2010), even though data are not consistent (Rabbitts et al. 2008). In a recent study by Wijeysundera and colleagues (Wijeysundera et al. 2012), the overall rate of 30-day events was 2.1 %. It demonstrated that elective noncardiac surgery could be performed reasonably safely in carefully selected patients once at least 6 months have elapsed since DES implantation and from 46 to 180 days after BMS implantation.

It is well known that antiplatelet therapy confers an increased risk of bleeding (Antithrombotic Trialists' Collaboration 2002; Yusuf et al. 2001). Conversely, the association between antiplatelet agents and perioperative bleeding risk has not been adequately addressed. The vast majority of the available data derives from registries or observational studies, which do not have sufficient statistical power.

A meta-analysis on low-dose aspirin on perioperative bleeding complications demonstrated that aspirin increased the frequency of bleeding complications by approximately 50 % (Burger et al. 2005). However, the definition used in the included studies was extremely heterogeneous and often did not use a standard definition. Moreover, when surgeons were blinded regarding aspirin application, they could not differentiate patients on aspirin from patients off aspirin just from bleeding behavior (Lindblad et al. 1993). The authors concluded that with the possible exception of intracranial neurosurgery and transurethral prostatectomy, where bleeding-related fatalities after aspirin ingestion were reported (Burger et al. 2005; Thurston and Briant 1993; Palmer et al. 1994), low-dose aspirin increases bleeding only quantitatively and does not move the bleeding complications toward a higher risk quality. Additionally, only few studies analyzed in the meta-analysis were randomized, and, therefore, low-dose aspirin might be considered just a risk indicator for increased comorbidity with an increased bleeding risk per se (Hui et al. 2002). Only one double-blind randomized trial has investigated the perioperative bleeding risk in patients undergoing noncardiac surgery while on 75 mg aspirin therapy (Oscarsson et al. 2010). No significant increase of bleeding events was identified in those patients taking aspirin as compared with those who were not on antiplatelet therapy. In Albadalejo's series, major and minor hemorrhagic complications were observed in 9.5 % patients. Most bleedings were at the surgical site (85.2 %) and were associated with repeat surgery in 18.5 % of patients. The death rate in patients with bleeding complications was 12.0 % (95 % CI 6.6–19.7). Another study (Artang and Dieter 2007) demonstrated a very low rate of excessive blood loss during surgery (1 %), whereas blood transfusion was required in

24 % of patients who continued vs. 20 % of those who discontinued antiplatelet therapy.

Data on the role of clopidogrel on perioperative bleeding risk are lacking. An increased hemorrhagic risk emerged in patients undergoing CABG while on clopidogrel therapy, which was reduced by stopping the drug at least 5 days prior to intervention (Firanescu et al. 2009; Fox et al. 2004; Berger et al. 2008; Kapetanakis et al. 2005; Mehta et al. 2006). In patients with femoral fracture, perioperative clopidogrel therapy does not seem to be associated with a significant increase of mortality and morbidity (Leonidou et al. 2011).

Prasugrel is a novel thienopyridine with a more rapid onset of action and a higher antiplatelet effect, as compared to clopidogrel, but has been associated with an increased bleeding risk (Wiviott et al. 2007a, b). In the TRITON-TIMI 38 trial, in the subgroup of patients undergoing CABG within 7 days after thienopyridine withdrawal, the number of CABG-related bleeding was fourfold higher in patients treated with prasugrel as compared to those treated with clopidogrel. Nevertheless, the risk of mortality was reduced (Wiviott et al. 2007b; Prasugrel 2009). Ticagrelor is a novel non-thienopyridine antiplatelet agent that inhibits the P2Y12 receptor, through a reversible binding mechanism of action. Like prasugrel, it is characterized by a more rapid onset of action and higher antiplatelet activity and clinical efficacy as compared to clopidogrel. Ticagrelor does not increase overall bleeding events, but is associated with a significant increase of non-CABG-related bleeding (Gurbel et al. 2009; Wallentin et al. 2009). Like in the TRITON-TIMI 38 (Held et al. 2011), also in the PLATO trial patients undergoing CABG within 7 days after discontinuation of antiplatelet therapy showed a significant decrease of overall and cardiovascular mortality in the ticagrelor group. Apparently, this protective effect was not due to a different hemorrhagic risk, which was similar in both groups (Held et al. 2011).

In patients undergoing surgery in whom discontinuation of antiplatelet therapy is required, prasugrel and ticagrelor should be stopped 7 and 5 days before intervention, respectively.

3.2 Clinical Implications

In recent years, international cardiological, anesthesiological, and hematological societies have proposed guidelines and joint position papers on the management of DAPT in patients undergoing noncardiac surgery (Task Force on Myocardial Revascularization of the ESC 2010; Chassot et al. 2007; Korte et al. 2011; Criteria ACCF/SCAI/STS/AATS/AHA/ASNC 2009 Appropriateness 2009; Brilakis et al. 2007; Riddell et al. 2007; Eagle et al. 2004; Grines et al. 2007). However, these recommendations provide little support with regard to managing antiplatelet therapy in the perioperative phase in case of urgent operations and/or high hemorrhagic risk patient. In particular, guidelines shared with orthopedics and cardiologists are lacking.

Elective surgical procedures ought to be postponed until after the initial requirement for DAPT is completed. Unfortunately, many procedures require a more urgent management according to the severity, and often the distinction between "deferrable" and "undeferrable" surgery is not a clear issue and can be misleading both for the surgeon and the patient.

The management of the risk ratio between bleeding and thrombosis requires the exact knowledge of risk stratification defined for each condition, paired with offering the minimal surgical impact. In this respect, it could be recommended that high-risk patients be referred to centers where the most minimally invasive therapies are available. These, coupled with a high-volume cardiological team, can allow the reduction of blood loss in case of maintenance of the antiplatelet therapy and permitting a prompt resumption of the antiplatelet drugs, if they had been discontinued.

3.3 Evidence-Based State of the Art

A consensus document on the optimal antiplatelet regimen in patients with coronary stents undergoing orthopedic interventions has been recently proposed by a multidisciplinary panel composed

Table 3.1 Stratification of orthopedic procedures according to bleeding risk

Low bleeding risk	
	Hand surgery
	Shoulder and knee arthroscopy
	Minor spine surgery
Intermediate bleeding risk	
	Prosthetic shoulder surgery
	Major spine surgery
	Knee surgery (anterior cruciate ligament, osteotomies)
	Foot surgery
High bleeding risk	
	Major prosthetic surgery (hip or knee)
	Major traumatology (pelvis, long bones)
	Fractures of the proximal femur in the elderly

Reproduced with permission from the Publisher, *Il Pensiero Scientifico Editore*

of orthopedics and cardiologists, who equally contributed to its creation (Rossini et al. 2012, 2014). The document was endorsed by the Italian Society of Orthopaedics and Traumatology (SIOT), Interventional Cardiology (GISE), and Cardiology (ANMCO). A stent thrombosis risk was graded considering procedural features, such as stent type, time from PCI to orthopedic surgery, and clinical aspects, such as concomitant diabetes, renal impairment, low cardiac ejection fraction, and age. Most orthopedic interventions were classified according to the bleeding risk (Table 3.1).

The present document is the first consensus to provide practical recommendations on the management of antiplatelet therapy in patients with coronary stents, undergoing diverse orthopedic interventions. Briefly, stent thrombosis risk is stratified in low, intermediate, and high (Table 3.2), and the most appropriate antiplatelet therapy and management is defined for each intervention, on the basis of the ischemic and hemorrhagic risk (Table 3.3).

This stratification allows to define in detail the optimal antiplatelet regimen which should be maintained in the perioperative period, thus avoiding an arbitrary management. Of note, it is important to define the ideal timing of the orthopedic intervention as elective procedures should be delayed until a low cardiac ischemic risk is reached.

Table 3.2 Definition of thrombotic risk in patients with coronary stents

Low risk	Intermediate risk	High risk
>6 months after PCI with BMS	>1 month <6 months after PCI with BMS	<1 month after PCI with BMS
>12 months after PCI with DES	>6 months <12 months after PCI with DES	<6 months after PCI with DES
	>12 months after complex PCI with DES (long stents, multiple stents, overlapping, small vessels, bifurcations, left main, last remaining vessel).	<12 months after complex PCI with DES (long stents, multiple stents, overlapping, small vessels, bifurcations, left main, last remaining vessel)

Reproduced with permission from the Publisher, *Il Pensiero Scientifico Editore*

PCI in ACS, previous stent thrombosis, LVEF <35 %, chronic renal failure, and diabetes mellitus increase the thrombotic risk. The use of second-generation DES might reduce the thrombotic risk. Patients submitted to CABG or with ACS medically treated are considered at high risk in the first month, at intermediate risk between the 1st and 6th month, and at low risk after 6 months. Patients treated with POBA are considered at high risk within the first 2 weeks, at intermediate risk between 2 and 4 weeks, and at low risk after 4 weeks

ACS acute coronary syndrome, *BMS* bare metal stent, *CABG* coronary artery by-pass graft, *DES* drug-eluting stent, *LVEF* left ventricular ejection fraction, *PCI* percutaneous coronary intervention, *POBA* plain old balloon angioplasty

3.4 Antiplatelet Therapy: To Stop or to Maintain?

The antiplatelet therapy (especially aspirin) has to be maintained whenever possible, especially when the ischemic risk is intermediate or high due to the extremely enhanced risk of ST. In case of withdrawal of the antiplatelet therapy in the perioperative phase, cardiologists recommend restarting the drugs as soon as possible after the intervention (ideally 24–48 h later), with a loading dose. In selected cases, such as patients with high ischemic and hemorrhagic risk, in whom the discontinuation of the oral antiplatelet therapy is necessary, the "bridge therapy" is advocated (Rossini et al. 2012, 2014). This consists of the intravenous, prolonged infusion of glycoprotein (GP) IIb/IIIa inhibitor (tirofiban or eptifibatide), a

Table 3.3 Perioperative antiplatelet therapy in patients with coronary stents undergoing orthopedic surgery

	Orthopedic surgery	Thrombotic risk		
		Low risk	Intermediate risk	High risk
Hemorrhagic risk	*Low risk*	ASA: continue	*Elective surgery*: postpone	*Elective surgery*: postpone
	Hand surgery	$P2Y_{12}$ receptor inhibitors	Non-deferrable surgery	Non-deferrable surgery
	Shoulder and knee arthroscopy	Discontinue 5 days before[a]	ASA: continue	ASA: continue
	Minor spine surgery l	Resume within 24–72 h, with a loading dose	$P2Y_{12}$ receptor inhibitors	$P2Y_{12}$ receptor inhibitors:
			Discontinue 5 days before[a]	Continue
			Resume within 24–72 h, with a loading dose[b]	
	Intermediate risk	ASA: continue	*Elective surgery*: postpone	Elective surgery: postpone
	Prosthetic shoulder surgery	$P2Y_{12}$ receptor inhibitors	Non-deferrable surgery	Non-deferrable surgery
	Major spine surgery	Discontinue 5 days before[a]	ASA: continue	ASA: continue
	Knee surgery (anterior cruciate ligament, osteotomies)	Resume within 24–72 h, with a loading dose	$P2Y_{12}$ receptor inhibitors:	$P2Y_{12}$ receptor inhibitors
	Foot surgery		Discontinue 5 days before[a]	Discontinue 5 days before[a]
			Resume within 24–72 h, with a loading dose[b]	Resume within 24–72 h, with a loading dose
				Bridge therapy with GPIIb/IIIa inhibitors[b]
	High risk	ASA: continue	*Elective surgery*: postpone	*Elective surgery*: postpone
	Major prosthetic surgery (hip or knee)	$P2Y_{12}$ receptor inhibitors	Non-deferrable surgery	Non-deferrable surgery
	Major traumatology (pelvis, long bones)	Discontinue 5 days before[a]	ASA: continue	ASA: continue
	Fractures of the proximal femur in the elderly	Resume within 24–72 h, with a loading dose	$P2Y_{12}$ receptor inhibitors	$P2Y_{12}$ receptor inhibitors
			Discontinue 5 days before[a]	Discontinue 5 days before[a,c]
			Resume within 24–72 h, with a loading dose[b]	Resume within 24–72 h, with a loading dose
				Bridge therapy with GPIIb/IIIa inhibitors[b]

Reproduced with permission from the Publisher, *Il Pensiero Scientifico Editore*
ASA aspirin
[a]7 days prior for prasugrel
[b]Collegial discussion of risk, even with family/patient
[c]In case of femur fracture, it may be appropriate to proceed immediately to surgery, despite dual antiplatelet therapy, without waiting for the 5-day suspension

potent antiplatelet drug which acts as the oral antiplatelet therapies, thus preventing ST. It is a short-acting drug given intravenously. Patients undergoing "bridge therapy" withdraw DAPT or only the second antiplatelet agent 5 days before surgery (7 days in case of therapy with prasugrel). The infusion of GP IIb/IIIa inhibitor starts 3 days before the intervention and is stopped 4 h before surgery (8 h in the case of creatinine clearance <30 ml min^{-1}). Oral antiplatelet therapy should be resumed within 24–48 h after the intervention. Of note, GP IIb/IIIa inhibitors are potent antiplatelet effects and are associated with an increased risk of bleeding during their infusion. Afterward, they might be contraindicated in patients with an active, clinically relevant bleeding. This therapy should be prescribed by cardiologists and administered in a cardiologic ward. "Bridge therapy" is currently off-label for perioperative period management of antiplatelet therapy (Douketis et al. 2008).

Conclusions

The risk of ST is significantly increased after premature discontinuation of DAPT. The management of the antiplatelet therapy in patients with coronary stents undergoing orthopedic procedures is still challenging and surely requires both an orthopedic and a cardiologic thorough assessment. It appears evident that the right direction is toward the application in clinical practice of the consensus documents available. The document endorsed by cardiologists, orthopedics, and anesthesiologists recommends to perioperatively discontinue the antiplatelet drugs if the known or assumed perioperative bleeding risks and their sequels are expected to be similar or more severe than the observed cardiovascular thrombotic risks after antiplatelet therapy withdrawal. A prospective case registry is now ongoing in Italy (the Surgery After Stenting (SAS) registry; ClinicalTrials.gov Identifier: NCT01997242), and its results might be a helpful tool to improve the DAPT patients' management. To potentially improve the quality of evidence derived from the *consensus document*, randomized studies could be considered merely from a methodological point of view. However, a comparison between surgery performed with versus without DAPT is not ethical for benign disease, due to the extremely increased risk of ST. Probably, the only possible comparison could be between traditional versus minimally invasive surgery during DAPT in high-risk cardiovascular patients.

References

ACCF/SCAI/STS/AATS/AHA/ASNC 2009 Appropriateness Criteria for Coronary Revascularization: a report by the American College of Cardiology Foundation Appropriateness Criteria Task Force, Society for Cardiovascular Angiography and Interventions, Society of Thoracic Surgeons, American Association for Thoracic Surgery, American Heart Association, and the American Society of Nuclear Cardiology Endorsed by the American Society of Echocardiography, the Heart Failure Society of America, and the Society of Cardiovascular Computed Tomography (2009) J Am Coll Cardiol 53(6): 530–553

Albaladejo P, Marret E, Samama CM, Collet JP, Abhay K, Loutrel O, Charbonneau H, Jaber S, Thoret S, Bosson JL, Piriou V (2011) Non-cardiac surgery in patients with coronary stents: the RECO study. Heart 97: 1566–1572

Antithrombotic Trialists' Collaboration (2002) Collaborative meta-analysis of randomised trials of antiplatelet therapy for prevention of death, myocardial infarction, and stroke in high risk patients. Br Med J 324:71–86

Anwaruddin S, Askari AT, Saudye H, Batizy L, Houghtaling PL, Alamoudi M, Militello M, Muhammad K, Kapadia S, Ellis SG (2009) Characterization of post-operative risk associated with prior drug-eluting stent use. JACC Cardiovasc Interv 2:542–549

Artang R, Dieter RS (2007) Analysis of 36 reported cases of late thrombosis in drug eluting stents placed in coronary arteries. Am J Cardiol 99:1039–1043

Berger JS, Frye CB, Harshaw Q, Edwards FH, Steinhubl SR, Becker RC (2008) Impact of clopidogrel in patients with acute coronary syndromes requiring coronary artery bypass surgery: a multicenter analysis. J Am Coll Cardiol 52:1693–1701

Berger PB, Kleiman NS, Pencina MJ, Hsieh WH, Steinhubl SR, Jeremias A, Sonel A, Browne K, Barseness G, Cohen DJ, EVENT Investigators (2010) Frequency of major noncardiac surgery and subsequent adverse events in the year after drug-eluting stent placement: results from the EVENT (Evaluation of Drug-Eluting Stents and Ischemic Events) Registry. JACC Cardiovasc Interv 3:920–927

Biondi-Zoccai GG, Lotrionte M, Agostoni P, Abbate A, Fusaro M, Burzotta F, Testa L, Sheiban I, Sangiorgi G (2006) A systematic review and metaanalysis on the hazards of discontinuing or not adhering to aspirin among 50,279 patients at risk for coronary artery disease. Eur Heart J 27:2667–2674

Brilakis ES, Banerjee S, Berger PB (2007) Perioperative management of patients with coronary stents. J Am Coll Cardiol 49:2145–2150

Burger W, Chemnitius JM, Kneissl GD, Rücker G (2005) Low-dose aspirin for secondary cardiovascular prevention, cardiovascular risks after its perioperative withdrawal versus bleeding risks with its continuation. Review and meta-analysis. J Intern Med 257:399–414

Chassot PG, Delabays A, Spahn DR (2007) Perioperative antiplatelet therapy: the case for continuing therapy in patients at risk of myocardial infarction. Br J Anaesth 99(3):316–328

Cruden NL, Harding SA, Flapan AD, Graham C, Wild SH, Slack R, Pell JP, Newby DE, Scottish Coronary Revascularisation Register Steering Committee (2010) Previous coronary stent implantation and cardiac events in patients undergoing noncardiac surgery. Circ Cardiovasc Interv 3:236–242

Douketis JD, Berger PB, Dunn AS, Jaffer AK, Spyropoulos AC, Becker RC et al (2008) The perioperative management of antithrombotic therapy. American College of Chest Physicians Evidence-based Clinical Practice Guidelines (8th edition). Chest 133:299–339

Eagle KA, Guyton RA, Davidoff R, Edwards FH, Ewy GA, Gardner TJ et al (2004) ACC/AHA 2004 guideline update for coronary artery bypass graft surgery: a report of the American College of Cardiology/American Heart Association Task Force on Practice Guidelines (Committee to Update the 1999 Guidelines for Coronary Artery Bypass Graft Surgery). Circulation 110:1168–1176

Ferreira-González I, Marsal JR, Ribera A, Permanyer-Miralda G, García-Del Blanco B, Martí G, Cascant P, Martín-Yuste V, Brugaletta S, Sabaté M, Alfonso F, Capote ML, De La Torre JM, Ruíz-Lera M, Sanmiguel D, Cárdenas M, Pujol B, Baz JA, Iñiguez A, Trillo R, González-Béjar O, Casanova J, Sánchez-Gila J, García-Dorado D (2010) Background, incidence, and predictors of antiplatelet therapy discontinuation during the first year after drug-eluting stent implantation. Circulation 122(10):1017–1025

Firanescu CE, Martens EJ, Schonberger JP, Soliman Hamad MA, van Straten AH (2009) Postoperative blood loss in patients undergoing coronary artery bypass surgery after preoperative treatment with clopidogrel. A prospective randomised controlled study. Eur J Cardiothorac Surg 36:856–862

Fox KA, Mehta SR, Peters R, Zhao F, Lakkis N, Gersh BJ, Yusuf S (2004) Benefits and risks of the combination of clopidogrel and aspirin in patients undergoing surgical revascularization for non-ST-elevation acute coronary syndrome: the Clopidogrel in Unstable angina to prevent Recurrent ischemic Events (CURE) Trial. Circulation 110:1202–1208

Grines CL, Bonow RO, Casey DE Jr, Gardner TJ, Lockhart PB et al; American Heart Association; American College of Cardiology; Society for Cardiovascular Angiography and Interventions; American College of Surgeons; American Dental Association; American College of Physicians (2007) Prevention of premature discontinuation of dual antiplatelet therapy in patients with coronary artery stents. A science advisory from the American Heart Association, American College of Cardiology, Society for Cardiovascular Angiography and Interventions, American College of Surgeons, and American Dental Association, with representation from the American College of Physicians. J Am Coll Cardiol 49:734–739

Gurbel PA, Bliden KP, Butler K, Tantry US, Gesheff T, Wei C, Teng R, Antonino MJ, Patil SB, Karunakaran A, Kereiakes DJ, Parris C, Purdy D, Wilson V, Ledley GS, Storey RF (2009) Randomized double-blind assessment of the ONSET and OFFSET of the antiplatelet effects of ticagrelor versus clopidogrel in patients with stable coronary artery disease: the ONSET/OFFSET study. Circulation 120:2577–2585

Held C, Asenblad N, Bassand JP, Becker RC, Cannon CP, Claeys MJ, Harrington RA, Horrow J, Husted S, James SK, Mahaffey KW, Nicolau JC, Scirica BM, Storey RF, Vintila M, Ycas J, Wallentin L (2011) Ticagrelor versus clopidogrel in patients with acute coronary syndromes undergoing coronary artery bypass surgery: results from the PLATO (Platelet Inhibition and Patient Outcomes) trial. J Am Coll Cardiol 57:672–684

Hui CK, Lai KC, Yuen MF, Wong WM, Lam SK, Lai CL (2002) Does withholding aspirin for one week reduce the risk of postsphincterotomy bleeding? Aliment Pharmacol Ther 16:929–936

Iakovou I, Schmidt T, Bonizzoni E, Ge L, Sangiorgi GM, Stankovic G, Airoldi F, Chieffo A, Montorfano M, Carlino M, Michev I, Corvaja N, Briguori C, Gerckens U, Grube E, Colombo A (2005) Incidence, predictors, and outcome of thrombosis after successful implantation of drug-eluting stents. JAMA 293(17):2126–2130

Kapetanakis EI, Medlam DA, Boyce SW, Haile E, Hill PC, Dullum MK, Bafi AS, Petro KR, Corso PJ (2005) Clopidogrel administration prior to coronary artery bypass grafting surgery: the cardiologist's panacea or the surgeon's headache? Eur Heart J 26:576–583

Korte W, Cattaneo M, Chassot PG, Eichinger S, von Heymann C, Hofmann N et al (2011) Peri-operative management of antiplatelet therapy in patients with coronary artery disease. Thromb Haemost 105:1–7

Leonidou A, Cam NB, Chambers IR (2011) Femoral neck fractures in patients on clopidogrel. The effect of delaying surgery and the introduction of the new SIGN guidelines. Surgeon 9:318–321

Lindblad B, Persson NH, Takolander R, Bergqvist D (1993) Does low dose acetylsalicylic acid prevent stroke after carotid surgery? A double-blind, placebo-controlled randomized trial. Stroke 24:1125–1128

Mangano DT, Multicenter Study of Perioperative Ischemia Research Group (2002) Aspirin and

mortality from coronary bypass surgery. N Engl J Med 347:1309–1317
Mehta RH, Roe MT, Mulgund J, Ohman EM, Cannon CP, Gibler WB, Pollack CV Jr, Smith SC Jr, Ferguson TB, Peterson ED (2006) Acute clopidogrel use and outcomes in patients with non-ST-segment elevation acute coronary syndromes undergoing coronary artery bypass surgery. J Am Coll Cardiol 48:281–286
Moschovitis A, Cook S, Meier B (2010) Percutaneous coronary interventions in Europe in 2006. EuroIntervention 6:189–194
Oscarsson A, Gupta A, Fredrikson M, Järhult J, Nyström M, Pettersson E, Darvish B, Krook H, Swahn E, Eintrei C (2010) To continue or discontinue aspirin in the perioperative period: a randomized, controlled clinical trial. Br J Anaesth 104:305–312
Palmer JD, Sparrow OC, Iannotti F (1994) Postoperative hematoma: a 5-year survey and identification of avoidable risk factors. Neurosurgery 35:1061–1064
Prasugrel (LY640315; CS-747) as an anti-thrombotic therapy in patients with acute coronary syndromes (ACS). NDA 22–307, EffientTM (prasugrel). Presentation to the Cardiovascular and Renal Drugs Advisory Committee. 3 Feb 2009. Available at http://www.fda.gov/ohrms/dockets/AC/09/slides/2009-4412s1-02-sponsor.pdf. Accessed 29 Mar 2012
Priebe HJ (2004) Triggers of perioperative myocardial ischaemia and infarction. Br J Anaesth 93:9–20
Rabbitts JA, Nuttall GA, Brown MJ, Hanson AC, Oliver WC, Holmes DR, Rihal CS (2008) Cardiac risk of noncardiac surgery after percutaneous coronary intervention with drug-eluting stents. Anesthesiology 109:596–604
Riddell JW, Chiche L, Plaud B, Hamon M (2007) Coronary stents and noncardiac surgery. Circulation 116:e378–e382
Roger VL, Go AS, Lloyd-Jones DM, Adams RJ, Berry JD, Brown TM, Carnethon MR, Dai S, de Simone G, Ford ES, Fox CS, Fullerton HJ, Gillespie C, Greenlund KJ, Hailpern SM, Heit JA, Ho PM, Howard VJ, Kissela BM, Kittner SJ et al (2011) Heart disease and stroke statistics – 2011 update: a report from the American Heart Association. Circulation 123:e18–e209
Rossini R, Capodanno D, Lettieri C, Musumeci G, Nijaradze T, Romano M, Lortkipanidze N, Cicorella N, Biondi Zoccai G, Sirbu V, Izzo A, Guagliumi G, Valsecchi O, Gavazzi A, Angiolillo DJ (2011) Prevalence, predictors, and long-term prognosis of premature discontinuation of oral antiplatelet therapy after drug eluting stent implantation. Am J Cardiol 107(2):186–194
Rossini R, Bramucci E, Castiglioni B, De Servi S, Lettieri C, Lettino M, Musumeci G, Visconti LO, Piccaluga E, Savonitto S, Trabattoni D, Buffoli F, Angiolillo DJ, Bovenzi F, Cremonesi A, Scherillo M, Guagliumi G, Società Italiana di Cardiologia Invasiva (GISE); Associazione Nazionale Medici Cardiologi Ospedalieri (ANMCO) (2012) Coronary stenting and surgery: perioperative management of antiplatelet therapy in patients undergoing surgery after coronary stent implantation. G Ital Cardiol (Rome) 13(7–8): 528–551
Rossini R, Musumeci G, Oltrona Visconti L, Bramucci E, Castiglioni B, De Servi S, Lettieri C, Lettino M, Piccaluga E, Savonitto S, Trabattoni D, Capodanno D, Buffoli F, Parolari A, Dionigi G, Boni L, Biglioli F, Valdatta L, Droghetti A, Bozzani A, Setacci C, Ravelli P, Crescini C, Staurenghi G, Scarone P, Francetti L, D'Angelo F, Gadda F, Comel A, Salvi L, Lorini L, Antonelli M, Bovenzi F, Cremonesi A, Angiolillo DJ, Guagliumi G (2014) Perioperative management of antiplatelet therapy in patients with coronary stents undergoing cardiac and non-cardiac surgery: a Consensus Document from Italian Cardiological, Surgical, and Anesthesiological Societies. EuroIntervention 10(1):38–46
Savonitto S, Caracciolo M, Cattaneo M, De Servi S (2011) Management of patients with recently implanted coronary stents on dual antiplatelet therapy who need to undergo major surgery. J Thromb Haemost 9(11): 2133–2142
Schouten O, van Domburg RT, Bax JJ, de Jaegere PJ, Dunkelgrun M, Feringa HH, Hoeks SE, Poldermans D (2007) Noncardiac surgery after coronary stenting: early surgery and interruption of antiplatelet therapy are associated with an increase in major adverse cardiac events. J Am Coll Cardiol 49:122–124
Task Force on Myocardial Revascularization of the European Society of Cardiology (ESC) and the European Association for Cardio-Thoracic Surgery (EACTS); European Association for Percutaneous Cardiovascular Interventions (EAPCI), Kolh P, Wijns W, Danchin N, Di Mario C, Falk V, Folliguet T, Garg S, Huber K, James S, Knuuti J, Lopez-Sendon J, Marco J, Menicanti L, Ostojic M, Piepoli MF, Pirlet C, Pomar JL, Reifart N, Ribichini FL, Schalij MJ, Sergeant P, Serruys PW, Silber S, Sousa Uva M, Taggart D (2010) Guidelines on myocardial revascularization. Eur Heart J 31(20):2501–2555. doi:10.1093/eurheartj/ehq277
Thurston AV, Briant SL (1993) Aspirin and post-prostatectomy haemorrhage. Br J Urol 71:574–576
Topol EJ (2002) Aspirin for bypass surgery: from taboo to new standard of care. N Engl J Med 347:1359–1360
van Kuijk JP, Flu WJ, Schouten O, Hoeks SE, Schenkeveld L, de Jaegere PP, Bax JJ, van Domburg RT, Serruys PW, Poldermans D (2009) Timing of noncardiac surgery after coronary artery stenting with bare metal or drug-eluting stents. Am J Cardiol 104:1229–1234
Wallentin L, Becker RC, Budaj A, Cannon CP, Emanuelsson H, Held C, Horrow J, Husted S, James S, Katus H, Mahaffey KW, Scirica BM, Skene A, Steg PG, Storey RF, Harrington RA, PLATO Investigators, Freij A, Thorsén M (2009) Ticagrelor versus clopidogrel in patients with acute coronary syndromes. N Engl J Med 361:1045–1057
Wijeysundera DN, Wijeysundera HC, Yun L, Wąsowicz M, Beattie WS, Velianou JL, Ko DT (2012) Risk of elective major noncardiac surgery after coronary stent insertion: a population-based study. Circulation 126(11):1355–1362

Wiviott SD, Trenk D, Frelinger AL, O'Donoghue M, Neumann FJ, Michelson AD, Angiolillo DJ, Hod H, Montalescot G, Miller DL, Jakubowski JA, Cairns R, Murphy SA, McCabe CH, Antman EM, Braunwald E, PRINCIPLE-TIMI 44 Investigators (2007a) Prasugrel compared with high loading and maintenance-dose clopidogrel in patients with planned percutaneous coronary intervention: the Prasugrel in Comparison to Clopidogrel for Inhibition of Platelet Activation and Aggregation-Thrombolysis in Myocardial Infarction 44 trial. Circulation 116:2923–2932

Wiviott SD, Braunwald E, Angiolillo DJ, Meisel S, Dalby AJ, Verheugt FW, Goodman SG, Corbalan R, Purdy DA, Murphy SA, McCabe CH, Antman EM, TRITON-TIMI 38 Investigators (2007b) Prasugrel versus clopidogrel in patients with acute coronary syndromes. N Engl J Med 357:2001–2015

Yusuf S, Zhao F, Mehta SR, Chrolavicius S, Tognoni G, Fox KK, CURE Trial Investigators (2001) Effects of clopidogrel in addition to aspirin in patients with acute coronary syndromes without ST-segment elevation. N Engl J Med 345:494–502

4 LMWHs: Are Still the Gold Standard in Arthroplasty? Arguments in Favor

Rosanna Abbate, Maddalena Pazzi, Lorenza Rossi, and Gabriele Cioni

Open Questions

- Why do we need pharmacologic thromboprophylaxis in arthroplasty procedures?
- LMWH vs. old and new anticoagulants: which one has a better thromboprophylaxis efficacy?
- LMWH vs. old and new anticoagulants: which one has an inferior bleeding rate?
- Which are the final recommendations based on the actual guidelines?

4.1 Introduction

The risk of venous thromboembolism following major orthopedic procedures, such as total hip and knee arthroplasty (THA, TKA) and surgical intervention of hip joint fractures, is well recognized and represents one of the major challenges in orthopedic practice. Orthopedic surgery is one of the most commonly performed surgical procedures in Western countries (United States and Europe) (National Center for Health Statistics 2010; Organisation for Economic Co-operation and Development 2010; Canadian Institute for Health Information 2008; Kurtz et al. 2005; Dixon et al. 2004), with an increasing number of arthroplasties of the hip and knee done worldwide per year with successful outcome (National Center for Health Statistics 2010).

The incidence of deep venous thrombosis when no prophylaxis is administered is 42–57 % with total hip arthroplasty and 41–85 % with total knee arthroplasty. Fatal PE (pulmonary embolism) occurs in 0.1–2 % of patients after hip THA and in 0.1–1.7 % of the patients with TKA (National Institute for Health and Clinical Excellence: Guidance 2010). It is defined that symptomatic VTE, which occurs in about 4 % of patients, is more frequent than other complications such as dislocation and postoperative infection. These figures clearly underline the need for effective and safe thromboprophylaxis.

In clinical practice, different current guidelines recommend routine post-procedural thromboprophylaxis by low-molecular-weight heparin (LMWH), vitamin K antagonists (VKA), or synthetic pentasaccharides (fondaparinux); other less common options include unfractionated heparin (UFH), aspirin, and mechanical prophylaxis. Recently, new oral anticoagulants (NOAC) are available in clinical practice.

In literature, several data were reported about the pharmacological properties and the well-established efficacy and safety of LMWH.

R. Abbate • M. Pazzi (✉) • L. Rossi
G. Cioni
Department of Experimental and Clinical Medicine, AOU Careggi, University of Florence, Largo Brambila 3, Florence 50134, Italy
e-mail: rosanna.abbate@unifi.it; maddalena.pazzi@gmail.com; gabriele.cioni@unifi.it

A. Baldini, P. Caldora (eds.), *Perioperative Medical Management for Total Joint Arthroplasty: How to Control Hemostasis, Pain and Infection*, DOI 10.1007/978-3-319-07203-6_4,

LMWH, derived from UFH by chemical or enzymatic degradation, is characterized by reduced anti-IIa activity in comparison to anti-Xa activity and by pharmacokinetic properties which offer more predictable antithrombotic effect than UFH, and due to a longer plasma half-life, LMWH may allow once-daily administration. Moreover, the reduced formation of heparin-induced antibodies and the reduced activation of osteoclasts account for lower incidence of HIT and lower risk of osteopenia in comparison to UHF.

Nevertheless, disadvantages include mainly parenteral administration, possibly implicating low patient compliance to therapy and, anyway, even if reduced in comparison to UFH, potential thrombocytopenia (Mismetti et al. 2004).

New oral anticoagulants, oral factor Xa inhibitors, and direct thrombin inhibitors are characterized by more predictable anticoagulant effects and by not requiring monitoring, but the costs are higher, and in case of bleeding, antidotes are not available.

4.2 Systematic Reviews and Meta-analysis of Interventional Studies for Preventing Venous Thromboembolism Post-total Hip Replacement and Post-total Knee Replacement

During the last twenty years, hundreds of interventional studies evaluated the efficacy and safety of the different antithrombotic drugs in preventing post-orthopedic surgery venous thromboembolism.

The availability of LMWH has represented a key point in clinical practice; so the antithrombotic drugs previously available, as well as those appeared successively, have to be compared to LMWH.

In 2012 and 2013, after the publication of the results obtained with the new oral anticoagulants, data of the randomized clinical trials (RCT) have been systematically reviewed and meta-analyzed.

The results of RCT, pooled and meta-analyzed, are the source from which guidelines and clinical recommendations. In this frame LMWH have been compared with different other antithrombotic drugs, but the direct comparison between all the "old" and all "new "molecules is presently not, and it is likely that it will be never, available.

The principal outcomes on which the analyses of the findings are founded commonly refer to any proximal DVT, symptomatic proven DVT or pulmonary embolism (PE), or fatal PE (as established by the American College of Chest Physicians – ACCP-Consensus Conference on Antithrombotic Therapy); or any proximal DVT, symptomatic proven PE, or death from any cause (as established by the European Committee for Proprietary Medicinal Products (CPMP)). As safety is concerned, major bleeding, bleeding requiring reoperation, fatal bleeding, and minor bleeding have been considered; moreover, many clinical trials considered also as safety outcome clinically relevant nonmajor bleeding, which actually remains difficult to define.

4.3 What Literature Says: LMWH Versus "Old" and "New" Anticoagulants

4.3.1 LMWH Versus UFH

Sobieraj et al. (2012) meta-analyzed 10 randomized controlled trials comparing LMWH to unfractionated heparin (UFH).

Compared with patients who received UFH, patients who received LMWH had fewer pulmonary embolism (OR 0.48, 95 % CI 0.24–0.95), a significantly decreased risk of total deep vein thrombosis (DVT) (RR 0.80, 95 % CI 0.65–0.99), especially proximal DVT (RR 0.60, 95 % CI 0.38–0.93) and less major bleeding (OR 0.57, 95 % CI 0.37–0.88), and heparin-induced thrombocytopenia events (OR 0.12, 95 % CI 0.03–0.43). Differences were not significant as regards mortality, symptomatic and asymptomatic DVT, distal DVT, and surgical site bleeding (Table 4.1).

Table 4.1 Risk ratios and 95 % CI endpoints of UFH, VKA, and fondaparinux compared with LMWH in orthopedic arthroplasty from two meta-analyses

	Sobieraj et al. (2012)		
	Proximal DVT (RR, 95 % CI)	**PE (OR, 95 % CI)**	**Major bleeding (OR, 95 % CI)**
LMWH vs. UFH	**0.60**[a] (0.38–0.93)	**0.48**[a] (0.24–0.95)	**0.57**[a] (0.37–0.88)
LMWH vs. VKA	0.63 (0.39–1.00)	1.11 (0.57–2.19)	**1.92**[a] (1.27–2.91)
	Yoshida et al. (2013)		
	Primary efficacy rates* (RR, 95 % CI)	**PE (RR, 95 % CI)**	**Major bleeding (RR, 95 % CI)**
Fondaparinux vs. enoxaparin	**0.50**[a] (0.39–0.63)	1.06 (0.36–3.12)	1.53 (0.92–2.55)

*Primary efficacy rate = any DVT, nonfatal PE, or all-cause mortality
[a]Statistically significant, $P < 0.05$ at least

When THR and TKR surgeries were considered separately, meta-analysis, by pooling seven studies, highlights the following evidences: patients undergoing THR and receiving LMWH had fewer total pulmonary embolism events versus UFH (OR 0.28, 95 % CI 0.13–0.62); both in THR (RR 0.75, 95 % CI 0.58–0.978 and RR 0.75, 95 % CI 0.58–0.96, respectively) and TKR surgeries (RR 0.75, 95 % CI 0.58–0.96 and RR 0.32, 95 % CI 0.13–0.82, respectively), patients had fewer total DVT and proximal events. As major bleeding concerns, patients undergoing THR surgery both had significantly fewer events (OR 0.54, 95 % CI 0.34–0.85) and less heparin-induced thrombocytopenia than patients receiving UFH.

4.3.2 LMWH Versus Warfarin

Sobieraj et al. (2012), in the meta-analysis previously mentioned, also compared vitamin K antagonists (VKA) to LMWH in patients undergoing orthopedic surgery by pooling seven studies. They found that patients who received LMWH had fewer total DVT (RR 0.66, 95 % CI 0.55–0.79) and distal DVT events (RR 0.56, 95 % CI 0.43–0.73) with no significant difference in proximal DVT risk (RR 0.63, 95 % CI 0.39–1.00) but reported increased major bleeding (OR 1.92, 95 % CI 1.27–2.91), minor bleeding (RR 1.23, 95 % CI 1.06–1.43), and surgical site bleeding events (OR 2.63, 95 % CI 1.31–5.28).

Major efficacy end points such as symptomatic venous thromboembolism (OR 1.00, 95 % CI 0.69–1.46), pulmonary embolism (OR 1.11, 95 % CI 0.57–2.19), and nonfatal pulmonary embolism (OR 1.00, 95 % CI 0.20–4.95) showed similar benefits of therapy with LMWH and VKA (Table 4.1).

In particular when THR and TKR surgery were considered, meta-analysis highlights the following evidences for patients receiving LMWH: (1) patients undergoing THR and TKR surgery had fewer total DVT events (RR 0.61, 95 % CI 0.44–0.84 and RR 0.71, 95 % CI 0.57–0.87, respectively) and fewer distal DVT (RR 0.48, 95 % CI 0.30–0.78 and RR 0.60, 95 % CI 0.44–0.81, respectively); (2) patients undergoing THR (OR 1.91, 95 % CI 1.11–3.29) and TKR surgery (OR 1.93, 95 % CI 1.01–3.67) had more major and minor bleeding; and (3) patients in THR surgery had more surgical site bleeding and major surgical site bleeding (OR 2.56, 95 % CI 1.04–6.30).

4.3.3 Enoxaparin Versus Fondaparinux

Four studies evaluating fondaparinux in comparison to enoxaparin were meta-analyzed by Yoshida et al. (2013).

When primary efficacy end-points (defined as the frequency of any DVT, nonfatal pulmonary embolism or death from any cause) were analyzed, the results showed that fondaparinux had a positive and statistically significant effect if compared with enoxaparin (mixed doses) (RR 0.50, 95 % CI 0.39–0.63).

Nevertheless, considering the secondary efficacy outcomes, fondaparinux showed no significant difference if compared with enoxaparin. More specifically, the incidence of proximal DVT resulted reduced, but not significantly (RR 0.44, 95 % CI 0.19–1.02) and no significant difference was found in relation to pulmonary embolism (RR 1.06, 95 % CI 0.36,3.12), symptomatic DVT events (R.R 1.59, 95 % CI 0.51–4.90). As concerns safety outcomes, fondaparinux exhibited a higher any bleeding risk compared with enoxaparin (RR 1.27, 95 % CI 1.04–1.55). Similar results were observed in minor and major bleedings where fondaparinux proved to be associated with a higher risk (RR 1.06, 95 % CI 0.69–1.64 and RR 1.53, 95 % CI 0.92–2.55 respectively). Nevertheless heterogeneity limited the strength of these results (Table 4.1).

4.3.4 LMWH Versus Factor Xa Inhibitors

Systematic reviews and meta-analyses, addressed to evaluate LMWH efficacy and safety in comparison to oral direct factor Xa inhibitors, considered as a class of drug (Neuman et al. 2012 and Sobieraj et al. 2012), comparing the single drug rivaroxaban (Gómez-Outes et al. 2012; Hamidi et al. 2013; Yoshida et al. 2013) and apixaban (Gómez-Outes et al. 2012; Hamidi et al. 2013), are available.

Neumann et al. (2012) conducted a meta-analysis of 22 randomized, controlled trials performed on 32,159 patients undergoing hip or knee replacement (female sex 44.6–72.5 %; mean age 57.8–67.6 years), comparing different doses of different factor Xa inhibitors versus LMWH. Factor Xa inhibitors considered by these authors were apixaban, rivaroxaban, and edoxaban; YM150; and LY1517717, TAK442, razaxaban, and betrixaban. These authors reported any outcomes regarding mortality at the end of prophylaxis or during the follow-up period, symptomatic DVT, nonfatal pulmonary embolism, major bleeding, intracranial bleeding, and bleeding leading to reoperation. Eleven trials comprised patients undergoing total hip replacement, ten undergoing knee replacement, and only one undergoing either procedure.

In most trials, the European-approved dosage of enoxaparin (40 mg daily) was the comparator instead of the US-approved dosage (30 mg twice daily). Regarding doses of factor Xa inhibitors, 12 studies evaluated several doses, including high doses. In eight of the ten trials evaluating a single dose of factor Xa inhibitors, the dose used was low.

Timing of prophylaxis differed from studies: in particular, rivaroxaban was started 6 h after surgery in the majority of studies; apixaban was started 12–24 h after surgery.

The duration of follow-up varied from less than 14 days in 9 trials, 30–70 days in 12 trials, and reached 90 days in one trial.

The pooled effect estimate did not suggest important differences between oral factor Xa inhibitors in comparison to LMWH for all-cause mortality in patients (n = 31,702) having THR or TKR (OR 1.27, 95 % CI 0.63–2.55); risk difference, 0 fewer deaths per 1,000 patients [95 % CI, 1 fewer to 1 more death] or at the end of follow-up (OR 0.95, 95 % CI 0.55–1.63); risk difference, 0 fewer deaths per 1,000 patients [CI, 2 fewer to 1 more deaths]; conversely, the risk for symptomatic DVT is decreased by 4 events per 1,000 patients (OR 0.46, 95 % CI 0.30–0.70).

Regarding nonfatal pulmonary embolism, no important difference between factor Xa inhibitors and LMWH (OR 1.07, 95 % CI 0.65–1.73); risk difference, 0 fewer events [CI, 1 fewer to 2 more events per 1,000 patients], was found.

Data with a moderate strength of evidence showed that factor Xa inhibitors could increase the risk of bleeding by two major events per 1,000 patients. In a subgroup analysis, higher, but not intermediate or lower, doses of factor Xa inhibitors were associated with increased risk for bleeding (OR 2.50, 95 % [CI 1.38–4.53]; P=0.02). The pooled effect estimate of bleeding that led to reoperation also increased (OR 1.62, 95 % CI 0.82–3.19).

In this meta-analysis, subgroup analysis showed an interaction between the doses used in the intervention group and the risk for major bleeding; high doses increased the risk for major bleeding (OR 2.50, 95 % CI 1.38–4.53); test for interaction across the 3 doses, P = 0.02 (Table 4.2).

According to Sobieraj's meta-analysis (2012) of ten trials, compared with patients receiving factor Xa inhibitors, patients who received LMWH

Table 4.2 Risk ratios and 95 % CI endpoints of NOAC compared with enoxaparin in orthopedic arthroplasty from two meta-analyses

	Gomez et al. (2012)			Yoshida et al. (2013)		
	Symptomatic venous thromboembolism (RR, 95 %, CI)	Clinically relevant bleeding (RR, 95 %, CI)	Net clinical endpoint[a] (RR, 95 %, CI)	Symptomatic DVT (RR, 95 %, CI)	PE (RR, 95 %, CI)	Major bleeding (RR, 95 %, CI)
Dabigatran 150 mg vs. enoxaparin	0.86 (0.31–2.35)	1.12 (0.89–1.40)	0.93 (0.63–1.37)	1.64 (0.07–40.29)	0.33 (0.07–1.46)	0.75 (0.46–1.21)
Dabigatran 220 mg vs. enoxaparin	0.70 (0.18–2.76)	1.12 (0.94–1.35)		0.71 (0.12–4.01)	1.14 (0.50–2.61)	1.08 (0.67–1.75)
Rivaroxaban vs. enoxaparin	**0.48**[b] (0.31–0.75)	**1.25**[b] (1.05–1.49)	0.88 (0.70–1.12)	**0.45**[b] (0.27–0.77)	0.75 (0.15–3.67)	1.88 (0.92–3.82)
Apixaban vs. enoxaparin	0.82, (0.41–1.64)	**0.82**[b] (0.69–0.98)	0.92 (0.68–1.23)	**0.38**[b] (0.16–0.90)	1.50 (0.20–11.40)	0.76 (0.43–1.33)

[a]Net clinical endpoint = symptomatic venous thromboembolism, major bleeding, death
[b]Statistically significant, $P < 0.05$ at least

had more major venous thromboembolism (OR 2.64, 95 % CI 1.82–3.84), pulmonary embolism (OR 2.50, 95 % CI 1.08–5.78), total DVT (RR 2.05, 95 % CI 1.68–2.50), symptomatic DVT (RR 1.66, 95 % CI 1.04–2.64), proximal DVT (OR 2.62, 95 % CI 1.95–3.51), and distal DVT events (RR 2.14, 95 % CI 1.84–2.50) but fewer major bleeding events (OR 0.65, 95 % CI 0.49–0.86).

In particular when THR and TKR surgeries were considered, meta-analysis highlights the following evidences: as concerns major VTE events, patients undergoing THR and TKR surgeries had fewer events than patients receiving LMWH (OR 3.97, 95 % CI 2.17–7.24 and OR 2.04, 95 % CI 1.26–3.30, respectively). Patients receiving LMWH had more total DVT events than patients receiving factor Xa inhibitors in THR surgery (OR 2.24, 95 % CI 1.79–2.80) and in TKR surgery (RR 1.81, 95 % CI 1.44–2.28). Considering proximal and distal DVT events, patients undergoing to THR and TKR surgeries had more events (RR 2.29, 95 % CI 1.24–4.28 and RR 1.39, 95 % CI 1.00–1.94, respectively).

As concerns the safety, in THR and TKR surgery, patients receiving LMWH experienced fewer major bleeding events (OR 0.65, 95 % CI 0.45–0.93 and OR 0.42, 95 % CI 0.22–0.78, respectively).

In the meta-analysis performed by Gòmez-Outes et al. (2012), the authors separately analyzed the prophylactic effects of apixaban (four trials) and rivaroxaban (eight trials) in comparison to LMWH. Rivaroxaban was associated with a significant reduction in risk of symptomatic venous thromboembolism compared to enoxaparin (RR 0.48, 95 % CI 0.31–0.75; $P = 0.001$); apixaban reduced the risk of symptomatic thromboembolism (RR 0.82, 95 % CI 0.41–1.64), but not significantly.

As concerns primary safety outcomes, rivaroxaban was associated with a significant increased risk of clinically relevant bleeding [RR 1.25, 95 % CI (1.05–1.49) $P = 0.01$, whereas apixaban was associated with a significantly reduced risk [RR 0.82, 95 % CI (0.69–0.98) $P = 0.03$] (Table 4.2).

No difference in relation to surgery type (THR vs. TKR) for symptomatic VTE or clinically relevant bleeding (major bleeding and clinically relevant nonmajor bleeding) was reported. No statistically significant differences were found between rivaroxaban and enoxaparin as well as between apixaban and enoxaparin on the net clinical endpoint (symptomatic venous thromboembolism, major bleeding, and death). Overall, the net clinical benefit of rivaroxaban and apixaban was higher, albeit not significantly higher in TKR surgery than in total replacement surgery (Table 4.3).

Yoshida et al. (2013) meta-analyzed three studies with rivaroxaban and three with apixaban compared to enoxaparin.

Table 4.3 Risk ratios and 95 % CI endpoints of NOAC compared with enoxaparin in THR and TKR surgery from two meta-analyses

		Hamidi et al. (2013)				Gómez-Outes et al. (2012)		
		Mortality	DVT	PE	Major bleeding	Symptomatic venous thromboembolism	Clinically relevant bleeding	Net clinical endpoint
Dabigatran vs. enoxaparin	THR	1.17 (0.04–36.25)	0.98 (0.78–1.22)	0.84 (0.25–2.77)	1.24 (0.83–1.86)	0.78 (0.05–12.35)	1.22 (0.95–1.58)	1.26 (0.80–1.98)
	TKR	1.06 (0.36–3.12)	0.97 (0.7–1.34)	0.66 (0.27–1.65)	0.89 (0.47–1.69)	0.56 (0.16–1.98)	1.01 (0.74–1.39)	0.71 (0.48–1.05)
Rivaroxaban vs. enoxaparin	THR	0.73 (0.29–1.8)	**0.21**[a] (0.14–0.32)	1.0 (0.07–15.28)	**2.23**[a] (1.06–4.67)	0.52 (0.18–1.45)	1.25 (0.90–1.75)	0.92 (0.60–1.41)
	TKR	0.62 (0.13–2.9)	**0.62**[a] (0.51–0.75)	0.50 (0.17–1.46)	1.61 (0.8–3.24)	**0.49**[a] (0.29–0.83)	1.29 (0.99–1.67)	0.85 (0.60–1.19)
Apixaban vs. enoxaparin	THR	na[b]				0.40 (0.13–1.27)	0.95 (0.75–1.19)	1.00 (0.60–1.66)
	TKR	na[b]				1.08 (0.56–2.06)	**0.71**[a] (0.55–0.91)	0.88 (0.62–1.26)

PE pulmonary embolism, *na* data not available
[a]Statistically significant, $P<0.05$ at least
[b]Net clinical endpoint = symptomatic venous thromboembolism, major bleeding, death

The primary efficacy rates, any DVT, nonfatal PE, or all-cause mortality, were significantly reduced by rivaroxaban (RR 0.50, 95 % CI 0.34–0.73) and not significantly by apixaban (RR 0.63, 95 % CI 0.39–0.31).

The incidence of proximal DVT was reduced not significantly by rivaroxaban (RR 0.34, 95 % CI 0.11, 1.07) and significantly by apixaban (RR 0.45, 95 % CI 0.27–0.75); rivaroxaban (RR 0.45, 95 % CI 0.27–0.77) and apixaban (RR, 0.38, 95 % CI 0.16–0.90) produced significantly lower frequencies of symptomatic DVT.

Bleeding risk was reduced in apixaban patients; in particular when risk of clinically relevant nonmajor bleeding and risk of any bleeding were considered, the difference was statistically significant (RR 0.88, 95 % CI 0.79, 0.99) (Table 4.2).

Hamidi et al. (2013) analyzed eight RCT comparing rivaroxaban to enoxaparin, five in THR and three in TKR patients : a significant decrease in DVT, both in THR (RR 0.21, 95 % CI 0.4–0.32) and TKR (RR 0.62, 95 % CI 0.51–0.75), was observed, with no significant difference in mortality and PE. A significant increase in major bleeding in THR patients (RR 2.23, 95 % CI 1.06–4.67), but not for TKR, was observed (Table 4.3).

4.3.5 LMWH Versus Dabigatran

Four systematic reviews (Gòmez-Outes et al. 2012; Sobieraj et al. 2012; Hamidi et al. 2013; Yoshida Rde et al. 2013) evaluated effects of dabigatran in comparison to LMWH in thromboprophylaxis.

In the meta-analysis by Gòmez-Outes et al. (2012), including four trials and comparing dabigatran, at the doses of 150 and 220 mg, with enoxaparin for thromboprophylaxis of THR or TKR, the difference of risk for symptomatic VTE (RR 0.70, 95 % CI 0.18–2.76 and RR 0.86, 95 % CI 0.31–2.35 for dabigatran 220 and 150 mg, respectively) and major bleeding events (RR 1.12, 95 % CI 0.92–1.38 and RR 1.12, 95 % CI 0.89–1.40 for dabigatran 220 and 150 mg, respectively) was not statistically different between dabigatran and enoxaparin. The risk of total VTE or all-cause death was similar to enoxaparin for dabigatran 220 mg dose, but it was higher (RR 1.21, 95 % CI 1.05–1.39) for dabigatran 150 mg dose. No statistically significant differences were found between dabigatran and enoxaparin on the net clinical endpoint (symptomatic venous thromboembolism, major bleeding, and death). The type of surgery did not influence the net clinical effect (Tables 4.2 and 4.3).

Sobieraj et al. (2012) analyzed five RCT, but did not separate different doses (150 and 220 mg) of dabigatran. Compared with patients receiving direct thrombin inhibitors patients who received LMWH had more major venous thromboembolism (RR 1.35, 95 % CI 1.07–1.69), total DVT (RR 1.31, 95 % CI 1.09–1.57), and proximal DVT events (RR 1.39, 95 % CI 1.03–1.87) without significantly negatively affecting bleeding (major bleeding RR 1.04, 95 % CI 0.76–1.42 and minor bleeding RR 1.03, 95 % CI 0.88–1.21).

Hamidi et al. (2013) pooled five RCT, analyzing separately THR and TKR, but not different doses. No difference between dabigatran and enoxaparin in mortality, PE, DVT, and major bleeding was found in THR and TKR patients.

In 2013 Yoshida et al. (2013) by meta-analyzing four trials found no statically significant differences between dabigatran (150 and 220 mg) and enoxaparin in primary efficacy rates (RR 1.2, 95 % CI 1.03–1.41 and RR 1.02, 95 % CI 0.86–1.2), proximal DVT (RR 1.17, 95 % CI 0.76–1.81 and RR 0.73 M 95 % CI 0.48–1.11), symptomatic DVT (RR 1.64, 95 % CI 0.07–40.49 and RR 0.71, 95 % CI 0.12–4.01), major pulmonary embolism rates (RR 0.33, 95 % CI 0.07–1.46 and RR 1.14, 95 % CI 0.50–2.61), or major bleeding (RR 0.75, 95 % CI 0.46–1.21 and RR 1.08, 95 % CI 0.67–1.75) (Table 4.2).

Major bleeding did not differ among drug classes when analyzed by surgery type.

4.4 Comments and New Perspectives

The results of the RCT and meta-analysis are the source of data for developing evidence-based guidelines and recommendations of professional colleges, as the *American College of Chest Physicians* (*ACCP*); (Garcia et al. 2012) academies, as the *American Academy of Orthopedic Surgeons* (*AAOS*); and national health institutions, as *NICE* (*National Institute for Health and Clinical Excellence*).

Different clinical experiences and professional involvement induce to focus prevailingly on the prevention of symptomatic pulmonary embolism and deep vein thrombosis or on the negative impact that bleeding could have on patients after total joint arthroplasty, i.e., focusing more on the efficacy or, alternatively, on safety.

Actually, LMWH resulted superior to UFH for efficacy and safety and to antivitamin K for efficacy, not definitely lower for efficacy when compared to fondaparinux.

As concerns NOAC, an overall evaluation of the net clinical endpoint (symptomatic venous thromboembolism, major bleeding, and death) shows that no clear-cut differences stand out between LMWH and dabigatran, rivaroxaban, and apixaban. Nevertheless, different analyses of data available indicate inferior efficacy of LMWH in comparison to rivaroxaban and lower safety in comparison to apixaban.

How do the authors of guidelines and recommendations interpret and transfer for our clinical practice these bulk of data and evidences?

NICE guidelines, delivered in 2010, did not recommend any specific prophylactic regimen after total joint arthroplasty and indicate LMWH, fondaparinux, and UFH as well as dabigatran and rivaroxaban, but not antivitamin K or ASA. Neither apixaban was recommended as ADVANCE studies were published in 2010, too.

Different are the recommendations proposed by the *AAOS in 2011*. In the AAOS Clinical Practice Guidelines (Mont and Jacobs 2011), as a direct result of the network meta-analyses performed on 112 high- or medium-quality randomized controlled trial, the panel declared that thromboprophylaxis has to be applied, but no specific antithrombotic drug can be indicated.

As concerns the *ACCP guidelines* (Falck-Ytter et al. 2012), 9th edition Guidelines on "Antithrombotic Therapy and Prevention of Thrombosis" in patients undergoing THR or TKR, the use of one of the following was recommended: low-molecular-weight heparin; fondaparinux; dabigatran, apixaban, and rivaroxaban; low-dose unfractionated heparin; adjusted-dose vitamin K antagonist; aspirin (all grade 1B); or an intermittent pneumatic compression device (IPCD) (grade 1C) for a minimum of 10–14 days. They suggest the use of low-molecular-weight heparin rather than the other agents and recommend as alternatives fondaparinux, apixaban, dabigatran, rivaroxaban, UFH (low dose) (all grade 2B), and adjusted-dose antivitamin K, or ASA (all grade 2C).

Another issue that has to be considered is the cost-effectiveness, which Hamidi et al. (2013) analyzed in a systematic review of the studies comparing subcutaneous enoxaparin to rivaroxaban and dabigatran for thromboprophylaxis after THR and TKR. For the cost-effectiveness evaluation of the three interventions, a decision tree was set up for the short-term prophylaxis (90-day postsurgery) including DVT, PE, and major bleedings. For the chronic phase, a Markov model was used, containing three health states: "symptoms-free patient, "post-thrombotic syndrome (PTS)," and "dead" and separately considering the two surgery types of patients," THR and TKR.

The results of economic evaluations, which calculated quality-adjusted life-years (QALYs) and lifetime costs were expressed as incremental cost-effectiveness ratios (ICERs) and net health benefit (NHB) and took into account also the disutility and costs related to injection of enoxaparin and to the patients requiring nurse assistance for injections during the period after hospital discharge.

The costs were calculated for diagnosing DVT or PE, for treating bleeding, DVT, or PE events or post-thrombotic syndrome.

Dabigatran and rivaroxaban decreased lifetime costs and effectiveness in terms of fewer QALYs gained relative to enoxaparin in both THR and TKR. Thus the ICER = incremental costs/incremental QALYs failed to provide strong indications on the most valuable prophylactic approach. Therefore no clear statement could be made for the choice of the most appropriate agent, in the light of the uncertainty of the most effective strategy.

In the overall evaluation of the drug to be administered for the prophylaxis of thromboembolism after surgery, in particular for prolonged prophylaxis, possibly determined by the presence of comorbidities in elderly patients, the adherence to therapy has to be considered. Nonadherence in outpatient thromboprophylaxis after major orthopedic surgery with LMWH or fondaparinux was investigated in a systematic review (Wilke and Müller 2010) which showed a nonadherence rate of 13–37 %. The disutility related to self-injection, or to injection by family members, or visiting nurses may be responsible, at least in part, of noncompliance. However, this may happen to some extent also in patients on OAC who may be unwilling to adhere to periodical INR checks. NOACS, which do not deserve INR monitoring and can be taken orally, could be associated with better adherence, especially if patients will be appropriately informed and motivated by clinicians.

Considering the present attention to personalize our clinical practice, the values and the preferences of patients cannot be neglected; patients undergoing symptomatic VTE after THR or TKR or bleedings related to thromboprophylaxis experience very often unforeseen and/or unpredicted unpleasant conditions. The perception by the patients of the relative disutility of thrombosis and hemorrhagic complications of thromboprophylaxis is poorly known and still a matter of debate. However, it is commonly considered that the disutility related to a VTE episode roughly equals that related to a clinically relevant bleeding (Guyatt et al. 2012).

Conclusions

In conclusion, although the strength of evidence in favor of LMWH for the efficacy and safety in comparison to "old" anticoagulants is moderate, in today's real world practice the indication for UFH or antivitamin K remains limited to patients with renal failure.

With regard to NOAC, in spite of no definite differences in terms of net clinical benefit, in the present trend toward a personalized medicine, those patients at high thrombotic and vascular risk might be better protected against thromboembolic events by rivaroxaban and apixaban. This evaluation can be particularly relevant when the clinical conditions of the patient suggest a prolonged prophylaxis. For the majority of patients, LMWH represents the gold standard therapy.

Key Points

- Pharmacologic thromboprophylaxis has to be applied.
- RCT comparing different antithrombotic drugs are nonhomogenous.
- LMWH favorably compare with UFH and antivitamin K.
- No clear-cut differences of the net clinical endpoint exist between enoxaparin and NOAC.

References

Canadian Institute for Health Information (2008) Hip and knee replacements in Canada 2007, annual report. Canadian Institute for Health Information, Ottawa

Dixon T, Shaw M, Ebrahim S, Dieppe P (2004) Trends in hip and knee joint replacement: socioeconomic inequalities and projections of need. Ann Rheum Dis 63:825–830. PMID: 15194578

Falck-Ytter Y, Francis CW, Johanson NA, Curley C, Dahl OE, Schulman S, Ortel TL, Pauker SG, Colwell CW Jr (2012) Prevention of VTE in orthopedic surgery patients antithrombotic therapy and prevention of thrombosis, 9th ed: American College of Chest Physicians Evidence-Based Clinical Practice Guidelines. Chest 141:e278S–e325S

Garcia DA, Baglin TP, Weitz JI, Samama MM, American College of Chest Physicians (2012) Parenteral anticoagulants: antithrombotic therapy and prevention of thrombosis, 9th ed: American College of Chest Physicians Evidence-Based Clinical Practice Guidelines. Chest 141(2 Suppl):e24S–e43S. doi:10.1378/chest.11-2291

Gómez-Outes A, Terleira-Fernández AI, Suárez-Gea ML, Vargas-Castrillón E (2012) Dabigatran, rivaroxaban, or apixaban versus enoxaparin for thromboprophylaxis after total hip or knee replacement: systematic review, meta-analysis, and indirect treatment comparisons. BMJ 344:e3675. doi:10.1136/bmj.e3675

Guyatt GH, Norris SL, Schulman S et al (2012) Methodology for the development of antithrombotic therapy and prevention of thrombosis guidelines: antithrombotic therapy and prevention of thrombosis, 9th ed: American College of Chest Physicians evidence-based clinical practice guidelines. Chest 141(2 Suppl):53S–70S

Hamidi V, Ringerike T, Hagen G, Reikvam A, Klemp M (2013) New anticoagulants as thromboprophylaxis after total hip or knee replacement. Int J Technol Assess Health Care 29(3):234–243. doi:10.1017/S0266462313000251. Epub 2013 Jun 17

Kurtz S, Mowat F, Ong K, Chan N, Lau E, Halpern M (2005) Prevalence of primary and revision total hip and knee arthroplasty in the United States from 1990 through 2002. J Bone Joint Surg Am 87:1487–1497. PMID: 15995115

Mismetti P, Laporte S, Zufferey P, Epinat M, Decousus H, Cucherat M (2004) Prevention of venous thromboembolism in orthopedic surgery with vitamin K antagonists: a meta-analysis. J Thromb Haemost 2:1058–1070. PMID: 15219187

Mont MA, Jacobs JJ (2011) AAOS clinical practice guideline: preventing venous thromboembolic disease in patients undergoing elective hip and knee arthroplasty. J Am Acad Orthop Surg 19(12):777–778

National Center for Health Statistics (2010) Health, United States, 2009: with special feature on medical technology. National Center for Health Statistics, Centers for Disease Control and Prevention, U.S. Department of Health and Human Services, Hyattsville

National Institute for Health and Clinical Excellence: Guidance (2010) Venous thromboembolism: reducing the risk of venous thromboembolism (deep vein thrombosis and pulmonary embolism) in patients admitted to hospital. National Clinical Guideline Centre – Acute and Chronic Conditions (UK). Royal College of Physicians (UK), London

Neuman I, Rada G, Claro JC, Carrasco-Labra A, Thorlund K, Akl EA, Bates SM, Guyatt GH (2012) Oral direct Factor Xa inhibitors versus low-molecular-weight heparin to prevent venous thromboembolism in patients undergoing total hip or knee replacement: a systematic review and meta-analysis. Ann Intern Med 156(10):710–719. doi:10.7326/0003-4819-156-10-201205150-00421. Epub 2012 Mar 12

Organisation for Economic Co-operation and Development (2010) Health at a glance: Europe 2010. OECD Publishing, Paris. Accessed at http://dx.doi.org/10.1787/health_glance-2010-en. Accessed on 25 Jan 2012

Sobieraj DM, Coleman CI, Tongbram V, Chen W, Colby J, Lee S, Kluger J, Makanji S, Ashaye A, White CM (2012) Comparative effectiveness of low-molecular weight heparins versus other anticoagulants in major orthopedic surgery: a systematic review and meta-analysis. Pharmacotherapy 32(9):799–808. doi:10.1002/j.1875-9114.2012.01106.x. Epub 2012 Jun 28

Wilke T, Müller S (2010) Nonadherence in outpatient thromboprophylaxis after major orthopedic surgery: a systematic review. Exp Rev Pharmacoecon Outcomes Res 10(6):691–700

Yoshida Rde A, Yoshida WB, Maffei FH, El Dib R, Nunes R, Rollo HA (2013) Systematic review of randomized controlled trials of new anticoagulants for venous thromboembolism prophylaxis in major orthopedic surgeries, compared with enoxaparin. Ann Vasc Surg 27(3):355–369. doi:10.1016/j.avsg.2012.06.010. Epub 2013 Jan 23

5 The Rationale for the Use of Multimodal Thromboprophylaxis with Limited Anticoagulation in Patients Undergoing Total Joint Replacement: Arguments Against LMWHs Being Still the Gold Standard

Erik Schnaser, Alejandro Gonzalez Della Valle, Nigel Sharrock, and Eduardo A. Salvati

Open Questions

- Which is the real thromboembolic risk after hip and knee arthroplasty in the year 2014?
- Mortality after hip and knee arthroplasty: is pulmonary embolism still the main cause?
- Which are the pillars of a multimodal approach for thromboprophylaxis?
- Is multimodal prophylaxis with aspirin safe to prevent thromboembolism after hip and knee arthroplasty in patients with no predisposing factors?

5.1 Historical Perspective on Venous Thromboembolism

In the 1970s, during the "early years" of modern total joint replacement (TJR), several investigators highlighted the dangers of postoperative pulmonary embolism (PE) and the importance of postoperative anticoagulation for prophylaxis (Coventry et al. 1973; Johnson and Charnley 1977; Johnson et al. 1977). Death associated with venous thromboembolism (VTE) occurred in 2.3–3.4 % of patients (Coventry et al. 1973; Johnson et al. 1977).

In 1977, Sir John Charnley reported the rate of symptomatic PE and mortality in his own series of 7959 total hip replacement (THR) patients operated on between 1962 and 1973. The rate of PE and fatal PE in patients who did not receive chemoprophylaxis was 15.2 and 2.3 %, respectively. The rates of these complications were drastically reduced to 7.9 and 1 %, respectively, in patients who received postoperative anticoagulation (Johnson et al. 1977). Likewise, Coventry et al. reported a significant reduction in the rate of fatal PE from 3.4 % in 58 THR patients who received no postoperative anticoagulation to 0.05 % in 1950 patients who received postoperative warfarin. The authors also highlighted that potent anticoagulants can produce serious bleeding complications (Coventry et al. 1973).

The majority of postoperative deaths were related to PE. In the previously mentioned study by Johnson and Charnley, 88 % of deaths attributable to PE were confirmed by autopsy (Johnson et al. 1977). Freidin et al. studied 1,324 patients

E. Schnaser • A. Gonzalez Della Valle (✉)
N. Sharrock • E.A. Salvati
Department of Orthopaedic Surgery, Hospital for Special Surgery, 535 East 70th Street, New York, NY 10021, USA
e-mail: gonzaleza@hss.edu

A. Baldini, P. Caldora (eds.), *Perioperative Medical Management for Total Joint Arthroplasty: How to Control Hemostasis, Pain and Infection*, DOI 10.1007/978-3-319-07203-6_5,

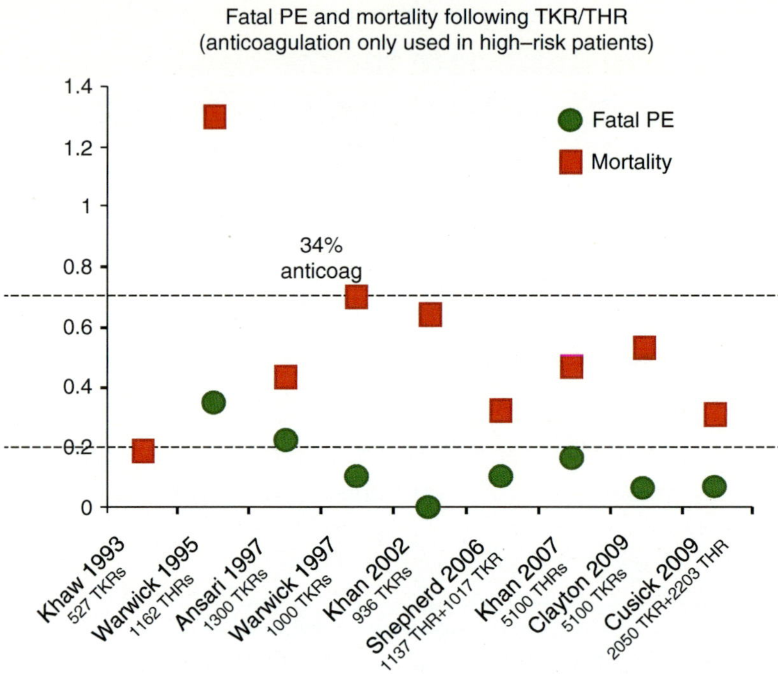

Fig. 5.1 Published rates of fatal PEs and all-cause mortality in patients undergoing hip or knee arthroplasty. This figure represents the lead author in the study, the year of publication, the number of patients, and procedure type on the *X*-axis and the corresponding rate on the *Y*-axis

who underwent THR surgery between 1969 and 1978 and received chemoprophylaxis with dextran. Nine out of the 16 patients (0.7 % of all patients and 56 % of all deaths) who died within the first 90 days of surgery were due to a PE (Fredin and Nillius 1982).

5.2 Thromboembolic Disease Following Elective Surgery in the Twenty-First Century

Despite the high rates of PE and fatal PE observed during the 1970s, there is abundant evidence suggesting that the rates of postoperative VTE and mortality have substantially diminished in the 1990s and in the twenty-first century, even when no routine anticoagulation is used. We recently reviewed nine studies reporting on all-cause mortality and fatal PE rates following an aggregate of 17,700 TJRs. The surgeries were performed in the 1990s and 2000s. Anticoagulants were not used or given only to high-risk patients. The all-cause mortality and fatal PE rates were extremely low (range 0.2–1.3 % and 0–0.35 %, respectively) (Fig. 5.1) (Khaw et al. 1993; Warwick et al. 1995; Ansari et al. 1997; Warwick and Whitehouse 1997; Shepherd and Mills 2006; Khan et al. 2002, 2007; Clayton et al. 2009; Cusick and Beverland 2009).

The low rates of postoperative mortality and fatal PE even when no routine anticoagulation is used are the result of substantial improvements in the understanting of VTE, anesthesia, surgery and perioperative care: In the 1960s and 1970s, surgical time averaged 3 hours, average bleeding was 1 liter, and surgeries were performed under general anesthesia; patients were mobilized after the first week and remained hospitalized for 2–3 weeks. At the present time, TJR has been perfected. In the hands of a specialized team, the surgical time does not exceed 60–75 min. When performed under hypotensive epidural anesthesia, there is minimal intraoperative bleeding. Patients are mobilized promptly after surgery and often remain hospitalized for 2–3 days (González Della Valle et al. 2006).

Our own institutional experience indicates that mortality and the proportion of deaths attributable to PE diminished systematically since the 1980s: The 30-day mortality rate following 5,874 TJRs performed in Hospital for Special Surgery between 1981 and 1985 using a general anesthetic was 0.4 % (23 of 5,874). Seven of 23 deaths (30 %) were attributed to a PE. With the introduction of regional anesthesia and no major changes in postoperative chemoprophylaxis, the 30-day mortality of 9,685 TJR patients operated between 1987 and 1991 was only 0.1 % (10 of 9,685). Moreover, only 2 of the 10 fatalities (20 %) were attributed to a PE (Sharrock et al. 1995a), though autopsies were not performed. Our most recent 90-day mortality rates following elective TJR surgery using "multimodal prophylaxis" are even lower and will be discussed below.

With the low rates of PE, fatal PE, and mortality observed by us and other investigators (Yassin et al. 2014), even when no routine anticoagulation is prescribed, the routine use of anticoagulants for prophylaxis must be questioned particularly in view of the risk of bleeding complications. This chapter will focus the historical development of our multimodal VTE prophylaxis protocol that minimizes the use of postoperative anticoagulants, the clinical results observed by us and other investigators, and on the historical aspects of traditional methods of VTE prophylaxis that we believe to be outdated.

5.3 Myths and Challenges Associated with Chemoprophylaxis

Based on the historically high rates of fatal PE, orthopedic surgeons specializing in TJR have always feared postoperative PE. Moreover, as PE is a thrombotic phenomenon, there has been a general belief that potent anticoagulation should be used routinely for prophylaxis. This practice is deeply rooted in the orthopaedic community. In the United States, warfarin has been the preferred form of chemoprophylaxis until the introduction of low-molecular-weight heparins in the 1990s and modern factor Xa inhibitors in the last decade. The routine use of potent anticoagulation for prophylaxis has been reinforced since the 1990s by guidelines conceived by a panel of experts and endorsed by the American College of Chest Physicians (Geerts et al. 2008). Guidelines were subsequently adopted and enforced by regulatory bodies like Centers for Medicare and Medicaid Services in the United States and the National Institute for Health and Care Excellence in the United Kingdom.

In addition, as PE has historically been regarded as a "preventable" complication, orthopedic surgeons have been compelled to routinely prescribe anticoagulants following surgery due to the need to comply with the previously mentioned guidelines, fear of litigation, and decreased reimbursement.

With the increased use of potent anticoagulation, the orthopedic community witnessed a raise in the number of postoperative bleeding complications. Local bleeding has resulted in excessive wound drainage, hematoma formation and infection leading to reoperation, and neurologic complications, among others. Systemic complications have resulted in substantial morbidity and rarely in fatal bleeding and heparin-induced thrombocytopenia (HIT). Leaders in the field of joint replacement surgery voiced their concern about the increase in bleeding complications associated with the routine use of anticoagulation for prophylaxis (Callaghan et al. 2005). The concerns of the orthopedic community and awareness of the commercial bias of the majority of authors of guidelines (Johanson 2011) have resulted in the recent reformulation of the ACCP guidelines (Falck-Ytter et al. 2012) and the development of guidelines for thromboprophylaxis by the American Academy of Orthopedic Surgeons (Jacobs et al. 2012) that advocate preoperative risk stratification of the thromboembolic risk (Bekşaç et al. 2006) and the use of effective anticoagulation in patients with a higher VTE risk.

5.4 The Framework and Scientific Basis for Multimodal Thromboprophylaxis

In the last four decades, efforts have been made to understand the pathogenesis of thromboembolic disease and perfect its prophylaxis. In our institution, a large body or clinical and applied research has been built since the 1970s (Salvati et al. 2007). The basic and applied investigations hereby discussed provided the basis for our "multimodal approach for thromboprophylaxis." The multimodal approach emphasizes nonpharmacological gestures to address the pillars of the Virchow's triad (Virchow 1856) and favors the use of safe, inexpensive aspirin for postoperative chemoprophylaxis in the majority of patients (approximately 80 %).

In the early 1970s, we observed that patients undergoing a THR had a more pronounced drop in the blood levels of antithrombin III than in patients undergoing general surgery. This study suggested that an intense activation of the clotting cascade occurred during THR. However, at that time, we were unable to determine the exact time of maximal thrombogenic activity (Gitel et al. 1979).

In the early 1990s, and with the advent of faster markers of thrombosis (Dahl 1997; Sharrock et al. 1995b), we demonstrated that thrombosis is strongly activated when the femoral canal is invaded and progressively increased with rasping and cementation, peaking at the time of femoral stem insertion (Sharrock et al. 1995b). The activation of the clotting cascade is triggered by intramedullary procoagulants that are forced from the femoral canal into the venous circulation during the femoral work. The effect is more pronounced with cemented fixation than with cementless fixation as a result of greater extravasation of intramedullary contents to the venous circulation caused by cement pressurization (Sharrock et al. 1995b).

The thrombogenic stimulus at the time of the femoral work is further compounded by venous stasis: The flow in the femoral vein is obstructed at the same time when the extreme limb position needed for these steps (flexion, abduction, and internal rotation in the posterolateral approach) (Binns and Pho 1990; Plánes et al. 1990; Stamatakis et al. 1977) kinks the femoral vein.

In order to obliterate thrombogenesis during the femoral work, we studied and implemented the administration of a bolus of intravenous unfractionated heparin (10–15 U/kg) immediately before femoral canal preparation. Our own investigations in the 1990s demonstrated that heparin effectively suppresses intraoperative fibrin formation (Sharrock et al. 1995b, 1999).

5.5 Multimodal Prophylaxis

Based on the results of the investigations performed in our and other institutions, the senior authors conceived a series of measures that are implemented by internists, anesthesiologists, surgeons, nurses, and physical therapists. Such measures are implemented *before, during, and after surgery* and are independent of the type for postoperative chemoprophylaxis. The measures aim at combating the pillars of Virchow's triad and when implemented together are known as "multimodal thromboprophylaxis." The measures include preoperative VTE risk stratification and discontinuation of procoagulant medications, the use of regional anesthesia (a bolus of intraoperative heparin is used before the femoral work in THR patients), expeditious surgery, postoperative use of pneumatic compression devices and rapid mobilization. When all these mentioned measures are observed, the use of aggressive postoperative anticoagulation becomes unnecessary. In fact, aspirin is our preferred form of chemoprophylaxis in the majority of patients with a low risk of VTE.

5.6 Preoperative Risk Stratification and Discontinuation of Procoagulant Medication

The most recognized clinical risk factors for VTE after TJA, in order of importance, include the diagnosis of hip fracture, malignancy, particularly if associated with chemotherapy, antiphospholipid syndrome, immobility or reduced mobility, history of VTE, tamoxifen and raloxifene therapy, American Society of Anesthesiologists (ASA) Physical Status Classification greater than 3, oral contraceptives, estrogen replacement therapy, stroke, atherosclerosis, advanced age, and obesity. The following risk factors are controversial: diabetes mellitus, certain cardiovascular conditions (congestive heart disease and atrial fibrillation), varicose veins, and smoking (Beksaç et al. 2006).

However, we observed that 50 % of patients who develop VTE after THR have no clinical predisposing factors. In a matched, controlled study, we defined that such patients with a low clinical risk of VTE may carry genetic predispositions that increase the risk of VTE. We identified the deficiency of antithrombin III (<75 %) and protein C (<70 %) and prothrombin gene (G20210A) mutation to be strong predisposing factors for postoperative VTE (Salvati et al. 2005). Preoperative genetic screening in conjunction with the identification of the recognized clinical risk factors can help determine the individual risk of postoperative VTE, and postoperative anticoagulation can be selected accordingly (Salvati et al. 2007).

5.7 Discontinuation of Procoagulant Medications

One of the most important gestures that can be done prior to surgery is the discontinuation of procoagulant drugs according to their known ½ life. In an effort to reduce postoperative bleeding complications, antiplatelet medication (clopidogrel, rivaroxaban, warfarin, etc.) should be stopped unless otherwise indicated by the patient's primary care physician or cardiologist.

5.8 Regional Anesthesia

Spinal anesthesia reduces blood loss and the prevalence of VTE by 40–50 % in comparison to general anesthesia (Salvati et al. 2007; Davis et al. 1989; Modig 1989; Modig et al. 1983; Prins and Hirsh 1990; Sculco and Ranawat 1975; Sharrock et al. 1993a, 1997; Sharrock and Salvati 1996; Wille-Jorgensen et al. 1989). Epidural anesthesia increases lower extremity blood flow, minimizing both venous stasis and thrombosis especially if low-dose epinephrine is used (Sharrock et al. 1993c; Sharrock and Salvati 1996; Sharrock et al. 1997; Bading et al. 1994; Mineo and Sharrock 1993). We have previously shown that a difference of 10 mmHg (50 versus 60 mmHg) in the mean arterial pressure, achieved through a high lumbar blockade (L1–2 or higher), has a measurable effect on intraoperative blood loss (Sharrock et al. 1993b). In addition, hypotensive anesthesia has been shown in prospective studies to be safe in the elderly patient population with comorbidities (Williams-Russo et al. 1999).

Our current protocol includes an epidural injection in the L1–L2 disk space of 2 % lidocaine with epinephrine (or 0.75 % bupivacaine) to ensure blockade to approximately L4. This is followed by intravenous infusion of epinephrine adjusted to maintain a mean arterial pressure between 50 and 60 mmHg to ensure hemodynamic stability. This approach allows the surgical team to proceed expeditiously on a bloodless field with excellent observation of the anatomic structures and without the delay produced by persistent bleeding. In a previously discussed retrospective study performed at our hospital, we observed that the 30-day mortality from a suspected PE after 15,559 TJRs declined from 0.12 % with the use of general anesthesia to 0.02 % with epidural anesthesia (Sharrock et al. 1995a).

5.9 Intraoperative Heparin During THR Surgery

During the early 1970s, we noticed patients undergoing THR were more susceptible to VTE than those who had other surgical procedures. Therefore, we began administering intraoperative unfractionated heparin intravenously and conducted three clinical trials. The heparin was administered at different times and in different doses. Venographic postoperative deep vein thrombosis (DVT) was reduced in all three studies in the heparin group in comparison to the control group (Sharrock et al. 1990; Huo et al. 1992a, b).

In the early 1990s, and with the advent of faster markers of thrombosis, we demonstrated that thrombogenesis is strongly activated as soon as the femoral canal is invaded, increasing progressively with rasping, cementation, and insertion of the femoral stem. Accordingly, we tested the efficacy of a low dose (1,000 U) of unfractionated heparin administered intravenously a few minutes before femoral preparation and found it suppressed fibrin formation during femoral preparation and insertion of the femoral component (Sharrock et al. 1995b). In a subsequent dose-response study, 10 U/kg of unfractionated heparin inhibited fibrin formation, whereas 20 U/kg completely suppressed fibrin formation (Sharrock et al. 1999).

The virtue of this single, small intravenous dose of unfractionated heparin, given a few minutes before femoral work when the thrombogenesis is maximally activated, is its short half-life (±30 min) so the risk of bleeding is minimal. With epidural hypotensive anesthesia, no additional intraoperative or postoperative bleeding is evident (Salvati et al. 2007).

5.10 Early Mobilization and Intermittent Pneumatic Compression

Patients with regional anesthesia do not recover active motion of the lower extremities for a few hours after surgery, which increases venous stasis. Thus, we apply intermittent pneumatic compression (IPC) early in the recovery room. We have shown that the application of IPC immediately after the operation increases the velocity and volume of venous flow, preventing or minimizing the formation and propagation of clots (Westrich et al. 2000). We evaluated the hemodynamic effects of several commercially available IPC devices in a crossover study involving ten patients who underwent TKR (Westrich et al. 1998). Newer pulsatile calf and pulsatile calf-foot IPC with a rapid inflation time produced the greatest increase in peak venous velocity, whereas sequential compression of the calf and thigh showed the greatest increase in venous volume. In a randomized, prospective study, we compared the rate of asymptomatic DVT in patients who were treated with or without IPC after joint replacement surgery. The rate of occlusive thrombi detected using MRV was 2 % (1 of 50) in the IPC group and 10 % (5 of 50) in the control group ($p=0.04$) (Ryan et al. 2002).

Active ankle dorsi-plantar flexion increases femoral venous flow by 50 % compared with baseline resting values (Markel et al. 1997). Thus, we strongly encourage such exercise throughout the entire recovery period. The postoperative pain relief provided by the patient-controlled analgesia facilitates early mobilization, which starts with the physical therapist on the day of surgery or in the morning of the first postoperative day.

5.11 Chemoprophylaxis

Aspirin is administered (325 mg twice daily) to patients with no predisposing factors for VTE and who mobilize promptly to provide mild suppression of thrombogenesis in the postoperative period. Aspirin also reduces the risk of heterotopic ossification (Bek et al. 2009).

Patients who are intolerant to aspirin or have a predisposition for VTE are given warfarin, which is initiated on the night of the surgical day aiming at obtaining an INR of 2 for 4–6 weeks.

Patients with an unusually high risk of VTE can be treated with low-molecular-weight heparin (LMWH) or an oral factor Xa inhibitor (Brown and Huo 2013). When the risk of VTE is high, we start both coumadin and LMWH postoperatively. If the epidural catheter is maintained for pain control, we delay the LMWH for 6 hours after its removal. The LMWH is discontinued after 3–4 days, once the patient's INR is >1.8. If the administration of LMWH is prolonged for 5 days or more, a platelet count is indicated in view of the risk of heparin-induced thrombocytopenia (HIT) (Warkentin and Greinacher 2004). The 2012 ACCP Guidelines recommend against the use of vena cava filters in patients who are not candidates for pharmacologic or mechanical prophylaxis (Falck-Ytter et al. 2012).

5.12 Clinical Results of Multimodal Thromboprophylaxis

In order to determine safety and efficacy of multimodal prophylaxis, we have published three studies evaluating a combined aggregate of 4,616 patients undergoing primary, elective THR or knee arthroplasty. All patients received multimodal thromboprophylaxis (González Della Valle et al. 2006; Gesell et al. 2013; Vulcano et al. 2012). All patients were followed for 90 days and none was lost. A total of 31 patients (0.6 %) were diagnosed with a symptomatic PE. None of these 31 patients died as a consequence of the PE during the follow-up period. Five patients (0.1 %) died during the initial 90 days. Three of the five patients received an autopsy which revealed arrhythmia in one patient, congestive heart failure in the second patient, and a myocardial infarction in the third patient. Consequently, the fatal PE rate ranged between 0 % (best-case scenario: assumes that none of the remaining two patients died of a PE) and 0.043 % (worse-case scenario: assumes that the remaining two patients without an autopsy died from a PE).

In addition, we addressed if multimodal prophylaxis with aspirin can be safely used in patients undergoing bilateral THR surgery, which carry a greater thrombogenic stimulus than unilateral surgery. We reviewed 644 consecutive patients who underwent one-stage bilateral THR, to determine the prevalence of VTE with two types of chemoprophylaxis. All patients received a similar multimodal prophylaxis protocol, which differed only in the postoperative chemoprophylaxis: 292 patients received Coumadin and 352 received aspirin. All patients were followed for a minimum of 3 months. There was no difference in the prevalence of VTE between the groups: 18 patients (6.16 %) in group 1 and 20 (5.68 %) in group 2. Four patients in each group developed a nonfatal PE (1.36 and 1.13 %, respectively). There were two deaths in each group, neither related to VTE. None of these differences were statistically significant (Beksaç et al. 2007).

5.13 How Does Multimodal Thromboprophylaxis Compare to Other Thromboprophylaxis Protocols?

In order to determine if multimodal thromboprophylaxis is as efficacious as other regimes that rely only on the routine administration of an anticoagulant, we performed a systematic review of peer-reviewed studies published between 1998 and 2007 that included a 6-week or 3-month incidence of all-cause mortality and symptomatic PE. In an aggregate of over 25,000 patients, we compared 3 different thromboprophylaxis protocols (Sharrock et al. 2008): Group A (15,839 patients) received potent, fast-acting anticoagulants such as LMWH, ximelagatran, fondaparinux, and rivaroxaban; group B (7,193 patients) received multimodal thromboprophylaxis (as outlined above); and group C (5,006 patients) received a slow-acting anticoagulant (warfarin). All-cause mortality was significantly lower in the multimodal group (0.19 %) when compared to the potent anticoagulation group (0.41 %) and the warfarin group (0.40 %). Similarly, the symptomatic PE rate was lower in the multimodal group (0.35 %) when compared to the potent anticoagulation group (0.59 %) and the warfarin group (0.52 %) (Fig. 5.2). We concluded that multimodal thromboprophylaxis is associated with the lowest all-cause mortality and PE rates after joint replacement in the lower extremity and that PE occurs despite the use of potent anticoagulation.

5.14 Pulmonary Embolism: No Longer the Leading Cause of Postoperative Mortality

In order to determine if PE continues to be the leading cause of death after TJR and if the proportion of deaths attributable to PE is lower when potent anticoagulants are used for prophylaxis, we conducted a second, larger systematic review.

The study consisted on a meta-analysis of 99,441 patients who underwent TJR. Among 373

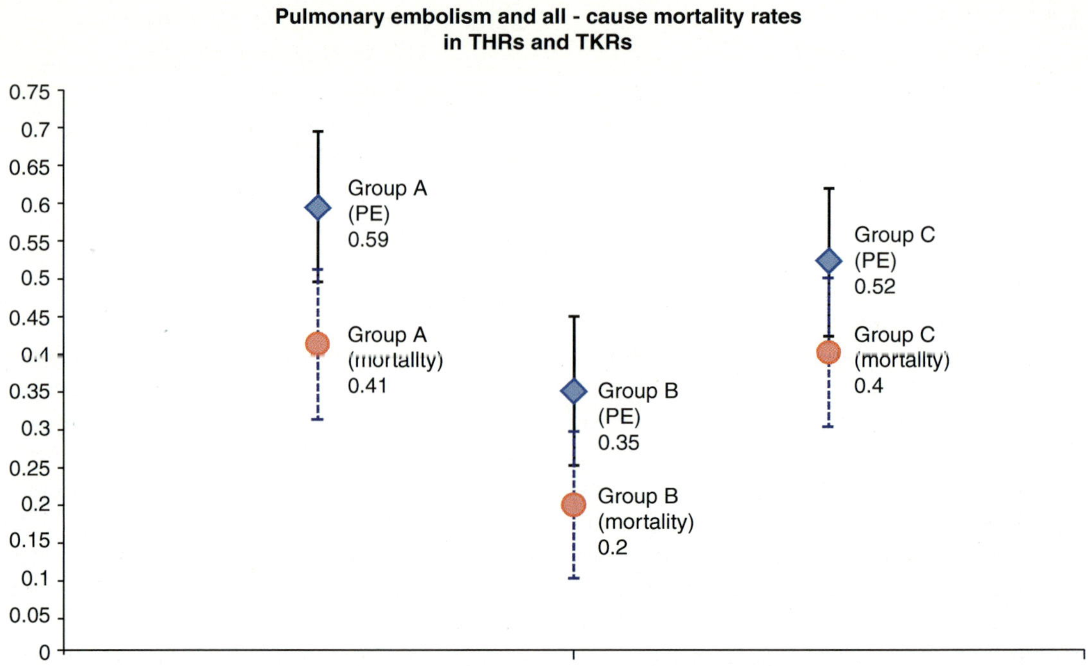

Fig. 5.2 Rates (events/100 patients) of PE and all-cause mortality stratified by prophylaxis modality. Group A = potent anticoagulation; group B = multimodal prophylaxis; group C = warfarin. *Error bars* demonstrate reported ranges from the literature (Adapted from Sharrock et al. (2008))

(0.38 %) deaths reported, the majority occurred due to cardiopulmonary complications unrelated to PE. PE was suspected to be responsible for only 25 % of the reported deaths (Poultsides et al. 2012). Moreover, the proportion of deaths due to PE was not affected by the type of postoperative chemoprophylaxis. In a large observational cohort study involving 93,840 patients from 307 hospitals, Bozic et al. showed that the overall 30-day mortality rate in patients undergoing TKR was 0.12 %. Patients received aspirin (5 %), warfarin (55.3 %), or injectable agents (39.6 %). No difference in mortality was seen between the three VTE prophylaxis groups (Bozic et al. 2010). Furthermore, the use of aspirin as chemoprophylaxis was associated with a lower adjusted risk for all VTE events compared to warfarin and a similar adjusted VTE risk compared to injectable agents. This study further highlights the fact that death after joint replacement is exceedingly rare and the multimodal approach is simple and efficacious in preventing VTE events.

5.15 Concerns with the Routine Use of Anticoagulants for Prophylaxis

A large number of patients undergoing TJR in the United States receive warfarin for postoperative thromboprophylaxis despite delayed effect, variable patient response, its narrow range of therapeutic efficacy, and a perplexing tendency to oscillate in and out of therapeutic target range. Effective prophylactic anticoagulation occurs only after a few days of administration, and there is no protection during the immediate postoperative period, when thrombogenesis is maximally activated. Warfarin has a number of drug interactions and with the current short hospital stay, it is difficult to achieve an adequate prophylactic level prior to discharge (Salvati and Lachiewicz 1976). In addition, the response to warfarin is affected by genetic mutations: Patients who are genetically predisposed to hyporespond to warfarin may be at an increased risk of VTE, whereas those who hyperrespond may be at an increased risk of bleeding (González Della Valle et al. 2009).

With regard to injectable agents, HIT can affect between 0.1 and 5 % of postoperative patients (Linkins et al. 2012). HIT is a prothrombotic disorder mediated by IgG antibodies that bind to conformational epitopes complexed with heparin. Typically, the platelet counts are only moderately reduced. Occasionally, patients do not have thrombocytopenia, but their platelet counts decrease by 50 % from pretreatment levels (Warkentin et al. 2003). There are two types of HIT: Type I is relatively common (10–20 %), nonimmune, and benign, with no ensuing bleeding or thrombotic complications. Platelet count drops but reverts to normal gradually without treatment. Type II is relatively rare (2–3 %) and is immune mediated. The platelet count falls to about 50,000/ul after 5–10 days of heparin therapy. Life-threatening conditions occur due to associated bleeding and/or thrombosis. The mortality rate may be as high as 40 %. Though routine monitoring of platelet count is controversial, we strongly recommend doing so in patients receiving heparin as the consequences of HIT can be devastating. Several case reports exist in the arthroplasty literature highlighting the dangers of HIT (Lilikakis et al. 2006; Chow et al. 2012; Craik and Cobb 2013; Ketha et al. 2013; Patterson et al. 1989).

5.16 Summary

Whereas the traditional strategy of routinely administering potent anticoagulation for prophylaxis is deeply rooted in the medical community, our experience supports a multimodal approach and aspirin which is both cost-efficient and safe in patients with no predisposing factors. Our opinion stems from four decades of clinical experience, the findings in our own patients, and evidence from other institutions.

Key Points

- The risk of VTE after hip and knee arthroplasty is currently low due to a number of preventive perioperative measures unrelated to postoperative chemoprophylaxis.
- The use of potent anticoagulants such as LMWH does not reduce the mortality rate associated with PE or any other cause after hip and knee arthroplasty.
- A multimodal protocol that includes aspirin as the sole chemoprophylactic agent is safe and effective to prevent thromboembolic complications for the majority of healthy patients undergoing hip and knee arthroplasty.
- Postoperative use of LMWH or warfarin or oral direct factor Xa inhibitors should be limited to patients with a high risk of postoperative VTE.

Acknowledgments This work was partially funded by the generous donation of Mr. Glenn Bergenfield and the Sidney Milton and Leoma Simon Foundation.

References

Ansari S, Warwick D, Ackroyd CE, Newman JH (1997) Incidence of fatal pulmonary embolism after 1,390 knee arthroplasties without routine prophylactic anticoagulation, except in high-risk cases. J Arthroplasty 12:599–602

Bading B, Blank SG, Sculco TP, Pickering TG, Sharrock NE (1994) Augmentation of calf blood flow by epinephrine infusion during lumbar epidural anesthesia. Anesth Analg 78:1119–1124

Bek D, Beksaç B, González Della Valle A, Sculco TP, Salvati EA (2009) Aspirin decreases the prevalence and severity of heterotopic ossification after 1-stage bilateral total hip arthroplasty for osteoarthrosis. J Arthroplasty 24:226–232

Beksaç B, González Della Valle A, Salvati EA (2006) Thromboembolic disease after total hip arthroplasty: who is at risk? Clin Orthop Relat Res 453: 211–224

Beksaç B, González Della Valle A, Anderson J, Sharrock NE, Sculco TP, Salvati EA (2007) Symptomatic thromboembolism after one-stage bilateral THA with

a multimodal prophylaxis protocol. Clin Orthop Relat Res 463:114–119
Binns M, Pho R (1990) Femoral vein occlusion during hip arthroplasty. Clin Orthop Relat Res 255:168–172
Brown TS and Huo MH (2013) New anticoagulants for thromboprophylaxis after total knee arthroplasty. Am J Orthop 42:424–429
Bozic KJ, Vail TP, Pekow PS, Maselli JH, Lindenauer PK, Auerbach AD (2010) Does aspirin have a role in venous thromboembolism prophylaxis in total knee arthroplasty patients? J Arthroplasty 274:1053–1060
Callaghan JJ, Dorr LD, Engh GA, Hanssen AD, Healy WL, Lachiewicz PF, Lonner JH, Lotke PA, Ranawat CS, Ritter MA, Salvati EA, Sculco TP, Thornhill TS, American College of Chest Physicians (2005) Prophylaxis for thromboembolic disease: recommendations from the American College of Chest Physicians – are they appropriate for orthopaedic surgery? J Arthroplasty 20:273–274
Chow VW, Abnousi F, Huddleston JI, Lin LH (2012) Heparin-induced thrombocytopenia after total knee arthroplasty, with subsequent adrenal hemorrhage. J Arthroplasty 27(1413):e15–e18
Clayton RA, Gaston P, Watts AC, Howie CR (2009) Thromboembolic disease after total knee replacement: experience of 5100 cases. Knee 16:18–21
Coventry MB, Nolan DR, Beckenbaugh RD (1973) "Delayed" prophylactic anticoagulation: a study of results and complications in 2,012 total hip arthroplasties. J Bone Joint Surg Am 55:1487–1492
Craik JD, Cobb AG (2013) Heparin-induced thrombocytopenia following hip and knee arthroplasty. Br J Haematol 161:255–261
Cusick LA, Beverland DE (2009) The incidence of fatal pulmonary embolism after primary hip and knee replacement in a consecutive series of 4253 patients. J Bone Joint Surg Br 91:645–648
Dahl OE (1997) The role of the pulmonary circulation in the regulation of coagulation and fibrinolysis in relation to major surgery. J Cardiothorac Vasc Anesth 11: 322–328
Davis FM, Laurenson VG, Gillespie WJ, Wells JE, Foate J, Newman E (1989) Deep vein thrombosis after total hip replacement. A comparison between spinal and general anaesthesia. J Bone Joint Surg Br 71: 181–185
Falck-Ytter Y, Francis CW, Johanson NA, Curley C, Dahl OE, Schulman S, Ortel TL, Pauker SG, Colwell CW Jr, American College of Chest Physicians (2012) Prevention of VTE in orthopedic surgery patients: Antithrombotic Therapy and Prevention of Thrombosis, 9th ed: American College of Chest Physicians Evidence-Based Clinical Practice Guidelines. Chest 141:e278S–e325S
Fredin HO, Nillius AS (1982) Fatal pulmonary embolism after total hip replacement. Acta Orthop Scand 53:407–411
Geerts WH, Bergqvist D, Pineo GF, Heit JA, Samama CM, Lassen MR, Colwell CW, American College of Chest Physicians (2008) Prevention of venous thromboembolism: American College of Chest Physicians Evidence-Based Clinical Practice Guidelines (8th Edition). Chest 133:381S–453S
Gesell MW, González Della Valle A, Bartolome Garcia S, Memtsoudis SG, Ma Y, Haas SB, Salvati EA (2013) Safety and efficacy of multimodal thromboprophylaxis following total knee arthroplasty: a comparative study of preferential aspirin vs. routine coumadin chemoprophylaxis. J Arthroplasty 28:575–579
Gitel SN, Salvati EA, Wessler S, Robinson HJ Jr, Worth MH Jr (1979) The effect of total hip replacement and general surgery on antithrombin III in relation to venous thrombosis. J Bone Joint Surg Am 61: 653–656
González Della Valle A, Serota A, Go G, Sorriaux G, Sculco TP, Sharrock NE, Salvati EA (2006) Venous thromboembolism is rare with a multimodal prophylaxis protocol after total hip arthroplasty. Clin Orthop Relat Res 444:146–153
González Della Valle A, Khakharia S, Glueck CJ, Taveras N, Wang P, Fontaine RN, Salvati EA (2009) VKORC1 variant genotypes influence warfarin response in patients undergoing total joint arthroplasty: a pilot study. Clin Orthop Relat Res 467:1773–1780
Huo MH, Salvati EA, Sharrock NE, Brien WW, Sculco TP, Pellicci PM, Mineo R, Go G (1992a) Intraoperative heparin thromboembolic prophylaxis in primary total hip arthroplasty. A prospective, randomized, controlled, clinical trial. Clin Orthop Relat Res 274:35–46
Huo MH, Salvati EA, Sharrock NE, Pellicci PM, Sculco TP, Go G, Mineo R, Brien WW (1992b) Intraoperative adjusted-dose heparin thromboembolic prophylaxis in primary total hip arthroplasty. Clin Orthop Relat Res 277:188–196
Jacobs JJ, Mont MA, Bozic KJ, Della Valle CJ, Goodman SB, Lewis CG, Yates AC Jr, Boggio LN, Watters WC 3rd, Turkelson CM, Wies JL, Sluka P, Hitchcock K (2012) American Academy of Orthopaedic Surgeons clinical practice guideline on: preventing venous thromboembolic disease in patients undergoing elective hip and knee arthroplasty. J Bone Joint Surg Am 94:746–747
Johanson NA (2011) Venous thromboembolism guidelines and prophylaxis. In: Glassman AH, Lachiewicz PF, Tanzer M (eds) Orthopaedic knowledge update 4: hip and knee reconstruction. American Academy of Orthopaedic Surgeons, Rosemont, USA
Johnson R, Charnley J (1977) Treatment of pulmonary embolism in total hip replacement. Clin Orthop Relat Res 124:149–154
Johnson R, Green JR, Charnley J (1977) Pulmonary embolism and its prophylaxis following the Charnley total hip replacement. Clin Orthop Relat Res 127:123–132
Ketha S, Smithedajkul P, Vella A, Pruthi R, Wysokinski W, Mcbane R (2013) Adrenal haemorrhage due to heparin-induced thrombocytopenia. Thromb Haemost 109:669–675
Khan A, Emberson J, Dowd GS (2002) Standardized mortality ratios and fatal pulmonary embolism rates

following total knee replacement: a cohort of 936 consecutive cases. J Knee Surg 15:219–222; discussion 222

Khan A, Kiryluk S, Fordyce MJ (2007) Fatal pulmonary embolism, death rates and standardised mortality ratios after primary total hip replacement in a joint replacement centre. Hip Int 17:59–63

Khaw FM, Moran CG, Pinder IM, Smith SR (1993) The incidence of fatal pulmonary embolism after knee replacement with no prophylactic anticoagulation. J Bone Joint Surg Br 75:940–941

Lilikakis AK, Papapolychroniou T, Macheras G, Michelinakis E (2006) Thrombocytopenia and intracerebral complications associated with low-molecular-weight heparin treatment in patients undergoing total hip replacement. A report of two cases. J Bone Joint Surg Am 88:634–638

Linkins LA, Dans AL, Moores LK, Bona R, Davidson BL, Schulman S, Crowther M, American College of Chest Physicians (2012) Treatment and prevention of heparin-induced thrombocytopenia: antithrombotic therapy and prevention of thrombosis, 9th ed: American College of Chest Physicians Evidence-Based Clinical Practice Guidelines. Chest 141:e495S–e530S

Markel DC, Urquhart B, Derkowska I, Salvati EA, Sharrock NE (1997) Effect of epidural analgesia on venous blood flow after hip arthroplasty. Clin Orthop Relat Res 334:168–174

Mineo R, Sharrock NE (1993) Pulse oximeter waveforms from the finger and toe during lumbar epidural anesthesia. Reg Anesth 18:106–109

Modig J (1989) Beneficial effects on intraoperative and postoperative blood loss in total hip replacement when performed under lumbar epidural anesthesia. An explanatory study. Acta Chir Scand Suppl 550:95–100: discussion 100–103

Modig J, Borg T, Karlstrom G, Maripuu E, Sahlstedt B (1983) Thromboembolism after total hip replacement: role of epidural and general anesthesia. Anesth Analg 62:174–180

Patterson BM, Marchand R, Ranawat C (1989) Complications of heparin therapy after total joint arthroplasty. J Bone Joint Surg Am 71:1130–1134

Plánes A, Vochelle N, Fagola M (1990) Total hip replacement and deep vein thrombosis. A venographic and necropsy study. J Bone Joint Surg Br 72: 9–13

Poultsides LA, González Della Valle A, Memtsoudis SG, Ma Y, Roberts T, Sharrock N, Salvati E (2012) Meta-analysis of cause of death following total joint replacement using different thromboprophylaxis regimens. J Bone Joint Surg Br 94:113–121

Prins MH, Hirsh J (1990) A comparison of general anesthesia and regional anesthesia as a risk factor for deep vein thrombosis following hip surgery: a critical review. Thromb Haemost 64:497–500

Ryan MG, Westrich GH, Potter HG, Sharrock N, Maun LM, Macaulay W, Katkin P, Sculco TP, Salvati EA (2002) Effect of mechanical compression on the prevalence of proximal deep venous thrombosis as assessed by magnetic resonance venography. J Bone Joint Surg Am 84-A:1998–2004

Salvati EA, Gonzalez Della Valle A, Westrich GH, Rana AJ, Specht L, Weksler BB, Wang P, Glueck CJ (2005) The John Charnley Award: heritable thrombophilia and development of thromboembolic disease after total hip arthroplasty. Clin Orthop Relat Res 441:40–55

Salvati EA, Lachiewicz P (1976) Thromboembolism following total hip replacement arthroplasty. The efficacy of dextran-aspirin and dextran-warfatin in prophylaxis. J Bone Joint Surg (Am) 58-A(7):921–925

Salvati EA, Sharrock NE, Westrich G, Potter HG, Gonzalez Della Valle A, Sculco TP (2007) The 2007 ABJS Nicolas Andry Award: three decades of clinical, basic, and applied research on thromboembolic disease after THA: rationale and clinical results of a multimodal prophylaxis protocol. Clin Orthop Relat Res 459:246–254

Sculco TP, Ranawat C (1975) The use of spinal anesthesia for total hip-replacement arthroplasty. J Bone Joint Surg Am 57:173–177

Sharrock NE, Salvati EA (1996) Hypotensive epidural anesthesia for total hip arthroplasty: a review. Acta Orthop Scand 67:91–107

Sharrock NE, Brien WW, Salvati EA, Mineo R, Garvin K, Sculco TP (1990) The effect of intravenous fixed-dose heparin during total hip arthroplasty on the incidence of deep-vein thrombosis: a randomized, double-blind trial in patients operated on with epidural anesthesia and controlled hypotension. J Bone Joint Surg Am 72:1456–1461

Sharrock NE, Mineo R, Go G (1993a) The effect of cardiac output on intraoperative blood loss during total hip arthroplasty. Reg Anesth 18:24–29

Sharrock NE, Mineo R, Urquhart B, Salvati EA (1993b) The effect of two levels of hypotension on intraoperative blood loss during total hip arthroplasty performed under lumbar epidural anesthesia. Anesth Analg 76:580–584

Sharrock NE, Ranawat CS, Urquhart B, Peterson M (1993c) Factors influencing deep vein thrombosis following total hip arthroplasty under epidural anesthesia. Anesth Analg 76:765–771

Sharrock NE, Cazan MG, Hargett MJ, Williams-Russo P, Wilson PD Jr (1995a) Changes in mortality after total hip and knee arthroplasty over a ten-year period. Anesth Analg 80:242–248

Sharrock NE, Go G, Harpel PC, Ranawat CS, Sculco TP, Salvati EA (1995b) The John Charnley Award. Thrombogenesis during total hip arthroplasty. Clin Orthop Relat Res 319:16–27

Sharrock NE, Go G, Williams-Russo P, Haas SB, Harpel PC (1997) Comparison of extradural and general anaesthesia on the fibrinolytic response to total knee arthroplasty. Br J Anaesth 79:29–34

Sharrock NE, Go G, Sculco TP, Salvati EA, Westrich GH, Harpel PC (1999) Dose response of intravenous heparin on markers of thrombosis during primary total hip replacement. Anesthesiology 90:981–987

Sharrock NE, González Della Valle A, Go G, Lyman S, Salvati EA (2008) Potent anticoagulants are associated with a higher all-cause mortality rate after hip and knee arthroplasty. Clin Orthop Relat Res 466:714–721

Shepherd A, Mills C (2006) Fatal pulmonary embolism following hip and knee replacement. A study of 2153 cases using routine mechanical prophylaxis and selective chemoprophylaxis. Hip Int 16:53–56

Stamatakis JD, Kakkar VV, Sagar S, Lawrence D, Nairn D, Bentley PG (1977) Femoral vein thrombosis and total hip replacement. Br Med J 2:223–225

Virchow R (1856) Neuer Fall von tödtlicher Embolie der Lungenarterien. Archiv f pathol Anat 10:225–228

Vulcano E, Gesell M, Esposito A, Ma Y, Memtsoudis SG, González Della Valle A (2012) Aspirin for elective hip and knee arthroplasty: a multimodal thromboprophylaxis protocol. Int Orthop 36:1995–2002

Warkentin TE, Greinacher A (2004) Heparin-induced thrombocytopenia: recognition, treatment, and prevention: the seventh ACCP conference on antithrombotic and thrombolytic therapy. Chest 126:311S–337S

Warkentin TE, Roberts RS, Hirsh J, Kelton JG (2003) An improved definition of immune heparin-induced thrombocytopenia in postoperative orthopedic patients. Arch Intern Med 163:2518–2524

Warwick DJ, Whitehouse S (1997) Symptomatic venous thromboembolism after total knee replacement. J Bone Joint Surg Br 79:780–786

Warwick D, Williams MH, Bannister GC (1995) Death and thromboembolic disease after total hip replacement. A series of 1162 cases with no routine chemical prophylaxis. J Bone Joint Surg Br 77:6–10

Westrich GH, Specht LM, Sharrock NE, Windsor RE, Sculco TP, Haas SB, Trombley JF, Peterson M (1998) Venous haemodynamics after total knee arthroplasty: evaluation of active dorsal to plantar flexion and several mechanical compression devices. J Bone Joint Surg Br 80:1057–1066

Westrich GH, Specht LM, Sharrock NE, Sculco TP, Salvati EA, Pellicci PM, Trombley JF, Peterson M (2000) Pneumatic compression hemodynamics in total hip arthroplasty. Clin Orthop Relat Res 372:180–191

Wille-Jorgensen P, Christensen SW, Bjerg-Nielsen A, Stadeager C, Kjaer L (1989) Prevention of thromboembolism following elective hip surgery. The value of regional anesthesia and graded compression stockings. Clin Orthop Relat Res 247:163–167

Williams-Russo P, Sharrock NE, Mattis S, Liguori GA, Mancuso C, Peterson MG, Hollenberg J, Ranawat C, Salvati E, Sculco T (1999) Randomized trial of hypotensive epidural anesthesia in older adults. Anesthesiology 91:926–935

Yassin M, Mitchell C, Diab M, Senior C (2014) The necessity of pharmacological prophylaxis against venous thromboembolism in major joint arthroplasty. Int Orthop 38:1073–1075

tive morbidity in fast-track hip and knee arthroplasty. Transfusion 54(3):717–26
Konig G, Hamlin BR, Waters JH (2013) Topical tranexamic acid reduces blood loss and transfusion rates in total hip and total knee arthroplasty. J Arthroplasty 28(9):1473–1476
Naylor JM, Adie S, Fransen M, Dietsch S, Harris I (2010) Endorsing single-unit transfusion combined with a restrictive haemoglobin transfusion threshold after knee arthroplasty. Qual Saf Health Care 19(3):239–243
Salpeter SR, Buckley JS, Chatterjee S (2014) Impact of more restrictive blood transfusion strategies on clinical outcomes: a meta-analysis and systematic review. Am J Med 127(2):124–131.e3
So-Osman C, Nelissen R, Brand R, Brand A, Stiggelbout AM (2011) Postoperative anemia after joint replacement surgery is not related to quality of life during the first two weeks postoperatively. Transfusion 51(1):71–81
So-Osman C, Nelissen R, Brand R, Faber F, Slaa RT, Stiggelbout A, Brand A (2013) The impact of a restrictive transfusion trigger on post-operative complication rate and well-being following elective orthopaedic surgery: a post-hoc analysis of a randomised study. Blood Transfus 11(2):289–295
Spahn DR (2010) Anemia and patient blood management in hip and knee surgery: a systematic review of the literature. Anesthesiology 113(2):482–495
Spahn DR, Vamvakas EC (2013) Is best transfusion practice alone best clinical practice? Blood Transfus 22:1–3
Sundhedsstyrelsen. www.sundhedsstyrelsen.dk (VEJ nr 10333 af 20/12/2007)
Vuille-Lessard E, Boudreault D, Girard F, Ruel M, Chagnon M, Hardy JF (2012) Postoperative anemia does not impede functional outcome and quality of life early after hip and knee arthroplasties. Transfusion 52(2):261–270
Weber EW, Slappendel R, Prins MH, van der Schaaf DB, Durieux ME, Strümper D (2005) Perioperative blood transfusions and delayed wound healing after hip replacement surgery: effects on duration of hospitalization. Anesth Analg 100(5):1416–1421
WHO (2008) Worldwide prevalence of anaemia 1993–2005. World Health Organization, Geneva

A Low Hemoglobin Transfusion Trigger Is Not Dangerous: Arguments Against

7

Grazia Gentilini and Alvaro Ringressi

Open Questions

- Is Hb level the best indicator for patients transfusion requirements?
- Is it recommendable to use a single indicator (e.g. Hb level) in the clinical practice?
- Can we identify the tissue hypoxia level in order to have a "personalized, more physiological trigger point"?

7.1 Introduction

It is common for clinicians to observe how concentrations of hemoglobin (Hb) as low as 4 or even 3 g/dl may be compatible with life and to see patients affected by chronic anemia who may afford some physical practice, with Hb levels just above 5 or 6 g/dl. On the other hand, we observe that not severely anemic patients can undergo serious ischemic complications. These experiences suggest that, depending on interpersonal variability in anemia tolerance, the range of Hb in which appropriateness of transfusion is uncertain is wide and that other indicators are needed to guide clinical decisions about blood transfusion.

This chapter makes a critical review of the available literature in order to provide a useful interpretation of the conclusions of different studies and metanalysis.

7.2 Discussion About Methodology Used in Clinical Studies

Most of our knowledge about blood transfusion outcomes and adverse effects is based on observational, often retrospective, studies. Indeed, studies addressing etiologies as well as monitoring of adverse effects correctly relies on such a methodology, provided an adequate analysis is conducted for establishing causative relationship, such as application of Bradford Hill criteria (Isbister et al. 2011). On the other hand, in order to address the question: "What is a safe transfusion trigger (in a determined cohort of patients)?" RCTs are needed and many have actually been carried out in the last decades. Most RCTs, applying maximal statistical rigor, are based on an intention-to-treat analysis, where randomized patients remain in respective arms, regardless of the actual treatment in the course of the study. The other possible methodological approach is the on-treatment analysis. Both methods are limited, being the latter susceptible to different kinds of bias, and the

G. Gentilini (✉) • A. Ringressi
Immunohematology and Transfusion Service, Azienda Ospedaliero-Universitaria Careggi, 3, L.go Brambilla, Florence 50134, Italy
e-mail: gentilinig@aou-careggi.toscana.it

A. Baldini, P. Caldora (eds.), *Perioperative Medical Management for Total Joint Arthroplasty: How to Control Hemostasis, Pain and Infection*, DOI 10.1007/978-3-319-07203-6_7,

first potentially burdened by a certain rate of protocol violation or deviation. Because of these limitations, some authors suggest that both analysis should usually be performed and reported, ultimately stating that "clinical research results remain an imperfect approximation of what will happen when a treatment is implemented in practice" (Blumberg et al. 2007).

In order to draw conclusion from RCTs about transfusion thresholds, a valuable meta-analysis is available, from the Cochrane Collaborative Group (Carson et al. 2012a). Some notations are to be brought, in order to place this issue in the correct framework. Risk of bias exists in most studies, also considering that blinding is practically impossible. Also, RCTs show a considerable heterogeneity with regard to the threshold used in the two arms, being in the "restrictive" arm 7–9 g/dl and extremely variable in the "liberal" one.

For ethical reasons, since blood transfusion is considered a life-sparing therapy, deviations from protocol in transfusion medicine trials have always been high, even though over the last few decades increased education to adhere to evidence-based programs and growing confidence of medical and surgery staffs with lower transfusion thresholds have permitted to improve the compliance with protocols within clinical trials in transfusion medicine. The rate of protocol deviation in some studies is so high that the primary outcome (rate of patients transfused and/or number of units infused) does not achieve a statistically significant difference between the two arms (see Carson et al. 2012a).

The rationale for blood transfusion is to restore oxygen delivery, in a symptomatic patient or in an asymptomatic one, assuming that the benefits will overweight the risks. In routine clinical practice, reliable indicators of tissue hypoxia are not available. Therefore, often blood units are delivered and administered *before*, and *in the fear of*, signs of hypoxia are developed, as well as with the aim to provide a reserve when further bleeding is anticipated. This behavior relies on known risks of perioperative course, given that myocardial infarction (MI) and overall cardiovascular deaths are the main causes of deaths after non-cardiac surgery (Lie et al. 2002; Mantilla et al. 2002). MI is present in 5 % of patients by 30 days of surgery, with some 2/3 of these not experiencing symptoms of ischemic injury (Devereaux et al. 2011). Besides renal failure, postoperative independent risk factor for MI is ongoing blood loss (idem), suggesting that for bleeding patients the time lag between checking Hb concentration and eventual transfusion, in everyday ward practice, may be unacceptably long. Translation of the best literature in everyday routine must take in account a number of factors also including organization, ultimately concerning patient's safety. Rosencher et al. (2012) have suggested that "we must now move on towards tailoring allogeneic blood transfusion administration to suit individual needs by adapting to ward routines, to logistical problems of obtaining blood in a timely fashion ad to the kinetics of bleeding for each procedure" and that "according to the kinetics of bleeding, the transfusion trigger should be different in the recovery room and the ward."

In most RCTs addressing safety of a low transfusion threshold, patients presenting CVD or bleeding at enrollment are excluded. Usually and correctly from an ethical standpoint, transfusion of symptomatic patients assigned to the restricted arm is permitted *within* the protocol, and in some studies the opinion of clinician about a not better defined benefit for the patients is not considered a deviation from protocol. Therefore, even when the average Hb concentration detected in the two arms diverge appropriately, a doubt arises that in the restrictive arm those patients who would potentially get harm from not transfusing have actually been transfused, ultimately determining a lower rate of adverse outcomes related to tissue hypoxia. Therefore, results may potentially imply misleading conclusions. In other cases, misunderstanding originates in the title: for example, Foss et al. (2009) studied ambulation after hip fracture surgery. These authors did not find significant difference between liberal and restrictive arms, and they observed, in the restrictive arm, a striking higher rate of cardiovascular complications and death.

Another issue that we have not engaged yet is related to the quality of blood products used in the

RCTs, in terms of leukoreduction and storage consequences. We will not examine this issue in detail, referring to proper studies and reviews. We only underline that some of the studies that have a relative weight in analysis leading to conclude that not transfusing over a certain threshold is better than doing have been performed with not-leukoreduced blood components. It is clearly established that leukoreduction modifies proinflammatory properties of RBC units, and their reduction can be associated with short-term mortality in some settings (Vamvakas 2003). Therefore, it appears reasonable to state that some studies, reproduced with different products, would carry different results. The influence of "age" of blood components on clinical outcomes after transfusion is still debated (Lelubre and Vincent 2013), but arguing against any unfavorable consequence appears not reasonable. When new media for conservation of RBC units, able to reduce or delay the comparison of storage lesions, will be licensed (at present, some are under investigation), risk/benefit ratio for blood transfusion shall be revisited.

Indeed, taking into account the evidence so far accessible, currently available guidelines are very cautious in their indications. Carson et al. (2012b) for the AABB state that "Practice guidelines are not intended as standards or absolute requirements and do not apply to all individual transfusion decision. Clinical decision is critical in the decision to transfuse." After indicating a Hb threshold of 8 g/dl or symptoms in postoperative surgical patients, these authors explain: "The panel believed that these *recommendations would probably apply to most postsurgical and medical patients, with the exception of those with the acute coronary syndrome.*"

7.3 Physiological Trigger Points

It has been clearly established that morbidity and mortality risks for young, healthy subjects are extremely low, in acute normovolemic anemia with Hb levels as low as 5 g/dl (see the other chapters from Gentilini and Ringressi and from Husted), for activation of adaptive phenomena. What ability of compensation exists in elderly and/or ill populations, which indexes can effectively guide the decision to transfuse, and what measures can be taken to reduce transfusion dependency in specific settings are still a matter of debate. In mixed surgery patients refusing transfusion, Carson et al. (2002) found that the odds of death in patients with a postoperative Hb ≤8 g/dl increased 2.5 times for each gram decrease in Hb level, after adjusting main confounding factors. A restrictive strategy in critical care, with a transfusion threshold as low as 7 g/l Hb, was associated with a favourable outcome in the benchmark paper by Hébert et al. (1999). Even if every medical staff must credit this, as well as several other papers bringing analogous conclusions for their groundbreaking indications, conclusive statements on transfusion appropriateness in every patient cannot be drawn on the basis of Hb level alone.

From a theoretical point of view, since blood transfusion therapy is administered as a fundamental support to oxygenation of tissues, a step forward in the direction of tailoring transfusion for specific patient's need has to take into account the physiology of oxygen supply to the cells (Fig. 7.1).

The index of availability of oxygen for the tissues/organs is DO_2 (oxygen delivery), that is, the product of cardiac output (CO) by the content of oxygen in arterial blood (CaO_2). This value can be obtained knowing the arterial hemoglobin saturation (SaO_2), since $CaO_2 = SaO_2 \times Hb \times 1.34$ (i.e., the oxygen-carrying capacity of Hb in

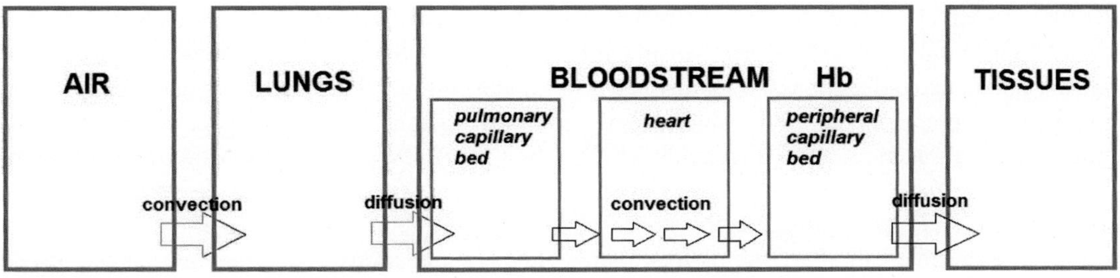

Fig. 7.1 Representation of the oxygen pathway, from air to tissues, in mammals

mlO_2/g Hb) + O_2 dissolved in plasma. The amount of dissolved gas is negligible when Hb concentration is not very low and air is inhaled.

In a healthy resting adult, DO_2 ranges from 800 to 1,200 ml/min, while global oxygen consumption (VO_2) is 200–300 ml/min. The oxygen extraction ratio (O_2ER), representing the ratio VO_2/DO_2, is thus 20–30 % and a large reserve exists for metabolic demand. When DO_2 is reduced for any reason affecting the oxygen pathway, enclosed acute normovolemic anemia, VO_2 remains mostly stable (unless fever, anxiety, or other causes of increased oxygen consumption are present), resulting an increased O_2ER. Lowering further the DO_2, a certain point is reached ($DO_{2\ CRIT}$), where VO_2 begins to decrease being O_2ER not increasable (value at peak 60–70 %). Then, oxygen is not sufficient anymore for the cell aerobic metabolism, hypoxia develops, and an anaerobic metabolism takes over, with a low production of ATP, unable to meet the tissue demand and lactate is released. Theoretically, $DO_{2\ CRIT}$ is one of the real, physiological trigger points. Therefore, we should be able to point at this key index, to guide any goal-directed therapy, including blood transfusion.

Nevertheless, it is to be considered that diverse $DO_{2\ CRIT}$ can coexist in an organism, because of reduced DO_2 and/or O_2ER at regional level, where an ischemic injury can develop in some organs, in the absence of global markers of hypoxia.

On the basis of what is described above, optimization of transfusion therapy would require reliable markers of hypoxia in tissues. Currently, because of the lack of validated, practicable markers of tissue hypoxia, we refer to surrogate ones. So, traveling back on the O_2 pathway (Fig. 7.1), the first element easy to derive (in quantitative terms) is hemoglobin concentration in blood. Therefore, it is obvious that, over last decades, a great effort has been put in research in the attempt to validate such an inexpensive and quickly obtainable indicator as a transfusion trigger. Nevertheless, the predictive value of determinate Hb levels as transfusion thresholds is high in patients who are young and without known comorbidities and become lower when other factors are present that can affect the oxygen pathway at any level.

A feasible index that can be integrated with Hb concentration is quantification of arterial hemoglobin saturation, (SaO_2), investigating the first part of the O_2 pathway, from inhaled air to diffusion toward pulmonary capillaries. SaO_2 measurement is effected by means of a pulse oximetry that gives a reliable esteem and is practicable in any ward.

Doing so, we still miss any information about the real amount of oxygen transferred to the tissues. As already mentioned, more refined indicators of tissue hypoxia, defined "physiological trigger points," have been developed to address more closely questions related with the oxygen utilization by the tissues, in order to guide a goal-directed therapy. On the basis of what is described above, ideal investigation on the critical part of O_2 pathway would require measurement of the key factor O_2ER. This is indirectly obtainable through measurement of mixed venous O_2 saturation (SvO_2), being $O_2ER = (SaO_2 - SvO_2)/SaO_2$. Targeting O_2ER for goal-directed therapy has shown, when integrated in an algorithm of treatment, its capability to guide clinical decision and to increase the rate of favorable outcomes (Donati et al. 2007). SvO_2 measurement requires pulmonary artery catheterization (PAC), by means of a Swan-Ganz catheter, but because of low feasibility and risks associated with this maneuver, it has been almost abandoned. Through a more practical central venous catheter, it is possible to measure the $ScvO_2$ (central venous O_2 saturation). $ScvO_2$ has been advocated to be close to SvO_2, only slightly overestimating, according to some authors (Reinhart et al. 2004), but presenting a more variable relationship (Dueck et al. 2005) and not fully substitutable to SvO_2, according to other authors (Chawla et al. 2004). Therefore, extending its use has required an entirely new step of validation as a marker of global tissue hypoxia and tool for goal-directed therapy. Most, but not all, studies pointing at $ScvO_2$ as fundamental indicator for monitoring clinical conditions and therapy have shown its effectiveness in diverse critical illness (see van Beest et al. 2011). Moreover, its perioperative use for goal-directed therapy in high-risk surgery has been found to be effective in predicting complications (Pearse et al. 2005a; Boyle et al. 2014) and in improving clinical outcomes

(Pearse et al. 2005b; recently reviewed by Arulkumaran et al. 2014). Therefore, $ScvO_2$ appears to be one of the best candidates to guide the goal-directed therapy in ICUs. Still, its intrinsic main limit is related to the requirement in invasive procedures, and currently it is not usable in most settings, such as in uncomplicated surgery.

Nevertheless, the value of $ScvO_2$ in monitoring goal-directed therapy in ICUs cannot overshadow other more "traditional" measures, such as blood pressure and heart rate monitoring, diuresis control, pulse oximetry, ECG, EEG, central venous pressure, serum lactate concentration, and other index obtained by hemo-gas analysis. However, it has to be considered that the rise in lactate is delayed in comparison to increased O_2ER (Donati et al. 2007). CO, assessed by thermodilution or by a less invasive ultrasound technique, is a central factor in evaluation of hemodynamics and therapy, since measures to support cardiac inotropy are critical for a favorable outcome.

In several studies performed in critical care settings such as fluid resuscitation and sepsis, focusing on the safety and effectiveness of goal-directed therapy, blood transfusion were administered according to an established protocol, usually Hb-based. It has been observed that monitoring and therapies based on global oxygenation indexes determine an improvement in clinical outcomes; we underline that this approach appears to entail an increase in blood transfusion rates (Rivers et al. 2001; Trzeciak et al. 2006). Thus, when transfusion therapy is guided by reliable indicators of tissue hypoxia, its beneficial effects appear to be maximized. On the other hand, in septic patients (Mazza et al. 2005; Fuller et al. 2012) as well as in unselected ICU population (Saugel et al. 2013), blood transfusion appears not to affect $ScvO_2$. What seems to emerge from these studies is that blood transfusion affects global indexes of hypoxia only in cases of severe dysfunction, while when RBC are administered on the base of Hb only, they may not exert any improvement and might be not beneficial at all.

Surprisingly enough, global oxygenation indexes have not been widely investigated as drivers for transfusion therapy; only a few published studies focus on transfusion "oxygenation" triggers. Targeting the potential utility of oxygen extraction ratio (O_2ER) as an adjunct to the hemoglobin (Hb) concentration for guiding RBC transfusion, it has been observed that, ultimately, ABT rate can be impressively affected, determining either a relevant reduction (by 40–43 %, according to Sehgal et al. 2001; Orlov et al. 2009) or an increase (de Oliveira et al. 2008) or no difference (Donati et al. 2007). An overlook at all the investigational work so far conducted on global oxygenation indexes as drivers for clinical decision about blood transfusion seems to suggest that the direction is correct, but the tools are limited, especially in the perspective of a wide clinical use. Limited results from controlled trials also suggest that application of more complex algorithms including multiple parameters, in the framework of specific clinical situations, may be more informative and useful for monitoring the balance between oxygen supply and tissue demand (Futier et al. 2010).

7.4 New Perspectives

More indicative and practical tools appear to be required to better address questions concerning tissue oxygenation and transfusion need. In this respect, we look with interest at the development of new, or renewed, technologies. Microdialysis, whose application has been widely studied in neurointensive care (Tisdall and Smith 2006), can produce information about multiple indicators, among which particularly valuable is the lactate/pyruvate ratio (L/P) as index of anaerobic metabolism (Waelgaard et al. 2012). It has been found related to the severity of illness in hemorrhagic shock (Ohashi et al. 2009) and sepsis (Dimopoulou et al. 2011) and as predictor of poor outcome (idem; Nikitas et al. 2013). Interestingly, L/P has been found to be significantly affected by blood transfusion (Kopterides et al. 2012) in critically ill patients.

Another interesting noninvasive technique is near-infrared spectroscopy (NIRS) that gives information about the saturation of Hb within the tissues (StO_2). Notwithstanding intrinsic limits, it has been suggested as a valuable mean for monitoring the situation of the microcirculation and the effects of therapies in some clinical settings, including non-cardiac surgery (Abdelmalak et al. 2013). In particular, NIRS utilization may result very informative for the evaluation of effects of RBC administration (Creteur et al. 2009; Dani et al. 2010; Yuruk et al. 2012).

Also, orthogonal polarization spectral (OPS) imaging is a noninvasive technique developed to investigate tissue microcirculation and is applied to sublingual district obtaining information about capillary density and blood flow. It has been shown that RBC transfusion has a variable effect in septic patients (Sakr et al. 2007), but in surgical patients, transfusion with fresh RBC causes an increase in the amount of perfused microvessels (Ayhan et al. 2013).

As a practical marker of anemia-induced tissue hypoxia, Hare et al. (2013) propose methemoglobin blood concentration, which may reflect activation of adaptive mechanisms which stimulate NO signaling. Nevertheless, at present, this hypothesis remains to be definitively proven.

In conclusion, in acute normovolemic anemic patients, currently available guidelines indicate RBC transfusion when Hb concentration drops under a determined threshold *or* in the presence of symptoms that reflect activation of compensatory mechanisms. This strong recommendation is consequent to analysis of results of RCTs that show inferiority, or not superiority, of a liberal transfusion strategy. In particular, in the postoperative management after hip surgery of high-risk patients (actually defined as having any of common cardiovascular risks factors in history), applying a protocol comparing restrictive versus liberal transfusion strategy has not modified the relevant rate of severe outcomes (an overall rate of 7.1 % of death was observed; Carson et al. 2011). Therefore, it appears that other strategies are to be explored in order to improve clinical outcomes in patients belonging to elderly and high-risk populations (i.e., most patients undergoing lower limb arthroplasty). Implementation of monitoring global indexes of tissue hypoxia, possibly by means of noninvasive techniques, should be considered as a future standard of care, even if cost-effectiveness evaluations are still lacking. Doing so, we will be able to restore oxygen delivery to hypoxic tissues, withiin a framework in which the management of every surgery patient, considering his/her centrality, is based on integration of knowledge, communication and formation skiils, also evaluations of organizational constrains. We define this process "Patient Tissue O_2 Supply Management."

Key Points

- Hb is chosen as transfusion trigger because so far experimental and clinical researches have not been able to address issues concerning a more "physiological" approach.
- Known and unknown comorbidities can be underestimated when considering a single indicator.
- Existing results from clinical research are dampened by intrinsic limitations.
- Strict implementation of recommendations concerning transfusion thresholds may be difficult to be applied in a clinical routine.
- A better blood product may feature a better benefit/cost ratio.
- New technologies, applied to noninvasive investigation of tissue oxygenation, may shortly be validated and constitute new standards for appropriateness of blood transfusion.

References

Abdelmalak BB, Cata JP, Bonilla A, You J, Kopyeva T, Vogel JD, Campbell S, Sessler DI (2013) Intraoperative tissue oxygenation and postoperative outcomes after major non-cardiac surgery: an observational study. Br J Anaesth 110(2):241–249

Arnold RC, Shapiro NI, Jones AE et al (2009) Multicenter study of early lactate clearance as a determinant of survival in patients with presumed sepsis. Shock 32(1):35

Arulkumaran N, Corredor C, Hamilton MA, Ball J, Grounds RM, Rhodes A, Cecconi M (2014) Cardiac complications associated with goal-directed therapy in high-risk surgical patients: a meta-analysis. Br J Anaesth 112(4):648–59

Axler O, Megarbane B, Lentschener C, Fernandez H (2003) Comparison of cardiac output measured with echocardiographic volumes and aortic Doppler methods during mechanical ventilation. Intensive Care Med 29:208

Ayhan B, Yuruk K, Koene S, Sahin A, Ince C, Aypar U (2013) The effects of non-leukoreduced red blood cell transfusions on microcirculation in mixed surgical patients. Transfus Apher Sci 49(2):212–222

Boyle MS, Bennett M, Keogh GW, O'Brien M, Flynn G, Collins DW, Bihari D (2014) Central venous oxygen saturation during high-risk general surgical procedures-relationship to complications and clinical outcomes. Anaesth Intensive Care 42(1):28–36

Blumberg N, Zhao H, Wang H, Messing S, Heal JM, Lyman GH (2007) The intention-to-treat principle in clinical trials and meta-analyses of leukoreduced blood transfusions in surgical patients. Transfusion 47(4):573–581

Brown JM (2002) Use of echocardiography for hemodynamic monitoring. Crit Care Med 30:1361

Carson JL, Noveck H, Berlin JA, Gould SA (2002) Mortality and morbidity in patients with very low postoperative Hb levels who decline blood transfusion. Transfusion 42(7):812–818

Carson JL, Terrin ML, Noveck H, Sanders DW, Chaitman BR, Rhoads GG, Nemo G, Dragert K, Beaupre L, Hildebrand K, Macaulay W, Lewis C, Cook DR, Dobbin G, Zakriya KJ, Apple FS, Horney RA, Magaziner J, FOCUS Investigators (2011) Liberal or restrictive transfusion in high-risk patients after hip surgery. N Engl J Med 365(26):2453–2462

Carson JL, Carless PA, Hebert PC (2012) Transfusion thresholds and other strategies for guiding allogeneic red blood cell transfusion. Cochrane Database Syst Rev (4):CD002042

Carson JL, Grossman JB, Kleinman S, Tinmouth AT, Marques MB, Fung MK, Holcomb JB, Illoh O, Kaplan LJ, Katz LM, Rao SV, Roback JD, Shander A, Tobian AAR, Weinstein R, Swinton McLaughlin LG, Djulbegovic B, for the Clinical Transfusion Medicine Committee of the AABB (2012b) Red blood cell transfusion: a clinical practice guideline from the AABB. Ann Intern Med 157:49

Casutt M, Seifert B, Pasch T, Schmid E, Turina M, Spahn DR (1999) Factors influencing the individual effects of blood transfusions on oxygen delivery and oxygen consumption. Crit Care Med 27(10):2194

Caveh M, Spahn DR (2007) Allogeneic red blood cell transfusion: physiology of oxygen transport. Best Pract Res Clin Anaesthesiol 21(2):163

Chawla LS, Zia H, Gutierrez G, Katz NM, Seneff MG, Shah M (2004) Lack of equivalence between central and mixed venous oxygen saturation. Chest 126(6):1891–1896

Creteur J, Neves AP, Vincent JL (2009) Near-infrared spectroscopy technique to evaluate the effects of red blood cell transfusion on tissue oxygenation. Crit Care 13(Suppl 5):S11

Dani C, Pratesi S, Fontanelli G, Barp J, Bertini G (2010) Blood transfusions increase cerebral, splanchnic, and renal oxygenation in anemic preterm infants. Transfusion 50(6):1220–1226

Dean JS, Douglas HR, Frederick BR, Pineo KL, Frederick G, Doig CJ, Laporta DP, Viner S, Passerini L, Devitt H, Kirby A, Jacka M (2003) A randomized, controlled trial of the use of pulmonary-artery catheters in high-risk surgical patients. N Engl J Med 348(1):5

de Oliveira CF, de Oliveira DS, Gottschald AF, Moura JD, Costa GA, Ventura AC, Fernandes JC, Vaz FA, Carcillo JA, Rivers EP, Troster EJ (2008) ACCM/PALS haemodynamic support guidelines for paediatric septic shock: an outcomes comparison with and without monitoring central venous oxygen saturation. Intensive Care Med 34(6):1065–75

Devereaux PJ, Xavier D, Pogue J, Guyatt G, Sigamani A, Garutti I, Leslie K, Rao-Melacini P, Chrolavicius S, Yang H, Macdonald C, Avezum A, Lanthier L, Hu W, Yusuf S, POISE (PeriOperative ISchemic Evaluation) Investigators (2011) Characteristics and short-term prognosis of perioperative myocardial infarction in patients undergoing noncardiac surgery: a cohort study. Ann Intern Med 154(8):523–528

Dimopoulou I, Nikitas N, Orfanos SE, Theodorakopoulou M, Vassiliadi D, Ilias I, Ikonomidis I, Boutati E, Maratou E, Tsangaris I, Karkouli G, Tsafou E, Diamantakis A, Kopterides P, Maniatis N, Kotanidou A, Armaganidis A, Ungerstedt U (2011) Kinetics of adipose tissue microdialysis-derived metabolites in critically ill septic patients: associations with sepsis severity and clinical outcome. Shock 35(4):343–8

Donati A, Loggi S, Preiser JC, Orsetti G, Münch C, Gabbanelli V, Pelaia P, Pietropaoli P (2007) Goal-directed intraoperative therapy reduces morbidity and length of hospital stay in high-risk surgical patients. Chest 132(6):1817–1824

Dueck MH, Klimek M, Appenrodt S, Weigand C, Boerner U (2005) Trends but not individual values of central venous oxygen saturation agree with mixed venous oxygen saturation during varying hemodynamic conditions. Anesthesiology 103:249–257

Foss NB, Kristensen MT, Jensen PS, Palm H, Krasheninnikoff M, Kehlet H (2009) The effects of liberal versus restrictive transfusion thresholds on ambulation after hip fracture surgery. Transfusion 49(2):227–234

Frykholm P, Andersson JL, Valtysson J, Silander HC, Hillered L, Persson L, Olsson Y, Yu WR, Westerberg G, Watanabe Y et al (2000) A metabolic threshold of irreversible ischemia demonstrated by pet in a middle cerebral artery occlusion-reperfusion primate mode. Acta Neurol Scand 102:18

Fuller BM, Gajera M, Schorr C, Gerber D, Dellinger RP, Parrillo J, Zanotti S (2012) Transfusion of packed red blood cells is not associated with improved central venous oxygen saturation or organ function in patients with septic shock. J Emerg Med. 2012 43(4):593–8

Futier E, Robin E, Jabaudon M, Guerin R, Petit A, Bazin JE, Constantin JM, Vallet B (2010) Central venous O_2 saturation and venous-to-arterial CO_2 difference as complementary tools for goal-directed therapy during high-risk surgery. Crit Care 14(5):R193. Epub 2010 Oct 29

Hampton DA, Schreiber MA (2013) Near infrared spectroscopy: clinical and research uses. Transfusion 53(Suppl 1):52S–58S

Hare MTG, Tsui AKY, Ozawa S, Shander A (2013) Anaemia: can we define haemoglobin thresholds for impaired oxygen homeostasis and suggest new strategies for treatment? Best Pract Res Clin Anaesthesiol 27:85

Harvey S, Harrison DA, Singer M, Ashcroft J, Jones CM, Elbourne D, Brampton W, Williams D, Young D, Rowan K (2005) Assessment of the clinical effectiveness of pulmonary artery catheters in management of patients in intensive care (PAC-MAN): a randomised controlled trial. Lancet 366:472

Hébert PC, Wells G, Blajchman MA, Marshall J, Martin C, Pagliarello G, Tweeddale M, Schweitzer I, Yetisir E (1999) A multicenter, randomized, controlled clinical trial of transfusion requirements in critical care. Transfusion Requirements in Critical Care Investigators, Canadian Critical Care Trials Group. N Engl J Med 340(6):409–417. Erratum in: N Engl J Med 1999;340(13):1056

Hebert PC, McDonald BJ, Tinmouth A (2004a) Clinical consequences of anemia and red cell transfusion in the critically ill. Crit Care Clin 20:225

Hebert PC, Van der Linden P, Biro G et al (2004b) Physiologic aspects of anemia. Crit Care Clin 20:187

Isbister JP, Shander A, Spahn DR, Erhard J, Farmer SL, Hofmann A (2011) Adverse blood transfusion outcomes: establishing causation. Transfus Med Rev 25(2):89–101

Ince C, Sinaasappel M (1999) Microcirculatory oxygenation and shunting in sepsis and shock. Crit Care Med 27:1369

Jones AE, Shapiro NI, Trzeciak S, Arnold RC, Claremont HA, Kline JA (2010) Lactate clearance vs central venous oxygen saturation as goals of early sepsis therapy. JAMA 303(8):739

Kopterides P, Bonovas S, Mavrou I, Kostadima E, Zakynthinos E, Armaganidis A (2009) Venous oxygen saturation and lactate gradient from superior vena cava to pulmonary artery in patients with septic shock. Shock 31:561

Kopterides P, Theodorakopoulou M, Nikitas N, Ilias I, Vassiliadi DA, Orfanos SE, Tsangaris I, Maniatis NA, Tsantes AE, Travlou A, Dimitriadis G, Armaganidis A, Ungerstedt U, Dimopoulou I (2012) Red blood cell transfusion affects microdialysis-assessed interstitial lactate/pyruvate ratio in critically ill patients with late sepsis. Intensive Care Med 38(11):1843–50

Kuo JA, Maher KO, Kirshbom PM, Mahle WT (2011) Red blood cell transfusion for infants with single-ventricle physiology. Pediatr Cardiol 32(4):461–468

Leal-Noval SR, Muñoz-Gómez M, Arellano-Orden V, Marín-Caballos A, Amaya-Villar R, Marín A, Puppo-Moreno A, Ferrándiz-Millón C, Flores-Cordero JM, Murillo-Cabezas F (2008) Impact of age of transfused blood on cerebral oxygenation in male patients with severe traumatic brain injury. Crit Care Med 36(4):1290–1296

Lelubre C, Vincent JL (2013) Relationship between red cell storage duration and outcomes in adults receiving red cell transfusions: a systematic review. Crit Care 17(2):R66

Leung JM, Weiskopf RB, Feiner J, Hopf HW, Kelley S, Viele M, Lieberman J, Watson J, Noorani M, Pastor D, Yeap H, Ho R, Toy P (2000) Electrocardiographic ST-segment changes during acute, severe isovolemic hemodilution in humans. Anesthesiology 93(4):1004–1010

Lie SA, Engesaeter LB, Havelin LI, Furnes O, Vollset SE (2002) Early postoperative mortality after 67,548 total hip replacements: causes of death and thromboprophylaxis in 68 hospitals in Norway from 1987 to 1999. Acta Orthop Scand 73(4):392–399

Lienhart A, Auroy Y, Péquignot F, Benhamou D, Warszawski J, Bovet M, Jougla E (2006) Survey of anesthesia-related mortality in France. Anesthesiology 105(6):1087–1097

Madjdpour C, Spahn DR, Weiskopf RB (2006) Anemia and perioperative red blood cell transfusion: a matter of tolerance. Crit Care Med 34(5 Suppl):S102–S108

Mantilla CB, Horlocker TT, Schroeder DR, Berry DJ, Brown DL (2002) Frequency of myocardial infarction, pulmonary embolism, deep venous thrombosis, and death following primary hip or knee arthroplasty. Anesthesiology 96(5):1140–1146. Erratum in: Anesthesiology 2002;97(2):531

Mazza BF, Machado FR, Mazza DD, Hassmann V (2005) Evaluation of blood transfusion effects on mixed venous oxygen saturation and lactate levels in patients with SIRS/sepsis. Clinics (Sao Paulo) 60(4):311–316. Epub 2005 Aug 29

Nguyen HB, Rivers EP, Knoblich BP et al (2004) Early lactate clearance is associated with improved outcome in severe sepsis and septic shock. Crit Care Med 32(8):1637

Nikitas N, Kopterides P, Ilias I, Theodorakopoulou M, Vassiliadi DA, Armaganidis A, Dimopoulou I (2013) Elevated adipose tissue lactate to pyruvate (L/P) ratio predicts poor outcome in critically ill patients with septic shock: a microdialysis study. Minerva Anestesiol 79(11):1229–37

Ohashi H, Kawasaki N, Fujitani S, Kobayashi K, Ohashi M, Hosoyama A, Wada T, Taira Y (2009) Utility of microdialysis to detect the lactate/pyruvate ratio in subcutaneous tissue for the reliable monitoring of hemorrhagic shock. J Smooth Muscle Res 45(6):269–78

Orlov D, O'Farrell R, McCluskey SA, Carroll J, Poonawala H, Hozhabri S, Karkouti K (2009) The clinical utility of an index of global oxygenation for guiding red blood cell transfusion in cardiac surgery. Transfusion 49:682

Pearse R, Dawson D, Fawcett J, Rhodes A, Grounds RM, Bennett ED (2005a) Early goal-directed therapy after major surgery reduces complications and duration of hospital stay. A randomised controlled trial. Crit Care 9:R687

Pearse R, Dawson D, Fawcett J, Rhodes A, Grounds RM, Bennett ED (2005b) Changes in central venous satura-

The postero-lateral approach was used on all patients undergoing THA. All patients undergoing TKA received a standard paramedical approach: a tourniquet was routinely used. Patients were assessed daily for any signs of DVT. All patients were given prophylaxis for DVT for 35 days postoperatively: a daily single dose of LMWH medication (Nadroparin, 0.4 mL) was given to 32 % of the patients, while a daily single dose of Fondaparinux was given to 78 % of the patients. Two hundred and thirty-four patients (9 %) were preoperatively taking warfarin because of a collateral pathology, so warfarin was suspended for 5 days preoperatively and replaced by a personalized dose of LMWH ("bridging anticoagulation") (Lohr et al. 1995). Warfarin was resumed in the early postoperative period (48–72 h).

Nadroparin is a porcine-derived LMWH which accelerates the inactivation of factor II and factor Xa when bound to antithrombin III (ATIII). Nadroparin halts the coagulation pathway by inhibiting the activation of thrombin (factor IIa) by factor Xa. The amplification of the fibrin clotting cascade is stopped once factors Xa and IIa are inactivated.

Fondaparinux (Arixtra) is a synthetic pentasaccharide anticoagulant. Apart from the O-methyl group at the reducing end of the molecule, the identity and sequence of the five monomeric sugar units contained in Fondaparinux are identical to a sequence of five monomeric sugar units which can be isolated after either chemical or enzymatic cleavage of the polymeric glycosaminoglycan heparin and heparan sulfate (HS). This monomeric sequence in heparin and HS is thought to form the high-affinity binding site for the natural anticoagulant factor, antithrombin III (ATIII). Binding of heparin/HS to ATIII has been shown to increase the anticoagulant activity of antithrombin III 1,000-fold. Fondaparinux potentiates the neutralizing action of ATIII on activated Factor ×300-fold.

All patients used an intermittent pneumatic boot compression device in the first 24 h postoperatively, while being monitored in a sub-intensive care unit and then during the hospital stay in all non-deambulatory situations. As in the preoperative period, assessment for postoperative DVT was carried out by color Doppler ultrasonography on postoperative day 4. The same angiologist, experienced in color Doppler ultrasonography, repeated the study in all cases. All patients wore below-the-knee elastic compression stockings for 35 days postoperatively. Statistical analysis was performed using Student's *t*-test.

8.1.1.2 Results

Preoperative Period

The preoperative ultrasound screening highlighted the presence of DVTs in 120 patients (4.5 %). Those patients were withdrawn from the operative schedule and began DVT treatment with personalized doses of LMWH. They then underwent TJA once the preoperative color Doppler ultrasonography revealed the absence of DVT (between 3 and 6 months).

Postoperative Period

The incidence (Table 8.1) of proximal or distal DVT in patients following TKA was found to be 4.8 % (26 patients). The incidence of proximal or distal DVT in patients following THA was found to be 3.2 % (69 patients). THA procedures showed more distal DVT (62 patients, 2.9 %) than proximal DVT (7 patients, 0.3 %). TKA procedures showed more distal DVT (21 patients, 3.9 %) than proximal DVT (5 patients, 0.9 %). No patients developed DVT in the contralateral limb.

Table 8.1 Incidence and location of ultrasonographically confirmed postoperative deep vein thrombosis (DVT)

Arthroplasty type	No. patients	Proximal DVT	Distal DVT	Total DVT
TKA	540	5 (0.9 %)	21 (3.9 %)	26 (4.8 %)
THA	2,138	7 (0.3 %)	62 (2.9 %)	69 (3.2 %)
Total	2,678			

TKA total knee arthroplasty, *THA* total hip arthroplasty

The difference of overall DVT between the groups was not statistically significant ($p=0.35$). The difference of isolated distal DVT between the groups also was not statistically significant ($p=0.71$). All DVTs were asymptomatic clinically.

All patients began DVT treatment with personalized doses of LMWH or Fondaparinux, according to the American College of Chest Physicians (ACCP) Evidence-Based Clinical Practice Guidelines (Gordon et al. 2012). None of the patients had a PE in the postoperative period. Patients with acute DVT did not receive a period of bed rest but walked as soon as possible to reduce the risk of post-thrombotic syndrome. All DVT patients wore below-the-knee elastic compression stockings until DVT resolution, as shown by final color Doppler ultrasound. All DVT patients had color Doppler ultrasonography for DVT evolution assessment on postoperative days 30, 60, 90, and 120 if needed.

8.1.1.3 Discussion

The presence of DVT in the lower extremities following TJA is considered a potentially life-threatening situation (Lotke et al. 1994). Prevention of DVT using duplex ultrasonography to avoid the complication of pulmonary embolism has shown its efficacy (Grady-Benson et al. 1994). The fundamental aid from preoperative color Doppler evaluation is to identify the location of a silent DVT. In fact, proximal DVTs are well known to be closely associated with increased risk of pulmonary embolism and are conventionally treated more aggressively with closer monitoring.

On the other hand, the role of distal DVT is less obvious. It was once thought to be quite benign (Doouss 1976), but it has also been reported to be associated with pulmonary embolism, especially when there is propagation of a distal DVT to a more proximal location (Masuda et al. 1998). Recently, Grady-Benson et al. (1994) used serial venous Doppler flow measurements to document a propagation rate of 24 % in the calf. DVT formation during TJA could be related to the flexion position of the lower limb during the procedure, or to the use of a tourniquet on the thigh causing stasis or surgical trauma to the surrounding vasculature during the release.

Unfortunately, Duplex ultrasonography as a non-invasive screening tool has not yet received universal acceptance (Davidson et al. 1992), despite promising reports (Ko et al. 2003). This study shows that preoperative Doppler ultrasonography prevents any false positive cases and forewarns the surgeon of an increased risk of DVT and need for prophylaxis. The preoperative ultrasound screening demonstrated a DVT in 4.5 % of our patients: without screening they were at risk of developing a perioperative pulmonary embolism. Therefore, in our hands, it is beneficial to carry out preoperative Doppler ultrasonography to detect any pre-existing DVT, especially in patients who are considered at high risk as shown in Table 8.2. In fact, preoperative and postoperative clinical findings alone are generally considered poor predictors of the presence of DVT (Lieberman and Pellegrini 1999). Once a DVT episode has been detected, surveillance with duplex scanning is also mandatory in determining efficacy and duration of therapeutic anticoagulation for DVT (Grady-Benson et al. 1994).

Table 8.2 High risks factors for deep vein thrombosis (DVT)

Old age
BMI >30
History of venous thromboembolism
Revision joint surgery
Congestive heart failure
Chronic rheumatic heart disease
Steroid/hormonal therapy
Anticoagulant therapy
Varicose veins
Prolonged immobilization
Malignancy
Factor V Leiden

Our study intentionally does not address the issues of the indication and timing of initiating anticoagulation therapy for patients undergoing TJA. Although the value of routine pharmacologic thromboprophylaxis in TJA has been questioned by a metanalysis (Murray et al. 1996), the majority of surgeons would still recommend some form of prophylaxis against DVT (Brookenthal et al. 2001) in consideration of the morbidity and mortality associated with postoperative DVT in THA and TKA. The authors of the current study recognize that venous thromboembolic events following primary hip and knee arthroplasty have decreased significantly over the past two decades, mainly because of new multidisciplinary approaches. Rapid postoperative mobilization, optimization of surgical techniques, and improved perioperative pain management (which includes the use of regional anesthesia) have all contributed to decreasing the DVT risk. At the author's institution we use pharmacologic and mechanical approaches for thromboprophylaxis after TJA as suggested by the 2012 American College of Chest Physicians (ACCP) Evidence-Based Clinical Practice Guidelines (Gordon et al. 2012) and the 2009 Tuscany Region Protocol for Thromboprophylaxis in Orthopaedic Surgery (www.regione.toscana.it). All patients undergoing a TJA procedure receive a form of pharmacologic thromboprophylaxis (LMWH or Fondaparinux) for 35 days postoperatively, use an intermittent pneumatic compression device during the hospital stay, and wear below-the-knee elastic compression stockings for 35 days postoperatively. The main difference from 2012 ACCP guidelines is that all our patients underwent Doppler ultrasonography screening preoperatively and postoperatively before hospital discharge. Doppler ultrasonography is historically a non-invasive procedure and provides good sensitivity (89 %) and specificity (100 %) for detecting DVT (Cronan et al. 1987). There is a lack of published data on the appropriateness of preoperative Doppler ultrasonography in patients undergoing TJA: Sisodia et al. (2013) recently reported 22.4 % preoperative asymptomatic DVTs in a group of patients awaiting TJA.

The current study supports the benefit of Doppler ultrasonography as a preoperative and postoperative investigation method in patients undergoing TJA.

8.2 Arguments Against Pre- and Postoperative US Screening for All TJA Patients

Marco Scardino, Federica Martorelli, and Antonino Gurgone

8.2.1 Introduction

Deep venous thrombosis (DVT), with thromboembolic complications which may lead to pulmonary embolism, is a serious disease and potentially fatal. This often complicates the clinical course of patients suffering with another disease, already hospitalized or no, but it also affects individuals in apparently good health.

The most important clinical objectives of an early and correct diagnosis and treatment are:

1. Reduce the morbidity and mortality associated with its acute manifestations
2. Reduce the incidence of recurrence of further acute events
3. Counteract the incidence of long term sequelae represented by the post-thrombotic (or post-phlebitic) syndrome

Venous thrombosis in the majority of cases involves the veins of the legs and, depending on the locations, is deep venous thrombosis if it involve the venous system subfascial and a superficial venous thrombosis if it involves overfascial veins (Fig. 8.1).

The incidence of pulmonary thromboembolism increases with age, aggressiveness of surgical procedures, and the length of hospital stay,

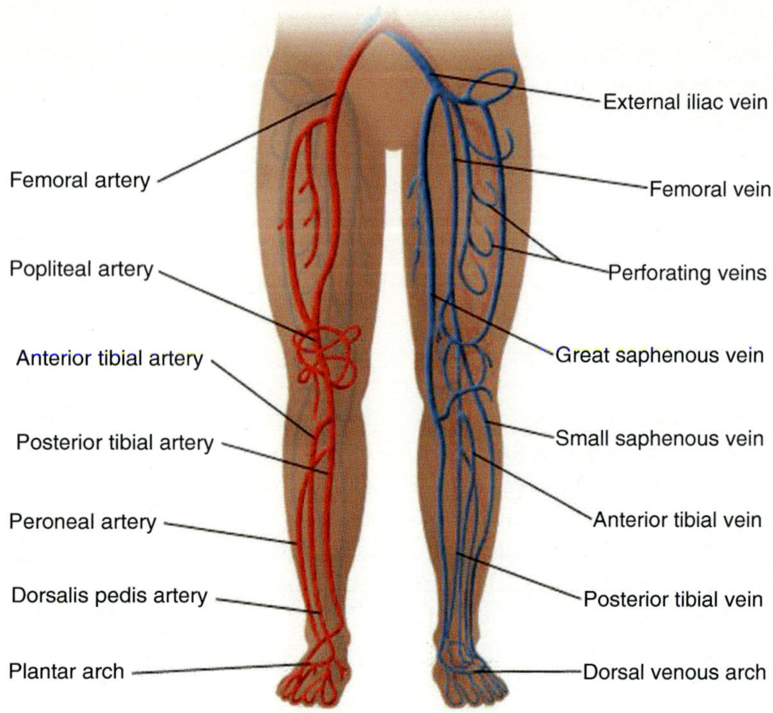

Fig. 8.1 Arterial and venous circulation of the legs (Courtesy of Bayer Pharma AG)

and is highest in patients treated in intensive care because of the overlap of these risk factors and prolonged immobility.

It is estimated that only in approximately 30 % of ambulatory patients in whom a clinical suspicion of DVT has been made is actually confirmed by objective investigations.

In the absence of prophylaxis, the incidence of DVT in the hospital population varies between 10 % in medical patients and 40–60 % in patients undergoing orthopedic major surgery (Turpie et al. 2002; Geerts et al. 2008; Cohen et al. 2007; Heit et al. 2005; Blann and Lip 2006).

8.2.2 Diagnosis

The clinical manifestations of DVT of the lower limbs are multiple (spontaneous pain, flushing, cyanosis, increased skin temperature, cramps, increase in the size of the limb, edema, development of collateral circulation, phlegmasia alba dolens, etc.). However, the clinical diagnosis of DVT is not accurate because it is based on symptoms and signs that, taken separately or together, are neither sensitive nor specific. Lack of a pathognomonic element requires that the diagnosis should be definitively confirmed by instrumental examination.

There are many factors associated with DVT, predisposing or precipitating, which influence the onset, evolution, and response to treatment. The main factors are history of previous episodes of DVT or pulmonary embolism, recent surgery, immobilization, age, concomitant neoplastic disease, heart failure, trauma with tissue disruption and/or fractures, estrogen hormone therapy, pregnancy, obesity, or thrombophilia genetically determined acquired. They form the basis for the distinction between idiopathic (absence of factors) and secondary (presence of one or more factors) DVT, which has implications as regards the choice of duration of treatment. The existence of predisposing conditions or triggers should be considered in each individual patient, because they contribute in varying degrees to define the risk profile. It is important to evaluate preoperatively whether the subject belongs to a category of high or low risk because this affects the predictive value of the assessment instrument which has been used to make the final diagnosis.

Determining the risk level is critical to the decision-making process regarding the diagnostic process to be reserved for an individual patient.

Different systems have been proposed in order to quantify the clinical probability of DVT in individual patients (Wells et al. 1997). Wells et al. developed a scoring system, which identifies three categories of clinical risk for DVT: high, medium, and low. This system combines medical records (neoplastic disease, limb immobilization, lower limb entrapment) and physical examination of the patient (pain, swelling, venous varicosities). This score has been validated in a cross-sectional study based on systematic comparison with venography as the standard diagnostic reference, and in a longitudinal study based on the occurrence of clinical events. In this way it has been demonstrated that it can minimize the use of invasive techniques (venography) or non-invasive (ultrasonography) without increasing the risk associated with false-negative diagnosis.

Risk stratification is an effective way to ensure a universally applied prophylactic.

The risk is generally based on a specific group of patients:

- Low risk: mobilized in minor surgery, medical patients who are totally mobilized, <10 % risk of developing DVT without prophylaxis
- Moderate risk: general surgery increased, urological and gynecological patients, medical patients who are not fully mobilized; 10–40 % risk of developing DVT without prophylaxis
- High risk: hip and knee arthroplasty, major trauma, 40–80 % risk of developing DVT without prophylaxis (Table 8.3).

Table 8.3 Wells score for prediction of DVT

Parameter	Score
Active cancer (treatment ongoing or within previous 6 months or palliative)	1
Paralysis, paresis, or recent plaster immobilization of lower extremities	1
Recently bedridden for more than 3 days or major surgery within 4 weeks	1
Localized tenderness along distribution of the deep vein system	1
Entire leg swollen	1
Calf swelling by more than 3 cm when compared with asymptomatic leg	1
Pitting edema	1
Collateral superficial veins	1
Alternative diagnosis as likely or greater than that of DVT	2

DVT, deep vein thrombosis.

Reproduced with permission from Wells et al. (1997)
A high score is 3 or more, a moderate score 1–2 and a low score 0

Ultrasonography (ultrasound B-mod, duplex scanning, and Doppler ultrasound) is a non-invasive method of choice for the diagnosis of proximal DVT of the lower limbs (by definition, thrombosis extended from the popliteal vein to the iliac- femoral segments). It has high diagnostic accuracy, convenience and ease of use, affordability, safety, and can be repeated without restrictions.

Allows the visualization of the venous system (venous wall and valvular) and the representation of the real-time flow in various ways (track spectral analysis, color Doppler, power Doppler) in static conditions or during dynamic maneuvers. The detailed US examination is performed with the patient in the supine position for the investigation of the proximal segment, in the prone position for the stretched hamstrings, and finally standing or sitting on the edge of the bed for the examination of distal deep veins (the distention of the veins promotes the display of anatomical details). You can browse directly and comprehensively the common femoral vein, deep femoral artery to the confluence with the municipality, the superficial femoral artery, the popliteal artery, the

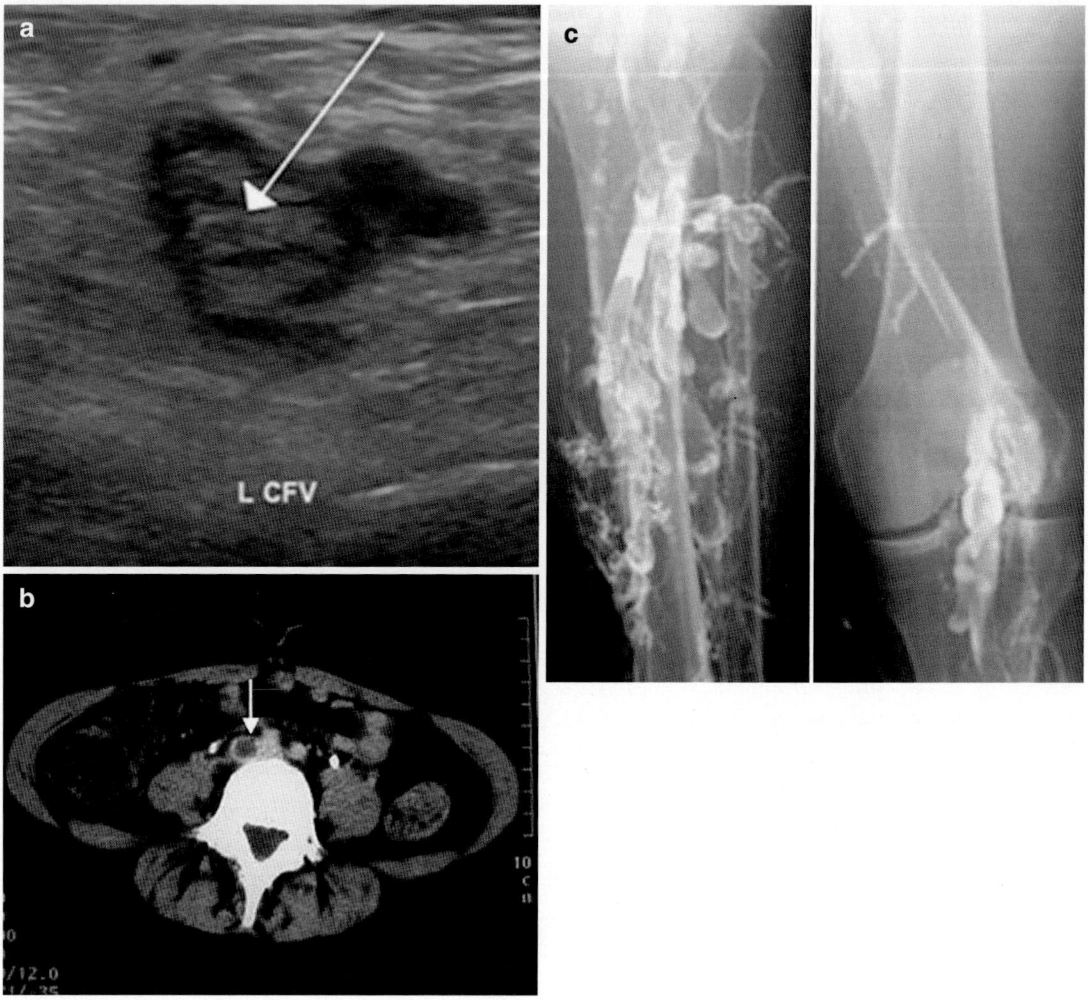

Fig. 8.2 Venous thrombosis as detected by ultrasound (**a**), CT-scan (**b**), and venogram (**c**)

underpopliteal, the confluence with the popliteal, and finally those in the calf. The exploration of the veins sottopoplitee calf is wasteful in terms of time, requiring a special skill of the examiner and the use of suitable up-to-date equipment. The Doppler component is essential for the study of valvular function and reflux syndrome (post-thrombotic).

The main diagnostic criterion for the presence or absence of DVT is the test of compression (compression ultrasonography = CUS), executed by applying light pressure with the probe on the venous tract examined, allowing you to determine whether the walls of the vein are collapsible: a completely compressible vein certainly does not contain thrombi (Fig. 8.2a–c).

It should be noted, however, and taking into account that for various reasons some sections are difficult compressible venous (superficial femoral artery in Hunter's canal, deep femoral, iliac vein, inferior vena cava), which may occur because of their anatomical location, their depth, sovrapposizione of structures osteotendinee, or finally to the presence of sclerotico tissue surrounding. The compression test is evaluated better in transverse scans and reaches high values of sensitivity and specificity with regard to the diagnosis of thrombosis in the proximal level. The diagnostic reliability is reduced distally, where it has a sensitivity of 33 %, a specificity of 91 %, and a positive predictive value of 58 %. The introduction of the color Doppler has undoubtedly increased the possibility of recognizing and properly reviewing the venous structures at the distal end. It should be stressed that, especially for the examination of the distal veins, the training and skills of the operator, as well as the use of suitable and latest equipment are key determinants of the quality of the survey results. US. Criteri additional diagnostic are the 'absence of the Doppler signal spontaneous and/ or induced and direct visualization of the thrombus. Complementary reliefs are obtained by evaluating the degree of echogenicity of the thrombus, its adhesion to the vessel wall (particularly the presence of a proximal end float), and its organization. The usefulness of ultrasonics in asymptomatic patients is good but in high risk patients (i.e., orthopedic patients in the postoperative phase) its use is very limited for a number of reasons. In these patients distal thrombosis predominates, and the method showed low sensitivity (47–59 %). The possibility that thrombi initially confined in the veins sottopoplitee may extend to the popliteal vein and thigh (in other words, a distal thrombosis becomes proximal) occurs in 13.3 % of cases. This makes it extremely important to repeat the US examination.

The D-dimers are fibrin degradation products; in normal subjects the half-life is approximately 48 h. Elevated plasma levels of D-dimers, in addition to the presence of thrombi (both venous and arterial) can frequently be caused by many other conditions in which there is formation of fibrin in the vascular spaces or resorption of degradation products from the extravascular spaces (subcutaneous haematomas, surgical wounds, skin necrosis, extensive burns, ascites, pleural effusions). An increase in the D-dimer is found frequently in a wide variety of clinical situations (CID, neoplasms, unstable angina, myocardial infarction, eclampsia, infections, liver and kidney diseases, surgery). The dosage of D-dimers therefore proved extremely sensitive (i.e., positive in many circumstances), but poorly specific for the presence of thrombi, and is used for the high negative predictive value.

The dosage of D-dimers in the diagnosis of DVT showed the highest diagnostic yield when facing symptomatic subjects (with high probability of DVT), but with negative CUS investigation. In these cases, a normal dosage of D-dimers may allow you to exclude the presence of DVT.

A high level allows a selection of the cases to be followed over time with sequential instrumental examinations, hoping to promptly the possible proximal extension of the disease recognize.

The finding of normal levels of D-dimers, even in the presence of a thrombotic process, is a phenomenon which, as already mentioned, can occur in a limited number of cases. This may be for several reasons: (1) ipofibrinolisis, (2) clinical symptoms appeared for more than 7–10 days, (3) use of insensitive methods, and (4) incorrect definition of the cut-off level (limit of abnormality). It is currently not recommended to use this test in asymptomatic patients at high risk, or in symptomatic patients hospitalized, since no validated cut-off values exist for these specific situations.

In a study of 59 patients undergoing knee replacement surgery, it is seen that the preoperative dosage of D-dimer is of no use in predicting the development of a DVT in those undergoing this surgery. In fact, at a cut-off of 500 ng/mL sensitivity, specificity and positive predictive value and negative concentration of preoperative D-dimer for the development of a subsequent DVT were, respectively, 58, 46, 55, and 50 %. There remains a high risk index as confirmed by a recent study of Shiojama et al. where a cut-off at 0.85 μg/mL preoperatively led to 42 % of patients diagnosed with a DVT.

Phlebography has, for many years, been the only reliable method for the identification of a venous thrombosis, and is still considered the reference standard (gold standard) for the diagnosis of DVT. However, given the different aspects of the method, such as invasiveness, possible unwanted side effects, lack of repeatability, and advances in US treatment, today venography is the second choice for examining symptomatic patients, while remaining first choice in the postoperative screening in asymptomatic patients.

The CT scan is widely used in the diagnosis of proximal DVT (pelvic, iliac) and in producing pictures of pulmonary embolism, with MRI indications superimposed on a CT scan giving specific sensitivity to the pelvic region (Andrews and Fleischer 2005; Zhu et al. 2010; Giannini et al. 2008; Patel et al. 2013; Dermody et al. 2011; Wells et al. 1997; Shimoyama et al. 2012; Chotanaphuthi et al. 2009; Stern et al. 2002; Saad and Saad 2007).

8.2.3 Discussion

The diagnosis of DVT is not always easy to make and can be complex and expensive. As we have seen, several authors have tried to create an algorithm for the diagnoses of DVT to try to prevent the complications that can be fatal, as in the case of massive pulmonary embolism.

However, some of our patients have undergone examination by Doppler ecocolor, which, although expensive, is non-invasive, although sometimes generating false negatives. We believe, according to the literature, that pre and postoperative ultrasound DVT screening should only be performed in patients classified at high risk for DVT. In the paper by Goodacre et al. (2006a), the authors not only estimate the diagnostic accuracy, clinical effectiveness and cost-effectiveness of each method, but also identify practical diagnostic algorithms for DVT.

Here is the conclusion of this work which took 4 years of data analysis in British hospitals.

"Diagnostic algorithms based on a combination of Wells score, D-dimer and ultrasound (with repeat if negative) are feasible at most UK hospitals and are among the most cost-effective. Use of repeat scanning depends on the level of willingness to pay for health improvement. Further diagnostic testing for patients with a low Wells score and negative D-dimer is unlikely to represent a cost-effective use of resources. Recommendations for research include the evaluation of the costs and outcomes of using the optimal diagnostic algorithms in routine practice, the development and evaluation of algorithms appropriate for specific groups of patients with suspected DVT, such as intravenous drug abusers, pregnant patients and those with previous DVT, the evaluation of the role of plethysmography, interaction with other diagnostic tests, outcome of low-risk patients with negative plethysmography and measurement of the costs of providing plethysmography, and methodological research into the incorporation of meta-analytic data into decision-analytic modelling."

Confirmation of the utility and rationalization of expenses using ultrasound in "How should we diagnose suspected deep-vein thrombosis?" (Goodacre et al. 2006b) identifies the most cost-effective strategy for the UK National Health Service with a systematic review, meta-analysis and cost-effectiveness analysis.

"At the thresholds for willingness to pay recommended by the National Institute for Clinical Excellence (£20,000–£ 30,000 per QALY), the optimal strategy was to discharge patients with a low or intermediate Wells score and negative D-dimer, limiting ultrasound to those with a high score or positive D-dimer. Strategies using radiological testing for all patients were only cost-effective at £40,000 per QALY or more." I think it useful to indicate, in consideration of the collected cases, our experience with the analysis of historical data. Our register is held for all of the work done by the team of Prof. Guido Grappiolo from 2008 to October 2013. The data collected refer a total of 5,430 pcs operated for replacement of hip and knee, but for only 4,120 pcs do we have a full record (Table 8.4). All these patients were operated on for elective orthopedic surgery with prosthetic ASA between one and three.

Table 8.4 Data collected from the author's own register and referring to patients operated for hip and knee replacements

Total	5,430
Male	2,520
Female	2,910
Primary cementless THA	2,515
Primary cemented THA	*80*
Revision THA	462
Revision THA- only the cup	378
Primary cemented TKA	700
Revision TKA	65

Age: 59 ± 15, BMI: 22 ± 3

The venous Doppler tests were performed on the basis of clinical risk stratification according to the method of Wells and based on the preoperative clinical data. During this time the Doppler tests performed preoperatively were 229; of these, 42 patients underwent preoperative safenectomy.

Six patients underwent Doppler saphenectomy performed as post-operative control. Another eight Doppler examinations were performed post-operatively where preoperative screening had not been done. For a total of 14 Doppler tests performed post operatively there was a diagnosis of SDVT in 2 cases and a single TAC examination was performed to rule out pulmonary embolism, with negative results.

None of the patients operated in our institution has developed a TVP post-thrombotic syndrome complicated by thrombosis or pulmonary problems.

All patients were subjected to early mobilization and pharmacological prophylaxis for prevention of TVP. The choice of drugs used were: Arixtra 5 g until January 2011, in February 2011 as drugs for the prophylaxis NAO, specifically Xarelto 10 mg in 1980 and pradaxa 110 mg pcs 790 pcs. One hundred and twenty patients have used nardroprarine 6000 UI, 200 Clexane 4000 U.I.

Analysis of the data shows that the choice of reserving the echo Doppler examination only for patients at high risk means we can limit the use of this type of screening without compromising patient safety when they undergo orthopedic prosthetic surgery. Our experience, which is confirmed by the literature, has been shown that ultrasound DVT screening for patients undergoing hip and knee arthroplasty procedure is a useful and cost/effective procedure only if combined with a clinical suspicion.

A separate chapter deals with the case of patients who have already developed a DVT in the past.

In addition to the high risk of PE and long-term complications, DVT is associated with an estimated risk of VTE (venous thromboembolism) recurrence of approximately 21 % within 5 years of the initial event. The risk of VTE recurrence appears greater if the initial event was unprovoked, or associated with persistent risk factors such as cancer rather than a transient risk factor like surgery (Hansson et al. 2000; Prandoni et al. 2007; Eichinger et al. 2010; Zhu et al. 2009).

Three important risk factors were identified and quantified in the Vienna Prediction Model (Prandoni et al. 2007):

- Initial proximal (rather than distal) DVT
- Male gender
- Elevated D-dimer concentration

Short-term (rather than long-term) duration of anticoagulation therapy is also associated with recurrence (Eichinger et al. 2010).

Patients with a previous history of VTE, malignancy or hematological abnormality which predisposes them to thrombus formation are also at high risk of recurrent VTE. Homozygous Factor V Leiden or heterozygous Factor V Leiden and the prothrombin G20210A mutation are examples of the types of hematological abnormalities which confer a heightened risk of VTE recurrence (Zhu et al. 2009).

Measurement of specific proteins involved in coagulation can help guide clinical decision-making, although this type of laboratory assessment is rarely done in clinical practice. For example, a high level of coagulation Factors VIII, IX, and XI signals an increased risk of VTE recurrence (Kyrle and Eichinger 2005).

In addition, a D-dimer concentration above 250 ng/mL measured 3 weeks after discontinuation of anticoagulation is associated with a 3.1-fold increased risk of VTE recurrence at 2 years (Eichinger et al. 2003).

Elevated P-selectin levels are also associated with VTE recurrence within the first year after an initial event (Vormittag et al. 2007). A high plasma level of soluble P-selectin (sP-selectin) is modulated by variations of the P-selectin gene and is a predictive biomarker for VTE recurrence in patients with a first episode of unprovoked VTE. However, the clinical applicability of P-selectin needs further investigation (Pabinger and Ay 2009).

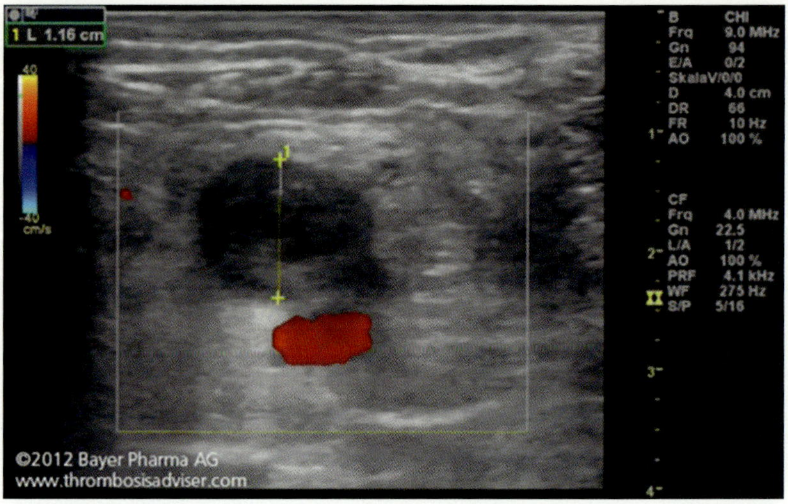

Fig. 8.3 Residual thrombus within the lumen at a distance of 3 months after the acute event (Courtesy of Bayer Pharma AG)

In these patients, is highly recommended to run a pre-operative screening with repeated dosing of D-dimer and repeated ultrasound (Fig. 8.3).

References

Andrews EJ, Fleischer C (2005) Sonography for deep venous thrombosis: current and future applications. Ultrasound Q 21:213–225

Blann AD, Lip GYH (2006) Venous thromboembolism. BMJ 332:215–219

Brookenthal KR, Freedman KB, Lotke PA et al (2001) A meta-analysis of thromboembolic prophylaxis in total knee arthroplasty. J Arthroplasty 16:293–300

Chotanaphuthi T, Heebthamai D, Taweewuthisub W, Thiengwittayaporn S, Roschan S, Kanchanaroek K (2009) Prediction of deep vein thrombosis after total knee arthroplasty with preoperative D-dimer plasma measurement. J Med Assoc Thai 92(Suppl 6):S6–S10

Clagett GP, Anderson FA, Heit J et al (1995) Prevention of venous thromboembolism. Chest 108:312S–334S

Clarke MT, Green JS, Harper WM et al (1997) Screening for deep vein thrombosis after total hip and knee replacement without prophylaxis. J Bone Joint Surg Br 79:787–791

Cohen AT, Agnelli G, Anderson FA et al (2007) Venous thromboembolism (VTE) in Europe. The number of VTE events and associated morbidity and mortality. Thromb Haemost 98:756–764

Cronan JJ, Dorfman GS, Scola FH et al (1987) Deep venous thrombosis: US assessment using vein compression. Radiology 162:191–194

Davidson BL, Elliott CG, Lensing AW (1992) Low accuracy of color Doppler ultrasound in the detection of proximal leg vein thrombosis in asymptomatic high-risk patients. The RD Heparin Arthroplasty Group. Ann Intern Med 117:735–738

Dermody M, Alessi-Chinetti J, Iafrati MD, Estes JM (2011) The utility of screening for deep venous thrombosis in asymptomatic, non-ambulatory neurosurgical patients. J Vasc Surg 53(5):1309–1315. doi:10.1016/j.jvs.2010.10.115. Epub 2011 Jan 7

Doouss TW (1976) The clinical significance of venous thrombosis of the calf. Br J Surg 63:377–378

Eichinger S, Minar E, Bialonczyk C et al (2003) D-dimer levels and risk of recurrent venous thromboembolism. JAMA 290:1071–1074

Eichinger S, Heinze G, Jandeck LM, Kyrle PA (2010) Risk assessment of recurrence in patients with unprovoked deep vein thrombosis or pulmonary embolism: the Vienna prediction model. Circulation 121:1630–1636

Francis CW, Pellegrini VD Jr, Totterman S et al (1997) Prevention of deep-vein thrombosis. J Bone Joint Surg Am 9:1365–1372

Geerts WH, Bergqvist D, Pineo GF et al (2008) Prevention of venous thromboembolism: American College of Chest Physicians evidence-based clinical practice guidelines (8th edition). Chest 133:381S–453S

Giannini M, Rollo HA, Maffei FH, Carvalho LR (2008) Advances in ultrasound techniques improve early detection of deep vein thrombosis. Int Angiol 27(6):466–474

Goodacre S, Sampson F, Stevenson M, Wailoo A, Sutton A, Thomas S, Locker T, Ryan A (2006a) Measurement of the clinical and cost-effectiveness of non-invasive diagnostic testing strategies for deep vein thrombosis. Health Technol Assess 10(15):1–168, iii–iv

Goodacre S, Stevenson M, Wailoo A, Sampson F, Sutton AJ, Thomas S (2006b) How should we diagnose suspected deep-vein thrombosis? QJM 99(6):377–388

Gordon H, Guyatt EA, Crowther M et al (2012) Antithrombotic therapy and prevention of thrombosis,

9th ed: American College of Chest Physicians Evidence-Based Clinical Practice Guidelines. Chest 141(2 Suppl):1S. doi:10.1378/chest.1412S1

Grady-Benson JC, Oishi CS, Hanson PB et al (1994) Postoperative surveillance for deep vein thrombosis with duplex ultrasonography after total knee arthroplasty. J Bone Joint Surg Am 11:1649–1657

Hansson PO, Sorbo J, Eriksson H (2000) Recurrent venous thromboembolism after deep vein thrombosis: incidence and risk factors. Arch Intern Med 160: 769–774

Heit JA, Cohen AT, Anderson FA, On behalf of the VTE Impact Assessment Group (2005) Estimated annual number of incident and recurrent, non-fatal and fatal venous thromboembolism (VTE) events in the US. Blood 106:910A

Ko PS, Chan WF, Siu TH et al (2003) Duplex ultrasonography after total hip or knee arthroplasty. Int Orthop 27:168–171

Kyrle PA, Eichinger S (2005) Deep vein thrombosis. Lancet 365:1163–1174

Lieberman JR, Pellegrini VD (1999) Orthopaedic knowledge update 6. American Academy of Orthopaedic Surgeon, Rosemont

Lohr JM, James KV, Deshmukh RM et al (1995) Calf vein thrombi are not a benign finding. Am J Surg 170:86–90

Lotke PA, Steinbery ME, Ecker ML (1994) Significance of deep vein thrombosis in the lower extremity after total joint arthroplasty. Clin Orthop 299:25–30

Masuda EM, Kessler DM, Kistner RL et al (1998) The natural history of calf vein thrombosis: lysis of thrombi and development of reflux. J Vasc Surg 28(1):67–73; discussion 73–74

McKenna R, Bachmann F, Kaushal SP et al (1976) Thromboembolic disease in patients undergoing total knee replacement. J Bone Joint Surg Am 58:928–932

Murray DW, Britton AR, Bulstrode CJ (1996) Thromboprophylaxis and death after total hip replacement. J Bone Joint Surg Br 78:863–870

National Institutes of Health Consensus Development Conference statement (1986) Prevention of venous and pulmonary thromboembolism. JAMA 256:744–749

Pabinger I, Ay C (2009) Biomarkers and venous thromboembolism. Arterioscler Thromb Vasc Biol 29:332–336

Parvizi J, Ghanem E, Joshi A et al (2007) Does "excessive" anticoagulation predispose to periprosthetic infection? J Arthroplasty 22(6 Suppl 2):24–28

Patel AP, Koltz MT, Sansur CA, Gulati M, Hamilton DK (2013) An analysis of deep vein thrombosis in 1277 consecutive neurosurgical patients undergoing routine weekly ultrasonography. J Neurosurg 118(3):505–509. Epub 2012 Dec 14

Planes A, Samama MM, Lensing AW et al (1999) Prevention of deep vein thrombosis after hip replacement. Thromb Haemost 81:22–25

Prandoni P, Noventa F, Ghirarduzzi A et al (2007) The risk of recurrent venous thromboembolism after discontinuing anticoagulation in patients with acute proximal deep vein thrombosis or pulmonary embolism. A prospective cohort study in 1,626 patients. Haematologica 92:199–205

Saad WE, Saad N (2007) Computer tomography for venous thromboembolic disease. Radiol Clin North Am 45:423–445

Shimoyama Y, Sawai T, Tatsumi S, Nakahira J, Oka M, Nakajima M, Jotoku T, Minami T (2012) Perioperative risk factors for deep vein thrombosis after total hip arthroplasty or total knee arthroplasty. J Clin Anesth 24(7):531–536. Epub 2012 Sep 21

Sisodia G, Garnet Fernando WS, Melton C et al. (2013) The incidence of pre-operative asymptomatic DVT among patients awaiting total knee arthroplasty or total hip arthroplasty. http://www.nlg.nhs.uk/services/radiology/The.incidence.of.preop.DVT.in.patients.awaiting.TKR.and.THR.pdf. Accessed 22 Dec 2013

Stern JB, Abehsera M, Grenet D et al (2002) Detection of pelvic vein thrombosis by magnetic resonance angiography in patients with acute pulmonary embolism and normal lower limb compression ultrasonography. Chest 122:115–121

Stulberg BN, Insall JN, Williams GW et al (1984) Deep vein thrombosis following total knee replacement. An analysis of six hundred and thirty-eight arthroplasties. J Bone Joint Surg Am 66:194–201

Turpie AGG, Chin BSP, Lip GYH (2002) Venous thromboembolism: pathophysiology, clinical features, and prevention. BMJ 325:887–890

Vormittag R, Panzer S, Ay C et al (2007) Soluble P-selectin and thrombosis risk of patients with a persistent lupus anticoagulant in a prospective study. Haematologica 92:327. Abstract 0878

Wells PS, Anderson DR, Bormanis J et al (1997) Value of assessment of pretest probability of deep-vein thrombosis in clinical management. Lancet 350:1795–1798

Westrich GH, Haas SB, Mosca P et al (2000) Meta-analysis of thromboembolic prophylaxis after total knee arthroplasty. J Bone Joint Surg Br 82(6): 795–800

Zhu T, Martinez I, Emmerich J (2009) Venous thromboembolism: risk factors for recurrence. Arterioscler Thromb Vasc Biol 29:298–310

Zhu R, Wei S, Wu S, Gong H, Chen X (2010) Early diagnosis of lower limb deep vein thrombosis after major orthopedic surgeries. Zhongguo Xiu Fu Chong Jian Wai Ke Za Zhi 24(6):730–734

Part II

Pain Control

What Works and What Does Not Work for Pain Control in Arthroplasty

9

Giorgio Danelli and Marco Gardini

> **Open Questions**
> - Which are the drawbacks of local wound infiltration analgesia?
> - Is patient-controlled analgesia still feasible?
> - Which is the level of evidence of each component of a multimodal analgesia protocol?
> - Regional anesthesia: single shots or continuous blocks?

9.1 Background

Proper management of postoperative pain is fundamental in delivering quality care to orthopedic surgery patients. The outcome of a satisfactory pain management affects hospital stay and time to patient remobilization. Lower limb surgeries, such as total hip arthroplasty (THA) and total knee arthroplasty (TKA), are common surgical procedures and both generate a substantial amount of postoperative pain and impact a large part of the elderly population. Up to 50 % of patients who undergo arthroplasty grade their pain as severe immediately after surgery and report that pain becomes significantly worse during rehabilitation (Hogan et al. 2009). Pain management contributes significantly to overall patient satisfaction after such procedures and an optimal pain control is associated with a better outcome and an early rehabilitation and mobilization. A multimodal analgesia is one of the mainstays of any fast-track protocol for arthroplasty surgery, and other key points, such as deep venous thrombosis prophylaxis and early mobilizations, are strongly related to pain control. The impact of the feasibility of a fast-track program on total joint replacement surgery has been studied and showed impressive advantages in terms of patient safety, satisfaction, rehabilitation, length of hospital stay, and cost (Ilfield et al. 2010). Continuous peripheral nerve block shows an early mobilization with fewer side effects in respect to epidural and opioid analgesia when maintained at least for the first 48 h after surgery (Capdevila et al. 1999, 2008).

Among regional anesthesia technique continuous femoral nerve block has a level I recommendation; however, in attempt of maintaining the muscular strength of quadriceps, recent studies suggest the use of the adductor nerve block that involve block of saphenous nerve, which has

G. Danelli
Department of Anesthesia,
Analgesia and Perioperative Medicine,
Istituti Ospitalieri di Cremona, Cremona, Italy

M. Gardini (✉)
Department of Anesthesia,
Intensive Care and Pain Therapy,
Azienda Ospedaliero-Universitaria di Parma, Parma, Italy
e-mail: ares982@hotmail.it

A. Baldini, P. Caldora (eds.), *Perioperative Medical Management for Total Joint Arthroplasty: How to Control Hemostasis, Pain and Infection*, DOI 10.1007/978-3-319-07203-6_9,

a lower analgesic efficacy but is not related with motor block (Kim et al. 2014). When the use of continuous nerve block is not feasible, local articular infiltration with local anesthetic may be a good option, although this technique showed a lesser analgesic efficacy and some concerns about infection risk (Chelly 2013).

When is not possible to use regional anesthesia techniques emerging evidences suggest the role of NMDA antagonist drugs: last evidences show the role of ketamine when used perioperatively in the prevention of chronic pain after total knee and hip replacement (Perrin 2009).

9.2 Systemic Analgesia

First of all, it is mandatory to pay attention with hemostasis during surgery before skin closure for reduction of postoperative hematoma, and it is necessary to underline the preoperative pain as an independent risk of acute postoperative pain.

Large doses of parenteral opioids, a mainstay in many pain management strategies, can be associated with significant adverse effects including constipation, nausea, vomiting, dizziness, urinary retention, and respiratory depression. In addition, opioid-induced respiratory depression and hypoxia are associated with myocardial ischemia, tachycardia, delirium, and delayed wound healing. Opioid effects and side effects are potentiated in the elderly due to modified volumes of distribution and reduced drug clearance and total joint arthroplasties. Traditionally, postoperative protocols for total joint arthroplasty were based on general anesthesia and parenteral patient-controlled analgesia (PCA). In recent years, efforts have centered on regional anesthesia along with multimodal analgesic protocols to improve early postoperative pain control, while decreasing the associated adverse effects. In 2004, the American Society of Anesthesiologists task force published the first set of guidelines dealing with perioperative pain management and from then strongly recommended the adoption of multimodal analgesia protocols for all surgical patients, including those undergoing orthopedic procedures (American Society of Anesthesiologists, 2004–2012). Multimodal analgesia involves using different classes of medications or analgesics with different receptors and other techniques, such as local injections, nerve blocks, and epidural infusions, in order to decrease the amount of opioid medication required postoperatively. Unless contraindicated, they recommended the routine use of perioperative non-opioid medications in addition to regional anesthetic techniques (Lachiewicz 2013) (Tables. 9.1 and 9.2).

9.3 Regional Anesthetic Techniques

Regional anesthesia has always been a stalemate in hip and knee joint replacement management. Its benefits include, other than lessening or avoidance of opioid drugs in the postoperative, better pain control, reduction in chronic pain occurrence, faster recovery and discharge rates, and thus reduction of immobilization-related severe adverse effects, such as thromboembolic events.

Lumbar epidural analgesia has been popular over the last decades as there is evidence for lower postoperative thromboembolic complications and other protective effects. Nevertheless, there is today little evidence for a decrease in perioperative mortality and morbidity in a low- to medium-risk population in relation to the use of perioperative epidural analgesia. Moreover, the widespread implementation of anticoagulant regimens may not only overcome the benefits of epidural analgesia on thromboembolic complications but also make around 30 % of the patients ineligible for the technique (Rawal 2012). The failure rate of the technique may reach 28 % (Hermanides et al. 2012). A previous systematic review in TKA comparing lumbar epidural blockade with systemic opioid analgesia reported better dynamic pain scores (Fowler et al. 2008). As the magnitude of pain relief must be weighed against the frequency of adverse events, patients who received epidural analgesia had more hypotension, urinary retention, and pruritus whereas systemic opioids caused more sedation, but no difference was found for the postoperative respiratory depression and nausea or

Table. 9.1 Systemic analgesics for total hip replacement

Drugs	Recommended?	Evidence level	Exceptions	Dosing and notes
Corticosteroids	No, lack of efficacy	Grade D		
NSAIDs	Yes, with acetaminophen and opioids in an opioid-sparing multimodal protocol	Grade A	Not suitable in patients with aspirin-sensitive asthma, increased bleeding risk, increased gastrointestinal morbidity (grade B)	Ketorolac 10 mg po or 30 mg ev Ketoprofen 100 mg po The ev administration should last max 48 h, then it is mandatory to switch to oral administration
COX2 selective inhibitors	Yes, with acetaminophen and opioids in an opioid-sparing multimodal protocol	Grade A	Careful use in patients with cardiovascular risk (grade B)	Parecoxib 40 mg ev Valdecoxib 20 mg or 40 mg po
Ketamine	Not yet, but it is being studied for suitable application in patients not eligible for locoregional anesthesia	Grade D		A morphine equianalgesic protocol would be 0.5 mg/kg ev followed by a 24 h infusion 2 mcg/kg/min (racemic formula)
Strong opioids	Yes, in a multimodal therapy and whenever applicable with a PCA protocol	Grade A	Intramuscular administration and transdermal administration are not recommended (grade A)	Morphine initial dose should be titrated in the recovery room and then given with PCA protocol (e.g., 1 mg with 8' lockout) for the following 48 h
Paracetamol	Yes, in a multimodal protocol as an opioid-sparing drug	Grade A	Dose reduction according to hepatic and renal level of impairment	Paracetamol 1 g po or ev every 6–8 h immediately following surgery

vomiting. Development and implementation of peripheral nerve blocks (PNBs) for THA and TKA anesthesia and analgesia evolved from an understanding of the sensory innervations to the hip and knee and progressively received greater attention along the development of nerve stimulation and ultrasound technique and technology. A working knowledge of the sensory distribution of the lower limb helps one understand how PNBs can be useful in managing pain after lower extremity procedures. Unfortunately, these blocks traditionally have been overlooked as anesthetic choices, as many anesthesiologists had no experience in using these techniques, and orthopedic surgeons lacked an understanding of the patient benefits they offered. However, a clear understanding of the anatomy of the pertinent nerve innervation of the lower limb, the technical and procedural aspects of block delivery, and the advantages and disadvantages of both PNBs and traditional methods of postoperative analgesia (e.g., spinal or epidural blocks) is of great importance. In recent years, however, single-injection and continuous PNBs have become part of the orthopedic postoperative analgesic approach, as they have been shown to optimize patient outcomes, satisfaction, and rehabilitation while minimizing complications and reducing costs and length of hospital stay (Hogan et al. 2009).

The lumbar plexus may be blocked with three distinct approaches. Block of the full lumbar plexus (femoral, lateral femoral cutaneous, and obturator) is accomplished with the psoas block. In comparison, the fascia iliaca and femoral approaches will reliably block the femoral but not the lateral femoral, cutaneous, and obturator nerves.

Selection of regional analgesic technique is dependent on the surgical site. For example, the psoas compartment approach to the lumbar plexus is preferable for surgery to the hip because it is the most proximal lumbar plexus technique and provides complete block of the lumbar plexus and the needle or catheter insertion site is distant from the surgical incision (allowing preoperative

Table 9.2 Systemic analgesics for total knee replacement

Drugs	Recommended?	Evidence level	Exceptions	Dosing and notes
Alpha-2 receptor ligands (clonidine)	No, lack of specific evidence	Grade D		
Gabapentinoids	No, lack of specific evidence	Grade D		
NSAIDs	Yes, with acetaminophen and opioids in an opioid-sparing multimodal protocol. More data should be provided for use in conjunction with locoregional techniques	Grade A	Not suitable in patients with aspirin-sensitive asthma, increased bleeding risk, increased gastrointestinal morbidity (grade B)	Ketorolac 10 mg po or 30 mg ev Ketoprofen 100 mg po The ev administration should last max 48 h, then it is mandatory to switch to oral administration
COX2 selective inhibitors	Yes, with acetaminophen and opioids in an opioid-sparing multimodal protocol. More data should be provided for use in conjunction with locoregional techniques	Grade A	Careful use in patients with cardiovascular risk (grade B)	Parecoxib 40 mg ev Valdecoxib 20 mg or 40 mg po
Corticosteroids	No, although a recent meta-analysis showed a pain reduction in patients treated with high doses preoperatively		Caution should be undertaken if high doses of corticosteroids are planned to be given	Preoperative use of low doses (<10 mg dexamethasone) are encouraged for PONV prevention but showed no effect on pain reduction
Ketamine	Not yet, but procedural-specific data are being collected for stronger recommendation	Grade D		A 48 h infusion at 2 mcg/kg/min (racemic formula) starting intraoperatively showed increased knee flexion during early rehabilitation vs. placebo and reduced chronic pain incidence after surgery
Strong opioids	Yes, in a multimodal therapy and whenever applicable with a PCA protocol	Grade A	Intramuscular and transdermal administrations are not recommended (grade A)	Morphine initial dose should be titrated in the PACU and then given with PCA protocol (e.g., 1 mg with 8' lockout) for the following 48 h. Extended release oral opioids are also encouraged since they show faster discharge rates when compared to intravenous administered opioids
Paracetamol	Yes, in a multimodal protocol as an opioid-sparing drug	Grade B	Dose reduction according to hepatic and renal level of impairment	Paracetamol 1 g po or ev every 6–8 h immediately following surgery

placement). However, for patients undergoing total knee replacement or for patients in whom a psoas approach may be contraindicated due to infection or existing coagulopathy, a more distal approach to the lumbar plexus (femoral or fascia iliaca blockade) is warranted (Horlocker 2011).

In total hip replacement surgery, continuous lumbar plexus block and continuous femoral nerve block with PCNB or continuous infusion protocols showed a higher extend of block and more successful analgesia in opposition to single shot techniques. Posterior lumbar plexus blocks (psoas sheath blocks) have a greater efficacy than distal lumbar plexus blocks (femoral nerve blocks) in total hip replacement and are recommended. However, they have a potential for more serious complications than the femoral block (plus supplementary obturator and lateral cutaneous nerve of thigh blocks). This recommendation must be balanced against risks of motor blockade and falls and the efficacy of systemic multimodal analgesia (Aguirre et al. 2012).

Each of the aforementioned nerve block techniques has complications. LPBs carry a risk for epidural or subarachnoid injection when the needle is introduced improperly. There is also the risk that the aorta and/or inferior vena cava will be pierced. Both occurrences can be prevented by performing frequent aspirations to ensure that no cerebrospinal fluid or blood is drawn during block administration. Each FNB and SNB combination has minimal complications. SNBs uncommonly cause self-limiting dysesthesias, and FNBs carry a very low risk of intravascular injection or hematoma formation. Adverse effects are shown to be minimized by ultrasound-guided technique when performing such blocks.

The true benefits of PNB emerge when these procedures are compared with traditional spinal or epidural anesthesia and PCA methods. PNB techniques reduce postoperative nausea and vomiting and are not associated with the urinary retention problems that often plague patients who receive neuraxial blocks and other standard analgesic techniques. Moreover, PNBs are associated with faster rehabilitation times and faster discharge rates. Although neuraxial anesthesia does decrease blood loss and transfusion needs in THA patients, it carries the well-known risk for life-threatening spinal hematoma formation and severe neurologic dysfunction. Lower extremity blocks can be safely used in patients who receive anticoagulation therapy, which is known to increase the risk for hematoma formation in patients undergoing spinal anesthesia. Unlike spinal, epidural, and patient-controlled analgesia, PNBs have not been reported to cause severe hypotension or respiratory depression.

Finally, the concept of multimodal pain control including local periarticular injection (LIA) has received increasing interest in the recent literature, and published results are promising in terms of improved perioperative pain control, reduced need for narcotic medications, and reduced associated side effects. Recent reports have used periarticular injections as a supplement to conventional pain control modalities including patient-controlled anesthesia (PCA) pumps and peripheral nerve blocks. In addition, most of the data reported have been on predischarge pain control and functional recovery. LIA technique is a promising, easy, and safe technique, which has proven its efficacy after TKA. The joint and surrounding tissues are infiltrated by the surgeon with a high volume of a local anesthetic solution mainly including ropivacaine, epinephrine, and some adjuvants like NSAIDs, clonidine, corticosteroid, or opioids. The placement of the injections is important, and the total volume should be divided into quarters, with one-quarter injected into the posterior capsule, one-quarter into the medial periosteum and medial capsule, one-quarter into the lateral periosteum and lateral capsule, and one-quarter into the soft tissues around the skin incision (Dalury et al. 2011). The results of several randomized clinical trials demonstrate excellent pain relief and functional recovery after THA and TKA in a multimodal protocol in conjunction with a minimally invasive approach (Figs. 9.3 and 9.4).

Table 9.3 Regional anesthesia techniques for total hip replacement

Technique	Recommended?	Evidence level	Exceptions	Dosing and notes
Epidural analgesia	Yes, with opioids (non-extended release formulations) especially in patients with increased cardiovascular risk	Grade B	Evaluation on preexistent bladder or neurological impairment; evaluation of independent and iatrogenic bleeding risk	*Bupivacaine, levobupivacaine, and ropivacaine* have a similar analgesic profile when started intraoperatively allowing peak concentration in the postoperative time
				Sufentanyl should be the opioid of choice for epidural administration, due to its pharmacokinetic properties. A dose of 0.5 mcg/ml in a ropivacaine 0.1 % solution has the same level of analgesia compared with increased doses (0.75 and 1 mcg/ml)
Posterior lumbar plexus block (psoas sheath block)	Yes, better efficacy than distal blocks	Grade A	Assessment of risk of prolonged motor blockade and risk of postoperative falls	*Catheter* techniques should be preferred over single shot techniques, and *PCA plus basal infusion* protocol showed better efficacy than continuous infusion alone. *Timing* of the infusion start should allow peak effect at the end of the surgery
Femoral nerve block	Yes, better safety profile than proximal block but lesser efficacy	Grade B	Assessment of risk of prolonged motor blockade and risk of postoperative falls	*Catheter* techniques should be preferred over single shot techniques, and *PCA plus basal infusion* protocol showed better efficacy than continuous infusion alone. *Timing* of the infusion start should allow peak effect at the end of the surgery
Spinal analgesia	Yes, as part of spinal anesthesia but only as morphine single injection	Grade B	A prior risk assessment of respiratory failure and depression is mandatory	Single bolus of *Morphine* 0.1–0.2 mg is recommended. Clonidine and short-acting opioids are not recommended
Wound infiltration	Yes, but only single shot, low concentration, and high volume solutions; more data are needed	Grade A	Since drains are not recommended, drain injections are not too	Solution should contain local anesthetic (e.g., ropivacaine 2 mg/ml), NSAID (e.g., ketorolac 30 mg), and vasoconstrictor (e.g., epinephrine 0.5 mg/ml)

Table 9.4 Regional anesthesia techniques for total knee replacement

Technique	Recommended?	Evidence level	Exceptions	Dosing and notes
Epidural analgesia	No, similar efficacy compared to femoral nerve block and worse safety profile	Grade B	Evaluation on preexistent bladder or neurological impairment; evaluation of independent and iatrogenic bleeding risk	If epidural analgesia is chosen, ketamine, clonidine, or tramadol are not recommended for epidural injection in TKA. It should be used a *PCEA* with short-acting opioid and local anesthetic
Femoral nerve block	Yes, actually the evidence is supporting this block not in conjunction with sciatic or obturator nerve block although data are being collected	Grade A	Training of both anesthesiologist and nursing personnel is necessary for the correct placement and follow up of the catheter. If this condition is not met, a single shot injection should be performed	*Catheter* techniques should be preferred over single shot techniques, and *PCA plus basal infusion* protocol showed better efficacy than continuous infusion alone. *Timing* of the infusion start should allow peak effect at the end of the surgery. Clonidine is not recommended for infusion
Adductor canal nerves block	Although more data should be collected, it proved be an effective alternative to femoral nerve block	Need more data	Since it is a single shot technique, an epidural or systemic analgesia should be provided for the block wearing off time	A *mid-thigh level* should be targeted for ultrasound-guided adductor canal block allowing coverage of medial, lateral, and anterior aspects of the knee. A *low-dose anesthetic* injection (e.g., bupivacaine 75 mg) showed sufficient analgesia while allowing good quadriceps motor strength
Intra-articular infiltration (LIA)	More data are needed to demonstrate efficacy in TKA	Grade D		High volume of the solution should be used. The solution should contain local anaesthetics (bupivacaine 200–400 mg or ropivacaine 200–300 mg), morphine (4–10 mg), corticosteroids (methyl-prednisolone 40 mg) or NSAIDs (ketorolac 30 mg), epinephrine (300 mg)

Key Points

- Quality orthopedic care standards include a proper management of postoperative pain.
- Satisfactory postoperative pain control translates into better rehabilitation outcomes, lesser complications, and faster discharge rates.
- Systemic analgesia should always be modeled in a multimodal pathway, personalizing therapy on patient's clinical aspects.
- Locoregional analgesic techniques are mandatory when not contraindicated, providing good to excellent pain control and faster mobilization times especially when performed with a continuous technique.
- The site of blockade may range from epidural to intra-articular, and choice should be made weighing benefits and particular risks both independent and patient related.

References

Aguirre J et al (2012) The role of continuous peripheral nerve blocks. Anesth Res Pract vol. 2012, Article ID 560879, 20 pages. doi:10.1155/2012/560879
American Society of Anesthesiologists Task Force on Acute Pain Management (2004) Practice guidelines for acute pain management in the perioperative setting: an updated report by the American Society of Anesthesiologists Task Force on Acute Pain Management. Anesthesiology 100:1573–1581
Capdevila X, Barthelet Y, Biboulet P et al (1999) Effects of perioperative analgesic technique on the surgical outcome and duration of rehabilitation after major knee surgery. Anesthesiology 91:8–15
Capdevila X et al (2008) Continuous peripheral nerve blocks in clinical practice. Curr Opin Anaesthesiol 21(5):619–23
Chelly JE (2013) Is the continuous saphenous block the right technique for postoperative pain management after total knee replacement? Reg Anesth Pain Med 38(5):461
Dalury DF et al (2011) Current and innovative pain management techniques in total knee arthroplasty. J Bone Joint Surg Am 93:1938–1943
Fowler SJ et al (2008) Epidural analgesia compared with peripheral nerve blockade after major knee surgery: a systematic review and meta-analysis of randomized trials. Br J Anaesth 100(2):154–164
Hermanides J et al (2012) Failed epidural: causes and management. Br J Anaesth. doi:10.1093/bja/aes214
Hogan MV, Grant R, Lee L (2009) Analgesia for total hip and knee arthroplasty: a review of lumbar plexus, femoral, and sciatic nerve blocks. Am J Orthop 38(8):E129–E133
Horlocker TT (2011) Regional anaesthesia in the patient receiving antithrombotic and antiplatelet therapy. Br J Anaesth 107(Suppl 1):i96–i106
Ilfield B et al (2010) Ultrasound-guided perineural catheter insertion: three approaches, but little illuminating data. Reg Anesth Pain Med 35(2):123–126
Kim DH et al (2014) Adductor canal block versus femoral nerve block for total knee arthroplasty: a prospective, randomized, controlled trial. Anesthesiology 120(3):540–550
Lachiewicz P (2013) The role of intravenous acetaminophen in multimodal pain protocols for perioperative orthopedic patients. Orthopedics 36:15–19
Perrin SB (2009) Intraoperative ketamine may influence persistent pain following knee arthroplasty under combined general and spinal anaesthesia: a pilot study. Anaesth Intensive Care 37(2):248–53
Rawal N (2012) Epidural technique for postoperative pain: gold standard no more? Reg Anesth Pain Med 37(3):310–317

Further Suggested Reading

Andersen LJ, Poulsen T, Krogh B, Nielsen T (2007) Postoperative analgesia in total hip arthroplasty: a randomized double-blinded, placebo-controlled study on preoperative and postoperative ropivacaine, ketorolac, and adrenaline wound infiltration. Acta Orthop 78:187–192
Aveline C, Roux AL, Hetet HL, Gautier JF, Vautier P, Cognet F, Bonnet F (2013) Pain and recovery after total knee arthroplasty: a twelve months follow-up after a prospective randomized study evaluating nefopam and ketamine for early rehabilitation. Clin J Pain. doi:10.1097/AJP.0000000000000033. [Epub ahead of print]
Barbosa Neto JO (2014) Methadone patient-controlled analgesia for postoperative pain: a randomized, controlled, double-blind study. J Anesth. doi:10.1007/s00540-013-1785-3
Blaudszun G, Lysakowski C, Elia N, Tramer MR (2012) Effect of perioperative systemic alpha 2 agonists on postoperative morphine consumption and. pain intensity: systematic review and meta-analysis of randomized controlled trials. Anesthesiology 116:1312–1322
Bonnet F et al. Prospect Working Group. www.postoppain.org
Buvanendran A et al (2003) Effects of perioperative administration of a selective cyclooxygenase 2 inhibitor on pain management and recovery of function after knee replacement a randomized controlled trial. JAMA 290:2411–2418
Goyal N, Parikh A, Austin M (2008) Pain management after total joint arthroplasty. Semin Arthro 19:226–230
Grosu I, Lavand'homme P (2013) Pain after knee arthroplasty: an unresolved issue. Knee Surg Sports Traumatol Arthrosc. doi:10.1007/s00167-013-2750-2
Horlocker TT, Kopp SL, Pagnano MW, Hebl JR (2006) Analgesia for total hip and knee arthroplasty: a multimodal pathway featuring peripheral nerve block. J Am Acad Orthop Surg 14:126–135
Kejisers R et al (2013) Local infiltration analgesia following total knee arthroplasty: effect on post-operative pain and opioid consumption – a meta-analysis. Knee Surg Sports Traumatol Arthrosc. doi:10.1007/s00167-013-2788-1
Khia SK et al (2013) Peri-articular steroid injection in total knee arthroplasty: a prospective, double blinded, randomized controlled trial. J Arthroplasty 28(4):620–623. doi:10.1016/j.arth.2012.07.034. Epub 2012 Oct 26
Lamplot J, Wagner E, Manning D (2014) Multimodal pain management in total knee arthroplasty a prospective randomized controlled trial. J Arthroplasty 29:329–334
Lunn TH, Kehlet H (2013) Perioperative glucocorticoids in hip and knee surgery – benefit vs. harm? A review

of randomized clinical trials. Acta Anaesthesiol Scand 57(7):823–834

Martinez V et al (2014) The analgesic efficiency of combined pregabalin and ketamine for total hip arthroplasty: a randomised, double-blind, controlled study. Anaesthesia 69:46–52

Memsoudis S (2014) Inpatient falls after total knee arthroplasty. The role of anesthesia type and peripheral nerve blocks. Anesthesiology 120:551–563

Memtsoudis S et al (2013) Perioperative comparative effectiveness of anesthetic technique in orthopedic patients. Anesthesiology 118:1046–1058

Parvataneni H et al (2007) Controlling pain after total hip and knee arthroplasty using a multimodal protocol with local periarticular injections. J Arthroplasty 22(6 Suppl):2

Paul J et al (2013) Gabapentin does not improve multimodal analgesia outcomes for total knee arthroplasty: a randomized controlled trial. Can J Anesth 60:423–431. doi:10.1007/s12630-013-9902-1

Pizzi LT, Toner R, Foley K et al (2012) Relation-ship between potential opioid-related ad-verse effects and hospital length of stay in patients receiving opioids after orthopedic surgery. Pharmacotherapy 32(6):502–514

Ranawat A, Ranawat C (2007) Pain management and accelerated rehabilitation for total hip and total knee arthroplasty. J Arthroplasty 22(7 Suppl):3

Richards P, Gimbel J, Minkowitz H et al (2013) Comparison of the efficacy and safety of dual-opioid treatment with morphine plus oxycodone versus oxycodone/acetaminophen for moderate to severe acute pain after total knee arthroplasty. Clin Ther 35:498–511

Richman JM, Liu SS, Courpas G, Wong R, Rowlingson AJ, McGready J, Cohen SR, Wu CL (2006) Does continuous peripheral nerve block provide superior pain control to opioids? A meta-analysis. Anesth Analg 102:248–257

Rosseland LA, Romundstad L (2013) Multimodal pain management with glucocorticoids: killing two birds with one stone or shooting sparrows with cannons? Acta Anaesthesiol Scand 57(7):819–822. doi:10.1111/aas.12139

Zoric L et al (2014) Single-shot intraoperative local anaesthetic infiltration does not reduce morphine consumption after total hip arthroplasty: a double-blinded placebo-controlled randomized study. Br J Anaesth 112:722–728. doi:10.1093/bja/aet439

Mental Preparation of the Patient to the Arthroplasty Procedure

10

Jonathan Lorenzo Chiti

Open Questions

- Is patient satisfaction after TKA surgery somehow related to their psychological profile?
- Is there anything other than optimal surgical technique that can be done to optimize patient satisfaction?
- Are all depressed patients alike?
- How do patient's expectancies affect outcomes?
- Can the stress of surgery be confronted with other means than medication?

10.1 Introduction

Pain is a physical sensation, like touch or cold. But it is particular in that it has an unpleasant quality and generates powerful emotional reactions in the family of fear. Such fear reactions are normal and have evident evolutionary value. Clinically such fear can be referred as anxiety. In our culture, much attention is placed upon the physical component of pain and less on the emotional aspect. But when patients talk about pain, they are usually referring to the level of "emotional unpleasantness" derived from that physical sensation, as that is what is most relevant to them. While it is obvious that pain has many physical causes, mechanical, biochemical and physiological as in osteoarthritis, or in the wake of surgery, it is also clear that emotional interpretation of the physical sensation of pain plays a crucial role in the "experience" of pain.

The classical approach to pain reduction is to reduce its physical causes via optimal surgical technique, anaesthesiological procedures and pharmacological management. This is, should be and will remain the high road to achieving the best results in orthopaedic surgery. However, it may also be interesting to approach the pain "experience" from the emotional side. This is useful for the average patient and even more so for emotionally fragile patients.

Anxiety and pain are thus in very close relationship and modulate each other in both directions. We suggest confronting the pain issue by confronting anxiety. A patient with little pain but a lot of anxiety might have a bad "pain experience" and not be satisfied with the treatment received.

The modulation of anxiety has relevance on pain reduction especially in the perioperative phase, but it may well have lasting effects months or years after the surgery. The risk of pain sensitisation suggests the importance of controlling pain at every level in early stages.

J.L. Chiti
Orthopaedic Unit, IFCA Clinic, Florence, Italy
e-mail: lorenzo.chiti@gmail.com

A. Baldini, P. Caldora (eds.), *Perioperative Medical Management for Total Joint Arthroplasty: How to Control Hemostasis, Pain and Infection*, DOI 10.1007/978-3-319-07203-6_10,

There are three main topics regarding anxiety modulation for pain control that we will describe: preoperative information, preoperative screening of mentally fragile patients and use of relaxation techniques.

10.2 Preoperative Information

It has long been recognised (Hayward 1975) that preoperative information enhances perceived control in patients, facilitates patients' active involvement in their care and therefore reduces anxiety and improves outcomes and satisfaction (Pellino 1997, 1998; Johansson et al. 2005; Walker 2007; Livbjerg et al. 2013). Inadequate information is likely to compromise patient satisfaction (Keulers et al. 2008). Adequate information provided to patients also aligns patients' expectations with their surgeons' (Ghomrawi et al. 2012), and appropriate expectations are key for patient satisfaction (Noble et al. 2006) although there is some controversy on this topic due to the different definitions of "expectations" (Haanstra 2012). The effect of preoperative education has been evaluated in many domains: pain, knowledge, anxiety, length of stay, self-efficacy and empowerment. It is hard to quantify the effect in each of these domains. Anxiety seems to be the element that gains the most improvement, and pain itself to a minor extent (McDonald et al. 2004; Johansson et al. 2005). Probably there are some subgroups in the patient population that will benefit the most from preoperative information, for example, those who mostly use denial as a coping strategy and those with the highest anxiety (Daltroy et al. 1998). There are many ways to convey information: via printed material, video, direct oral explanation, conference and web-based material (Gautschi et al. 2010; Jlala et al. 2010; Ihedioha et al. 2013); it is not clear which is the best manner or timing (Jlala et al. 2010). Some authors recommend that there be a moment of verbal transmission with a question-and-answer session at the end. Preoperative information should be offered prior to admission for at that stage patients are already anxious and do not retain as much information (Hughes 2002).

10.3 Preoperative Psychological Screening

In an effort to interpret the reasons that compromise outcomes in the percentage of unsatisfied TKA patients, the importance of the psychological profile has been long advocated. Depression, pain and disability are clearly statistically linked. Depressed patients preoperatively have worse results after TKA surgery in terms of pain, functionality and satisfaction (Hirschmann et al. 2013; Duivenvoorden et al. 2013; Singh et al. 2013, 2014). Among depression and pain/dysfunction, it is not obvious though which is the cause and which is the effect. Some authors argue that depression is likely to be the effect rather than the cause of knee pathology at least to some extent (Blackburn et al. 2012). Pérez-Prieto et al. recently showed that although it is true that depressed patients have worse outcomes after TKA surgery, as a group they also start from worse pain and function levels preoperatively and the degree of improvement is the same as for non-depressed patients. They conclude that it is equally worthwhile for the depressed to undergo TKA surgery as for the non-depressed. To some extent the surgery will also cure the depression (Pérez-Prieto et al. 2014). Actually "depression" is too broad a concept, for it has often been used as a synonym of "poor mental health". The SF 36 mental health subscales have been used extensively for the purpose of evaluating the psychological condition of surgical patients, but this tool seems not to be sensitive enough. Many authors recommend additional use of other scoring scales like the HAD (Hospital Anxiety and Depression scale) or other specific scales (Fosså et al. 2002; Ulvik et al. 2008).

We are interested in identifying those patients that have modifiable psychological conditions preoperatively that, if treated, might avoid the compromising of outcomes or at least might modulate correct expectations. Postoperative anxiety is a recognized risk factor for persistent post-surgical pain (Pinto et al. 2013b). Pain catastrophizing, an aspect of anxiety, seems to be a more specific trait element that can be recognized in patients. Pain catastrophising can be described as a tendency to magnify or exaggerate the threat value or seriousness of the pain sensations (Sullivan 1995). It has been proven to predict post-surgical pain severity at 6 weeks (Sullivan et al. 2009) to 6 months (Riddle et al. 2010) and has been linked to residual long-term pain after TKA (Bonnin et al. 2011; Vissers et al. 2012). Preoperative optimism is an indicator that has been evaluated and in a sense is the opposite of the pain catastrophising tendency. The optimistic patient believes that they and/or the surgery will change their condition and control their pain. Optimism as measured with the IPQ-R (Revised Illness Perception Questionnaire) and with the LOT-R (Life Orientation Test - Revised) is associated with augmented pain tolerance for diminished pain sensitivity. It has been shown to modulate acute pain (Pinto et al. 2013a). Sullivan et al. analysed "Behavioral Outcome Expectancies" as an indicator of the motivation to heal and found they where a predictor of pain and function 1 year after TKA surgery (Sullivan et al. 2011). Behavioural outcome expectancies express the confidence the patient has in returning to proper function (i.e. "How likely is it that 1 month following surgery you will have resumed your household responsibilities?"), they are likely more mediated by motivational factors. They differ from "Response" expectancies (i.e. "How likely is it that 1 month following surgery your pain will be reduced?"), which don't imply a direct role of the patient and therefore essentially automatic or passive. Such observations seem confirmed by experiences in other settings where Anticipated Pain predicted postoperative pain scores, as suggesting a self-fulfilling prophecy (Logan et al. 2005). It seems that if patients have a positive outlook on the experience of surgery and its results, it is more likely that they will actually obtain good results. This might be because an optimistic mind creates the conditions for the best recovery or because patients have a good perception of their health after all and can to some extent predict what will happen to them. In both cases it is a good idea to investigate the patient's point of view because it is likely to be quite accurate. To date probably the most effective tool for the psychological screening of TKA patients is the Pain Catastrophizing Scale.

10.4 Relaxation Techniques

If the problem is anxiety, it is plausible to imagine relaxation as a solution. There have been several attempts to produce relaxation in the perioperative setting. It is an interesting field though still relatively unexplored and can potentially offer complementary tools for the optimal management of the surgical patient. Such tools might be especially valuable in patients that cannot metabolically tolerate heavy pain medication. There are obvious advantages like non-invasiveness and non-toxicity. The costs can span from inexpensive to very expensive depending on the method and on the time spent by health-care professionals devoted to it. To date there are very few certainties in this field, and the results are promising but modest. The difficulties of applying such methods, aside from the cost issue, are that in confronting the psychological side of patients, it is difficult to standardize treatment, since varying individual tastes, culture and belief systems are involved.

Generally speaking, in the realm of relaxation techniques, there are two main objectives that are sought. One is distraction from the "drama" of surgery and the connected fears: "diversion therapy". The other is to modify the physical symptoms of anxiety by directly controlling some of them (i.e. breathing exercises) or by triggering a pleasant mind state (i.e. imagining a peaceful scene). Methods often combine both objectives. Many relaxation techniques have been proposed: progressive muscle relaxation, music, guided imagery, awareness, attention control, hypnosis, humour and others.

The moment of surgery and the days after are inherently stressful. Some patients might not be able to cope with the intensity of these experience. Such intensity demands attention but because of the fear and aversion to the situation the patients' mind might seek distraction in other thoughts. The mind goes back and forth from the intensity of fear to shallow distraction and back to fear again, thus potentiating such fear in the intimate knowledge of not being able to meet it fully. Such situations are very frustrating and energy consuming. Any effective way of aiding these patient should either help in meeting fully with the intensity of the moment or provide solid distraction so to avoid the back and forth of the mind above described. Better to rest the attention on something else than one's emotion with some continuity than spiralling in fear and fear-avoidance mechanism. The goal of helping the patient to meet fully with their fear experience is very noble but quite ambitious and broad. It is likely that the TKA perioperative phase is not the appropriate setting either. A much better choice is the second option of providing occasions of solid distraction. This is the logic of distraction as a relaxation technique objective.

Anxiety creates a set of physical modifications such as increased muscle tension, heart rate, blood pressure, respiratory rate and others. Saying that anxiety "creates" reveals a belief that the mind governs the body, but actually the two sets of phenomena simply happen together like a two-sided coin with the psychological side and the physical side. It is possible to modify the psychological side by operating on the physical. Some physical symptoms are partially voluntarily modifiable and have been the terrain of relaxation techniques. Muscle tension and breathing rate are examples (Seers et al. 2008). In both these techniques, the attention is focused on the body (and thus diverted from one's anxiety). Through alternated contraction and relaxation of muscle groups with applied awareness to the muscle activity, a lowering of muscle tension of the body at rest is achieved. Similarly, with breathing exercises, the patient actively controls the breath, depth and rhythm of breathing. At the end of the exercise, changes in breathing rhythm are noted and persist.

Some techniques approach the coin directly on the psychological side. In guided imagery, patients are invited to imagine scenes and objects that are supposed to trigger positive mind states. Music, that brings a certain emotional atmosphere with it is used for such properties. Hypnosis is a procedure by which the patient is invited to imagine an altered subjective experience and feel it as real (Tefikow et al. 2013). Some advocate the use of humour as a complementary therapy; humour has been proven to increase pain tolerance (Weisenberg et al. 1995; Walker 2002).

Music for relaxation has been extensively used in many different settings. Two different subtypes of music application have been described: "music medicine", which is the use of pre-recorded standardized music delivered via an audio device, and "music therapy", which refers to a tailored music experience prepared by a trained music therapist (Bradt 2009). The first is cheaper and more practical has been applied more often and represents an interesting option for its easy applicability. Music combines the capacity of diverting attention and that of inducing emotional states of well-being. It has been shown to have effects on anxiety, satisfaction, pain, mood and vital signs (Bradt 2009; Evans 2002; Nilsson 2008) in many different settings and patient populations (Binns-Turner et al. 2011; Bradt et al. 2013a, b; Kleiber 2012; Lin et al. 2011). Research though is not yet conclusive on the topic (Nilsson 2008).

The use of "relaxation tapes", with a combination of instructions for breath awareness and control and suggestion of peaceful images, share with music the same easy application and have been used with some success in several settings including total joint replacement (Collins et al. 1997; Topcu et al. 2012; Thomas et al. 2010; Ko et al. 2011; Lin et al 2011, Lin 2012; Rejeh et al. 2013). Regarding "relaxation tapes" it must be said that there is no consensus on how long it should last, how many times a day it should be played and, most of all, what type of instructions it should contain.

The results of the above-mentioned studies are quite modest. In our opinion they all share the limitation of no preoperative training in relaxation. The expectation of having patients relax almost on command with no preparation is very optimistic. The ability to relax is teachable and learnable, but it is likely that patients undergoing surgery are unskilled in this capacity unless they are trained in advance. Recent culture has not assigned much value to the ability to relax, and many people have forgotten how to do so. It is unreasonable to expect people, elderly more often than not, to learn to relax instantly with a 20 min tape, on the very day of their operation. In an analogy with childbearing, it would be more reasonable to teach relaxation to patients in advance the same way women are prepared to give birth in a series of lessons well before delivery.

It is likely that in the near future, a variety of complementary relaxation programs will develop. Some programs will be cost-effective with standardized interventions based on music or relaxation tapes, while others will be individually tailored, time consuming and more expensive. Likely this type of intervention will be appreciated by patients for its "human" and non-invasive quality and will higher global satisfaction.

Key Points

- Postoperative anxiety heavily conditions pain and patient satisfaction in TKA.
- Preoperative information modulates expectations and provides a feeling of control to patients regardless of their level of pain postoperatively.
- Trait anxiety and pain catastrophising tendencies can be screened preoperatively so as to dedicate more attention to specific patients with a worse preoperative prognosis.
- Relaxation techniques are a non-invasive complementary way to reduce anxiety and therefore improve patient satisfaction.

References

Binns-Turner PG et al (2011) Perioperative music and its effects on anxiety, hemodynamics, and pain in women undergoing mastectomy. AANA J 79(4 Suppl): S21–S27

Blackburn J et al (2012) Does preoperative anxiety and depression predict satisfaction after total knee replacement? Knee 19(5):522–524

Bonnin MP et al (2011) What are the factors of residual pain after uncomplicated TKA? Knee Surg Sports Traumatol Arthrosc 19(9):1411–1417

Bradt J (2009) Music for stress and anxiety reduction in coronary heart disease patients. Cochrane Database Syst Rev

Bradt J et al (2013a) Music for stress and anxiety reduction in coronary heart disease patients. Cochrane Database Syst Rev (12):CD006577

Bradt J et al (2013b) Music interventions for preoperative anxiety. Cochrane Database Syst Rev (6):CD006908

Collins JA et al (1997) Effects of relaxation intervention in phase II cardiac rehabilitation: replication and extension. Heart Lung 26(1):31–44

Daltroy H et al (1998) Preoperative education for total hip and knee replacement patients. Arthritis Care Res 11(6):469–478

Duivenvoorden T et al (2013) Anxiety and depressive symptoms before and after total hip and knee arthroplasty: a prospective multicentre study. Osteoarthritis Cartilage 21(12):1834–1840

Evans D (2002) The effectiveness of music as an intervention for hospital patients: a systematic review. J Adv Nurs 37(1):8–18

Fosså SD et al (2002) Short Form 36 and Hospital Anxiety and Depression Scale. A comparison based on patients with testicular cancer. J Psychosom Res 52(2):79–87

Gautschi OP et al (2010) Web-based audiovisual patient information system – a study of preoperative patient information in a neurosurgical department. Acta Neurochir (Wien) 152(8):1337–1341

Ghomrawi HM et al (2012) Predictors of discordance in expectations of total hip arthroplasty between patients and surgeons. In: 2012 AAOS Annual Meeting, San Francisco

Haanstra TM (2012) Systematic review: do patient expectations influence treatment outcomes in total knee and total hip arthroplasty? Health Qual Life Outcomes 10:152

Hayward J (1975) Information – a prescription against pain. Royal College of Nursing, London, UK

Hirschmann MT et al (2013) The unhappy total knee arthroplasty (TKA) patient: higher WOMAC and lower KSS in depressed patients prior and after TKA. Knee Surg Sports Traumatol Arthrosc 21(10): 2405–2411

Hughes S (2002) The effects of giving patients preoperative information. Nurs Stand 16(28):33–37

Ihedioha U et al (2013) Patient education videos for elective colorectal surgery: results of a randomized controlled trial. Colorectal Dis 15(11):1436–1441

Jlala HA et al (2010) Effect of preoperative multimedia information on perioperative anxiety in patients undergoing procedures under regional anaesthesia. Br J Anaesth 104(3):369–374

Johansson K et al (2005) Preoperative education for orthopaedic patients: systematic review. J Adv Nurs 50(2):212–223

Keulers BJ et al (2008) Surgeons underestimate their patients' desire for preoperative information. World J Surg 32(6):964–970

Kleiber C (2012) Adolescents' perceptions of music therapy following spinal fusion surgery. J Clin Nurs 22(3-4):414–422

Ko YL et al (2011) The effect of using a relaxation tape on pulse, respiration, blood pressure and anxiety levels of surgical patients. J Clin Nurs 21(5):689–697

Lin PC (2012) An evaluation of the effectiveness of relaxation therapy for patients receiving joint replacement surgery. J Clin Nurs 21(5-6):601–608
Lin PC et al (2011) Music therapy for patients receiving spine surgery. J Clin Nurs 20(7-8):960–968
Livbjerg AE et al (2013) Pre-operative patient education is associated with decreased risk of arthrofibrosis after total knee arthroplasty: a case control study. J Arthroplasty 28(8):1282–1285
Logan DE et al (2005) Is postoperative pain a self-fulfilling prophecy? Expectancy effects on postoperative pain and patient-controlled analgesia use among adolescent surgical patients. J Pediatr Psychol 30(2):187–196
McDonald S et al (2004) Pre-operative education for hip or knee replacement. Cochrane Database Syst Rev (1):CD003526
Nilsson U (2008) The anxiety- and pain-reducing effects of music interventions: a systematic review. AORN J 87(4):780–807
Noble PC et al (2006) The John Insall Award: patient expectations affect satisfaction with total knee arthroplasty. Clin Orthop Relat Res 452:35–43
Pellino TA (1997) Relationships between patient attitudes, subjective norms, perceived control, and analgesic use following elective orthopedic surgery. Res Nurs Health 20(2):97–105
Pellino TA (1998) Perceived control mediates the relationship between pain severity and patient satisfaction. J Pain Symptom Manage 15(2):110–116
Pérez-Prieto D et al (2014) Influence of depression on total knee arthroplasty outcomes. J Arthroplasty 29(1): 44–47
Pinto PR et al (2013a) Predictors of acute postsurgical pain and anxiety following primary total hip and knee arthroplasty. J Pain 14(5):502–515
Pinto PR et al (2013b) Risk factors for moderate and severe persistent pain in patients undergoing total knee and hip arthroplasty: a prospective predictive study. PLoS One 8(9):e73917
Rejeh N et al (2013) Effect of systematic relaxation techniques on anxiety and pain in older patients undergoing abdominal surgery. Int J Nurs Pract 19(5):462–470
Riddle DL et al (2010) Preoperative pain catastrophizing predicts pain outcome after knee arthroplasty. Clin Orthop Relat Res 468(3):798–806
Seers K et al (2008) Effectiveness of relaxation for postoperative pain and anxiety: randomized controlled trial. J Adv Nurs 62(6):681–688
Singh JA et al (2013) Medical and psychological comorbidity predicts poor pain outcomes after total knee arthroplasty. Rheumatology (Oxford) 52(5):916–923
Singh JA et al (2014) Predictors of pain medication use for arthroplasty pain after revision total knee arthroplasty. Rheumatology (Oxford) [Epub ahead of print]
Sullivan JL (1995) PCS the pain catastrophizing scale, user manual. Departments of Psychology, Medicine, and Neurology School of Physical and Occupational Therapy McGill University Montreal, Quebec H3A 1B1
Sullivan M et al (2009) Psychological determinants of problematic outcomes following Total Knee Arthroplasty. Pain 143(1–2):123–129
Sullivan M et al (2011) The role of presurgical expectancies in predicting pain and function one year following total knee arthroplasty. Pain 152(10):2287–2293
Tefikow S Efficacy of hypnosis in adults undergoing surgery or medical procedures: A meta-analysis of randomized controlled trials – Clinical Psychology Review
Thomas KM et al (2010) Is guided imagery effective in reducing pain and anxiety in the postoperative total joint arthroplasty patient? Orthop Nurs 29(6): 393–399
Topcu SY et al (2012) Effect of relaxation exercises on controlling postoperative pain. Pain Manag Nurs 13(1):11–17
Ulvik B et al (2008) Comparison of the Short Form 36 and the Hospital Anxiety and Depression Scale measuring emotional distress in patients admitted for elective coronary angiography. Heart Lung 37(4):286–295
Vissers MM et al (2012) Psychological factors affecting the outcome of total hip and knee arthroplasty: a systematic review. Semin Arthritis Rheum 41(4): 576–588
Walker JA (2002) Emotional and psychological preoperative preparation in adults. Br J Nurs 11(8):567–575
Walker JA (2007) What is the effect of preoperative information on patient satisfaction? Br J Nurs 16(1):27–32
Weisenberg M et al (1995) Humor as a cognitive technique for increasing pain tolerance. Pain 63:207–212

Superficial intraoperative injection

Marcaine 0.5 % (5 mg/cc)	200–400 mg
Saline	22 cc

In a recent prospective, multicenter study, pain and satisfaction were investigated in 424 patients undergoing TKA by 15 surgeons in 14 hospitals. Combining intra-articular injections with nerve blocks provided the best pain relief for the first 48 h, and these modalities with epidural anesthesia yielded higher patient satisfaction at 2 weeks after surgery (Chang and Cho 2012). Interestingly, one recent investigation of posterior approach THA with regional anesthesia found no improvement for patients receiving periarticular local anesthetic in regard to postoperative pain, length of hospital stay, or mobility (Dobie et al. 2012). An injection of a new drug with liposome-encapsulated bupivacaine may deliver local anesthesia to the tissues for 96 h (Exparel 2014). This is a drug with theoretical benefits but no published studies yet for TJA.

The patient's own centrifuged blood to create platelet-rich plasma (PRP) has been used on and in joint replacement incisions to potentially improve healing. However, one recent study shows no difference in total knee arthroplasties treated with PRP in regard to blood loss, passive range of motion, narcotic requirement, or length of hospital stay (DiIorio et al. 2012).

11.4 Postoperative Care

Scheduled postoperative pain medications and anti-inflammatories are the hallmark of any postoperative pathway. These medications work better than having only "as-needed" or "rescue" dosing, and these doses should be given before therapy sessions to help the patients mobilize. Recovery protocols differ, depending on the patient demands and the priorities of the joint replacement center.

11.4.1 Standard Protocol

The following schedule would be considered a standard protocol and could be customized for a 1- or 2-day length of stay.

Day of surgery	
2 h preop	Patient arrives
1 h preop	Preemptive pain/nausea medications (celecoxib, pregabalin, oxycodone continuous release, acetaminophen, possible scopolamine patch)
Surgery	General or spinal anesthesia including intra-articular injection
2 h post-op	Transfer out of recovery room to joint replacement floor
On floor	Attempt out of bed for a walk with therapist
19:00	Pregabalin, oxycodone CR, acetaminophen, prn Ambien or Benadryl
Overnight	Short-acting narcotics as needed
Postoperative day #1	
06:00	Out of bed to recliner with towel roll under ankle, ice on surgery site
07:00	Celecoxib, pregabalin, oxycodone CR, acetaminophen
08:00	Individual therapy
12:00	Group lunch
12:30	Short-acting narcotic
13:30	Group therapy
17:00	Dinner in room
19:00	Pregabalin, oxycodone CR, acetaminophen, prn Ambien or Benadryl
Overnight	Short-acting narcotics as needed
Postoperative day #2	
Similar to post-op day #1 with therapy focus on stairs/car/curb (Figs. 11.1–11.6) and discharge home at 15:00. Postoperative outpatient therapy starts on postoperative day #3 for gait training, range of motion, and strengthening	

11.4.2 Total Hip Replacement Protocol with No Postoperative Physical Therapy

A Danish study recently looked at "fast-track" THA with a preoperative "optimization time" of 8 weeks or less and hospital time of 4 days or less

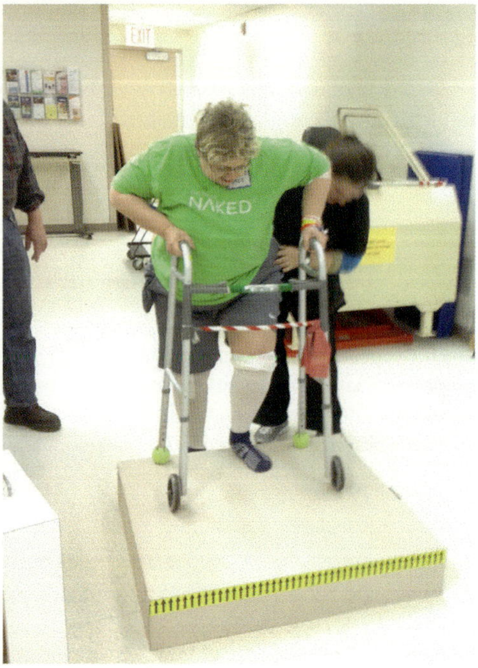

Fig. 11.1 Going up a curb

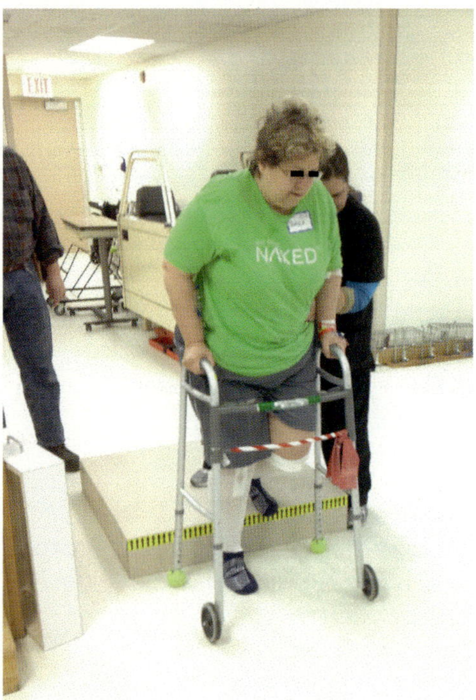

Fig. 11.2 Going down a curb

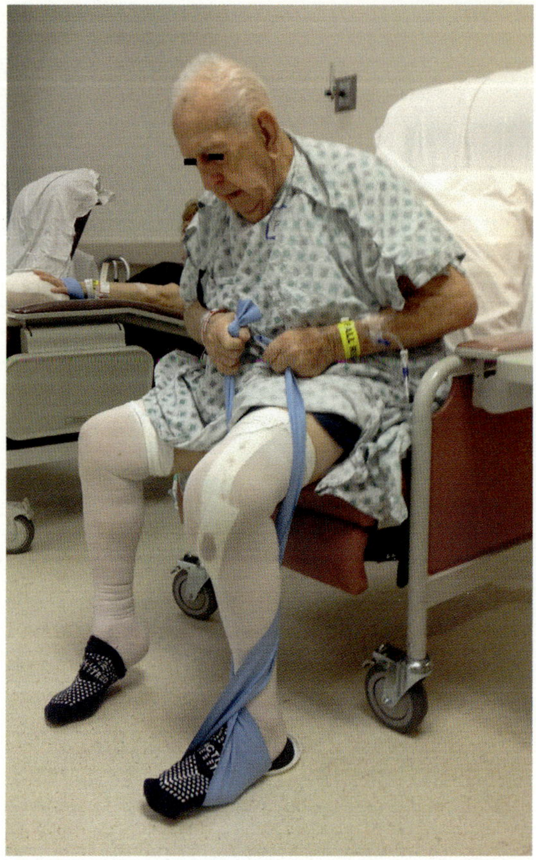

Fig. 11.3 Flexion exercises

with no formal postoperative physical therapy. This THA group achieved health-related quality-of-life scores (HRQOL) equal to that of an age- and sex-matched section of the general population at 3 months postoperatively. This could call into question the need for any postoperative therapy at all for THA (Larsen et al. 2010).

11.4.3 Surgery Center Total Joint Replacement: Same-Day Protocol

A new trend is for same-day discharge from surgery centers which requires yet another level of forethought and care coordination with motivated

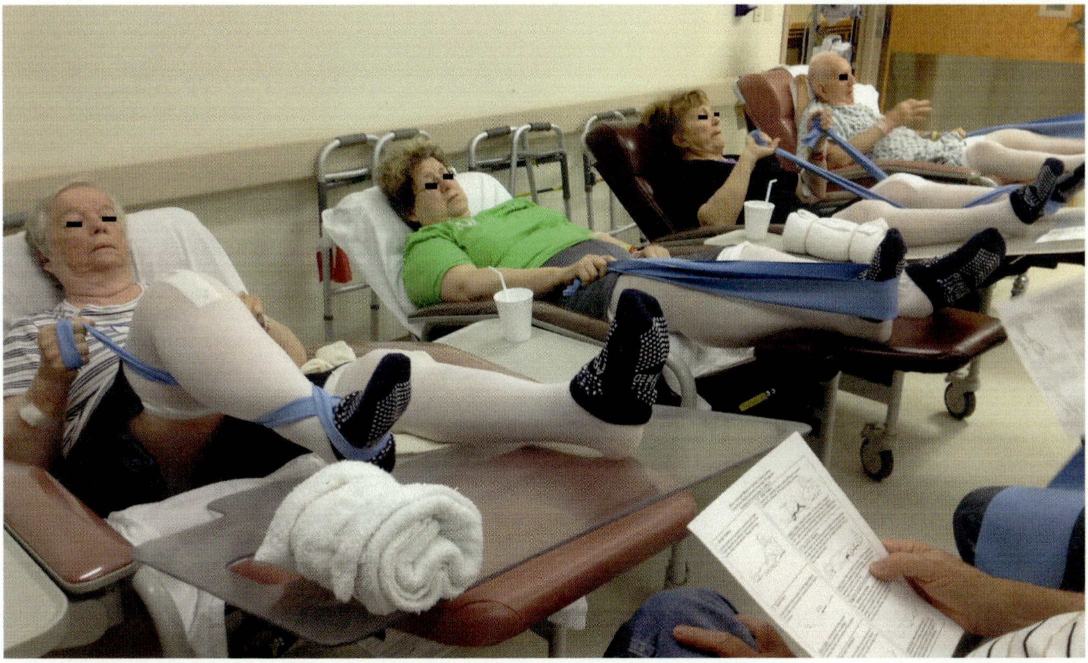

Fig. 11.4 Group therapy

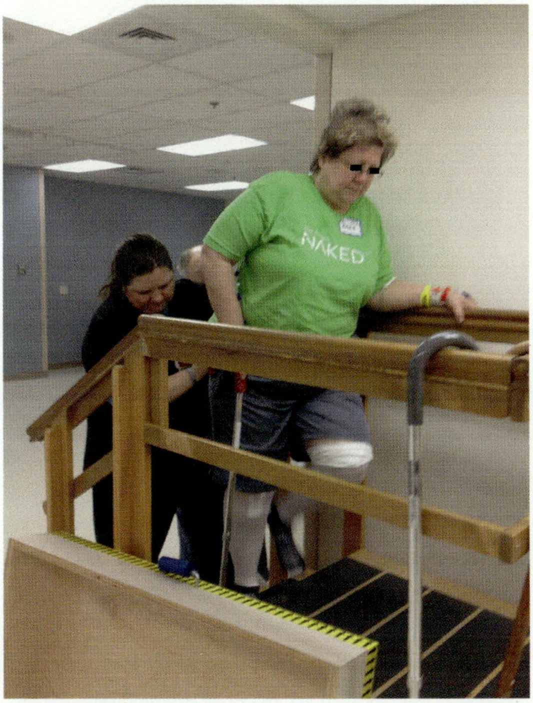

Fig. 11.5 Working on stairs

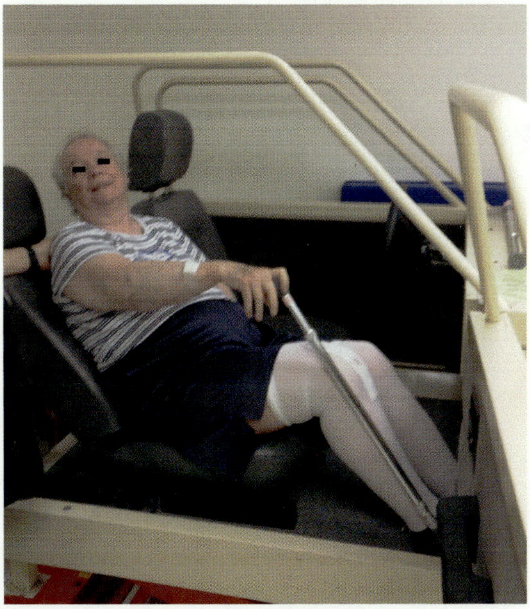

Fig. 11.6 Getting out of the practice car

and healthy patients. One surgeon has described a protocol involving careful patient selection and education with short-acting spinals for hips and adductor canal blocks for knees with general anesthesia, tranexamic acid, liposome bupivacaine, IV acetaminophen, IV steroids, and celecoxib. Unicondylar knee replacement may be an appropriate starting point when considering these protocols (Berend 2013).

11.4.4 Other Medications and Options

PCA is a method that can take pressure off of the floor nurses and can be popular with patients. However, many major centers are attempting to decrease narcotic use in postoperative patients to decrease side effects, and PCA use among these centers is less popular than in the past. Ketorolac is a very effective anti-inflammatory but only two doses should be used given the risks of gastrointestinal bleeding and nephrotoxicity.

Conclusion

Pain control is the reason patients come to see an orthopedic surgeon, and we are experts at correcting the bony anatomy and recreating functional joint surfaces. However, to provide more complete care to our surgical patients, we need to surround ourselves with the right protocols and specialists to manage the pain that accompanies these procedures. The best joint replacement centers will use a team approach to accomplish this task, but it is the surgeons who dictate the expectations and need to take control of the process. Patients will comply when told in advance what the expectations are, so each joint replacement center can decide upon their unique metrics and goals. These goals determine preferred anesthesia methods, lengths of stay, and discharge dispositions. This chapter provides a snapshot of where we are in the rapidly advancing field of total joint arthroplasty protocols in 2014, and new ideas on the horizon will make for better TJA recoveries in the future.

Key Points

- A team approach is essential to accomplish a fast recovery path after hip and knee arthroplasty.
- Patients need to be informed by the surgeons in detail what to expect and which their expectations should be.
- The surgeon should set in advance the goals that the patients should achieve during their functional recovery.
- The multimodal pain control begins preoperatively in the holding area and is continued intra- and postoperatively, taking care to keep all drugs employed below their side effect risk level.

Acknowledgments The author thanks Barbara and George Cromwell.

References

Berend K (2013) Innovations in pain management in TJA. VuMedi website
Bican O, Jacovides C, Palido L, Saunders C, Parvisi J (2011) Total knee arthroplasty in patients with fibromyalgia. J Knee Surg 24(4):265–271
Bono J, Robbins C, Mehio A, Aghazadeh M, Talmo C (2012) Pharmacologic pain management before and after total joint replacement of the hip and knee. Clin Geriatr Med 28:459–470
Booth R (2005) Podium presentation
Chan E-Y, Fransen M, Sathappan S, Chua N, Chan Y-H, Chua N (2013) Comparing the analgesia effects of single-injection and continuous femoral nerve blocks with patient controlled analgesia after total knee arthroplasty. J Arthroplasty 28:608–613
Chang C, Cho W-S (2012) Pain management protocols, peri-operative pain and patient satisfaction after total knee replacement. J Bone Joint Surg Br 94-B: 1511–1516
Dalury D, Leiberman J, MacDonald S (2011) Current and innovative pain management techniques in total knee arthroplasty. J Bone Joint Surg Am 93:1938–1943
Del Gaizo D (2013) Total hip or knee replacement in patients with chronic pain. N C Med J 74(3):218–220
DiIorio T, Burkholder J, Good R, Parvizi J, Sharkey P (2012) Platelet-rich plasma does not reduce blood loss or pain or improve range of motion after TKA. Clin Orthop Relat Res 470:138–143
Dobie I, Bennett D, Spence D, Murray J, Beverland D (2012) Periarticular local anesthesia does not improve

pain or mobility after THA. Clin Orthop Relat Res 470:1958–1965

Exparel website (2014)

Horlocker T (2010) Pain management in total joint arthroplasty: a historical review. Orthopedics 33(9 Suppl): 14–19

Larsen K, Hansen T, Soball K, Kehlet H (2010) Patient-reported outcome after fast-track hip arthroplasty: a prospective cohort study. Health Qual Life Outcomes 8:144

Liu S, Buvanendran A, Rathmell J, Sawhney M, Bae J, Moric M, Perros S, Pope A, Poultsides L, Della Valle C, Shin N, McCartney C, Ma Y, Shah M, Wood M, Manion S, Sculco T (2012) Predictors for moderate to severe acute postoperative pain after total hip and knee replacement. Int Orthop 36: 2261–2267

Macfarlane A, Prasad G, Chan V, Brull R (2009) Does regional anaesthesia improve outcome after total hip arthroplasty? A systematic review. Br J Anaesth 103: 335–345

Meftah M, Wong A, Nawabi D, Yun R, Ranawat A, Ranawat C (2012) Pain management after total knee arthroplasty using a multimodal approach. Orthopedics 35(5):e660–e664

Ng F-Y, Chiu K-Y, Yan C, Ng K-F (2012) Continuous femoral nerve block versus patient-controlled analgesia following total knee arthroplasty. J Orthop Surg 20(1):23–26

Perlas A, Kirkham K, Billing R, Tse C, Brull R, Gandhi R, Chan V (2013) The impact of analgesic modality on early ambulation following total knee arthroplasty. Reg Anesth Pain Med 38:334–339

Renner B, Walter G, Strauss J, Fromm M, Zacher J, Brune K (2012) Preoperative administration of etoricoxib in patients undergoing hip replacement causes inhibition of inflammatory mediators and pain relief. Eur J Pain 16:838–848

12 Cost-Effectiveness of the Various Modalities for Pain Control

Sandrine Wiramus, David Delahaye, Sébastien Parratte, Jacques Albanese, and Jean-Noël Argenson

Open Questions

- Which are the pharmacological means to be used in a cost-effective multimodal treatment for pain control?
- Are peripheral nerve blocks cost-effective?
- Which is the most efficient technique for peripheral nerve blocks in total knee arthroplasty?
- Is there a role for local infiltration analgesia in the ideal multimodal protocol for pain control?

S. Wiramus • J. Albanese
Department of Anaesthesiology, Hôpital de la Conception, Aix-Marseille University, 147 boulevard Baille, Marseille, 13005, France
e-mail: sandrine.wiramus@ap-hm.fr; jacques.albanese@ap-hm.fr

D. Delahaye (✉)
Department of Anaesthesiology, Hôpital Sainte-Marguerite, Aix-Marseille University, 270 boulevard de Sainte Marguerite, Marseille 13009, France
e-mail: david.delahaye@ap-hm.fr

S. Parratte • J.-N. Argenson
Department of Orthopedic Surgery, Institute for Locomotion, Aix-Marseille University, 270 boulevard de Sainte Marguerite, Marseille 13009, France
e-mail: sebastien.parratte@ap-hm.fr; jean-noel.argenson@ap-hm.fr

12.1 Introduction

Over the past 10 years, the number of patients receiving a primary arthroplasty surgery or arthroplasty recovery has increased by almost 150 % (Cram et al. 2012). A reduction of hospital length of stay has been observed following the development of the so-called minimally invasive surgery. Unfortunately, several authors using these techniques reported a significantly increased number of readmissions (Barrack et al. 2009).

In July 2000, the Joint Commission on Accreditation of Healthcare Organizations (JCAHO) introduced a new standard for pain management, declaring the pain level to be the "fifth vital sign" (Reuben and Buvanendran 2007). The commission stated that acute and chronic pain are major causes of patient displeasure in the United States health-care system, leading to slower recovery times, creating a burden for patients and their families, and increasing costs (Reuben and Buvanendran 2007). This statement is particularly true after total joint arthroplasty (Mahomed et al. 2002). Patients have high expectations regarding the outcomes of total hip arthroplasty (THA): over 75 % expect to be completely pain-free when only 40 % expect to be unlimited in their usual activities (Mahomed et al. 2002). Furthermore the postoperative pain and the length of recovery are two of the most important patient's concerns after total hip arthroplasty (Trousdale et al. 1999). Previous studies have shown that

A. Baldini, P. Caldora (eds.), *Perioperative Medical Management for Total Joint Arthroplasty: How to Control Hemostasis, Pain and Infection*, DOI 10.1007/978-3-319-07203-6_12,

postoperative pain is correlated with the quality of patient's long-term recovery (Liu and Wu 2007). To limit the surgical trauma and improve patient's recovery after arthroplasty, minimally invasive approaches have been introduced during the last decade to become a standard of care in THA (Malik and Dorr 2007). The most important factor related to the development of MIS is the development of improved perioperative pain management protocols (Nuelle and Mann 2007). Reduction in postoperative pain and hospital length of stay, carlier hospital discharge directly to home and improved patient's satisfaction have been observed (Liu and Wu 2007; Malik and Dorr 2007; Nuelle and Mann 2007; Pagnano et al. 2006). Following this trend, multimodal analgesic protocols including initially peripheral nerve blocks and more recently intra-articular anaesthetic injections have been more widely used (Liu and Wu 2007; Malik and Dorr 2007; Nuelle and Mann 2007; Pagnano et al. 2006). The goal of this paper is to evaluate the cost related to the different anaesthetic protocols.

12.2 Principles of Analgesia

In a recent study evaluating pain during the postoperative days after different surgical techniques, prosthetic replacement surgery appears to be one of the most painful surgeries. Visual analogue (pain) scale (VAS) greater than 5–6 during the first postoperative day (Gerbershagen et al. 2013) has been reported. The authors concluded that there is the need for an adequate perioperative support concerning analgesia.

In France, three protocols published by the French Society of Anaesthesiology and Intensive Care Medicine (SFAR) (Comité douleur-anesthésie locorégionale et le comité des référentiels de la Sfar 2008a; Fuzier et al. 2008) and two about regional anaesthesia (Fuzier et al. 2007) serve as guidelines for the management of perioperative pain in orthopaedic surgery. This analgesia is based on the concept of multimodal analgesia described by Kehlet in 1993 (Kehlet and Dahl 1993). The principle is to use combine agents or analgesic to optimize the balance between efficiency and side effects. In postoperative pain management, sensitization plays also an important role. This central hyperalgesic component contributes to increase pain intensity, especially under dynamic conditions. It maintains and sustains independently of peripheral nociceptive stimuli and generates postsurgical chronic pain. This central component can be treated or prevented with anti-hyperalgesic drugs without anti-nociceptive effects. These drugs are synergistic with conventional analgesics.

Each of these techniques has a specific cost, and it's important to analyse the cost-efficiency of the different analgesic techniques.

12.3 Cost of Multimodal Analgesia

12.3.1 Systemic Analgesia

12.3.1.1 Non-opioid Analgesia

The combination of several non-opioid drugs allows additive or synergistic analgesia and therefore reduced the need for opioids and consecutively their secondary and side effects (Marret et al. 2009).

Thus, it's recommended to use acetaminophen and nonsteroidal anti-inflammatory drugs, in the absence of contraindication and nefopam in combination with opioids (Marret et al. 2009). But a recent study reports that nefopam provides no additional analgesic effect in a multimodal analgesia (Remérand et al. 2013). Rebound effects of nefopam and ketamine could be the cause. Otherwise, the eviction of nefopam could reduce some postoperative side effects like acute retention of urine.

The costs of these different treatments are summarized in Table 12.1.

Ketamine

At low doses, ketamine, a non-competitive antagonist (on non-methyl-D-aspartate, NMDA), is able to limit the awareness of the central nervous system in painful animals, in healthy volunteers exposed to various models of pain and in postoperative patients. In fact, a study reported a significant decrease of the postoperative pain level and

Table 12.1 Cost of multimodal systemic analgesia: intravenous (IV) and per os (dollars)

Drugs	Cost IV	Cost per os	Cost/day IV	Cost/day per os
Paracetamol (1 g)	$1.12	$0.03	$4.47	$0.11
Ketoprofen (100 mg)	$0.98	$0.21	$2.94	$0.41
Nefopam	$0.62	$0.62	$3.73	$3.73
Ketamine 50 mg (8 mg/h)	$1.55		($5.94)	
Gabapentin (300 mg)		$0.12		$0.37

better functional recovery in patients undergoing TKA after low dose of ketamine intravenously (Adam et al. 2005). It also allows a reduction in morphine consumption after THA (Remérand et al. 2009). Ketamine is more effective with a preoperative bolus (0.1–0.5 mg/kg) followed by a continuous infusion during 48 h (2 μg/kg/min or above 5–12 mg/h). Ketamine decreases the postoperative pain in limiting both postoperative hyperalgesia after the surgical trauma and intraoperative use of high doses of opioids. This limits the use of analgesics, reduces morphine tolerance and improves the overall quality of analgesia in postoperative period (Bell et al. 2005). The cost of 50 mg of ketamine is above 1.5 dollars.

Gabapentin

Before surgery, gabapentin not only reduces morphine consumption but also the postoperative pain at rest and in dynamic conditions (Clarke et al. 2009b; Dahl et al. 2004; Hurley et al. 2006). It also improves functional recovery after orthopaedic surgery (Ménigaux et al. 2005) and prevents pruritus induced by intrathecal morphine in patients undergoing lower extremity surgery under spinal anaesthesia (Sheen et al. 2008). It's mainly due to a presynaptic blockage of calcium channel voltages dependent resulting in an anti-hyperalgesic effect. However, recent studies have shown that the effectiveness of gabapentin given preoperatively in THA (Clarke et al. 2009a) or in TKA (Paul et al. 2013) may not be as high as initially described. Currently French recommendations concerning postoperative analgesia propose to use gabapentin premedication without exceeding one daily dose of 800 mg to avoid side effects like sedation or dizziness. The cost of 300 mg gabapentin per os is $0.13.

Intravenous Lidocaine

It has been shown that the use of low doses of intravenous lidocaine before and after THA did not improve postoperative analgesia (Martin et al. 2008). Lidocaine is probably recommended for analgesia in abdominal surgery, but not in orthopaedic surgery.

12.3.1.2 Opioid Analgesia

Prosthetic joint replacement surgery is considered like a moderate to severe painful surgery, and the use of opioids called « strong » (level III of WHO) is recommended, including the use of controlled analgesia with an opioid pump device. The cost of this system is about $4,917 (amortized over 5 years with $1,530 per year and used about 260 days per year with finally an approximate daily cost of $5.9). Annual maintenance is approximately $546 and disposables such as injectable morphine are $0.9 (100 mg/10 ml), a charging pump ($18) and an adapter ($4). All disposables bring the daily cost of these morphine pumps at $29. It must be added to the nurse working time which is estimated around $16 for the installation. In conclusion the total cost for a morphine pump is about $45. The oral treatment can be provided by morphine sulphate with a total cost of $0.14 daily for 10 mg.

12.3.2 Intrathecal and Epidural Analgesia

According to the French recommendations in 2007 (Fuzier et al. 2007), epidural analgesia provides the same analgesia than peripheral nerve blocks but a better analgesia at rest and especially during mobilization than analgesia with drugs alone. However, epidural analgesia is not without risks or side effects, and the risk to benefit ratio is clearly in favour of peripheral blocks for the management of post-arthroplasty analgesia. The central blocks can induce arterial hypotension, acute retention of urine, infectious complications and headaches. They have a small benefit in terms of morbidity and mortality and a low profitability on convalescence: therefore, epidural analgesia is not indicated after lower limb arthroplasty (Fletcher and Jayr 2009). However, indications should be discussed in each case.

The cost of epidural analgesia over a period of 72 h is as follows: aseptic surgical equipment (sterile gloves, coat, operative field and compresses) ($5.1), analgesia catheter Perifix® ($11.3), tools for fixing the catheter to the skin ($2.6), syringe of 20 ml ($0.13), a vial of 20 ml of ropivacaine 0.2 % ($1.8) and a vial of 400 mg in 200 ml of ropivacaine ($9.8/ 24 h, $29.5/ 72 h): the cost of epidural analgesia for 72 h is estimated at $50, plus the cost of nursing time. That brings the final cost at a total of $16.8 per day.

Spinal anaesthesia may be used for arthroplasty surgery of the lower limb as well as to start postoperative analgesia. Indeed the use of adjuvants, such as clonidine, or liposoluble opioids can potentiate the action of local anaesthetics. The postoperative analgesic effect does not exceed 12–14 h, and the use of high doses quickly exposes to many side effects (sedation, pruritus, nausea and vomiting, acute urinary retention, hypotension). Despite a low cost, estimated at $10.5, the profitability of spinal anaesthesia in terms of postoperative analgesia seems minimal because of many side effects and a short analgesia.

12.3.3 Peripheral Analgesia

12.3.3.1 Blocks and Perineural Catheters Devices

Indications, Feasibility and Cost

According to French expert recommendations (Fuzier et al. 2007), it is recommended to use peripheral blocks for postoperative analgesia of arthroplasty surgery compared with epidural analgesia. The benefit of analgesia with peripheral blocks is also true with intravenous patient-controlled analgesia with morphine pump. Indeed perineural blocks minimize the sympathetic response to surgery, reduced postoperative pain especially during mobilization, improve analgesia during the postoperative period and increase patient's satisfaction.

Table 12.2 Cost of peripheral analgesia (dollars)

Ultrasound-guided nerve block	Cost of treatment	Cost of treatment per day
Single-shot injection	$20.85	$20.85
Perineural catheter (72 h)	$77.72	$25.91

The cost of a single ultrasound-guided peripheral nerve block injection is estimated at $20.85 including the needle, aseptic equipment, injection equipment, local anaesthetic and a set of protection of the ultrasound probe. The cost of this technique of analgesia with continuous injection of ropivacaine for 72 h is estimated at $77 (Table 12.2).

Today, it's not mandatory to use ultrasound for a peripheral nerve block (single injection or catheterization). Indeed, the evaluation of the cost-effectiveness of locoregional analgesia ultrasound guided versus neurostimulation has not yet been evaluated. The cost of an ultrasound is around $54 630 plus the prices of disposables (ultrasound gel, sterile protection of ultrasound probes, plus the cost of maintenance), while a neurostimulator costs about $1,161. Up to now, the superiority of ultrasound compared with neurostimulation on the success of locoregional anaesthesia has not been demonstrated. There is however several advantages for ultrasound: a direct visualization of the needle and of the surrounding tissue and the dissemination of local anaesthetic. Ultrasound helps to decrease time required to perform the nerve blocks, the number of needle's redirection and the number of vascular punctures and decrease the setting time of nerve blocks (Casati et al. 2007; Domingo-Triadó et al. 2007; Marhofer et al. 1998; Soeding et al. 2005). Ultrasound also allows a better understanding of the anatomical variations. There is also a decrease of complications due to systemic toxicity of local anaesthetic (Barrington and Kluger 2013). It also improves patient's satisfaction by reducing the discomfort of the nerve research by neurostimulation (Koscielniak-Nielsen et al. 2002) and by decreasing pain in trauma patient (Casati et al. 2007; Soeding et al. 2005). The impact on the risk of postoperative neuropathy is less clear, but a trend in favour of ultrasonographic techniques has been outlined (Orebaugh et al. 2012). Thus, the cost of an ultrasound remains the main limitation compared to standard neurostimulation techniques. However, a study published in 2004 reported the same cost for an infraclavicular block under ultrasound and neurostimulation (the introduction of a catheter costs only 13.90 dollars more with ultrasound) (Sandhu et al. 2004). Another study published in 2012 compared the cost- effectiveness of the analgesia produced by an ultrasound-guided popliteal sciatic catheter inserted with the same block by neurostimulation approach. The use of ultrasound is associated with a higher probability of success and reduced the costs about 84.7 % (Ehlers et al. 2012).

Hip Arthroplasty

For postoperative analgesia, a femoral nerve block with a single injection is recommended (Comité douleur-anesthésie locorégionale et le comité des référentiels de la Sfar 2008b).

Knee Arthroplasty

The debate is over: the French guidelines recommend the use of a femoral perineural catheter, probably associated with a single-injection sciatic nerve block (Comité douleur-anesthésie locorégionale et le comité des référentiels de la Sfar 2008b; Eledjam and viel 2013), while an European working group (PROSPECT Group) recommend neither a single injection nor a continuous infusion femoral nerve block because of too much heterogeneity among studies (Fischer et al. 2008).

If the implementation of a femoral nerve block, at least as a single injection, seems obvious to improve the management of acute and chronic pain after TKA, the effect of a sciatic block has to be demonstrated. Indeed, Wegener et al. (2013) did not find any significant difference in terms of functional recovery, and acute and chronic pain in patients who underwent TKA with a continuous femoral block alone or combined with a single or continuous injection sciatic nerve block. Sinha et al. (2012) found an improvement of postoperative acute pain in patients with a femoral catheter associated with a sciatic block or elective tibial block.

Thus, peripheral nerve blocks after arthroplasty surgery improve management of acute and chronic pain (Liu et al. 2012), reduce postoperative morphine consumption and improve patient's satisfaction (Fischer et al. 2008). However, the locoregional anaesthesia leads to postoperative quadriceps paresis whatever the concentration and volume of the local anaesthetic (Bauer et al. 2012). It may alter the initial functional recovery and increase the number of falls (Johnson et al. 2013).

12.3.3.2 Infiltration of Local Anaesthetic

In 2011, Kehlet performed a review of literature about analgesic infiltration after hip and knee arthroplasty (Kehlet and Andersen 2011).

This approach was first described by Bianconi et al. in 2003 (Bianconi et al. 2003): patients undergoing THA or TKA with continuous infiltration of ropivacaine in scar had better pain control than those receiving only systemic analgesia. Kerr and Kohan, in a case study of 325 patients, reported an excellent pain control after systematic periarticular infiltration with a mixture of ropivacaine associated with ketorolac and adrenaline (Kerr and Kohan 2008). Rostlund and Kehlet also described an excellent analgesia after infiltration of high doses of long-acting local anaesthetic: there was no motor block, a low morbidity and a length of hospital stay reduced (Röstlund and Kehlet 2007).

Despite positive results in many studies, the apparent simplicity and safety of the technique, Kehlet points to several methodological errors and a lack of comparison with other analgesic techniques such as peripheral nerve blocks (Kehlet and Andersen 2011). In conclusion, there is little evidence to support the use of analgesic infiltration after THA. On the contrary after TKA, the scientific data support the use of intraoperative infiltration of long-acting local anaesthetic, but not the use of a catheter for continuous infiltration of the scar. Few current data support the use of NSAIDs or adrenaline in mixtures of analgesic infiltration, although a recent study advocates the use of ketorolac (Andersen et al. 2013b).

A recent meta-analysis of Keijsers et al. (2013) concludes that infiltration of local anaesthetic improves postoperative analgesia and reduces morphine consumption on the first postoperative day after a TKA when compared to placebo. However, in a review of Fowler and Christellis (2013), the authors report that the equivalence in terms of analgesia and functional outcome is not clear between infiltration and peripheral nerve blocks. This is confirmed by the study of Carli et al. (2010): a better management of pain and improved functional recovery initially and at 6 weeks with continuous perineural femoral techniques. Otherwise many studies describe earlier and more effective ambulation when infiltration is performed as compared to a continuous femoral block (Chaumeron et al. 2013; Perlas et al. 2013; Rivière et al. 2012). A local analgesic infiltration reduces pain after TKA in the same manner as peripheral nerve block, but without motor block. However, volumes and therefore doses of local anaesthetic are more important than with locoregional anaesthesia exposing them to a potential systemic toxicity.

In addition, the duration and effectiveness of analgesia by infiltration remain insufficient compared with a continuous femoral nerve block. The latest studies report states that the combination of a catheter on the adductor feeder (continuous block of the saphenous nerve) and a local periarticular infiltration provides equivalent analgesia to a continuous femoral nerve block (Andersen et al. 2013a). It's associated with earlier ambulation and a less functional impairment of quadriceps (Jæger et al. 2013b; Jaeger et al. 2013a; Kwofie et al. 2013). However, other studies are needed before recommending this technique.

Moreover, it has also been proposed to use a liposomal bupivacaine to extend the analgesic effect of local anaesthetic. An animal study published in 2012 (Ohri et al. 2012) reported a duration of sensory block of about 40 h and a motor block about 36 h after sciatic nerve block. Thus, the use of the liposomal bupivacaine would improve analgesia by extending the duration of sensory block. If the duration of motor block is increased as well, it would compromise the initial functional recovery. It would be interesting to use this liposomal bupivacaine by infiltration as it has been recently described. However, the cost of around $283 per vial is a main limitation.

Conclusion

The control of postoperative pain after arthroplasty surgery is closely linked to the concept of multimodal analgesia. It combines first systemic drugs analgesia represented by paracetamol, NSAIDs, gabapentin and ketamine, associated or not with opioid analgesia. This approach is cost-effective too. In addition, locoregional analgesia may play a role. The recommendations on which type of locoregional analgesia are still not completely clear, especially those regarding knee arthroplasty procedures. However, the cost-effectiveness study of these techniques has shown that the use of ultrasonographic techniques for perineural analgesia may be valuable. The most significant point is that the cost of the multimodal analgesia is minimal and largely compensated by the savings obtained through a shorter hospital stay.

Key Points

- Postoperative pain control is overall a cost-effective practice to be implemented in every arthroplasty service.
- Systemic drug analgesia and locoregional anaesthesia are the pillar of a multimodal pain control regimen.
- Cost-effectiveness of different locoregional anaesthesia techniques is still under scrutiny.
- Peripheral nerve block has a clear role in multimodal analgesia. The efficacy and safety of continuous perineural infusion of anaesthetics remain to be

determined. Further studies are required before finalizing the recommendations for different techniques of local anaesthetic infiltrations.

References

Adam F, Chauvin M, Du Manoir B, Langlois M, Sessler DI, Fletcher D (2005) Small-dose ketamine infusion improves postoperative analgesia and rehabilitation after total knee arthroplasty. Anesth Analg 100:475–480

Andersen HL, Gyrn J, Møller L, Christensen B, Zaric D (2013a) Continuous saphenous nerve block as supplement to single-dose local infiltration analgesia for postoperative pain management after total knee arthroplasty. Reg Anesth Pain Med 38:106–111

Andersen KV, Nikolajsen L, Haraldsted V, Odgaard A, Søballe K (2013b) Local infiltration analgesia for total knee arthroplasty: should ketorolac be added? Br J Anaesth 111:242–248

Barrack RL, Barnes CL, Burnett RS, Miller D, Clohisy JC, Maloney WJ (2009) Minimal incision surgery as a risk factor for early failure of total knee arthroplasty. J Arthroplasty 24(4):489–498

Barrington MJ, Kluger R (2013) Ultrasound guidance reduces the risk of local anesthetic systemic toxicity following peripheral nerve blockade. Reg Anesth Pain Med 38:289–297

Bauer M, Wang L, Onibonoje OK, Parrett C, Sessler DI, Mounir-Soliman L, Zaky S, Krebs V, Buller LT, Donohue MC, Stevens-Lapsley JE, Ilfeld BM (2012) Continuous femoral nerve blocks: decreasing local anesthetic concentration to minimize quadriceps femoris weakness. Anesthesiology 116:665–672

Bell RF, Dahl JB, Moore RA, Kalso E (2005) Peri-operative ketamine for acute post-operative pain: a quantitative and qualitative systematic review (Cochrane review). Acta Anaesthesiol Scand 49:1405–1428

Bianconi M, Ferraro L, Traina GC, Zanoli G, Antonelli T, Guberti A, Ricci R, Massari L (2003) Pharmacokinetics and efficacy of ropivacaine continuous wound instillation after joint replacement surgery. Br J Anaesth 91:830–835

Carli F, Clemente A, Asenjo JF, Kim DJ, Mistraletti G, Gomarasca M, Morabito A, Tanzer M (2010) Analgesia and functional outcome after total knee arthroplasty: periarticular infiltration vs continuous femoral nerve block. Br J Anaesth 105:185–195

Casati A, Danelli G, Baciarello M, Corradi M, Leone S, Di Cianni S, Fanelli G (2007) A prospective, randomized comparison between ultrasound and nerve stimulation guidance for multiple injection axillary brachial plexus block. Anesthesiology 106:992–996

Chaumeron A, Audy D, Drolet P, Lavigne M, Vendittoli P-A (2013) Periarticular injection in knee arthroplasty improves quadriceps function. Clin Orthop 471:2284–2295

Clarke H, Pereira S, Kennedy D, Andrion J, Mitsakakis N, Gollish J, Katz J, Kay J (2009a) Adding gabapentin to a multimodal regimen does not reduce acute pain, opioid consumption or chronic pain after total hip arthroplasty. Acta Anaesthesiol Scand 53:1073–1083

Clarke H, Pereira S, Kennedy D, Gilron I, Katz J, Gollish J, Kay J (2009b) Gabapentin decreases morphine consumption and improves functional recovery following total knee arthroplasty. Pain Res Manag 14:217–222

Cram P, Lu X, Kates SL, Singh JA, Li Y, Wolf BR (2012) Total knee arthroplasty volume, utilization, and outcomes among Medicare beneficiaries, 1991-2010. JAMA 308:1227–1236

Dahl JB, Mathiesen O, Møiniche S (2004) "Protective premedication": an option with gabapentin and related drugs? A review of gabapentin and pregabalin in the treatment of post-operative pain. Acta Anaesthesiol Scand 48:1130–1136

Comité douleur-anesthésie locorégionale et le comité des référentiels de la Sfar, (2008a) Formalized recommendations of experts 2008. Management of postoperative pain in adults and children. Ann Fr Anesth Rèanim 27:1035–1041

Comité douleur-anesthésie locorégionale et le comité des référentiels de la Sfar, (2008b) Formalized recommendations of experts 2008. Management of postoperative pain in adults and children. Ann Fr Anesth Rèanim 27:1035–1041

Domingo-Triadó V, Selfa S, Martínez F, Sánchez-Contreras D, Reche M, Tecles J, Crespo MT, Palanca JM, Moro B (2007) Ultrasound guidance for lateral midfemoral sciatic nerve block: a prospective, comparative, randomized study. Anesth Analg 104:1270–1274, tables of contents

Ehlers L, Jensen JM, Bendtsen TF (2012) Cost-effectiveness of ultrasound vs nerve stimulation guidance for continuous sciatic nerve block. Br J Anaesth 109:804–808

Eledjam JJ, viel E (2013) Les blocs périphériques des membres chez l'adulte. Recommandadtions pour la pratique clinique de la Société Française d'Anesthésie et de Réanimation

Fischer HBJ, Simanski CJP, Sharp C, Bonnet F, Camu F, Neugebauer EAM, Rawal N, Joshi GP, Schug SA, Kehlet H, PROSPECT Working Group (2008) A procedure-specific systematic review and consensus recommendations for postoperative analgesia following total knee arthroplasty. Anaesthesia 63:1105–1123

Fletcher D, Jayr C (2009) Indications for postoperative epidural analgesia. Ann Fr Anesth Rèanim 28:e95–e124

Fowler SJ, Christelis N (2013) High volume local infiltration analgesia compared to peripheral nerve block for hip and knee arthroplasty-what is the evidence? Anaesth Intensive Care 41:458–462

Fuzier R, Cuvillon P, Delcourt J, Lupescu R, Bonnemaison J, Bloc S, Theissen A, Berthou P, Malassine P, Richez A-S (2007) Peripheral nerve block in orthopaedic surgery: multicentric evaluation of practicing professionals and impact on the activity of the recovery room. Ann Fr Anesth Rèanim 26:761–768

Fuzier R, Belbachir A, Gall O, Keïta H (2008) comité douleur et anesthésie locorégionale de Société française d'anesthésie et de réanimation, 2008. Postoperative analgesia in "particular situations". Practical recommendations. Ann Fr Anesth Rèanim 27:966–968

Gerbershagen HJ, Aduckathil S, van Wijck AJM, Peelen LM, Kalkman CJ, Meissner W (2013) Pain intensity on the first day after surgery: a prospective cohort study comparing 179 surgical procedures. Anesthesiology 118:934–944

Hurley RW, Cohen SP, Williams KA, Rowlingson AJ, Wu CL (2006) The analgesic effects of perioperative gabapentin on postoperative pain: a meta-analysis. Reg Anesth Pain Med 31:237–247

Jaeger P, Nielsen ZJK, Henningsen MH, Hilsted KL, Mathiesen O, Dahl JB (2013a) Adductor canal block versus femoral nerve block and quadriceps strength: a randomized, double-blind, placebo-controlled, crossover study in healthy volunteers. Anesthesiology 118:409–415

Jæger P, Zaric D, Fomsgaard JS, Hilsted KL, Bjerregaard J, Gyrn J, Mathiesen O, Larsen TK, Dahl JB (2013b) Adductor canal block versus femoral nerve block for analgesia after total knee arthroplasty: a randomized, double-blind study. Reg Anesth Pain Med 38:526–532

Johnson RL, Kopp SL, Hebl JR, Erwin PJ, Mantilla CB (2013) Falls and major orthopaedic surgery with peripheral nerve blockade: a systematic review and meta-analysis. Br J Anaesth 110:518–528

Kehlet H, Andersen LØ (2011) Local infiltration analgesia in joint replacement: the evidence and recommendations for clinical practice. Acta Anaesthesiol Scand 55:778–784

Kehlet H, Dahl JB (1993) The value of "multimodal" or "balanced analgesia" in postoperative pain treatment. Anesth Analg 77:1048–1056

Keijsers R, van Delft R, van den Bekerom MPJ, de Vries DCAA, Brohet RM, Nolte PA (2013) Local infiltration analgesia following total knee arthroplasty: effect on post-operative pain and opioid consumption-a meta-analysis. Knee Surg Sports Traumatol Arthrosc, Nov 30. [Epub ahead of print]

Kerr DR, Kohan L (2008) Local infiltration analgesia: a technique for the control of acute postoperative pain following knee and hip surgery: a case study of 325 patients. Acta Orthop 79:174–183

Koscielniak-Nielsen ZJ, Rotbøll-Nielsen P, Rassmussen H (2002) Patients' experiences with multiple stimulation axillary block for fast-track ambulatory hand surgery. Acta Anaesthesiol Scand 46:789–793

Kwofie MK, Shastri UD, Gadsden JC, Sinha SK, Abrams JH, Xu D, Salviz EA (2013) The effects of ultrasound-guided adductor canal block versus femoral nerve block on quadriceps strength and fall risk: a blinded, randomized trial of volunteers. Reg Anesth Pain Med 38:321–325

Liu SS, Wu CL (2007) The effect of analgesic technique on postoperative patient-reported outcomes including analgesia: a systematic review. Anesth Analg 105:789–808

Liu SS, Buvanendran A, Rathmell JP, Sawhney M, Bae JJ, Moric M, Perros S, Pope AJ, Poultsides L, Della Valle CJ, Shin NS, McCartney CJL, Ma Y, Shah M, Wood MJ, Manion SC, Sculco TP (2012) A cross-sectional survey on prevalence and risk factors for persistent postsurgical pain 1 year after total hip and knee replacement. Reg Anesth Pain Med 37:415–422

Mahomed NN, Liang MH, Cook EF, Daltroy LH, Fortin PR, Fossel AH, Katz JN (2002) The importance of patient expectations in predicting functional outcomes after total joint arthroplasty. J Rheumatol 29:1273–1279

Malik A, Dorr LD (2007) The science of minimally invasive total hip arthroplasty. Clin Orthop 463:74–84

Marhofer P, Schrögendorfer K, Wallner T, Koinig H, Mayer N, Kapral S (1998) Ultrasonographic guidance reduces the amount of local anesthetic for 3-in-1 blocks. Reg Anesth Pain Med 23:584–588

Marret E, Beloeil H, Lejus C (2009) What are the benefits and risk of non-opioid analgesics combined with postoperative opioids? Ann Fr Anesth Rèanim 28:e135–e151

Martin F, Cherif K, Gentili ME, Enel D, Abe E, Alvarez JC, Mazoit JX, Chauvin M, Bouhassira D, Fletcher D (2008) Lack of impact of intravenous lidocaine on analgesia, functional recovery, and nociceptive pain threshold after total hip arthroplasty. Anesthesiology 109:118–123

Ménigaux C, Adam F, Guignard B, Sessler DI, Chauvin M (2005) Preoperative gabapentin decreases anxiety and improves early functional recovery from knee surgery. Anesth Analg 100:1394–1399, table of contents

Nuelle DG, Mann K (2007) Minimal incision protocols for anesthesia, pain management, and physical therapy with standard incisions in hip and knee arthroplasties: the effect on early outcomes. J Arthroplasty 22:20–25

Ohri R, Blaskovich P, Wang JC-F, Pham L, Nichols G, Hildebrand W, Costa D, Scarborough N, Herman C, Strichartz G (2012) Prolonged nerve block by microencapsulated bupivacaine prevents acute postoperative pain in rats. Reg Anesth Pain Med 37:607–615

Orebaugh SL, Kentor ML, Williams BA (2012) Adverse outcomes associated with nerve stimulator-guided and ultrasound-guided peripheral nerve blocks by supervised trainees: update of a single-site database. Reg Anesth Pain Med 37:577–582

Pagnano MW, Hebl J, Horlocker T (2006) Assuring a painless total hip arthroplasty: a multimodal approach emphasizing peripheral nerve blocks. J Arthroplasty 21:80–84

Paul JE, Nantha-Aree M, Buckley N, Cheng J, Thabane L, Tidy A, DeBeer J, Winemaker M, Wismer D, Punthakee D, Avram V (2013) Gabapentin does not improve multimodal analgesia outcomes for total knee arthroplasty: a randomized controlled trial. Can J Anaesth 60:423–431

Perlas A, Kirkham KR, Billing R, Tse C, Brull R, Gandhi R, Chan VWS (2013) The impact of analgesic modality on early ambulation following total knee arthroplasty. Reg Anesth Pain Med 38:334–339

Remérand F, Le Tendre C, Baud A, Couvret C, Pourrat X, Favard L, Laffon M, Fusciardi J (2009) The early and delayed analgesic effects of ketamine after total hip arthroplasty: a prospective, randomized, controlled, double-blind study. Anesth Analg 109:1963–1971

Remérand F, Le Tendre C, Rosset P, Peru R, Favard L, Pourrat X, Laffon M, Fusciardi J (2013) Nefopam after total hip arthroplasty: role in multimodal analgesia. Orthop Traumatol Surg Res 99:169–174

Reuben SS, Buvanendran A (2007) Preventing the development of chronic pain after orthopaedic surgery with preventive multimodal analgesic techniques. J Bone Joint Surg Am 89:1343–1358

Rivière C, Chaumeron A, Rivière C, Lacasse M-Ê, Audy D, Drolet P, Lavigne M, Vendittoli P-A (2012) Bloc analgésique crural continu versus infiltration périarticulaire lors PTG: une étude randomisée et en double insu. Rev Chir Orthop Traumatol 98:S292

Röstlund T, Kehlet H (2007) High-dose local infiltration analgesia after hip and knee replacement–what is it, why does it work, and what are the future challenges? Acta Orthop 78:159–161

Sandhu NS, Sidhu DS, Capan LM (2004) The cost comparison of infraclavicular brachial plexus block by nerve stimulator and ultrasound guidance. Anesth Analg 98:267–268

Sheen MJ, Ho S-T, Lee C-H, Tsung Y-C, Chang F-L (2008) Preoperative gabapentin prevents intrathecal morphine-induced pruritus after orthopedic surgery. Anesth Analg 106:1868–1872

Sinha SK, Abrams JH, Arumugam S, D'Alessio J, Freitas DG, Barnett JT, Weller RS (2012) Femoral nerve block with selective tibial nerve block provides effective analgesia without foot drop after total knee arthroplasty: a prospective, randomized, observer-blinded study. Anesth Analg 115:202–206

Soeding PE, Sha S, Royse CE, Marks P, Hoy G, Royse AG (2005) A randomized trial of ultrasound-guided brachial plexus anaesthesia in upper limb surgery. Anaesth Intensive Care 33:719–725

Trousdale RT, McGrory BJ, Berry DJ, Becker MW, Harmsen WS (1999) Patients' concerns prior to undergoing total hip and total knee arthroplasty. Mayo Clin Proc 74:978–982

Wegener JT, van Ooij B, van Dijk CN, Karayeva SA, Hollmann MW, Preckel B, Stevens MF (2013) Long-term pain and functional disability after total knee arthroplasty with and without single-injection or continuous sciatic nerve block in addition to continuous femoral nerve block: a prospective, 1-year follow-up of a randomized controlled trial. Reg Anesth Pain Med 38:58–63

Pain After Knee Arthroplasty: An Ongoing Battle

13

Irina Grosu, Patricia Lavand'homme, and Emmanuel Thienpont

Open Questions

- How significant is the incidence of moderate-to-severe postoperative pain in TKA?
- Who is at risk for postoperative persistent pain after TKA?
- How do we identify patients who will catastrophise postoperative pain?
- Which is the role of non-opioids adjuvants for pain control?
- What does prehabilitation means?

13.1 Introduction

Pain, either acute or chronic, is the most frequent reason for patients to look for medical help and is probably one of the most common clinical problems faced by orthopaedic surgeons, especially those performing (knee) arthroplasty (Cross et al. 2006). A recent prospective cohort study compared 179 surgical procedures in 50,523 patients. The 40 procedures with the highest pain scores included 22 orthopaedic procedures on the extremities (Gerbershagen et al. 2013). Total knee arthroplasty (TKA) carries a high risk of severe acute postoperative pain with immediate implications on the patients' recovery and their ability to participate in fast-track rehabilitation programmes (Carli et al. 2010a). The persistence of pain after surgical procedures or trauma has become a major focus of interest and its prevention now represents a challenge for caregivers as an index for health cares' quality (Apfelbaum et al. 2003; Grosu and de Kock 2011). Although many studies have demonstrated improved pain, function and quality of life after TKA, up to 20% of the patients are actually not satisfied, chronic postsurgical pain (CPSP), present at 6 months and later, being the principal cause of dissatisfaction (Carli et al. 2010a). Therefore, real efforts should be made to improve perioperative pain management for TKA (Carli et al. 2010a). However, pain is a multifactorial and complex process that is defined as "an unpleasant sensory and emotional experience associated with actual or potential tissue damage" (Merskey 1994). The only way to develop effective strategies aiming to improve acute postoperative pain and to prevent the development of persistent pain is to better understand the mechanisms involved in pain after TKA and its risk factors (Grosu et al. 2014).

I. Grosu (✉) • P. Lavand'homme • E. Thienpont
Department of Anesthesiology,
Cliniques Universitaires St Luc,
Avenue Hippocrate, Brussels, 1200, Belgium
e-mail: irina.grosu@uclouvain.be;
patricia.lavandhomme@uclouvain.com;
emmanuel.thienpont@uclouvain.be

A. Baldini, P. Caldora (eds.), *Perioperative Medical Management for Total Joint Arthroplasty: How to Control Hemostasis, Pain and Infection*, DOI 10.1007/978-3-319-07203-6_13,

13.2 Pain Mechanisms in TKA

13.2.1 Incisional Pain

Incisional pain is a common form of acute pain resulting from nociceptive, ischaemic and inflammatory mechanisms as well as nerve damage. Different tissues, i.e. bone, viscera and muscle, display unique responses to incision (Brennan 2011). Tissue injury and local inflammation induce an enhanced response to subsequent noxious stimuli (*hyperalgesia*) and innocuous stimuli (*allodynia*). This exaggerated response is caused partly by sensitisation of the peripheral nociceptors (*peripheral sensitisation*) and partly by initiation of a facilitated state of pain processing into the spinal cord and higher in the central nervous system (*central sensitisation*) (Woolf 2011). Hyperalgesia participates to postoperative pain as enhanced pain is perceived not only at the wound site (*primary hyperalgesia*) but also at a distance of the operation site (*secondary hyperalgesia*).

The development of experimental models of incisional pain, both in animal (Brennan 2011) and in humans (Andersen et al. 2009), has strongly improved our understanding of postoperative pain. Firstly, these models have shown the major contribution of the peripheral sensitisation process in acute postoperative pain in contrast with chronic inflammatory or neuropathic models where central sensitisation predominates. Deep tissue lesions particularly account for the increased spontaneous activity of nociceptors and hence spinal sensitisation process. Therefore, reducing the amount of deep tissue injury rather than the length of the skin incision allows to decrease postoperative pain and opioid use as demonstrated after hip surgery (Ogonda et al. 2005). Furthermore, the use of adapted minimally invasive surgical approaches has shown faster recovery in TKA (Thienpont 2013a, b). Secondly, there is a prominent role of peripheral nociceptive afferents not only in initiating but also in maintaining central nervous system sensitisation across the perioperative period. This explains the deceiving short-lived benefits of "pre-emptive analgesia" observed in clinical practice.

Thirdly, the peripheral nociceptive inputs trigger a prolonged increase in the excitability and synaptic efficacy of neurons in central nociceptive pathways. In other words, nociceptive inputs from the wound are amplified by central mechanisms, a phenomenon called *central sensitisation or pain memory* (Woolf 2011). Although central sensitisation participates to the postoperative pain experience, it seems to play an even more striking role in the persistence of pain after surgery. As demonstrated in animal models and also in human volunteers, when it has fully developed, central sensitisation may even become independent of peripheral inputs (Kawamata et al. 2002). The aforementioned findings argue for the use of perioperative preventive-protective strategies to prevent the development of central sensitisation, hence the risk to develop chronic postsurgical pain.

13.2.2 Peripheral Sensitisation After TKA

Tissue trauma induces both local and systemic inflammatory responses that are proportional to the severity of the injury. These inflammatory processes are considered essential for the recovery from the injury although some aspects might be potentially detrimental because released inflammatory mediators may also act on distant organs (kidneys, heart and brain) (Nicholson and Hall 2011). As incisional pain relies on peripheral sensitisation processes, local inflammation drives postoperative pain. Besides the inflammatory mediators released from damaged cells (histamine, bradykinin, etc.), immune cells attracted to the site of injury (polymorphonuclear cells (PMNs), macrophages, etc.) release proinflammatory cytokines (TNF-α, IL-1β, IL-6) which in turn increase from 10- to 80-fold the intracellular expression of inducible cyclooxygenase (COX)-2 in monocytes, macrophages, fibroblasts, chondrocytes and endothelial cells. It is now admitted that constitutive COX-1 is responsible for the initial production of prostaglandins (PGs) and inducible COX-2 is activated with the progression of inflammatory reaction (Khan et al. 2007). After 6 h, it seems that the role of COX-2 is ended, and the subsequent release of local PGs is related to COX-1 (Muscara et al. 2000). Among the prostaglandins released, prostaglandin E2 (PGE2) plays a key role by acting as a pro-nociceptive and hyperalgesic mediator to sensitise both the central and the peripheral nervous systems. Indeed, PGE2 modulates nociceptive signals at multiple sites in the pain pathway. High levels of PGE2 in the wound are correlated not only with postoperative pain but also with poor recovery after major orthopaedic surgery (Buvanendran et al. 2006). These high levels of PGE2 may already be present in patients who will undergo major joint surgery as demonstrated for other inflammatory mediators (IL 1, TNF alpha, IL 6) found routinely in synovial fluids of patients suffering from inflammatory joint diseases (Omoigui 2007a, b).

Furthermore, recent advances highlighted a less known component of the local inflammatory reaction, which is the resolution of inflammation, a both pro-resolving and anti-inflammatory process that occurs spontaneously and results in the recovery of acute inflammation. Resolution of acute inflammation is an active process, which involves pro-resolving lipid mediators, like lipoxins, protectins, maresins and resolvins (Serhan et al. 2008). Resolvin D1, aspirin-triggered resolvin D1 and resolvin E1 are a new family of pro-resolution mediators, biosynthesised from the omega-3 fatty acids by the action of several enzymes, COX-2 being one of them. Interestingly and with possible implications on the postoperative management, it has been shown in a rat model of inflammation that the COX-2 inhibitor NS-398 reduced inflammation at 2 h but enhanced it at 48 h (Gilroy et al. 1999; Xu et al. 2010). Resolvins exert their anti-inflammatory actions by promoting the phagocytic activity of macrophages and via peripheral and central actions (Xu et al. 2010).

Besides inflammatory mediators, incision in animal models also induced an increase in local lactate concentration to which the nociceptors exhibit greater sensitivity. This suggests that an ischaemic-like signal might contribute to incisional pain (Xu and Brennan 2011).

In the perioperative period, local inflammation is accompanied by a marked systemic response, i.e. the stress response to surgery, involving neuroendocrine and inflammatory components. Cortisol level is augmented, and C-reactive protein (CRP) concentration increases 24 h after surgery and peaks around 48 and 72 h (Bagry et al. 2008). Interleukin-6 (IL-6) is the most reliable marker of the stress response to surgery as IL-6 concentrations correlate with the degree of tissue injury. In patients undergoing unilateral or bilateral TKA, significantly higher IL-6 levels were found after bilateral TKA (Kugisaki et al. 2009).

13.2.3 Central Sensitisation After TKA

Within 3–6 h after tissue injury, peripheral nociceptive inputs from the surgical area will drive the spinal expression of COX-1 (in microglial cells) as well as that of COX-2 (in neurons). The spinal inflammatory reaction enhances the production of excitatory neurotransmitters (NTM) like glutamate and substance P in the spinal cord and reduces the effectiveness of inhibitory NTM like glycine (Buvanendran et al. 2012). Activation of N-methyl-D-aspartate (NMDA) receptors by glutamate, an excitatory neurotransmitter, plays an important role in the induction and maintenance of central sensitisation and the development of chronic pain. Besides the production of excitatory transmitters by spinal neurons, recent findings also point to the role of glial cells, i.e. microglia (central "immune cells") and astrocytes ("supportive cells" of neurons) present in the spinal cord and the brain in the genesis of central sensitisation in a context of inflammatory pain. Glial production of proinflammatory cytokines like TNF-α and IL-1β drives central sensitisation by increasing excitatory processes and by decreasing inhibitory ones in dorsal horn neurons (Kawasaki et al. 2008). After TKA, central inflammatory reaction in the central nervous system goes along with peripheral inflammation at the wound site. Their additive effects account for the severity of postoperative pain. It is worth noting also that numerous patients undergoing major orthopaedic procedures experience moderate-to-severe preoperative pain for months and sometimes years before surgery. Hyperalgesia and the presence of both peripheral and central states of sensitisation have been demonstrated in patients suffering from painful knee osteoarthritis (Arendt-Nielsen et al. 2010; Suokas et al. 2012). Interestingly, these pathological processes of somatosensory perception may normalise following successful surgical treatment as found in pain-free patients after TKA (Kosek and Ordeberg 2000b; Skou et al. 2013).

13.3 Postoperative Pain After TKA

13.3.1 Incidence and Characteristics of Acute Pain After TKA

Besides suffering and discomfort, severe unrelieved postoperative pain delays rehabilitation, increases the length of hospital stay and is currently considered as the most striking risk factor for the development of persistent postsurgical pain. Despite the variety of analgesic protocols and techniques developed in order to improve postoperative pain control, the prevalence of moderate-to-severe postoperative pain has remained unchanged for more than 10 years (Breivik and Stubhaug 2008). During the first 24 h after surgery, around 30 % of the patients, both hospitalised and ambulatory patients, report severe pain (visual analogue scale (VAS) score of 6 or higher on a scale from 0 (no pain) to 10 (the worst pain possible)), particularly during mobilisation (Fletcher et al. 2008). Almost 15 % of the patients still present with moderate or severe pain on days 3 and 4, emphasising the need for more efficacious analgesia protocols (Table 13.1) (Sommer et al. 2008). As a matter of fact, the percentage of patients with severe pain after TKA is even greater than reported for all surgical patients together or for patients who have undergone hip arthroplasty (Thomas et al. 1998; Wylde et al. 2011c). More importantly, the severity of pain seems to remain very constant after TKA by contrast with the rapid decrease observed in postoperative pain severity after hip arthroplasty.

As the goal of TKA is usually to improve patient's mobility, it is important to assess postoperative pain associated with rehabilitation and therefore to make a distinction between pain at rest (PAR or stimulus-independent pain) and movement-evoked pain (MEP or stimulus-dependent pain). Although MEP is only reported in less than 40 % of published clinical trials, these articles suggest that MEP is 95–226 % more intense than PAR in the first 3 postoperative days. In a recent systematic review, MEP after TKA was found to be 95, 150 and 156 % more intense than PAR in the first, second and third postoperative day, respectively (Srikandarajah and Gilron 2011). Such findings raise important concerns. First, distinct mechanisms underlie MEP and PAR, which will respond differently to analgesic treatment. By example, although opioids are relatively ineffective to alleviate MEP in the early postsurgical period, they still remain the standard rescue drug for moderate-to-severe postoperative pain. Second, besides deleterious effects upon the patient's functional recovery, especially in fast-track rehabilitation protocols with early mobilisation, MEP as poorly relieved pain might enhance central sensitisation process and thereby might increase the risk for persistent postsurgical pain.

Table 13.1 Incidence of moderate-to-severe pain[a] after TKA by comparison with all surgeries in a general population

	Day 1	Day 3	Day 30	3 months and over	Neuropathic features
All surgeries	30 %	12 %	8–10 %	18.3 %	24 % (7–51 %)
TKA	58 %	45 %	52 % 16 % severe pain	20 % (10–34 %)	6 %

[a]Moderate-to-severe pain: defined as a pain score >4 on a scale from 0 to 10 (0, no pain; 10, worst pain). Acute postoperative pain (day 1 and day 3), subacute pain (day 30) and chronic postsurgical pain (3 months and later)

As many as 44–57 % of the patients are woken by pain during the first 3 days after TKA (Wylde et al. 2011c). In turn, sleep deprivation reduces pain thresholds yielding to a vicious circle. Sleep disturbance and postoperative pain are independent predictors of persistent functional limitations at 1 and 3 months after TKA (Cremeans-Smith et al. 2006).

13.3.2 Predictive Factors for Severe Postoperative Pain

Several studies have been dedicated to find predictive risk factors for severe acute postoperative pain after various surgical procedures. Targeting patients at risk for severe acute pain should allow adopting specific measures directed to provide more appropriate perioperative analgesic protocols for these selected patients.

Kalkman et al. were among the first authors to stress the preoperative factors accounting for severe postoperative pain immediately after recovery from anaesthesia: younger age, female gender, level of preoperative pain, incision size and type of surgery (Kalkman et al. 2003). A recent systematic review highlights preoperative pain, anxiety, age and type of surgery as significant predictors of severe postoperative pain during hospital stay after heterogeneous surgical procedures (Ip et al. 2009). More focused on TKA, Thomas et al. had already demonstrated that female gender, younger age and high preoperative pain severity were strongly involved not only in acute postoperative pain severity but also in satisfaction after major orthopaedic procedures (Thomas et al. 1998).

Preoperative pain at the surgical site concerns a large number of the patients referred for surgery (63 % of patients, duration more than 1 year for 36 % of them) (Fletcher et al. 2008) and is documented as an important predictor in several large studies (Kalkman et al. 2003; Sommer et al. 2010). Patients addressed for TKA are particularly concerned because 40 % of patients justify their decision by the desire to reduce pain and 95 % of patients undergoing TKA suffer from osteoarthritis, a painful, degenerative condition (Singh et al. 2008). Preoperative arthritic pain may act as an "algesic priming" for patients going through surgery with both physiological and psychological implications. Preoperative pain related to continuous and intense nociceptive inputs from damaged joints may have sensitised the central nervous system, a status that will be further enhanced or at least maintained by the peripheral sensitisation process from the surgical wound (Woolf 2012). Severe and long-lasting preoperative pain, e.g. osteoarthritis, causes abnormalities of somatosensory perception and modifies the balance between endogenous excitatory and inhibitory processing of pain modulation (Arendt-Nielsen et al. 2010; Kosek and Ordeberg 2000a). Moreover, the presence of chronic pain before surgery is often associated with a chronic intake of analgesics including opioids and antidepressant and anxiolytic drugs that may influence the central sensitisation process (Aubrun et al. 2008). Exposure to *opioids* induces a state of central sensitisation called "opioid-induced hyperalgesia" which is responsible for the expression of augmented responses to both noxious and innocuous stimuli (Simonnet and Rivat 2003). Hyperalgesia related to opioid use has an additive effect on incisional hyperalgesia caused by the surgical trauma. Intraoperative administration of high doses of opioids worsen postoperative pain as shown in experimental models and in patients (Simonnet and Rivat 2003), and chronic preoperative consumption of opioids is associated with a modified pain perception (decreased nociceptive thresholds) and modified endogenous pain modulation (Chen et al. 2009). The perioperative analgesic management of these patients is usually difficult.

Pain is not only limited to nociceptive inputs reaching the central nervous system but also includes a *complex psychological experience*. Psychological states can either exacerbate or inhibit the nociceptive perception. Emotional and attentional mechanisms of pain processing already known to play a role in chronic pain conditions have recently attracted interest in trauma and perioperative conditions (Chen et al. 2009). Obviously, there is a vulnerable population who presents with reduced ability to cope with pain, to anticipate pain and to control pain when confronted with (Chen et al. 2009). Pain *hypervigilance*, a strong attentional bias towards pain defined as an automatic prioritisation of pain, conscious or not, aimed to avoid physical threat, is a powerful predictor of acute postoperative pain (Lautenbacher et al. 2009). Presurgical *anxiety* and psychological distress are often reported as predictive factors of postoperative pain intensity (Ip et al. 2009; Pinto et al. 2012). *Pain castastrophisation* is an important cognitive and emotional factor in the experience of pain. Catastrophisation of pain is defined as a negative orientation to aversive stimuli involving rumination about painful sensations, magnification of the threat value of pain and perceived inability to control pain. High catastrophisation is predictive of greater postoperative pain specifically pain at day 2 and later after TKA (Roth et al. 2007). Pinto et al. have recently suggested that pain catastrophising may act as a mediator in the relationship between presurgical anxiety and acute postsurgical pain (Pinto et al. 2012).

The current data regarding the *influence of gender* on immediate and persistent pain after TKA are contradictory (Roth et al. 2007). Women report higher pain severity at lower thresholds and have less tolerance to noxious stimulation than males, the greatest sex differences being noted in mechanical pain tests that could be of importance for patients undergoing TKA (Hurley and Adams 2008). However, the difference in pain perception between males and females decreases with advancing age, to become nonsignificant in volunteers older than 40 years old. Women display higher catastrophisation personalities than men, what might account for the gender difference observed in the postoperative pain experience (Edwards et al. 2006; Keefe et al. 2000).

Genetic background certainly has an influence on pain perception as well as on the metabolism of analgesic drugs and the efficacy of their postoperative analgesic effect (Allegri et al. 2012). Interindividual differences in the modulation of endogenous pain perception and modulation place patients at more or less risk to present with severe pain. Preoperative *assessment of pain* sensitivity by application of quantitative sensory testing may predict to some extent the degree of postoperative pain and the probability to develop persistent pain (Edwards 2005). Patients who preoperatively display enhanced activity of their endogenous excitatory processes of pain modulation (i.e. who have a positive temporal summation of nociceptive stimuli and clinical correlate to a spinal windup phenomenon which relies on NMDA receptor activation) will have higher postoperative pain (Weissman-Fogel et al. 2009). Patients who suffer from a preoperative chronic pain condition like fibromyalgia, irritable bowel syndrome and osteoarthritis show hyperactivity of endogenous pain processing, i.e. significant facilitation of temporal summation (Arendt-Nielsen et al. 2010).

13.4 Persistent Postsurgical Pain After TKA

13.4.1 Incidence, Characteristics and Evolution

A large European survey mentions a 19 % incidence of chronic pain in the population, 3 % of the individuals reporting surgery as the initial cause of their chronic pain (Breivik et al. 2006). For 22 % of the patients who consult in pain clinics, surgery is the origin of their chronic pain (Crombie et al. 1998). Joint arthroplasties are highly successful when judged by prosthesis-related outcomes (clinical evaluation and radiographic appearance), and several outcome studies have reported improved function and health-related quality of life. However, one in five patients (i.e. 19 %) undergoing primary TKA is not satisfied with the outcome (Bourne et al. 2010), and chronic postsurgical pain appears to be the primary predictor of dissatisfaction (Scott et al. 2010).

Chronic postsurgical pain (*CPSP*) has been defined by the International Association for the Study of Pain (IASP) as pain that develops after a surgical intervention and that lasts at least 2 months, with other causes for the pain having been excluded (e.g. infection, recurrence of malignancy) as well as pain from a condition preceding the surgery (Merskey 1994). The time frame of 2 months has been strongly debated because the exact duration of postoperative inflammatory processes still remains undetermined. Actually, one may consider CPSP as pain lasting more than 3–6 months (often beyond 6 months) after surgery. CPSP is a prevalent problem involving all types of surgical procedures including minor ones. The incidence varies between 10 and 50 % according to the type of procedure, but more worrisome is the fact that 2–10 % of these patients present with moderate-to-severe pain, which strongly affects their daily quality of life (Kehlet et al. 2006). Johansen et al. reported a prevalence between 6.2 and 18.3 % of moderate-to-severe pain in the area of surgery 3–36 months after the procedure (Johansen et al. 2012). While most patients usually recover and experience pain relief within 3 months after TKA (Vilardo and Shah 2011), about 20 % (10–34 %) of the patients are left with an unfavourable long-term pain outcome according to a recent systematic review (Table 13.1) (Beswick et al. 2012).

The large variability in reported incidences of persistent pain after TKA can be explained by the various definitions used for CPSP. Pain is often reported as an element of functional knee scores (i.e. WOMAC, KOOS) instead of using specific chronic pain questionnaires (i.e. McGill Pain Questionnaire, Brief Pain Inventory). It is also important to consider that pain identified by functional scores, reported during specific activities, may not totally reflect CPSP. Intermittent and intense pain at rest or during the night may also exist and usually has a major negative impact on the daily quality of life (Beswick et al. 2012).

The nature of CPSP remains unclear because inflammatory mechanisms play an important role even in the development of neuropathic pain. Iatrogenic neuropathic pain caused by incision and nerve injury is thought to be the most common cause of CPSP (Kehlet et al. 2006). The average prevalence of neuropathic pain after surgery is around 24 % with a large range from 6 % to more than 50 % in thoracic procedures (e.g. breast surgery and thoracotomy) (Table 13.1). Chronic pain of neuropathic origin is usually associated with higher pain intensity (average visual analogue scale (VAS) score around 7–8/10) than non-neuropathic chronic pain (Torrance et al. 2006). Johansen et al. observed at 4 months to 3 years after knee surgery that 66 % of patients self-reported knee pain was associated with sensory disturbances, 22 % with hypoesthesia and 12 % with hyperesthesia in an area at or close to the incision. The presence of hyperalgesia close to the scar is associated with an increased risk of severe CPSP (odds ratio 6.3). Due to the lack of use of adequate questionnaires, the nature of CPSP after TKA has been rarely questioned. It seems that the incidence of CPSP of a neuropathic origin is rare after TKA, 6 % at 1 year and later (Haroutiunian et al. 2013; Liu et al. 2012; Wylde et al. 2011b). The causes of nerve injury after TKA do not only involve direct surgical trauma of the infrapatellar branch of the saphenous nerve (84 %) or more exceptional the peroneal nerve (Henningsen et al. 2013) but may also be caused by the tourniquet during the procedure or peripheral nerve blocks used for perioperative analgesia (Kinghorn et al. 2012). Not all nerve lesions will cause pain, and CPSP associated with nerve injury will only develop in predisposed individuals (Lavand'homme 2011). Reflex sympathetic dystrophy (RSD), also called complex regional pain syndrome type 1 (CRPS-1), is a pain disorder associated with autonomic dysfunction and characterised by a disproportionate level of pain. CRPS-1 seems to occur more frequently after trauma or surgery of the lower limb. Harden et al. highlighted that "CRPS-like" phenomena, which diagnostic criteria include abnormal sensory modalities like hyperalgesia and allodynia, may affect up to 13–20 % of the patients during the first year after TKA. CRPS-like phenomena, in the early postoperative period, might also be the result of delayed postsurgical healing and persistent inflammatory reaction that would not normally merit the diagnosis of CRPS (Harden et al. 2003). Experimental studies support that hypothesis as focal nerve inflammation induces neuronal signs consistent with symptoms of early CRPS (Bove 2009). Burns et al. reviewed the medical records of 1,280 patients who underwent TKA for osteoarthritis and found a very low incidence of CRPS, as low as 0.7 %. More importantly, when managed early, patients complicated with CRPS after TKA have a similar prognosis to patients with uncomplicated TKA (Burns et al. 2006).

Today, it is still unclear whether a distinct transition period exists between acute and chronic pain after surgery or trauma. Subacute pain, which can last for several weeks after the surgery, is now recognised as a neglected area of clinical investigation. Poorly relieved subacute pain after surgery not only has a negative psychological impact but also might contribute to maintain a state of central sensitisation, which in turn might facilitate the persistence of pain (Lavand'homme 2011). According to Andersen et al., 52 % of patients report moderate pain, and 16 % report severe pain at rest 30 days after TKA, while pain when moving affects as much as 78 % of the patients (Table 13.1). Using the recent concept of pain trajectories (Chapman et al. 2011), Morze et al. have examined the weekly resolution of knee pain during the first 3 months after TKA (Morze et al. 2013). Clearly, all patients are not equal in facing pain and recovery, and 25 % of the patients still have worst average pain score of 4.9/10 by week 12 after surgery. The overall time taken to reduce worst pain was 6 weeks in 52 % of the patients but could be as long as 12 weeks for 32 % of the patients.

The unexplained painful TKA with no obvious cause remains a challenge for the surgeon (Hofmann et al. 2011). Surgical exploration is rarely advised, and only 45 % of the patients have problems related to their implant (Mont et al. 1996). Revision TKA for unexplained knee pain might harm even more. Between 4 and 22 months after surgery, 38 % of patients suffer from daily life disturbing pain after revision arthroplasty, and 40 % of these patients use analgesics (Puolakka et al. 2010). At 2 and 5 years after a TKA revision, pain is still reported three times more frequently than after a primary arthroplasty (Singh et al. 2008).

However, it is encouraging to see that the incidence of CPSP after TKA seems to be falling down since the 1990s, when 22 % of patients experienced pain at 7 years (Murray and Frost 1998) and as much as 51 % at 1 year (Dickstein et al. 1998). Such evolution underlines the progresses that have been realised in perioperative care, both in surgical and anaesthetic management, of these patients. Further improvements are still needed, mainly based on individualised and tailored management thanks to targeting patients at risk and promoting effective perioperative treatments.

13.4.2 Predictive Factors of Persistent Pain and Poor Recovery

Predisposition to chronic pain is multifactorial and includes the severity of postoperative pain, which is the most striking risk factor, pre-existing pain and psychological factors such as catastrophising and hypervigilance to pain (Kehlet et al. 2006). Predictive factors of CPSP do not really differ from those involved in the risk of severe acute postoperative pain.

Early severe postoperative pain is an important predictor for CPSP after TKA (Puolakka et al. 2010). If the degree of pain during the first postoperative week ranges from moderate to severe, the risk to develop persistent pain is 3–10 times higher compared with patients complaining of mild pain during the same period (Puolakka et al. 2010). Not only poorly relieved postoperative pain contributes to central nervous system sensitisation, but it also has a negative impact on the psychological aspects of recovery in predisposed individuals.

Preoperative pain, either at the operative site or elsewhere, is a known risk factor (Liu et al. 2012; Puolakka et al. 2010; Wylde et al. 2011b) for both severe postoperative pain and CPSP. Current research is ongoing to assess and to target by tailored treatments the endogenous pain modulatory processes.

Negative psychosocial conditions like preoperative anxiety and catastrophisation are regularly found in the history of patients suffering from CPSP (Kehlet et al. 2006). The impact of preoperative psychological factors on the persistence of pain after surgery or trauma has received a growing attention (Lautenbacher et al. 2010).

A recent systematic review has demonstrated that, effectively, low preoperative mental health and pain catastrophising influence the outcome after TKA in terms of function and pain scores (Vissers et al. 2012). Surprisingly, those factors have shown only limited impact on the outcome after total hip arthroplasty. Recent results support the fact that high, if not unrealistic, expectations of TKA are common and should be moderated to maintain patient satisfaction (Hepinstall et al. 2011). From a clinical point of view, patients with a low preoperative pain score (assessed by WOMAC score) are 2.4 times more likely to be dissatisfied with their operation (Bourne et al. 2010). Morze et al. found that the rate of decline of worst postsurgical pain was slower in patients who reported lower preoperative pain scores (6 % per week versus 13 %) (Morze et al. 2013).

Other common risk factors to develop CPSP are younger age and female gender (Kehlet et al. 2006). Those factors have been incriminated in several large retrospective studies from 1 to 5 years after TKA (Liu et al. 2012; Singh et al. 2008). Female sex as predictive factor for CPSP after TKA might be supported by the fact that women usually wait much longer than men before having surgery, despite greater reported disability (Petterson et al. 2007). Waiting longer before having surgery signifies living longer with the aggravating preoperative pain, which is another known predictive factor of CPSP after TKA (Puolakka et al. 2010; Singh et al. 2008).

Finally, the genetic background of the patient also affects the sensitivity to pain as well as the metabolism of analgesic drugs. Some protective phenotypes have been described (France et al. 2009) but at the present, no genotype screening to identify populations at risk is available.

13.4.3 Risks Associated with the Treatment of CPSP

Whereas numerous studies have assessed the incidence and the risk factors for persistent pain after TKA, very few reports have investigated the real consequences of chronic postsurgical pain in these patients, particularly the impact of long-term analgesic use (Steyaert and Lavand'homme 2013). According to published clinical reports, 56 % of patients were still under analgesics at 30 days after TKA (Andersen et al. 2009), 40 % of patients after 4 months (Puolakka et al. 2010) and around 25 % of patients about 2 years later (Carroll et al. 2012).

Nonsteroidal anti-inflammatory drugs (NSAIDs) are very effective in alleviating pain after orthopaedic procedures. Alam et al. (2012) found that elderly patients who started taking NSAIDs within 7 days of surgery were almost four times more likely to become long-term NSAIDs users. Aside from the risks of gastrointestinal ulcers and bleeding or renal insufficiency, chronic use of NSAIDs carries a non-negligible cardiovascular risk for stroke and myocardial infarction. Recently, the American Geriatric Society has recommended the use of opioid analgesics for elderly patients (Kuehn 2009) instead of NSAIDs. Opioids are not innocent either and there have been some alarming reports in the last years. In a propensity-matched cohort study, Solomon et al. (2010) compared the safety of opioids and NSAIDs in more than 12,000 elderly patients with arthritis where patients on opioids had an increased relative risk for many safety events (fractures, cardiovascular events, hospitalisations) compared with NSAIDs. It is mandatory to keep in mind that the initiation of a short-term opioid therapy may lead to longer-term use after discharge in some patients. Elderly patients receiving an opioid prescription after surgery seem to be 44 % more likely to become long-term opioid users compared to patients who did not receive opioids (Alam et al. 2012). Andersen et al. highlighted the fact that 56 % of patients are still on opioids, including 36 % taking strong opioids, 30 days after TKA (Andersen et al. 2009). Carroll et al. found that 6 % of the patients started taking new opioids more than 150 days after surgery and about a quarter of patients, having undergone total hip or knee arthroplasty, were still taking opioids at the end of the follow-up period 2 years later (Carroll et al. 2012). Interestingly, postoperative pain duration and severity only account for 48 % variance in that long-lasting opioid intake, while preoperative factors like legitimate prescribed opioid use, self-perceived risk of addiction and depressive symptoms are better predictors of prolonged opioid use (Carroll et al. 2012). It is mandatory that caregivers involved in the management of patients undergoing TKA take their responsibilities for the prescription of analgesics in these patients: better identification of the patients who are at risk of needing prolonged postoperative opioids, adaptation of perioperative treatments to reduce the need for opioids to a minimum (preventive analgesia, i.e. multimodal analgesia with regional analgesia and anti-hyperalgesics) and closer follow-up of patients after their discharge (Steyaert and Lavand'homme 2013).

13.5 Perioperative Management of Patients Undergoing TKA

The combination of modern surgical techniques and perioperative anaesthetic/analgesic management is aiming to produce a "reasonably pain-free postoperative patient" to facilitate early rehabilitation and to prevent the development of persistent pain. However, facing the clinical reality, it turns out that the task remains complicated despite the use of *multimodal balanced analgesia*. Recent developments in our understanding of incisional pain have prompted to change the old concept of pre-emptive analgesia forwards to the more accurate concepts of *preventive and protective analgesia* (Bromley 2006). Experimental models of incisional pain as well as clinical studies have shown deceiving results with only short-term benefits of pre-emptive treatments (Pogatzki-Zahn and Zahn 2006). First, the wound itself is able to maintain and to reinitiate the sensitisation processes when the effects of treatment abate what implicates a prominent role of postoperative nociceptive stimuli from the wound and the need for a long-lasting postoperative pain control. Second, the existence of preoperative pain may have already triggered central sensitisation in some patients, thereby blunting the benefits of pre-emptive treatments (Aida et al. 2000). That later point argues for an optimal control of preoperative pain in patients who will undergo a knee arthroplasty.

Thereby, pre-emptive analgesia has evolved to the concept of *preventive analgesia*, a broader definition, which involves any perioperative analgesic and anti-hyperalgesic treatments aimed to control central nervous system sensitisation and to reduce the development of persistent postsurgical pain. In preventive analgesia, both the duration and the efficacy of the treatment are more important than the timing of administration of the drugs. Recent clinical studies have highlighted the fact that an optimal control of preoperative, perioperative and postoperative pain is mandatory to ensure the success of preventive analgesia. In the future, progresses made in the assessment of endogenous mechanisms of pain processing should allow to improve even more the preventive-protective analgesia by an individualisation of analgesic and anti-hyperalgesic perioperative treatments (Lavand'homme 2011; Yarnitsky 2010).

13.5.1 Less Invasive Surgery and Rapid Recovery Protocols for TKA

Minimally invasive (MI) techniques gained popularity in the last decade. Minimally invasive TKA is a technique that focuses on using a smaller skin incision, avoiding patella eversion and quadriceps-sparing approaches (Arnout et al. 2009; Khanna et al. 2009; Thienpont 2013a, b). Less tissue damage should reduce the release of inflammatory mediators and its cascade. The length of the skin incision in TKA is proportional with the surface area of sensory change in the front of the knee, which is related to the inability to kneel following surgery (Hassaballa et al. 2012). MI-TKA leads to reduced length of stay (LOS), reduced pain and more rapid rehabilitation (Niki et al. 2009). Although the learning curve of such new techniques seems to be substantial, the benefits in terms of need for opioids and need for rehabilitation and LOS are significant (King et al. 2007). The reduction of tissue damage, the decrease in tourniquet time as well as the reduction of the duration of the surgical procedure may also play a role in postoperative recovery

(Niki et al. 2009). Despite that tourniquet use does not have a direct impact on knee pain and analgesics use, tourniquet however induces thigh pain (Wakankar et al. 1999). Quadriceps muscle strength is the parameter, which correlates the best with postoperative functional performance (Khanna et al. 2009). MI-TKA drastically reduces the direct quadriceps damage. In opposite, tourniquet-induced ischaemia represents a substantial contributor to intraoperative muscle damage (Appell et al. 1993). A recent systematic review of the literature showed that as a group, patients undergoing MI-TKA tend to have decreased postoperative pain, rapid recovery of quadriceps function, improved range of motion and shorter LOS (Khanna et al. 2009).

In order to facilitate early discharge from the hospital and more rapid return to the normal daily activities, the concept of fast-track surgery has been developed. Fast-track surgery integrates new modalities in surgery, anaesthesia and nutrition, enforcing early mobilisation and rehabilitation. Along with the use of minimally invasive techniques, the choice of anaesthesia and analgesia techniques has to be adapted, a choice which relies on multimodal balanced techniques allowing a subsequent opioid-sparing effect (White et al. 2007).

13.5.2 Multimodal Analgesia in Modern Perioperative Pain Management

The aim of multimodal analgesia is to minimise the need for opioid analgesics (Kehlet and Dahl 1993). Although opioids remain very effective analgesics, their well-known side effects like sedation, nausea and vomiting and respiratory depression may prevent rapid rehabilitation. Furthermore, opioids may also induce hyperalgesia (also called "opioid-induced hyperalgesia") and acute tolerance that enhances postoperative pain.

Nonsteroidal anti-inflammatory drugs (NSAIDs) and acetaminophen (paracetamol) are commonly associated drug combinations used for multimodal analgesia. Recent meta-analyses have shown that the significant 30–50 % opioid dose-sparing effect of non-selective NSAIDs is associated with a 30 % reduction in opioid-related side effects like postoperative nausea and vomiting and sedation (Elia et al. 2005; Marret et al. 2005). Selective inhibitors of cyclooxygenase 2 (COX-2) also display a 35 % opioid-sparing effect (Straube et al. 2005). However, non-selective and selective NSAIDs are contraindicated in one patient out of five because of the risks of gastrointestinal bleeding or renal insufficiency. For those patients, paracetamol then represents an alternative. Paracetamol has complex analgesic effects, which rely on central endocannabinoid and serotoninergic mechanisms and perhaps on a COX-3 inhibition (Mallet et al. 2008). By itself it demonstrates only a weak opioid-sparing effect of around 20 % not associated with a reduction of opioids' side effects (Remy et al. 2005).

Corticosteroids represent the "ultimate anti-inflammatory drugs" (Turan and Sessler 2011) and are used in rheumatic disease for their local anti-inflammatory properties. In the perioperative setting, they are often administered for their anti-emetic effect as a preventive strategy for postoperative nausea and vomiting. A recent meta-analysis has demonstrated that a small dose of perioperative dexamethasone (0.1–0.2 mg/kg) reduced postoperative pain at rest and during mobilisation up to 24 h postoperatively, as well as opioid consumption (Waldron et al. 2013). Corticosteroids have previously proven their efficiency in reducing postoperative pain after spine surgery, hip replacement and TKA. A high dose of 40 mg dexamethasone before anaesthesia significantly prevented dynamic pain until 24 h after elective hip replacement (Kardash et al. 2008). In patients undergoing elective TKA, preoperative high dose of methylprednisolone 125 mg significantly reduced pain during walking up to 32 h after surgery (Lunn et al. 2011). The postoperative opioid requirements were also reduced as well as nausea and vomiting. Postoperatively, inflammatory parameters like CRP concentrations were lower. These patients reported less postoperative fatigue although the sleep quality was worse on the first night. Other authors have assessed the modulatory effect of a low dose of hydrocortisone (two doses of 100 mg given at 8 h apart) in patients undergoing bilateral TKA (Jules-Elysee et al. 2012, 2011). The decreased inflammatory response as measured by 40 % reduction in IL-6 production was associated with higher postoperative haemodynamic stability, lowered pain scores and improved knee motion. It is interesting to note that administration of corticosteroids 1 day after surgery may help to control pain even better than regular NSAIDs. Romundstad et al. have assessed the time course and magnitude of the analgesic effect of 125 mg methylprednisolone in patients with moderate-to-severe pain 1 day after orthopaedic surgery (Romundstad et al. 2004). Methylprednisolone analgesic effect was as effective as the effect of 30 mg ketorolac but lasted longer and provided higher opioid-sparing effect up to 72 h after administration. Very few studies have evaluated the benefit of combining NSAIDs with corticosteroids to improve postoperative pain. It seems that such combination may demonstrate superior analgesic effect as reported after knee arthroscopic surgery in patients receiving a low dose of 8 mg dexamethasone and a COX-2 selective inhibitor (Dahl et al. 2012). Finally, experimental data found a preventive effect of intraoperative systemic corticosteroids on the development of persistent neuropathic pain (Liu et al. 2012). Further studies are needed in order to define the optimal doses of corticosteroids to improve postoperative pain as well as the potential long-term benefits. Moreover, although no serious adverse effects have been reported, the safety aspects and implications on the glycaemic profile, risk of infections and wound healing remain largely unknown.

13.5.3 Non-opioid Adjuvants

Systemic administration of alpha-2 adrenergic agonists clonidine and dexmedetomidine decreases postoperative opioid consumption, pain intensity and nausea (Blaudszun et al. 2012). The major site of action of α2-adrenergic agonists is the spinal cord, and both their analgesic and anti-hyperalgesic effects result from spinal administration either epidurally or intrathecally. Alpha-2 adrenergic agonists also act locally on peripheral nerve endings and potentiate local anaesthetics effect in peripheral nerve blocks (Marhofer et al. 2013). Intra-articular injection of clonidine demonstrated local anti-inflammatory effect during knee arthroscopic surgery (Gentili et al. 2001). Alpha-2 adrenergic agonists also possess interesting anxiolytic and sedative effects (Crassous et al. 2007). Although they do not induce respiratory depression, they cause hypotension, which may interfere with rehabilitation process (Blaudszun et al. 2012).

Ketamine is an old anaesthetic drug used in clinical practice since the 1960s. The main working mechanism of action of ketamine is not clear but relies on a noncompetitive antagonism of excitatory neurotransmission (NMDA receptors) and potentially on an interaction with opioid, monoaminergic, cholinergic, purinergic and adenosine receptor systems. These multiple interactions account for the various clinical effects observed such as anaesthesia, analgesia, anti-hyperalgesia, induction of psychiatric symptoms (schizophrenia-like) or positive effects on depressive moods. Ketamine also has anti-inflammatory properties as it avoids an exacerbated proinflammatory reaction (De Kock et al. 2013). It influences the immune system and is able to regulate very early local inflammatory processes as it reduces the release of proinflammatory cytokines without affecting the production of anti-inflammatory ones. These anti-inflammatory properties of the drug may be involved in its anti-hyperalgesic effect. Several meta-analyses have highlighted the benefits of intraoperative use of low doses of ketamine (median dose 0.4 mg/kg; range 0.1–1.6 mg/kg). At that dose, a reduction of postoperative pain scores, both at rest and during mobilisation, as well as a 30–55 % reduction in postoperative opioid requirements has been demonstrated. The greatest efficacy of perioperative ketamine administration is observed in painful procedures including thoracic, upper abdomen and major orthopaedic surgeries (Laskowski et al. 2011). After TKA performed under general anaesthesia combined with a femoral nerve block, a single bolus dose of ketamine 0.5 mg/kg significantly reduced opioid use and facilitated rehabilitation (Adam et al. 2005). In TKA under general anaesthesia but without femoral nerve block, ketamine (bolus dose of 0.2 mg/kg followed by an infusion of 60–120 μg/kg/h) administered over 48 h had a significant opioid-sparing effect and decreased pain intensity at both rest and mobilisation (Aveline et al. 2009). Patients receiving ketamine infusion achieved earlier rehabilitation progresses and hospital discharge (Aveline et al. 2009).

Gabapentinoids (*gabapentin and pregabalin*) are primarily used in the treatment of epilepsia and chronic neuropathic pain syndromes. Gabapentin and its analogue pregabalin have been designed as analogues of γ-aminobutyric acid, but their mechanism of action mostly relies on binding to α2-δ subunit of voltage-gated calcium channels in the central nervous system, preventing the release of several excitatory neurotransmitters like glutamate. Pregabalin, the second generation of calcium channel α2-δ ligands, offers the advantages linked to a more reliable pharmacokinetic profile with a rapid dose-independent absorption. Thereby, pregabalin will be more suitable for a short-term use like the perioperative period, a single preoperative dose of 300 mg oral pregabalin displaying a sufficient central nervous system bioavailability to reach anti-hyperalgesic therapeutic levels within 6 h post-administration (Buvanendran et al. 2003). For a few years, both drugs have been used as part of multimodal analgesia in the perioperative setting where they help to reduce postoperative pain and opioid consumption (around 30 %) as well as opioid-related side effects like nausea and vomiting. More recently, they have also demonstrated promising anti-hyperalgesic effects, which might reduce the risk of persistent pain after surgery (Zhang et al. 2011). As a matter of fact, a preoperative dose of 300 mg pregabalin followed by a twice-daily dose of 150 mg during 14 days reduced the incidence of chronic neuropathic pain after TKA (0 % at 3 and 6 months versus 8.7 and 5.2 %, respectively) (Buvanendran et al. 2010). Patients who received pregabalin treatment required less oral opioids when hospitalised and had greater active flexion on the first 30 days (Buvanendran et al. 2010). Side effects of perioperative gabapentinoids involve greater sedation, dizziness and blurred vision (diplopia). The promising results obtained so far with pregabalin reinforce the need for further studies aimed to determine optimal doses and duration of administration.

13.5.4 Locoregional Anaesthesia

The supposed superiority of locoregional anaesthesia and analgesia over general anaesthesia and systemic analgesia for the perioperative management of various surgical procedures including orthopaedic surgery is currently debated, especially in the context of fast-track or enhanced recovery protocols (Carli et al. 2011; Harsten et al. 2013). For TKA, some authors strongly believe that spinal anaesthesia, continuous peripheral nerve blocks and/or wound infiltration represents the recommended standard to achieve the goals of fast-track surgery (Carli et al. 2010a; Memtsoudis et al. 2013). That might not be true anymore for two reasons. First, the drugs and techniques used for general anaesthesia and systemic analgesia have changed these last years, along with the use of less invasive surgical techniques. Modern general anaesthesia seems to favour a more comfortable recovery in terms of nausea, vomiting and dizziness, to reduce pain and morphine consumption pain and to result in shorter LOS (Harsten et al. 2013). Second, regional analgesic techniques provide statistically superior analgesia compared with systemic opioids. However, the benefits of locoregional techniques have been previously, almost exclusively, examined in terms of postoperative analgesia, while other significant clinical outcomes, e.g. performance-based outcomes, should be assessed besides pain intensity in order to determine the success of a chosen technique (Bernucci and Carli 2012). The benefits of locoregional techniques may not be so relevant when considering the later outcomes, which are now considered of major interest in the patient's rehabilitation process.

Besides an analgesic effect related to nerve conduction block preventing the noxious stimuli from the wound to reach and to further sensitise the central nervous system, locoregional analgesia also modulates the inflammatory response caused by tissue destruction. This beneficial anti-inflammatory effect partly relies on the use of local anaesthetics, which, in addition to blocking nerve conduction, are known to have a variety of anti-inflammatory actions. Inhibition of phagocytosis in macrophages or leucocytes, decrease in adhesion of polymorphonuclear granulocytes and reduction in platelet aggregation are well-known effects of local anaesthetics (Cullen and Haschke 1974; Hu and Muscoplat 1980). A newly discovered anti-inflammatory mechanism is the inhibition of the proton channels of microglia, which are known to play a crucial role in regulating inflammatory responses in the central nervous system (Matsuura et al. 2012).

Lumbar epidural analgesia has been popular over the last decades as there is evidence for lower postoperative thromboembolic complications and other protective effects (Rawal 2012). Nevertheless, there is today little evidence for a decrease in perioperative mortality and morbidity in a low- to medium-risk population in relation to the use of perioperative epidural analgesia. Moreover, the widespread implementation of anticoagulant regimens may not only overcome the benefits of epidural analgesia on thromboembolic complications but also make around 30 % of the patients ineligible for the technique. The failure rate of the technique may reach 28 %. Systemic review of the literature has shown that epidural analgesia provides superior analgesia to systemic opioids at rest and with activities whatever the type of surgery (Liu and Wu 2007). This clinical superiority of epidural analgesia may occur only with mobilisation through the first postoperative day. A previous systematic review in TKA comparing lumbar epidural blockade with systemic opioid analgesia reported better dynamic pain scores in the epidural group although limited to the first 6 h (Choi et al. 2003). As the magnitude of pain relief must be weighed against the frequency of adverse events, patients who received epidural analgesia had more hypotension, urinary retention and pruritus, whereas systemic opioids caused more sedation, but no difference was found for the postoperative respiratory depression or nausea and vomiting (Choi et al. 2003).

Peripheral nerve blocks (*PNB*) of the major nerves supplying the lower limb represent an attractive alternative to epidural analgesia. With the development of ultrasounds (US), peripheral nerve blocks have regained interest among the anaesthesiologists. Although nerve injuries lasting longer than 1 year are rare, their frequency with both US guidance techniques and nerve stimulator (NS) guidance techniques seems to be similar (Orebaugh et al. 2012). However, US-guided peripheral blocks are associated with a significant increase in the success rate when compared with NS techniques only or other methods (Gelfand et al. 2011) as is the US-guided peripheral nerve catheter placement which proves also a lower risk for accidental vascular puncture when compared with NS-alone guidance (Schnabel et al. 2013). The development of enhanced echogenic needles in the last years has contributed to the improvement of peripheral nerve blocks' safety and efficacy (Hebard and Hocking 2011).

The most popular analgesic technique after TKA remains the femoral nerve block (FNB) (also referred to as "3-in-1 block"), either single-shot or continuous infusion (United Kingdom, France). For major knee surgery, a femoral nerve block provides postoperative analgesia which is comparable with that obtained with an epidural technique but with an improved side effect profile, i.e. less hypotension, pruritus and urinary retention (Fowler et al. 2008). A preoperative single-shot FNB reduces postoperative opioid use and significantly decreases pain scores with activity, but not at rest, up to 48 h after surgery by comparison with systemic opioids (Paul et al. 2010). The addition of a continuous perineural infusion of local anaesthetic in the postoperative period does not seem to enhance the analgesic benefits observed after a single-shot injection (Paul et al. 2010).

The sensory innervation of the knee is complex and involves the femoral nerve along with contributions from the sciatic and obturator nerves at the posterior and medial aspects. Consequently, a peripheral block of the sciatic nerve may be added to the classical FNB in the aim to improve postoperative analgesia, such combination remaining less invasive and associated with fewer serious complications than the use of a lumbar plexus block. The addition of sciatic nerve block could improve the quality of analgesia during the first 24 h by reducing posterior knee and calf pain (Cappelleri et al. 2011; Cook et al. 2003; Wegener et al. 2011). However, the addition of a sciatic block does not result in better pain scores or lesser opioid consumption than the use of a single-shot FNB alone (Abdallah and Brull 2011; Fowler 2009; Fowler et al. 2008; Paul et al. 2010). The FNB is not always complete, as it does not constantly produce analgesia of the obturator nerve. Nevertheless, although the obturator nerve is far more consistently involved with a lumbar plexus block technique than with an inguinal FNB technique, the obturator block, like the sciatic one, does not seem to translate into improved patient recovery or pain reduction (Bergeron et al. 2009; Macalou et al. 2004). Compared with systemic analgesics, the use of FNB allows faster rehabilitation and reduces time to discharge (Macfarlane et al. 2009). Despite the reduction of local knee inflammation (Martin et al. 2008) and in some extent of the systemic inflammatory reaction (Bagry et al. 2008) associated with the use of locoregional anaesthesia, the impact on patient's outcomes is disappointing. Better postoperative analgesia does not lead to better knee function as observed by an improved knee range of motion that usually does not extend long after the block's completion. Better postoperative analgesia does not translate into improved long-term pain reduction after TKA neither. Patients receiving a 48 h continuous FNB achieved better knee flexion in the first 6 days after TKA but not further on (no significant functional difference observed at 3 months) (Kadic et al. 2009). Within the concept of preventive analgesia, some authors have extended the duration of analgesia to 4 days by discharging patients at home with femoral catheter and infusion pumps. The results of the study did not show that extending an overnight continuous FNB to 4 days improves or worsens subsequent health quality of life, assessed by WOMAC scores, between 7 days and 12 months after TKA (Ilfeld et al. 2008; Ilfeld et al. 2011). Other authors have examined the impact of a more complete knee block by adding a 48 h sciatic block to the continuous FNB. They did not find improved postoperative outcomes in terms of long-term pain or functional disability (Wegener et al. 2011).

It is important to keep in mind that these blocks bear some complications which may interfere with the rehabilitation process (Richman et al. 2006). A large retrospective analysis including 1,190 patients found an overall complication rate of 1.5 % when using femoral nerve catheters to provide analgesia after TKA, and a rate of 0.7 % falls (Feibel et al. 2009). The FNB reduces the maximum voluntary isometric contraction (MVIC) of the quadriceps femoris muscle at hour 6 by 84 % (Charous et al. 2011) and strength of the quadriceps muscle by almost 50 % (Jaeger et al. 2013); hence, quadriceps weakness is present during continuous FNB and sometimes may persist after single-shot injection. A causality relationship between continuous FNB and the risk of falling has been highlighted (Ilfeld et al. 2010; Sharma et al. 2010). Although neurological complications are usually less disastrous after PNB than after neuraxial block, they should not be ignored. The rate of neuropathy attributable to PNB is between 0.1 % (Schug 2007) and 1.94 % (Widmer et al. 2013), and large series report a rate of 0.2 % permanent nerve injury associated with the use of femoral nerve catheters in TKA (Feibel et al. 2009). Surprisingly, in a large series of screened patients, the incidence was significantly higher in females (females = 2.5 %, males = 0.83 %) and in patients receiving a single-shot block (single shot = 2.66 %, femoral catheter = 0.93 %) (Widmer et al. 2013).

To overcome the undesirable quadriceps weakness, which results from the FNB, some authors have proposed the administration of local anaesthetics into the adductor canal (i.e. Hunter's canal) as it should produce an almost pure sensory block. Adductor canal blockade (ACB) not only seemed to reduce morphine consumption and pain but also significantly enhanced early ambulation ability after TKA (Jenstrup et al. 2012; Perlas et al. 2013). However, in a recent study performed on young healthy volunteers, the authors showed that quadriceps strength was reduced by 8 % in patients with ACB when compared with placebo (Jaeger et al. 2013). Further clinical trials are needed in order to determine the place of the adductor canal block in the panel of analgesic techniques after TKA (Jaeger et al. 2013).

Because of the prominent role of the wound in the initiation and maintenance of sensitisation processes after a surgical incision, going back to the periphery is logical, and intra-wound analgesic techniques have received recently increased attention. Posterior capsular infiltration added to FNB reduces pain scores and leads to better active extension of the knee in the first postoperative 12 h (Krenzel et al. 2009). However, intra-articular analgesic injection alone does not improve patient's pain, satisfaction or range of motion (Joo et al. 2011). In contrast, *local infiltration analgesia* (*LIA*) technique is a promising, easy and safe technique, which has proven its efficacy after TKA (Carli et al. 2010b; Kehlet and Andersen 2011; Kerr and Kohan 2008; McCartney and McLeod 2011). The joint and surrounding tissues are infiltrated by the surgeon with a high volume of a local anaesthetic solution mainly including ropivacaine (low-toxicity local anaesthetic), epinephrine and some adjuvants like NSAIDs, clonidine, corticosteroid or opioids (Kerr and Kohan 2008; Maheshwari et al. 2009). In LIA technique, intracapsular and intra-articular infiltrations seem to have the same effect, and the subcutaneous infiltration of the tissues also plays an important role (Andersen et al. 2010b). Although the duration of effect of LIA technique concerns the first 6–12 h (Andersen et al. 2008) compared to intrathecal morphine, LIA demonstrates better analgesic effect, allowing earlier mobilisation and resulting in shorter hospital stay (Essving et al. 2011). Trials comparing LIA with epidural analgesia (Andersen et al. 2010a; Spreng et al. 2010) are also in favour of the local technique. A recent study suggests that LIA should be considered as an alternative to a femoral nerve block as it provides equivalent pain control without a negative impact on quadriceps function (Chaumeron et al. 2013). A continuous saphenous nerve block in addition to single-dose LIA may offer even better pain relief, but the possible quadriceps weakness induced by this peripheral block needs to be further investigated (Andersen et al. 2013). The available data support intraoperative use of the local infiltration technique but not postoperative use of wound catheter in orthopaedic procedures (Kehlet and Andersen 2011), one of the concerns with an indwelling catheter being the risk of infections. Future pharmacological developments regarding extended-release local anaesthetics will certainly bring promising results in the context of LIA technique (Bramlett et al. 2012).

There is currently a lack of studies regarding the impact of LIA on long-term outcomes after TKA. A large trial is ongoing to evaluate whether the use of LIA might reduce the severity of pain at 12 months after TKA (Wylde et al. 2011a). Despite its proven efficacy, more studies are necessary in order to determine the volume and concentration of the local anaesthetic solution as well as the adjuvants to be added to improve both the quality and the duration of action. A single study including 100 patients who underwent unilateral TKA has previously examined the effect of adding a corticosteroid, 40 mg triamcinolone, to the LIA mixture (Sean et al. 2011). Patients who received periarticular triamcinolone displayed lower pain scores and better range of motion, an effect which was significant from postoperative day 2 until 6 months after TKA but not later (follow-up at 2 years). Finally, as aforementioned, all the analgesic techniques have to be part of a multimodal analgesic regimen in order to achieve maximal analgesic benefits with minimal side effects.

13.5.5 Innovative Other Techniques

Cryotherapy gained in popularity these last years, and it was believed to be an interesting method of diminishing pain and maybe local inflammation after knee replacement. Lowering the temperature around the knee couyld also prolonge the effect of the local anaesthetic if LIA was performed during the surgery, but these beliefs were not confirmed by studies. Most studies noted no difference in range of motion of the operative knee, a small decrease in swelling and blood loss with cold compression (Adie et al. 2012; Markert 2011).

Capsaicin, a product derived from chilli pepper, causes local nervous desensitisation when applied topically by its binding with transient receptor potential vanilloide 1 (TRPV 1) receptors only present on nociceptive afferent fibres, hence inducing a pure sensory block without motor block. So far, clinical studies with highly purified forms of capsaicin instilled in the surgical wound reported only a modest positive effect on early postoperative pain. Wound infiltration with capsaicin after TKA showed promising results in terms of pain scores and opioid use, but this new technique needs more investigation prior to a clinical use (Hartrick et al. 2011).

13.5.6 The Concept of Prehabilitation

A new developing concept is prehabilitation. Prehabilitation is an intervention to enhance functional capacity in anticipation of a forthcoming physiological stressor (Carli et al. 2010a). Optimising functional exercise resulted in positive results in terms of fewer postoperative complications, shorter LOS and better quality of life for patients following prehabilitation programmes before cardiac or abdominal surgery (Carli and Zavorsky 2005). Light physical exercise may induce an anti-inflammatory preconditioning that protects against exacerbated inflammatory stress consecutive to surgery

Preoperative increase in quadriceps strength was thought to result in less postoperative pain and better, faster functional recovery after TKA. The published results so far are poor and discordant, and more trials should be done in order to determine the efficient prehabilitation programme. Increasing quadriceps strength preoperatively is achievable with short-term prehabilitation programmes (Swank et al. 2011), but the results seem to have small or no influence on the postoperative pain and function (McKay et al. 2012; Topp et al. 2009).

One of the problems of prehabilitation is the weak adherence to the programme (Carli et al. 2010a), but this could be solved with techniques like preoperative neuromuscular electrical stimulation at home, a technique that seems to have a good result in increasing preoperative quadriceps strength and also in producing a less functional degradation at 6 and 12 weeks after TKA (Walls et al. 2010).

Conclusion

The origin of pain after TKA is nociceptive, inflammatory, ischaemic and neuropathic. Once the inflammatory cascade is launched, peripheral and central sensitisations occur, which are processes that can contribute to the severity of acute postoperative pain or to its possible persistence (CPSP).

Despite the progress made in the understanding of pain mechanisms and the improvement of anaesthesia and analgesia techniques, severe acute postoperative pain and severe persistent pain after TKA touch a big percentage of patients. Recognising the risk factors for severe acute pain and for persistent pain after TKA could allow specific, more aggressive perioperative management for patients at risk.

General and spinal anaesthesias are both suitable when performing TKA. Modern general anaesthesia techniques allow a rapid, comfortable recovery, although spinal anaesthesia remains the gold standard for many centres across the world.

Epidural analgesia, although an effective technique, presents many side effects that limit early rehabilitation, especially in the setting of fast-track protocols. Peripheral nerve blocks, in single-shot or continuous infusion, are a tempting alternative, but quadriceps weakness and neurologic complications have to be taken into account when performing these techniques. Sciatic and obturator nerve blocks do not seem to bring a consistent and significant benefit when added to femoral nerve block, which remains a good postoperative analgesia strategy. With less quadriceps weakness, Hunter's canal block is a promising technique, but more studies are needed in order to define its place among the others. LIA is the easiest to perform and the safest analgesia technique that provides good quality analgesia after TKA.

The chosen postoperative analgesia protocol must be part of a multimodal regimen. NSAIDs and acetaminophen reduce significantly the opioid need and side effects and are the corner stone of every multimodal analgesia regimen. Alpha-2 agonists, adrenaline, corticosteroids and other drugs can be added to the local anaesthetic solution in order to increase its efficacy and duration.

A multimodal analgesia protocol should also include, whenever possible, perioperative corticosteroids and gabapentinoids, for their preventive analgesia effect along with diminishing the risk of developing persistent pain.

Although pain after TKA still remains an unresolved issue, recent progresses in understanding the mechanisms of pain and in developing new techniques allow better preventive and treatment strategies which translate in better pain control and rehabilitation.

Key Points

- Pain after total knee arthroplasty is still difficult to be controlled, despite advances in techniques and use of new drugs.
- Pain mechanism should be understood and addressed by multimodal means.
- There is a relationship between acute and chronic pain after arthroplasty procedures. This is another reason to address the onset of moderate-to-severe postoperative pain.

References

Abdallah FW, Brull R (2011) Is sciatic nerve block advantageous when combined with femoral nerve block for postoperative analgesia following total knee arthroplasty? A systematic review. Reg Anesth Pain Med 36:493–498

Adam F, Chauvin M, Du Manoir B, Langlois M, Sessler DI, Fletcher D (2005) Small-dose ketamine infusion improves postoperative analgesia and rehabilitation after total knee arthroplasty. Anesth Analg 100:475–480

Adie S, Kwan A, Naylor JM, Harris IA, Mittal R (2012) Cryotherapy following total knee replacement. Cochrane Database Syst Rev (9):CD007911

Aida S, Fujihara H, Taga K, Fukuda S, Shimoji K (2000) Involvement of presurgical pain in preemptive analgesia for orthopedic surgery: a randomized double blind study. Pain 84:169–173

Alam A, Gomes T, Zheng H, Mamdani MM, Juurlink DN, Bell CM (2012) Long-term analgesic use after low-risk surgery: a retrospective cohort study. Arch Intern Med 172:425–430

Allegri M, Clark MR, De Andres J, Jensen TS (2012) Acute and chronic pain: where we are and where we have to go. Minerva Anestesiol 78:222–235

Andersen LO, Husted H, Otte KS, Kristensen BB, Kehlet H (2008) High-volume infiltration analgesia in total knee arthroplasty: a randomized, double-blind, placebo-controlled trial. Acta Anaesthesiol Scand 52:1331–1335

Andersen LO, Gaarn-Larsen L, Kristensen BB, Husted H, Otte KS, Kehlet H (2009) Subacute pain and function after fast-track hip and knee arthroplasty. Anaesthesia 64:508–513

Andersen KV, Bak M, Christensen BV, Harazuk J, Pedersen NA, Soballe K (2010a) A randomized, controlled trial comparing local infiltration analgesia with epidural infusion for total knee arthroplasty. Acta Orthop 81:606–610

Andersen LO, Husted H, Kristensen BB, Otte KS, Gaarn-Larsen L, Kehlet H (2010b) Analgesic efficacy of intracapsular and intra-articular local anaesthesia for knee arthroplasty. Anaesthesia 65:904–912

Andersen HL, Gyrn J, Moller L, Christensen B, Zaric D (2013) Continuous saphenous nerve block as supplement to single-dose local infiltration analgesia for postoperative pain management after total knee arthroplasty. Reg Anesth Pain Med 38:106–111

Apfelbaum JL, Chen C, Mehta SS, Gan TJ (2003) Postoperative pain experience: results from a national survey suggest postoperative pain continues to be undermanaged. Anesth Analg 97:534–540, table of contents

Appell HJ, Gloser S, Duarte JA, Zellner A, Soares JM (1993) Skeletal muscle damage during tourniquet-induced ischaemia. The initial step towards atrophy after orthopaedic surgery? Eur J Appl Physiol Occup Physiol 67:342–347

Arendt-Nielsen L, Nie H, Laursen MB, Laursen BS, Madeleine P, Simonsen OH, Graven-Nielsen T (2010) Sensitization in patients with painful knee osteoarthritis. Pain 149:573–581

Arnout N, Victor J, Cleppe H, Soenen M, Van Damme G, Bellemans J (2009) Avoidance of patellar eversion improves range of motion after total knee replacement: a prospective randomized study. Knee Surg Sports Traumatol Arthrosc 17:1206–1210

Aubrun F, Valade N, Coriat P, Riou B (2008) Predictive factors of severe postoperative pain in the postanesthesia care unit. Anesth Analg 106:1535–1541, table of contents

Aveline C, Gautier JF, Vautier P, Cognet F, Hetet HL, Attali JY, Leconte V, Leborgne P, Bonnet F (2009) Postoperative analgesia and early rehabilitation after total knee replacement: a comparison of continuous low-dose intravenous ketamine versus nefopam. Eur J Pain 13:613–619

Bagry H, de la Cuadra Fontaine JC, Asenjo JF, Bracco D, Carli F (2008) Effect of a continuous peripheral nerve block on the inflammatory response in knee arthroplasty. Reg Anesth Pain Med 33:17–23

Bergeron SG, Kardash KJ, Huk OL, Zukor DJ, Antoniou J (2009) Functional outcome of femoral versus obturator nerve block after total knee arthroplasty. Clin Orthop Relat Res 467:1458–1462

Bernucci F, Carli F (2012) Functional outcome after major orthopedic surgery: the role of regional anesthesia redefined. Curr Opin Anaesthesiol 25:621–628

Beswick AD, Wylde V, Gooberman-Hill R, Blom A, Dieppe P (2012) What proportion of patients report long-term pain after total hip or knee replacement for osteoarthritis? A systematic review of prospective studies in unselected patients. BMJ Open 2:e000435

Blaudszun G, Lysakowski C, Elia N, Tramer MR (2012) Effect of perioperative systemic alpha2 agonists on postoperative morphine consumption and pain intensity: systematic review and meta-analysis of randomized controlled trials. Anesthesiology 116:1312–1322

Bourne RB, Chesworth BM, Davis AM, Mahomed NN, Charron KD (2010) Patient satisfaction after total knee arthroplasty: who is satisfied and who is not? Clin Orthop Relat Res 468:57–63

Bove GM (2009) Focal nerve inflammation induces neuronal signs consistent with symptoms of early complex regional pain syndromes. Exp Neurol 219: 223–227

Bramlett K, Onel E, Viscusi ER, Jones K (2012) A randomized, double-blind, dose-ranging study comparing wound infiltration of DepoFoam bupivacaine, an extended-release liposomal bupivacaine, to bupivacaine HCl for postsurgical analgesia in total knee arthroplasty. Knee 19:530–536

Breivik H, Stubhaug A (2008) Management of acute postoperative pain: still a long way to go! Pain 137:233–234

Breivik H, Collett B, Ventafridda V, Cohen R, Gallacher D (2006) Survey of chronic pain in Europe: prevalence, impact on daily life, and treatment. Eur J Pain 10:287–333

Brennan TJ (2011) Pathophysiology of postoperative pain. Pain 152:S33–S40

Bromley L (2006) Pre-emptive analgesia and protective premedication. What is the difference? Biomed Pharmacother 60:336–340

Burns AW, Parker DA, Coolican MR, Rajaratnam K (2006) Complex regional pain syndrome complicating total knee arthroplasty. J Orthop Surg (Hong Kong) 14:280–283

Buvanendran A, Kroin JS, Tuman KJ, Lubenow TR, Elmofty D, Moric M, Rosenberg AG (2003) Effects of perioperative administration of a selective cyclooxygenase 2 inhibitor on pain management and recovery of function after knee replacement: a randomized controlled trial. JAMA 290:2411–2418

Buvanendran A, Kroin JS, Berger RA, Hallab NJ, Saha C, Negrescu C, Moric M, Caicedo MS, Tuman KJ (2006) Upregulation of prostaglandin E2 and interleukins in the central nervous system and peripheral tissue during and after surgery in humans. Anesthesiology 104:403–410

Buvanendran A, Kroin JS, Della Valle CJ, Kari M, Moric M, Tuman KJ (2010) Perioperative oral pregabalin reduces chronic pain after total knee arthroplasty: a prospective, randomized, controlled trial. Anesth Analg 110:199–207

Buvanendran A, Kroin JS, Della Valle CJ, Moric M, Tuman KJ (2012) Cerebrospinal fluid neurotransmitter changes during the perioperative period in patients undergoing total knee replacement: a randomized trial. Anesth Analg 114:434–441

Cappelleri G, Ghisi D, Fanelli A, Albertin A, Somalvico F, Aldegheri G (2011) Does continuous sciatic nerve block improve postoperative analgesia and early rehabilitation after total knee arthroplasty? A prospective, randomized, double-blinded study. Reg Anesth Pain Med 36:489–492

Carli F, Zavorsky GS (2005) Optimizing functional exercise capacity in the elderly surgical population. Curr Opin Clin Nutr Metab Care 8:23–32

Carli F, Charlebois P, Stein B, Feldman L, Zavorsky G, Kim DJ, Scott S, Mayo NE (2010a) Randomized clinical trial of prehabilitation in colorectal surgery. Br J Surg 97:1187–1197

Carli F, Clemente A, Asenjo JF, Kim DJ, Mistraletti G, Gomarasca M, Morabito A, Tanzer M (2010b) Analgesia and functional outcome after total knee arthroplasty: periarticular infiltration vs continuous femoral nerve block. Br J Anaesth 105:185–195

Carli F, Kehlet H, Baldini G, Steel A, McRae K, Slinger P, Hemmerling T, Salinas F, Neal J (2011) Evidence basis for regional anesthesia in multidisciplinary fast-track surgical care pathways. Reg Anesth Pain Med 36:63–72

Carroll I, Barelka P, Wang CK, Wang BM, Gillespie MJ, McCue R, Younger JW, Trafton J, Humphreys K, Goodman SB, Dirbas F, Whyte RI, Donington JS, Cannon WB, Mackey SC (2012) A pilot cohort study of the determinants of longitudinal opioid use after surgery. Anesth Analg 115:694–702

Chapman CR, Donaldson GW, Davis JJ, Bradshaw DH (2011) Improving individual measurement of postoperative pain: the pain trajectory. J Pain 12:257–262

Charous MT, Madison SJ, Suresh PJ, Sandhu NS, Loland VJ, Mariano ER, Donohue MC, Dutton PH, Ferguson EJ (2011) Ilfeld BM Continuous femoral nerve blocks: varying local anesthetic delivery method (bolus versus basal) to minimize quadriceps motor block while maintaining sensory block. Anesthesiology 115: 774–781

Chaumeron A, Audy D, Drolet P, Lavigne M, Vendittoli PA (2013) Periarticular injection in knee arthroplasty improves quadriceps function. Clin Orthop Relat Res 471:2284–2295

Chen L, Malarick C, Seefeld L, Wang S, Houghton M, Mao J (2009) Altered quantitative sensory testing outcome in subjects with opioid therapy. Pain 143:65–70

Choi PT, Bhandari M, Scott J, Douketis J (2003) Epidural analgesia for pain relief following hip or knee replacement. Cochrane Database Syst Rev (3):CD003071

Cook P, Stevens J, Gaudron C (2003) Comparing the effects of femoral nerve block versus femoral and sciatic nerve block on pain and opiate consumption after total knee arthroplasty. J Arthroplasty 18:583–586

Crassous PA, Denis C, Paris H, Senard JM (2007) Interest of alpha2-adrenergic agonists and antagonists in clinical practice: background, facts and perspectives. Curr Top Med Chem 7:187–194

Cremeans-Smith JK, Millington K, Sledjeski E, Greene K, Delahanty DL (2006) Sleep disruptions mediate the relationship between early postoperative pain and later functioning following total knee replacement surgery. J Behav Med 29:215–222

Crombie IK, Davies HT, Macrae WA (1998) Cut and thrust: antecedent surgery and trauma among patients attending a chronic pain clinic. Pain 76:167–171

Cross WW 3rd, Saleh KJ, Wilt TJ, Kane RL (2006) Agreement about indications for total knee arthroplasty. Clin Orthop Relat Res 446:34–39

Cullen BF, Haschke RH (1974) Local anesthetic inhibition of phagocytosis and metabolism of human leukocytes. Anesthesiology 40:142–146

Dahl V, Spreng UJ, Waage M, Raeder JC (2012) Short stay and less pain after ambulatory anterior cruciate ligament (ACL) repair: COX-2 inhibitor versus glucocorticoid versus both combined. Acta Anaesthesiol Scand 56:95–101

De Kock M, Loix S, Lavand'homme P (2013) Ketamine and peripheral inflammation. CNS Neurosci Ther 19:403–410

Dickstein R, Heffes Y, Shabtai EI, Markowitz E (1998) Total knee arthroplasty in the elderly: patients' self-appraisal 6 and 12 months postoperatively. Gerontology 44:204–210

Edwards RR (2005) Individual differences in endogenous pain modulation as a risk factor for chronic pain. Neurology 65:437–443

Edwards RR, Smith MT, Stonerock G, Haythornthwaite JA (2006) Pain-related catastrophizing in healthy women is associated with greater temporal summation of and reduced habituation to thermal pain. Clin J Pain 22:730–737

Elia N, Lysakowski C, Tramer MR (2005) Does multimodal analgesia with acetaminophen, nonsteroidal antiinflammatory drugs, or selective cyclooxygenase-2 inhibitors and patient-controlled analgesia morphine offer advantages over morphine alone? Meta-analyses of randomized trials. Anesthesiology 103:1296–1304

Essving P, Axelsson K, Aberg E, Spannar H, Gupta A, Lundin A (2011) Local infiltration analgesia versus intrathecal morphine for postoperative pain management after total knee arthroplasty: a randomized controlled trial. Anesth Analg 113:926–933

Feibel RJ, Dervin GF, Kim PR, Beaule PE (2009) Major complications associated with femoral nerve catheters for knee arthroplasty: a word of caution. J Arthroplasty 24:132–137

Fletcher D, Fermanian C, Mardaye A, Aegerter P (2008) A patient-based national survey on postoperative pain management in France reveals significant achievements and persistent challenges. Pain 137:441–451

Fowler SJ (2009) Incidence of severe complications after central neuraxial block. Br J Anaesth 102:882; author reply 882–883

Fowler SJ, Symons J, Sabato S, Myles PS (2008) Epidural analgesia compared with peripheral nerve blockade after major knee surgery: a systematic review and meta-analysis of randomized trials. Br J Anaesth 100:154–164

France CR, Taddio A, Shah VS, Page MG, Katz J (2009) Maternal family history of hypertension attenuates neonatal pain response. Pain 142:189–193

Gelfand HJ, Ouanes JP, Lesley MR, Ko PS, Murphy JD, Sumida SM, Isaac GR, Kumar K, Wu CL (2011) Analgesic efficacy of ultrasound-guided regional anesthesia: a meta-analysis. J Clin Anesth 23:90–96

Gentili M, Enel D, Szymskiewicz O, Mansour F, Bonnet F (2001) Postoperative analgesia by intraarticular clonidine and neostigmine in patients undergoing knee arthroscopy. Reg Anesth Pain Med 26:342–347

Gerbershagen HJ, Aduckathil S, van Wijck AJ, Peelen LM, Kalkman CJ, Meissner W (2013) Pain intensity on the first day after surgery: a prospective cohort study comparing 179 surgical procedures. Anesthesiology 118:934–944

Gilroy DW, Colville-Nash PR, Willis D, Chivers J, Paul-Clark MJ, Willoughby DA (1999) Inducible cyclooxygenase may have anti-inflammatory properties. Nat Med 5:698–701

Grosu I, de Kock M (2011) New concepts in acute pain management: strategies to prevent chronic postsurgical pain, opioid-induced hyperalgesia, and outcome measures. Anesthesiol Clin 29:311–327

Grosu I, Lavand'homme P, Thienpont E (2014) Pain after knee arthroplasty: an unresolved issue. Knee Surg Sports Traumatol Arthrosc 22(8):1744–1758. doi:10.1007/s00167-013-2750-2

Harden RN, Bruehl S, Stanos S, Brander V, Chung OY, Saltz S, Adams A, Stulberg SD (2003) Prospective examination of pain-related and psychological predictors of CRPS-like phenomena following total knee arthroplasty: a preliminary study. Pain 106:393–400

Haroutiunian S, Nikolajsen L, Finnerup NB, Jensen TS (2013) The neuropathic component in persistent postsurgical pain: a systematic literature review. Pain 154:95–102

Harsten A, Kehlet H, Toksvig-Larsen S (2013) Recovery after total intravenous general anaesthesia or spinal anaesthesia for total knee arthroplasty: a randomized trial. Br J Anaesth 111:391–399

Hartrick CT, Pestano C, Carlson N, Hartrick S (2011) Capsaicin instillation for postoperative pain following total knee arthroplasty: a preliminary report of a randomized, double-blind, parallel-group, placebo-controlled, multicentre trial. Clin Drug Investig 31:877–882

Hassaballa M, Artz N, Weale A, Porteous A (2012) Alteration in skin sensation following knee arthroplasty and its impact on kneeling ability: a comparison of three common surgical incisions. Knee Surg Sports Traumatol Arthrosc 20:1983–1987

Hebard S, Hocking G (2011) Echogenic technology can improve needle visibility during ultrasound-guided regional anesthesia. Reg Anesth Pain Med 36:185–189

Henningsen MH, Jaeger P, Hilsted KL, Dahl JB (2013) Prevalence of saphenous nerve injury after adductor-canal-blockade in patients receiving total knee arthroplasty. Acta Anaesthesiol Scand 57:112–117

Hepinstall MS, Rutledge JR, Bornstein LJ, Mazumdar M, Westrich GH (2011) Factors that impact expectations before total knee arthroplasty. J Arthroplasty 26: 870–876

Hofmann S, Seitlinger G, Djahani O, Pietsch M (2011) The painful knee after TKA: a diagnostic algorithm for failure analysis. Knee Surg Sports Traumatol Arthrosc 19:1442–1452

Hu WS, Muscoplat CC (1980) Lidocaine: effect on phagocytosis and purification of monocytes in bovine peripheral blood. Am J Vet Res 41:447–449

Hurley RW, Adams MC (2008) Sex, gender, and pain: an overview of a complex field. Anesth Analg 107: 309–317

Ilfeld BM, Le LT, Meyer RS, Mariano ER, Vandenborne K, Duncan PW, Sessler DI, Enneking FK, Shuster JJ, Theriaque DW, Berry LF, Spadoni EH, Gearen PF (2008) Ambulatory continuous femoral nerve blocks decrease time to discharge readiness after tricompartment total knee arthroplasty: a randomized, triple-masked, placebo-controlled study. Anesthesiology 108:703–713

Ilfeld BM, Duke KB, Donohue MC (2010) The association between lower extremity continuous peripheral nerve blocks and patient falls after knee and hip arthroplasty. Anesth Analg 111:1552–1554

Ilfeld BM, Shuster JJ, Theriaque DW, Mariano ER, Girard PJ, Loland VJ, Meyer S, Donovan JF, Pugh GA, Le LT, Sessler DI, Ball ST (2011) Long-term pain, stiffness, and functional disability after total knee arthroplasty with and without an extended ambulatory continuous femoral nerve block: a prospective, 1-year follow-up of a multicenter, randomized, triple-masked, placebo-controlled trial. Reg Anesth Pain Med 36:116–120

Ip HY, Abrishami A, Peng PW, Wong J, Chung F (2009) Predictors of postoperative pain and analgesic consumption: a qualitative systematic review. Anesthesiology 111:657–677

Jaeger P, Nielsen ZJ, Henningsen MH, Hilsted KL, Mathiesen O, Dahl JB (2013) Adductor canal block versus femoral nerve block and quadriceps strength: a randomized, double-blind, placebo-controlled, cross-over study in healthy volunteers. Anesthesiology 118:409–415

Jenstrup MT, Jaeger P, Lund J, Fomsgaard JS, Bache S, Mathiesen O, Larsen TK, Dahl JB (2012) Effects of adductor-canal-blockade on pain and ambulation after total knee arthroplasty: a randomized study. Acta Anaesthesiol Scand 56:357–364

Johansen A, Romundstad L, Nielsen CS, Schirmer H, Stubhaug A (2012) Persistent postsurgical pain in a general population: prevalence and predictors in the Tromso study. Pain 153:1390–1396

Joo JH, Park JW, Kim JS, Kim YH (2011) Is intra-articular multimodal drug injection effective in pain management after total knee arthroplasty? A randomized, double-blinded, prospective study. J Arthroplasty 26:1095–1099

Jules-Elysee KM, Lipnitsky JY, Patel N, Anastasian G, Wilfred SE, Urban MK, Sculco TP (2011) Use of low-dose steroids in decreasing cytokine release during bilateral total knee replacement. Reg Anesth Pain Med 36:36–40

Jules-Elysee KM, Wilfred SE, Memtsoudis SG, Kim DH, YaDeau JT, Urban MK, Lichardi ML, McLawhorn AS, Sculco TP (2012) Steroid modulation of cytokine release and desmosine levels in bilateral total knee replacement: a prospective, double-blind, randomized controlled trial. J Bone Joint Surg Am 94: 2120–2127

Kadic L, Boonstra MC, DEWM MC, Lako SJ, VANE J, Driessen JJ (2009) Continuous femoral nerve block after total knee arthroplasty? Acta Anaesthesiol Scand 53:914–920

Kalkman CJ, Visser K, Moen J, Bonsel GJ, Grobbee DE, Moons KG (2003) Preoperative prediction of severe postoperative pain. Pain 105:415–423

Kardash KJ, Sarrazin F, Tessler MJ, Velly AM (2008) Single-dose dexamethasone reduces dynamic pain after total hip arthroplasty. Anesth Analg 106:1253–1257, table of contents

Kawamata M, Watanabe H, Nishikawa K, Takahashi T, Kozuka Y, Kawamata T, Omote K, Namiki A (2002) Different mechanisms of development and maintenance of experimental incision-induced hyperalgesia in human skin. Anesthesiology 97:550–559

Kawasaki Y, Zhang L, Cheng JK, Ji RR (2008) Cytokine mechanisms of central sensitization: distinct and overlapping role of interleukin-1beta, interleukin-6, and tumor necrosis factor-alpha in regulating synaptic and neuronal activity in the superficial spinal cord. J Neurosci 28:5189–5194

Keefe FJ, Lefebvre JC, Egert JR, Affleck G, Sullivan MJ, Caldwell DS (2000) The relationship of gender to pain, pain behavior, and disability in osteoarthritis patients: the role of catastrophizing. Pain 87: 325–334

Kehlet H, Andersen LO (2011) Local infiltration analgesia in joint replacement: the evidence and recommendations for clinical practice. Acta Anaesthesiol Scand 55:778–784

Kehlet H, Dahl JB (1993) The value of "multimodal" or "balanced analgesia" in postoperative pain treatment. Anesth Analg 77:1048–1056

Kehlet H, Jensen TS, Woolf CJ (2006) Persistent postsurgical pain: risk factors and prevention. Lancet 367:1618–1625

Kerr DR, Kohan L (2008) Local infiltration analgesia: a technique for the control of acute postoperative pain following knee and hip surgery: a case study of 325 patients. Acta Orthop 79:174–183

Khan AA, Iadarola M, Yang HY, Dionne RA (2007) Expression of COX-1 and COX-2 in a clinical model of acute inflammation. J Pain 8:349–354

Khanna A, Gougoulias N, Longo UG, Maffulli N (2009) Minimally invasive total knee arthroplasty: a systematic review. Orthop Clin North Am 40:479–489, viii

King J, Stamper DL, Schaad DC, Leopold SS (2007) Minimally invasive total knee arthroplasty compared with traditional total knee arthroplasty. Assessment of the learning curve and the postoperative recuperative period. J Bone Joint Surg Am 89:1497–1503

Kinghorn K, Ellinas H, Barboi AC, Dolinski SY (2012) Case scenario: nerve injury after knee arthroplasty and sciatic nerve block. Anesthesiology 116:918–923

Kosek E, Ordeberg G (2000a) Abnormalities of somatosensory perception in patients with painful osteoarthritis normalize following successful treatment. Eur J Pain 4:229–238

Kosek E, Ordeberg G (2000b) Lack of pressure pain modulation by heterotopic noxious conditioning stimulation in patients with painful osteoarthritis before, but not following, surgical pain relief. Pain 88:69–78

Krenzel BA, Cook C, Martin GN, Vail TP, Attarian DE, Bolognesi MP (2009) Posterior capsular injections of ropivacaine during total knee arthroplasty: a randomized, double-blind, placebo-controlled study. J Arthroplasty 24:138–143

Kuehn BM (2009) New pain guideline for older patients: avoid NSAIDs, consider opioids. JAMA 302:19

Kugisaki H, Sonohata M, Komine M, Tsunoda K, Someya S, Honke H, Mawatari M, Hotokebuchi T (2009) Serum concentrations of interleukin-6 in patients following unilateral versus bilateral total knee arthroplasty. J Orthop Sci 14:437–442

Laskowski K, Stirling A, McKay W, Lim HJ (2011) A systematic review of intravenous ketamine for postoperative analgesia. Can J Anaesth 58:911–923

Lautenbacher S, Huber C, Kunz M, Parthum A, Weber PG, Griessinger N, Sittl R (2009) Hypervigilance as predictor of postoperative acute pain: its predictive potency compared with experimental pain sensitivity, cortisol reactivity, and affective state. Clin J Pain 25:92–100

Lautenbacher S, Huber C, Schofer D, Kunz M, Parthum A, Weber PG, Roman C, Griessinger N, Sittl R (2010) Attentional and emotional mechanisms related to pain as predictors of chronic postoperative pain: a comparison with other psychological and physiological predictors. Pain 151:722–731

Lavand'homme P (2011) The progression from acute to chronic pain. Curr Opin Anaesthesiol 24:545–550

Liu SS, Wu CL (2007) The effect of analgesic technique on postoperative patient-reported outcomes including analgesia: a systematic review. Anesth Analg 105:789–808

Liu SS, Buvanendran A, Rathmell JP, Sawhney M, Bae JJ, Moric M, Perros S, Pope AJ, Poultsides L, Della Valle CJ, Shin NS, McCartney CJ, Ma Y, Shah M, Wood MJ, Manion SC, Sculco TP (2012) A cross-sectional survey on prevalence and risk factors for persistent postsurgical pain 1 year after total hip and knee replacement. Reg Anesth Pain Med 37:415–422

Lunn TH, Kristensen BB, Andersen LO, Husted H, Otte KS, Gaarn-Larsen L, Kehlet H (2011) Effect of high-dose preoperative methylprednisolone on pain and recovery after total knee arthroplasty: a randomized, placebo-controlled trial. Br J Anaesth 106:230–238

Macalou D, Trueck S, Meuret P, Heck M, Vial F, Ouologuem S, Capdevila X, Virion JM, Bouaziz H (2004) Postoperative analgesia after total knee replacement: the effect of an obturator nerve block added to the femoral 3-in-1 nerve block. Anesth Analg 99:251–254

Macfarlane AJ, Prasad GA, Chan VW, Brull R (2009) Does regional anesthesia improve outcome after total knee arthroplasty? Clin Orthop Relat Res 467:2379–2402

Maheshwari AV, Blum YC, Shekhar L, Ranawat AS, Ranawat CS (2009) Multimodal pain management after total hip and knee arthroplasty at the Ranawat Orthopaedic Center. Clin Orthop Relat Res 467:1418–1423

Mallet C, Daulhac L, Bonnefont J, Ledent C, Etienne M, Chapuy E, Libert F, Eschalier A (2008) Endocannabinoid and serotonergic systems are needed for acetaminophen-induced analgesia. Pain 139:190–200

Marhofer D, Kettner SC, Marhofer P, Pils S, Weber M, Zeitlinger M (2013) Dexmedetomidine as an adjuvant to ropivacaine prolongs peripheral nerve block: a volunteer study. Br J Anaesth 110:438–442

Markert SE (2011) The use of cryotherapy after a total knee replacement: a literature review. Orthop Nurs 30:29–36

Marret E, Kurdi O, Zufferey P, Bonnet F (2005) Effects of nonsteroidal antiinflammatory drugs on patient-controlled analgesia morphine side effects: meta-analysis of randomized controlled trials. Anesthesiology 102:1249–1260

Martin F, Martinez V, Mazoit JX, Bouhassira D, Cherif K, Gentili ME, Piriou P, Chauvin M, Fletcher D (2008) Antiinflammatory effect of peripheral nerve blocks after knee surgery: clinical and biologic evaluation. Anesthesiology 109:484–490

Matsuura T, Mori T, Hasaka M, Kuno M, Kawawaki J, Nishikawa K, Narahashi T, Sawada M, Asada A (2012) Inhibition of voltage-gated proton channels by local anaesthetics in GMI-R1 rat microglia. J Physiol 590:827–844

McCartney CJ, McLeod GA (2011) Local infiltration analgesia for total knee arthroplasty. Br J Anaesth 107:487–489

McKay C, Prapavessis H, Doherty T (2012) The effect of a prehabilitation exercise program on quadriceps strength for patients undergoing total knee arthroplasty: a randomized controlled pilot study. PM R 4:647–656

Memtsoudis SG, Sun X, Chiu YL, Stundner O, Liu SS, Banerjee S, Mazumdar M, Sharrock NE (2013) Perioperative comparative effectiveness of anesthetic technique in orthopedic patients. Anesthesiology 118:1046–1058

Merskey H (1994) International Association for the Study of Pain. Task Force on Taxonomy. Part III: Pain Terms, A Current List with Definitions and Notes on Usage (pp 209-214). Classification of Chronic Pain, Second Edition, IASP Task Force on Taxonomy, edited by H. Merskey and N. Bogduk, ISAP Press, Seattle, 1994. http://www.iasp-pain.org

Mont MA, Serna FK, Krackow KA, Hungerford DS (1996) Exploration of radiographically normal total knee replacements for unexplained pain. Clin Orthop Relat Res 331:216–220

Morze CJ, Johnson NR, Williams G, Moroney M, Lamberton T, McAuliffe M (2013) Knee pain during the first three months after unilateral total knee arthroplasty: a multi-centre prospective cohort study. J Arthroplasty 28:1565–1570

Murray DW, Frost SJ (1998) Pain in the assessment of total knee replacement. J Bone Joint Surg Br 80:426–431

Muscara MN, McKnight W, Asfaha S, Wallace JL (2000) Wound collagen deposition in rats: effects of an NO-NSAID and a selective COX-2 inhibitor. Br J Pharmacol 129:681–686

Nicholson G, Hall GM (2011) Effects of anaesthesia on the inflammatory response to injury. Curr Opin Anaesthesiol 24:370–374

Niki Y, Mochizuki T, Momohara S, Saito S, Toyama Y, Matsumoto H (2009) Is minimally invasive surgery in total knee arthroplasty really minimally invasive surgery? J Arthroplasty 24:499–504

Ogonda L, Wilson R, Archbold P, Lawlor M, Humphreys P, O'Brien S, Beverland D (2005) A minimal-incision technique in total hip arthroplasty does not improve early postoperative outcomes. A prospective, randomized, controlled trial. J Bone Joint Surg Am 87:701–710

Omoigui S (2007a) The biochemical origin of pain–proposing a new law of pain: the origin of all pain is inflammation and the inflammatory response. Part 1 of 3–a unifying law of pain. Med Hypotheses 69:70–82

Omoigui S (2007b) The biochemical origin of pain: the origin of all pain is inflammation and the inflammatory response. Part 2 of 3 – inflammatory profile of pain syndromes. Med Hypotheses 69:1169–1178

Orebaugh SL, Kentor ML, Williams BA (2012) Adverse outcomes associated with nerve stimulator-guided and ultrasound-guided peripheral nerve blocks by supervised trainees: update of a single-site database. Reg Anesth Pain Med 37:577–582

Paul JE, Arya A, Hurlburt L, Cheng J, Thabane L, Tidy A, Murthy Y (2010) Femoral nerve block improves analgesia outcomes after total knee arthroplasty: a meta-analysis of randomized controlled trials. Anesthesiology 113:1144–1162

Perlas A, Kirkham KR, Billing R, Tse C, Brull R, Gandhi R, Chan VW (2013) The impact of analgesic modality on early ambulation following total knee arthroplasty. Reg Anesth Pain Med 38:334–339

Petterson SC, Raisis L, Bodenstab A, Snyder-Mackler L (2007) Disease-specific gender differences among total knee arthroplasty candidates. J Bone Joint Surg Am 89:2327–2333

Pinto PR, McIntyre T, Almeida A, Araujo-Soares V (2012) The mediating role of pain catastrophizing in the relationship between presurgical anxiety and acute postsurgical pain after hysterectomy. Pain 153:218–226

Pogatzki-Zahn EM, Zahn PK (2006) From preemptive to preventive analgesia. Curr Opin Anaesthesiol 19: 551–555

Puolakka PA, Rorarius MG, Roviola M, Puolakka TJ, Nordhausen K, Lindgren L (2010) Persistent pain following knee arthroplasty. Eur J Anaesthesiol 27: 455–460

Rawal N (2012) Epidural technique for postoperative pain: gold standard no more? Reg Anesth Pain Med 37:310–317

Remy C, Marret E, Bonnet F (2005) Effects of acetaminophen on morphine side-effects and consumption after major surgery: meta-analysis of randomized controlled trials. Br J Anaesth 94:505–513

Richman JM, Liu SS, Courpas G, Wong R, Rowlingson AJ, McGready J, Cohen SR, Wu CL (2006) Does continuous peripheral nerve block provide superior pain control to opioids? A meta-analysis. Anesth Analg 102:248–257

Romundstad L, Breivik H, Niemi G, Helle A, Stubhaug A (2004) Methylprednisolone intravenously 1 day after surgery has sustained analgesic and opioid-sparing effects. Acta Anaesthesiol Scand 48:1223–1231

Roth ML, Tripp DA, Harrison MH, Sullivan M, Carson P (2007) Demographic and psychosocial predictors of acute perioperative pain for total knee arthroplasty. Pain Res Manag 12:185–194

Schnabel A, Meyer-Friessem CH, Zahn PK, Pogatzki-Zahn EM (2013) Ultrasound compared with nerve stimulation guidance for peripheral nerve catheter placement: a meta-analysis of randomized controlled trials. Br J Anaesth 111:564–572

Schug SA (2007) Peripheral nerve blockade carries only a minimal risk of permanent neurological complications. Anaesth Intensive Care 35:11–12

Scott CE, Howie CR, MacDonald D, Biant LC (2010) Predicting dissatisfaction following total knee replacement: a prospective study of 1217 patients. J Bone Joint Surg Br 92:1253–1258

Sean VW, Chin PL, Chia SL, Yang KY, Lo NN, Yeo SJ (2011) Single-dose periarticular steroid infiltration for pain management in total knee arthroplasty: a prospective, double-blind, randomised controlled trial. Singapore Med J 52:19–23

Serhan CN, Chiang N, Van Dyke TE (2008) Resolving inflammation: dual anti-inflammatory and pro-resolution lipid mediators. Nat Rev Immunol 8: 349–361

Sharma S, Iorio R, Specht LM, Davies-Lepie S, Healy WL (2010) Complications of femoral nerve block for total knee arthroplasty. Clin Orthop Relat Res 468:135–140

Simonnet G, Rivat C (2003) Opioid-induced hyperalgesia: abnormal or normal pain? Neuroreport 14:1–7

Singh JA, Gabriel S, Lewallen D (2008) The impact of gender, age, and preoperative pain severity on pain after TKA. Clin Orthop Relat Res 466:2717–2723

Skou ST, Graven-Nielsen T, Rasmussen S, Simonsen O, Laursen MB, Arendt-Nielsen L (2013) Widespread sensitization in patients with chronic pain after revision total knee arthroplasty. Pain 154:1588–1594

Solomon DH, Rassen JA, Glynn RJ, Garneau K, Levin R, Lee J, Schneeweiss S (2010) The comparative safety of opioids for nonmalignant pain in older adults. Arch Intern Med 170:1979–1986

Sommer M, de Rijke JM, van Kleef M, Kessels AG, Peters ML, Geurts JW, Gramke HF, Marcus MA (2008) The prevalence of postoperative pain in a sample of 1490 surgical inpatients. Eur J Anaesthesiol 25:267–274

Sommer M, de Rijke JM, van Kleef M, Kessels AG, Peters ML, Geurts JW, Patijn J, Gramke HF, Marcus MA (2010) Predictors of acute postoperative pain after elective surgery. Clin J Pain 26:87–94

Spreng UJ, Dahl V, Hjall A, Fagerland MW, Raeder J (2010) High-volume local infiltration analgesia combined with intravenous or local ketorolac + morphine compared with epidural analgesia after total knee arthroplasty. Br J Anaesth 105:675–682

Srikandarajah S, Gilron I (2011) Systematic review of movement-evoked pain versus pain at rest in postsurgical clinical trials and meta-analyses: a fundamental distinction requiring standardized measurement. Pain 152:1734–1739

Steyaert A, Lavand'homme P (2013) Postoperative opioids: let us take responsibility for the possible consequences. Eur J Anaesthesiol 30:50–52

Straube S, Derry S, McQuay HJ, Moore RA (2005) Effect of preoperative Cox-II-selective NSAIDs (coxibs) on postoperative outcomes: a systematic review of randomized studies. Acta Anaesthesiol Scand 49: 601–613

Suokas AK, Walsh DA, McWilliams DF, Condon L, Moreton B, Wylde V, Arendt-Nielsen L, Zhang W (2012) Quantitative sensory testing in painful osteoarthritis: a systematic review and meta-analysis. Osteoarthritis Cartilage 20:1075–1085

Swank AM, Kachelman JB, Bibeau W, Quesada PM, Nyland J, Malkani A, Topp RV (2011) Prehabilitation before total knee arthroplasty increases strength and function in older adults with severe osteoarthritis. J Strength Cond Res 25:318–325

Thienpont E (2013a) Faster quadriceps recovery with the far medial subvastus approach in minimally invasive total knee arthroplasty. Knee Surg Sports Traumatol Arthrosc 21:2370–2374

Thienpont E (2013b) Faster recovery after minimally invasive surgery in total knee arthroplasty. Knee Surg Sports Traumatol Arthrosc 21:2412–2417

Thomas T, Robinson C, Champion D, McKell M, Pell M (1998) Prediction and assessment of the severity of post-operative pain and of satisfaction with management. Pain 75:177–185

Topp R, Swank AM, Quesada PM, Nyland J, Malkani A (2009) The effect of prehabilitation exercise on strength and functioning after total knee arthroplasty. PM R 1:729–735

Torrance N, Smith BH, Bennett MI, Lee AJ (2006) The epidemiology of chronic pain of predominantly neuropathic origin. Results from a general population survey. J Pain 7:281–289

Turan A, Sessler DI (2011) Steroids to ameliorate postoperative pain. Anesthesiology 115:457–459

Vilardo LS, Shah M (2011) Chronic pain after hip and knee replacement. Tech Reg Anesth Pain Manag 15:110–115

Vissers MM, Bussmann JB, Verhaar JA, Busschbach JJ, Bierma-Zeinstra SM, Reijman M (2012) Psychological factors affecting the outcome of total hip and knee arthroplasty: a systematic review. Semin Arthritis Rheum 41:576–588

Wakankar HM, Nicholl JE, Koka R, D'Arcy JC (1999) The tourniquet in total knee arthroplasty. A prospective, randomised study. J Bone Joint Surg Br 81:30–33

Waldron NH, Jones CA, Gan TJ, Allen TK, Habib AS (2013) Impact of perioperative dexamethasone on postoperative analgesia and side-effects: systematic review and meta-analysis. Br J Anaesth 110:191–200

Walls RJ, McHugh G, O'Gorman DJ, Moyna NM, O'Byrne JM (2010) Effects of preoperative neuromuscular electrical stimulation on quadriceps strength and functional recovery in total knee arthroplasty. A pilot study. BMC Musculoskelet Disord 11:119

Wegener JT, van Ooij B, van Dijk CN, Hollmann MW, Preckel B, Stevens MF (2011) Value of single-injection or continuous sciatic nerve block in addition to a continuous femoral nerve block in patients undergoing total knee arthroplasty: a prospective, randomized, controlled trial. Reg Anesth Pain Med 36:481–488

Weissman-Fogel I, Granovsky Y, Crispel Y, Ben-Nun A, Best LA, Yarnitsky D, Granot M (2009) Enhanced presurgical pain temporal summation response predicts post-thoracotomy pain intensity during the acute postoperative phase. J Pain 10:628–636

White PF, Kehlet H, Neal JM, Schricker T, Carr DB, Carli F (2007) The role of the anesthesiologist in fast-track surgery: from multimodal analgesia to perioperative medical care. Anesth Analg 104:1380–1396, table of contents

Widmer B, Lustig S, Scholes CJ, Molloy A, Leo SP, Coolican MR, Parker DA (2013) Incidence and severity of complications due to femoral nerve blocks performed for knee surgery. Knee 20:181–185

Woolf CJ (2011) Central sensitization: implications for the diagnosis and treatment of pain. Pain 152:S2–S15

Woolf CJ (2012) Central sensitization: implications for the diagnosis and treatment of pain. Pain 152:S2–S15

Wylde V, Gooberman-Hill R, Horwood J, Beswick A, Noble S, Brookes S, Smith AJ, Pyke M, Dieppe P, Blom AW (2011a) The effect of local anaesthetic wound infiltration on chronic pain after lower limb joint replacement: a protocol for a double-blind randomised controlled trial. BMC Musculoskelet Disord 12:53

Wylde V, Hewlett S, Learmonth ID, Dieppe P (2011b) Persistent pain after joint replacement: prevalence, sensory qualities, and postoperative determinants. Pain 152:566–572

Wylde V, Rooker J, Halliday L, Blom A (2011c) Acute postoperative pain at rest after hip and knee arthroplasty: severity, sensory qualities and impact on sleep. Orthop Traumatol Surg Res 97:139–144

Xu J, Brennan TJ (2011) The pathophysiology of acute pain: animal models. Curr Opin Anaesthesiol 24:508–514

Xu ZZ, Zhang L, Liu T, Park JY, Berta T, Yang R, Serhan CN, Ji RR (2010) Resolvins RvE1 and RvD1 attenuate inflammatory pain via central and peripheral actions. Nat Med 16:592–597, 591p following 597

Yarnitsky D (2010) Conditioned pain modulation (the diffuse noxious inhibitory control-like effect): its relevance for acute and chronic pain states. Curr Opin Anaesthesiol 23:611–615

Zhang J, Ho KY, Wang Y (2011) Efficacy of pregabalin in acute postoperative pain: a meta-analysis. Br J Anaesth 106:454–462

Pain Management in Total Knee Arthroplasty: A Surgeon-Anesthesiologist Cooperation

14

Paolo Adravanti, Giuseppe Calafiore, and Aldo Ampollini

Open Questions

- How anesthesiologists and orthopedics surgeon should interact in pain management?
- Which patients need more attention to achieve a satisfactory pain control?
- Which components of the multimodal therapy are utilized in the daily practice?
- How should we manage pain after discharge?

14.1 Introduction

Outcome after knee replacement is significantly influenced by the choice of analgesic therapy to control pain and bleeding, both of which can interfere with the recovery of knee joint function. Pain needs to be effectively controlled in the days immediately after the procedure and over the following months. Effective pain control reduces complications and permits early rehabilitation, increasing patient satisfaction and diminishing the risk of chronic joint pain.

In order to achieve these goals, the multimodal approach to pain management requires three stages which should be guided by the cooperation between the orthopedic surgical team and the anesthesiologist:

1. Preoperative stage: placement of a peripheral nerve block or an epidural catheter
2. Intraoperative stage: intra-articular injection of local anesthetics for pain control and reduction of bleeding
3. Postoperative stage: continuous infusion of analgesics

14.2 Patient Characteristics

Various patient-related characteristics must be considered when selecting the analgesic protocol for the pre-, intra-, and postoperative stages:

14.2.1 Psychological Aspects

- Depression and anxiety can increase pain perception (Ayers et al. 2013)
- Being adequately informed about the intervention and the rehabilitation pathway helps the patient to contextualize the situation and reduce pain perception, as well as the development of arthrofibrosis (Livbjerg et al. 2013)

P. Adravanti (✉) • G. Calafiore • A. Ampollini
Department of Orthopaedics, "Città di Parma" Clinic, Piazza Maestri 5, Parma 43100, Italy
e-mail: info@paoloadravanti.com; gcalafiore@hotmail.com; info@aldoampollini.com

A. Baldini, P. Caldora (eds.), *Perioperative Medical Management for Total Joint Arthroplasty: How to Control Hemostasis, Pain and Infection*, DOI 10.1007/978-3-319-07203-6_14,

14.2.2 Sex, Age, and Ethnic Origin

- Female sex is associated with better response to narcotic drugs.
- Patients aged over 65 years had a better response to pain therapy than younger patients (Trousdale et al. 1999).
- Differences in pain perception in relation to ethnicity have been documented (Carragee et al. 1999; Davidhizar and Giger 2004). Pain perception and response to analgesics are associated with individual differences in enzymatic degradation of drugs (Anderson et al. 2009). For example, response to codeine is 5 % lower in blacks as compared to whites.

14.2.3 Pain Intensity and Joint Deformity

- Patients presenting with severe preoperative pain will experience greater postoperative pain unless they are adequately prepared with home-based analgesic therapy before the operation (Katz et al. 1992; Bridenbaugh 1994).
- Severe joint deformities, ankylosis, or other conditions, including reduced preoperative ROM or previous revision surgeries, require more aggressive surgical treatment that can cause greater postoperative pain (Noiseux et al. 2014).

14.3 Preoperative Anesthesiologist Assessment and Pain Therapy

Given the myriad factors that concur in good pain management, the anesthesiologist plays a key role in selecting the protocol to be applied in the situations described above. Unfortunately, time and attention to preoperative assessment shortly before the operation are frequently insufficient, often precluding administration of therapy that could provide long-lasting coverage. Establishing a tailored pain management protocol is of paramount importance. Pain service protocols after arthroplasty should then be adjusted on the basis of the patient's type, needs, and comorbidities.

14.4 Multimodal Anesthesia

14.4.1 Preoperative Therapy

There is solid documentation supporting a better response to intra- and postoperative pain after the administration of analgesics in the immediate preoperative period (Mullaji et al. 2010; Lin et al. 2013; Weng and Wijeysundera 2007). The functional recovery is also affected in a statistically significant way. The most commonly used drugs are celecoxib, meloxicam, oxycodone, acetaminophen, pregabalin, and gabapentin.

14.4.2 Perioperative Therapy: Peripheral Nerve Blocks and Epidural Catheter

The complication rate of epidural catheter placement following spinal anesthesia is 0.3 % (Swenson et al. 2006) (Table 14.1). However, pain control is strongly influenced by accurate catheter positioning (Salinas et al. 2006) and requires close monitoring during hospitalization (Horlocker et al. 1994; Jeng et al. 2010). The use of a femoral nerve block and sciatic nerve block, alone or combined (Cook et al. 2003; Weber et al. 2002), as compared with the risk of common complications such as loss of quadriceps strength (Widmer et al. 2012) and nerve damage (Horlocker et al. 1994; Jeng et al. 2010), has been reported to accelerate rehabilitation and reduce postoperative opiate consumption. However, the incidence of postoperative falls is around 3 % (Pelt et al. 2014). The complications are higher in obese patients if the duration of infusion lasts longer than 48 h (Wasserstein et al. 2013).

In contrast, recent systematic reviews and meta-analyses of the literature (Fowler et al. 2008; Fischer et al. 2008; Paul et al. 2010) found little difference in pain reduction in patients who received good postoperative continuous infusion therapy.

Table 14.1 Multiple potential problems

Motor block
Contralateral leg numbness
Ileus pressure phenomenon
Pruritus
Epidural hematoma
Nausea and vomiting
Technical issues

Table 14.2 Common drugs used for intraoperative injections

Bupivacaine
Ropivacaine
Morphine sulfate
Epinephrine
Methylprednisolone acetate
Cefuroxime
Ketorolac
Fentanyl
Pregabalin
Ibuprofen

Unlike peripheral nerve or sciatic nerve blockage, saphenous nerve block is not associated with complications such as loss of quadriceps strength since it acts only on sensory and not on motor nerves (Kim et al. 2014). In general, the use of saphenous nerve block has been shown to be equally effective in postoperative pain control, with fewer complications. And though a more complex procedure, there is a growing body of evidence for its greater efficacy and reliability in joint prosthesis surgery.

14.4.3 Perioperative Therapy: Intra-articular Injection

Intra-articular injection of drugs to reduce bleeding and manage postoperative pain is an established procedure for which a variety of protocols and drugs are available (Ranawat and Ranawat 2007; Kelley et al. 2013; Mullaji et al. 2010) (Table 14.2). Numerous studies have shown that local anesthetic infiltration can reduce pain and bleeding for about 4 h during the postoperative period and the need for analgesic drugs for 4 weeks postoperatively. Its effectiveness is directly related to the injection technique, which should be performed before and then again after prosthesis positioning (Ranawat and Ranawat 2007) in the intra- and extra-articular regions. The right execution allows a significant improvement of postoperative pain and a better functional recovery (Ranawat and Ranawat 2007).

14.4.4 Postoperative Therapy: Multimodal Analgesia

Maintenance of postoperative infusion therapy is essential for good pain management during the postoperative period. The use of morphine alone has been generally abandoned because of the numerous complications associated with the administration of high doses. Under one of the commonly used protocols, combination therapy involves continuous infusion of several different drugs at different times to create a synergistic effect between them, with optimal pain control and fewer side effects (Dalury et al. 2011).

The recent literature shows that multimodal analgesia allows a better pain control than PCA (Lamplot et al. 2014).

14.5 Pain Management at Discharge

Analgesic therapy prescribed at discharge should be selected by the anesthesiologist and should consider the following aspects:

- Side effects noted during hospitalization
- Pharmacologic response to the drugs administered
- Complications noted during hospitalization
- Subjective pain perception

Aggressive analgesic therapy is essential for ensuring patient satisfaction and accelerating rehabilitation and joint function recovery. Patients who have received aggressive continuous analgesic therapy have reported significantly better postoperative improvement than those who used analgesics only as needed (Pati et al. 1994).

Conclusions

Close cooperation between anesthesiologists and surgeons is essential for the application of effective analgesic protocols.

A multimodal approach for pain control serves to modulate the nociceptive response on different pain pathways, peripheral and central, reducing the consumption of opiate which is one of the main responsible for postoperative side effects.

The literature shows that the protocols should be standardized and should take into account the different subjective and objective patient's characteristics. Preoperative pain therapy, perioperative intra-articular injections, epidural catheter, and postoperative infusion therapy have been shown to improve the clinical outcome, as well as the patient's satisfaction.

The use of peripheral nerve block is still debated. Basing on benefits and complications of these procedures, there is a growing body of evidence for a greater efficacy in joint prosthesis surgery of the saphenous nerve block, although it is a more complex procedure preoperative

Key Points

- Patient characteristics and severe joint deformities or comorbidities can significantly influence the choice of pain management strategies.
- Thorough assessment by the anesthesiologist and appropriate preemptive analgesia are key to manage postoperative pain.
- Multimodal anesthesia, with particular reference to pain management, has been shown to provide optimal pain control during the immediate- and long-term postoperative periods, by virtue of the synergic effect of the drugs administered.
- Monitoring of analgesic therapy also after discharge is essential for accelerating joint functional recovery.

References

Anderson KO, Green CR, Payne R (2009) Racial and ethnic disparities in pain: causes and consequences of unequal care. J Pain 10(12):1187–1204

Ayers DC, Franklin PD, Ring DC (2013) The role of emotional health in functional outcome after orthopaedic surgery: extending the biopsychosocial model to orthopaedics: AOA critical issues. J Bone Joint Surg Am 95:e165

Bridenbaugh PO (1994) Preemptive analgesia-is it clinically relevant? Anesth Analg 78:203–204

Carragee J, Vittum D, Truong T, Burton D (1999) Pain control and cultural norms and expectations after closed femoral shaft fractures. Am J Orthop (Belle Mead NJ) 28(2):97–102

Cook P, Stevens J, Gaudron C (2003) Comparing the effects of femoral nerve block versus femoral and sciatic nerve block on pain and opiate consumption after total knee arthroplasty. J Arthroplasty 18:583–586

Dalury DF, Lieberman JR, MacDonald SJ (2011) Current and innovative pain management techniques in total knee arthroplasty. J Bone Joint Surg Am 93(20): 1938–1943

Davidhizar R, Giger JN (2004) A review of the literature on care of clients in pain who are culturally diverse. Int Nurs Rev 51(1):47–55

Fischer HBJ, Simanski CJP, Sharp C et al (2008) A procedure-specific systematic review and consensus recommendations for postoperative analgesia following total knee arthroplasty. Anesthesia 63:1105–1123

Fowler SJ, Symons J, Sabato S et al (2008) Epidural analgesia compared with peripheral nerve blockade after major knee surgery: a systematic review and meta-analysis of randomized trials. Br J Anaesth 100:154–164

Horlocker T, Cabanela ME, Wedel DJ (1994) Does postoperative epidural analgesia increase the risk of peroneal nerve palsy after total knee arthroplasty? Anesth Analg 79:495–500

Jeng L, Torrillo TM, Rosenblatt MA (2010) Complications of peripheral nerve blocks. Br J Anaesth 105(Suppl 1): i97–i107

Katz J, Kavanagh BP, Sandler AN et al (1992) Preemptive analgesia. Clinical evidence of neuroplasticity contributing to postoperative pain. Anesthesiology 77(3): 439–446

Kelley TC, Adams MJ, Mulliken BD (2013) Efficacy of multimodal perioperative analgesia protocol whit periarticular medication injection in total knee arthroplasty: a randomized, double-blinded study. J Arthroplasty 28:1274–1277

Kim DH, Lin Y, Goytizolo EA et al (2014) Adductor canal block versus femoral nerve block for total knee arthroplasty: a prospective, randomized, controlled trial. Anesthesiology 120(3):540–550

Lamplot JD, Wagner ER, Manning DW (2014) Multimodal pain management in total knee arthroplasty: a prospective randomized controlled trial. J Arthroplasty 29:329–334

Lin J, Zhang L, Yang H (2013) Perioperative administration of selective cyclooxygenase-2 inhibition for postoperative pain management in patient after total knee arthroplasty. J Arthroplasty 28:207–213

Livbjerg AE, Froekjaer S, Simonsen O, Rathleff MS (2013) Preoperative patient education is associated whit decreased risk of arthrofibrosis after total knee arthroplasty: a case control study. J Arthroplasty 28:1282–1285

Mullaji A, Kanna R, Shetty GM et al (2010) Efficacy of periarticular injection of bupivacaine, fentanyl, and methylprednisolone in total knee arthroplasty: a prospective, randomized trial. J Arthroplasty 25:851

Noiseux NO, Callaghan JJ, Clark CR (2014) Preoperative predictors of pain following total knee arthroplasty. J Arthroplasty 29:1383–1387

Pati AB, Perme DC, Trail M et al (1994) Rehabilitation parameters in total knee replacement patients undergoing epidural vs. conventional analgesia. J Orthop Sports Phys Ther 19:88–92

Paul J, Arya A, Hurlburt L et al (2010) Femoral nerve block improves analgesia outcomes after total knee arthroplasty: a meta-analysis of randomized controlled trials. Anesthesiology 113:1144–1162

Pelt CE, Anderson AW, Anderson M (2014) Postoperative falls after total knee arthroplasty in patients with a femoral nerve catheter: can we reduce the incidence? J Arthroplasty 29:1154–1157

Ranawat AS, Ranawat CS (2007) Pain management and accelerated rehabilitation for total hip and total knee arthroplasty. J Arthroplasty 22(7 Suppl 3):12–15

Salinas FV, Liu SS, Mulroy MF (2006) The effect of single- injection femoral nerve block versus continuous femoral nerve block after total knee arthroplasty on hospital length of stay and long-term functional recovery within an established clinical pathway. Anesth Analg 102:1234

Swenson JD, Bay N, Loose E et al (2006) Outpatient management of continuous peripheral nerve catheters placed using ultrasound guidance: an experience in 620 patients. Anesth Analg 103:1436

Trousdale RT, McGrory BJ, Berry DJ et al (1999) Patients' concerns prior to undergoing total hip and total knee arthroplasty. Mayo Clin Proc 74(10):978–982

Wasserstein D, Farlinger C et al (2013) Risk factor for inpatient falls after primary total knee arthroplasty. J Arthroplasty 28:1121–1124

Weber A, Fournier R, Van Gessel E, Gamulin Z (2002) Sciatic nerve block and the improvement of femoral nerve block analgesia after total knee replacement. Eur J Anaesthesiol 19:834–836

Weng PW, Wijeysundera DN (2007) Use of gabapentin for perioperative pain control – a meta-analysis. Pain Res Manag 12:85–92

Widmer BJ, Scholes CJ, Pattullo G et al (2012) Is femoral nerve block necessary during total knee arthroplasty: a randomized controlled trial. J Arthroplasty 27:1800–1805

Dealing with Pain in a "Fast-Track" Protocol: The Experience of a European Professional

15

Henrik Husted

Open Questions

- Which factor is more influential on pain reduction after THA and TKA: preoperative optimization of comorbidities, patient information, or prehabilitation?
- Which type of anesthesia is optimal for a fast-track protocol?
- Should LIA become a standard of care for a fast-track protocol?
- Is it possible to manage postoperative pain without opioids?
- Which is the role of the nurse staff in a fast-track protocol?

15.1 Introduction

Fast-track total hip and knee arthroplasty (THA and TKA) is a dynamic ongoing optimization of both clinical and organizational enhancement in order to optimize patient outcome. The entity is leading to faster postoperative recovery, earlier achievement of functional milestones, a reduction of perioperative morbidity and mortality, shorter length of stay (LOS) in hospital, and secondarily improved economy (Husted 2012; Kehlet and Wilmore 2008). The ultimate goal is to achieve the risk- and pain-free operation. Focus should be on improving patient outcome: first, we make it better, and then we make it faster. The concept combines optimized patient outcome and economic savings, thus making it the "right track." Patients can have an optimized stay, a shorter recovery, and be more satisfied and from an economic point of view, patients can have a shorter more streamlined stay allowing more patients to be operated on using the same number of beds. So, in an increasingly competitive and economic stressful environment with increasing numbers of procedures and reduced financial support and reimbursement, fast track allows for better patient treatment while being more cost-effective.

Efficient pain treatment is one of the five cornerstones of fast track – along with early mobilization, organizational optimization, a revision of traditions, and using updated care principles. Efficient pain treatment is essential and a prerequisite for early mobilization (hence, reducing complications associated with non-mobilization) again allowing for earlier fulfillment of functional discharge criteria and short LOS. Effective pain treatment includes preoperative evaluation of the patient (including information and verbal modulation of pain perception), choice of anesthesia, choice of intraoperative analgesia (local infiltration analgesia, LIA), and choice of postoperative pain treatment.

H. Husted
Orthopedic Department, Hvidovre University Hospital of Copenhagen, Kettegaard Alle 30, Hvidovre 2650, Denmark
e-mail: henrikhusted@dadlnet.dk

A. Baldini, P. Caldora (eds.), *Perioperative Medical Management for Total Joint Arthroplasty: How to Control Hemostasis, Pain and Infection*, DOI 10.1007/978-3-319-07203-6_15,

15.2 Preoperative Evaluation of the Patient

A prerequisite for enhanced recovery after hip and knee arthroplasty is optimization of the patient with comorbidities, and several factors have to be considered. The patient has to be prepared properly for the forthcoming anesthesia and surgery. Preoperative optimization of comorbidities may reduce pain from other locations than the operated joint and hence improve overall function (Ayers et al. 2013). A number of medical and psychological comorbidities have been identified to be associated with increased postoperative pain in TKA; among these are low back pain, pain in the contralateral joint, heart disease, depression, and anxiety (Singh and Lewallen 2013).

Also, patients with comorbidities have been shown to stay longer in hospital (to take longer to fulfill functional discharge criteria) and to be less satisfied with pain treatment – indicating a need for special attention (Husted et al. 2008; Williams et al. 2007). However, patients with comorbidities should not be excluded from fast-track surgery as these patients cannot only follow a fast track, but this large subgroup of patients has been shown to benefit the most from optimized treatment (Dowsey et al. 1999; Jørgensen et al. 2013).

Preoperative information should cover specific topics, i.e., pain, to ensure that the patients know what to expect and what is expected of them. Provision of preoperative information can alleviate anxiety regarding the upcoming anesthesia (Jlala et al. 2010) and surgical procedure but not regarding postoperative pain in general (McDonald et al. 2004). Also, in support of this, a recent review found no consistency in the association between patients' preoperative expectations and treatment outcomes for TKA and THA including pain, function, and satisfaction (Haanstra et al. 2012). However, another review concluded that pain catastrophizing and low preoperative mental health have an influence on outcome after TKA: in follow-ups shorter than 1 year, patients with pain catastrophizing reported more pain postoperatively, and in long-term follow-up, lower preoperative mental health was associated with lower scores on function and pain (SF 12 and SF 36). For THA, only limited, conflicting, or no evidence was found (Vissers et al. 2012). As also the most recent review on the potential influence of preoperative education on postoperative pain found only 1 of 13 studies with a reduction in postoperative pain following preoperative education compared to the noneducation group, it seems that preoperative education is of little if any value to reduce postoperative pain (Louw et al. 2013). Preoperative identification of pain catastrophizers/high-pain responders could allow for a more aggressive pain treatment protocol in these specific cases, but efforts so far have failed to identify these patients by simple means (Lunn et al. 2013a).

The effect of physical prehabilitation on pain has been studied in a few studies. For patients waiting to have a TKA, there was no effect on pain, function, walking speed, or muscle strength, whereas patients waiting for a THA had less pain and better function following an exercise program for 3–8 weeks (Gill and McBurney 2013). The effect of prehabilitation on postoperative pain following TKA was not significant (and neither was there any effect on stiffness, ROM, strength, or function) (Silkman Baker and McKeon 2012). There are no studies specifically addressing prehabilitation in THA and postoperative pain, but although a study found hip extensor and flexor muscle strength and endurance to be associated with postoperative limping, there was no association between the severity of limping and pain – indicating little chance of a pain-reducing effect of prehabilitation in THA (Horstmann et al. 2013).

15.3 Choice of Anesthesia

Fast-track anesthesia should be safe, minimize the impact of the surgical stress response, and facilitate the transition from surgical anesthesia to fast postoperative ambulation (within 1–2 h). However, all safety studies so far are performed with a conventional setup. Studies comparing neuraxial block (spinal, epidural) versus general anesthesia (GA) have found regional analgesia to result in lower 30-day mortality, less in-hospital complications, less bleeding, and less deep venous thromboembolism (DVT) and may also give a reduction in operating room (OR) time (Mauermann et al. 2006; Memtsoudis et al. 2013). Only GA and spinal analgesia are recommended for TKA, whereas both spinal and epidural are recommended for THA by the PROSPECT group (www.postoppain.org) and is found to be safe in a large consecutive series (Pumberger et al. 2013).

There is only one published study in fast-track TKA comparing GA and spinal anesthesia focusing on early functional recovery. GA resulted in shorter LOS, less nausea and vomiting and dizziness, less pain after 6 h, and less use of opioids, and patients were able to walk earlier and were also more preferred by patients (Harsten et al. 2013). The best choice of anesthesia for fast-track THA and TKA is thus debatable: GA may facilitate improved early functional recovery including less pain and opioid use, whereas spinal analgesia may have a better safety profile – studies on safety in fast-track THA and TKA using GA are lacking.

15.4 Choice of Intraoperative Analgesia

Surgical pain originates from the surgical wound and a rational approach to perioperative pain treatment has been directed toward the use of local infiltration analgesia (LIA) at the site of surgery. LIA has gained popularity due to the simplicity, low price, effectiveness of the technique, and the fact that the quadriceps strength remains unaffected thus facilitating early ambulation. Most of the more than 25 published randomized studies, of which only few are placebo controlled, have insufficient design hindering interpretation and do not allow comparison with other analgesic techniques. There is little evidence to support the use of LIA in THA either intraoperatively (Lunn et al. 2011a) or with a continuous postoperative wound infusion (Andersen et al. 2011; Solovyova et al. 2013) – *when* used in conjunction with multimodal opioid-sparing analgesia. In TKA, the data support the intraoperative use of the LIA technique (Andersen et al. 2008a), but there are limited data supporting the use of wound catheter administration. The analgesic effect is prolonged by using a compression bandage (Andersen et al. 2008b). LIA is effective in providing immediate pain relief – without motor blocking – allowing immediate mobilization postoperatively. This could result in less thromboembolic episodes and allow for early functional recovery (Husted et al. 2010). Various drugs are used for LIA, mostly bupivacaine and ropivacaine providing low pain scores for 6–8 h, but a new liposomal form of bupivacaine may provide this effect for up to 72 h which could further facilitate early postoperative recovery.

Peripheral nerve blocks may also like LIA reduce postoperative pain effectively but with accompanying motor problems making early mobilization difficult and risky (7 % falls) (Ilfeld et al. 2010). Also, pain and function is not improved beyond 24 h by a femoral block (Ilfeld et al. 2011) and hence will not ease early functional recovery beyond the first postoperative day. A new modality in the form of an adductor canal block may be promising in preserving quad control better than a femoral nerve block with equivalent pain control – but also technically demanding and time consuming (Jæger et al. 2013).

Steroids in the form of methylprednisolone (125 mg) have been found to be extremely potent in reducing postoperative pain in both THA and especially in TKA for 24–32 h following a single shot given during the operation (Lunn et al. 2011b, 2013b). Early functional recovery is also facilitated by less opioid use, less nausea, and less fatigue.

15.5 Choice of Postoperative Pain Treatment

Postoperative pain following fast-track THA (LOS <3 days) with a standardized multimodal opioid-sparing regime is at acceptable levels with concomitant low use of opioids in >95 % of patients before day 10 (Andersen et al. 2009). Pain following TKA is more pronounced: 52 % of patients reported moderate pain, and 16 % severe pain when walking 1 month after surgery with a concomitant increase in the use of strong opioids (56 % used weak or strong opioids on day 30) (Andersen et al. 2009). In a fast-track setting, it has been shown that 90 % of the TKA patients are able to walk independently on the first postoperative day and all managed to walk on postoperative day 2 with a maximum of moderate pain intensity (Holm et al. 2010). Still, pain is a challenge also in the early postoperative phase as a study found pain to be one of the three main clinical reasons (the others being dizziness and muscle weakness) for patients to be hospitalized following fast-track THA and TKA after 24 and 48 h (Husted et al. 2011).

The key to successful pain treatment in fast-track THA and TKA is multimodal opioid-sparing analgesia, where different drugs are combined to produce a synergistic pain-reducing effect with few side effects and with a low need for opioids (and as rescue medication) only. This has lead to the avoidance of delirium (Krenk et al. 2012) and a reduction of postoperative cognitive dysfunction with a reduction of postoperative pain to preoperative levels by day 5–9 (Krenk et al. 2013). No or only reduced use of opioids are the goal as opioids may slow recovery by its side effects (dizziness, sedation, nausea). A number of different drugs can be used to reduce both pain and the need for opioids, spanning from paracetamol and NSAIDs/COX-2 inhibitors over ketamine, alpha-2 agonists, serotonin-specific reuptake inhibitors (SSRI), to gabapentinoids, and more will come. Paracetamol and a COX-2 inhibitor have been shown to reduce pain and the need for opioids (Maund et al. 2011) and COX-2 inhibitors also in addition to reduce inflammation and increase range of motion (ROM) (Schroer et al. 2011) without compromising prosthetic fixation (Meunier et al. 2009). Gabapentinoids have been shown efficient in reducing postoperative pain across specialties (Tiippana et al. 2007) but in a recent study in TKA failed to reduce pain or opioid use (Paul et al. 2013). Procedure-specific dose-response studies are warranted.

Specific combinations of the abovementioned drugs could facilitate early functional recovery as a combination of paracetamol, a COX-2 inhibitor, and gabapentin allowed for the initiation of progressive strength training the day after surgery with resisted leg presses and knee extensions and reduced pain during two weeks of training (Jakobsen et al. 2012).

15.6 Other Considerations Regarding Pain Reduction

Fast track also includes a revision of traditions – as some may not be evidence based and cause more harm than good, i.e., result in more pain. An example of this is the use of a tourniquet in TKA, which may result in more postoperative pain and impaired ROM (without compromising fixation) compared to not using a tourniquet (Ledin et al. 2012). Cooling is also often used to reduce pain or opioid use – but has not been shown to do this clinically relevant (Adie et al. 2012).

An organizational example to reduce pain is seen when care is delivered by specialized staff members in relational coordination: postoperative pain was reduced and functioning improved resulting in shorter LOS (Gittell et al. 2000).

Conclusion

Optimized pain treatment in fast track is the key to early mobilization, less mortality and morbidity, shorter convalescence, earlier achievement of functional milestones, and shorter LOS. Patients should be informed preoperatively on pain and comorbidities optimized. The best choice of anesthesia is not yet determined as studies on safety with GA in fast track are lacking which results in still recommending spinal analgesia as the safer modality. Other modalities to reduce pain and opioid consumption include LIA, peripheral nerve blocks, and the use of steroids. Postoperative pain treatment should be multimodal and opioid sparing, and a variety of drugs can be combined. Staff should work in relational coordination. Finally, potentially harmful non-evidence-based traditions should be critically revised. Applying these enhancements should result in a less painful and safer perioperative outcome with LOS of 1–2 days for the majority of unselected patients.

Key Points

- Preoperative optimization of comorbidities may reduce postoperative pain, whereas information and prehabilitation does not.
- Spinal analgesia is safer than GA, whereas GA may reduce postoperative pain and facilitate early recovery.
- LIA and steroids may reduce pain.
- Postoperative pain treatment should be multimodal and opioid sparing.
- A revision of traditions may improve outcome and relational coordination between staff members reduce pain

References

Adie S, Kwan A, Naylor JM, Harris IA, Mittal R (2012) Cryotherapy following total knee replacement. Cochrane Database Syst Rev (9):CD007911

Andersen LØ, Husted H, Otte KS, Kristensen BB, Kehlet H (2008a) High-volume infiltration analgesia in total knee arthroplasty: a randomized, double-blind, placebo-controlled trial. Acta Anaesthesiol Scand 52(10):1331–1335

Andersen LØ, Husted H, Otte KS, Kristensen BB, Kehlet H (2008b) A compression bandage improves local infiltration analgesia in total knee arthroplasty. Acta Orthop 79(6):806–811

Andersen LØ, Gaarn-Larsen L, Kristensen BB, Husted H, Otte KS, Kehlet H (2009) Subacute pain and function after fast-track hip and knee arthroplasty. Anaesthesia 64(5):508–513

Andersen LØ, Otte KS, Husted H, Gaarn-Larsen L, Kristensen B, Kehlet H (2011) High-volume infiltration analgesia in bilateral hip arthroplasty. A randomized, double-blind placebo-controlled trial. Acta Orthop 82(4):423–426

Ayers DC, Li W, Oatis C, Rosal MC, Franklin PD (2013) Patient-reported outcomes after total knee replacement vary on the basis of preoperative coexisting disease in the lumbar spine and other nonoperatively treated joints: the need for a musculoskeletal comorbidity index. J Bone Joint Surg Am 95(20): 1833–1837

Dowsey MM, Kilgour ML, Santamaria NM, Choong PF (1999) Clinical pathways in hip and knee arthroplasty: a prospective randomised controlled study. Med J Aust 170:59–62

Gill SD, McBurney H (2013) Does exercise reduce pain and improve physical function before hip or knee replacement surgery? A systematic review and meta-analysis of randomized controlled trials. Arch Phys Med Rehabil 94(1):164–176

Gittell JH, Fairfield KM, Bierbaum B, Head W, Jackson R, Kelly M, Laskin R, Lipson S, Siliski J, Thornhill T, Zuckerman J (2000) Impact of relational coordination on quality of care, postoperative pain and functioning, and length of stay: a nine-hospital study of surgical patients. Med Care 38(8):807–819

Haanstra TM, van den Berg T, Ostelo RW, Poolman RW, Jansma EP, Cuijpers P, de Vet HC (2012) Systematic review: do patient expectations influence treatment outcomes in total knee and total hip arthroplasty? Health Qual Life Outcomes 10:152

Harsten A, Kehlet H, Toksvig-Larsen S (2013) Recovery after total intravenous general anaesthesia or spinal anaesthesia for total knee arthroplasty: a randomized trial. Br J Anaesth 111(3):391–399

Holm B, Kristensen MT, Myhrmann L, Husted H, Andersen LØ, Kristensen B, Kehlet H (2010) The role of pain for early rehabilitation in fast track total knee arthroplasty. Disabil Rehabil 32(4):300–306

Horstmann T, Listringhaus R, Brauner T, Grau S, Mündermann A (2013) Minimizing preoperative and postoperative limping in patients after total hip arthroplasty: relevance of hip muscle strength and endurance. Am J Phys Med Rehabil 92(12):1060–1069

Husted H (2012) Fast-track hip and knee arthroplasty: clinical and organizational aspects. Acta Orthop Suppl 83(346):1–39

Husted H, Holm G, Jacobsen S (2008) Predictors of length of stay and patient satisfaction after hip and knee replacement surgery: fast-track experience in 712 patients. Acta Orthop 79:168–173

Husted H, Otte KS, Kristensen BB, Ørsnes T, Wong C, Kehlet H (2010) Low risk of thromboembolic complications after fast-track hip and knee arthroplasty. Acta Orthop 81(5):599–605

Husted H, Lunn TH, Troelsen A, Gaarn-Larsen L, Kristensen BB, Kehlet H (2011) Why still in hospital after fast-track hip and knee arthroplasty? Acta Orthop 82(6):679–684

Ilfeld BM, Duke KB, Donohue MC (2010) The association between lower extremity continuous peripheral nerve blocks and patient falls after knee and hip arthroplasty. Anesth Analg 111(6):1552–1554

Ilfeld BM, Shuster JJ, Theriaque DW, Mariano ER, Girard PJ, Loland VJ, Meyer S, Donovan JF, Pugh GA, Le LT, Sessler DI, Ball ST (2011) Long-term pain, stiffness, and functional disability after total knee arthroplasty with and without an extended ambulatory continuous femoral nerve block: a prospective, 1-year follow-up of a multicenter, randomized, triple-masked, placebo-controlled trial. Reg Anesth Pain Med 36(2):116–120

Jæger P, Zaric D, Fomsgaard JS, Hilsted KL, Bjerregaard J, Gyrn J, Mathiesen O, Larsen TK, Dahl JB (2013) Adductor canal block versus femoral nerve block

for analgesia after total knee arthroplasty: a randomized, double-blind study. Reg Anesth Pain Med 38(6): 526–532
Jakobsen TL, Husted H, Kehlet H, Bandholm T (2012) Progressive strength training (10 RM) commenced immediately after fast-track total knee arthroplasty: is it feasible? Disabil Rehabil 34(12):1034–1040
Jlala HA, French JL, Foxall GL, Hardman JG, Bedforth NM (2010) Effect of preoperative multimedia information on perioperative anxiety in patients undergoing procedures under regional anaesthesia. Br J Anaesth 104(3):369–374
Jørgensen CC, Kehlet H, Lundbeck Foundation Centre for Fast-track Hip and Knee Replacement Collaborative Group (Soeballe K, Hansen TB, Husted H, Laursen MB, Hansen LT) (2013) Role of patient characteristics for fast-track hip and knee arthroplasty. Br J Anaesth 110(6):972–980
Kehlet H, Wilmore DW (2008) Evidence-based surgical care and the evolution of fast-track surgery. Ann Surg 248:189–198
Krenk L, Rasmussen LS, Hansen TB, Bogø S, Søballe K, Kehlet H (2012) Delirium after fast-track hip and knee arthroplasty. Br J Anaesth 108(4):607–611
Krenk L, Jennum P, Kehlet H (2013) Activity, sleep and cognition after fast-track hip or knee arthroplasty. J Arthroplasty 28(8):1265–1269
Ledin H, Aspenberg P, Good L (2012) Tourniquet use in total knee replacement does not improve fixation, but appears to reduce final range of motion. Acta Orthop 83(5):499–503
Louw A, Diener I, Butler DS, Puentedura EJ (2013) Preoperative education addressing postoperative pain in total joint arthroplasty: review of content and educational delivery methods. Physiother Theory Pract 29(3):175–194.
Lunn TH, Husted H, Solgaard S, Kristensen BB, Otte KS, Kjersgaard AG, Gaarn-Larsen L, Kehlet H (2011a) Intraoperative local infiltration analgesia for early analgesia after total hip arthroplasty: a randomized, double-blind, placebo-controlled trial. Reg Anesth Pain Med 36(5):424–429
Lunn TH, Kristensen BB, Andersen LØ, Husted H, Otte KS, Gaarn-Larsen L, Kehlet H (2011b) Effect of high-dose preoperative methylprednisolone on pain and recovery after total knee arthroplasty: a randomized, placebo-controlled trial. Br J Anaesth 106(2): 230–238
Lunn TH, Gaarn-Larsen L, Kehlet H (2013a) Prediction of postoperative pain by preoperative pain response to heat stimulation in total knee arthroplasty. Pain 154(9):1878–1885
Lunn TH, Andersen LØ, Kristensen BB, Husted H, Gaarn-Larsen L, Bandholm T, Ladelund S, Kehlet H (2013b) Effect of high-dose preoperative methylprednisolone on recovery after total hip arthroplasty: a randomized, double-blind, placebo-controlled trial. Br J Anaesth 110(1):66–73
Mauermann WJ, Shilling AM, Zuo Z (2006) A comparison of neuraxial block versus general anesthesia for elective total hip replacement: a meta-analysis. Anesth Analg 103(4):1018–1025
Maund E, McDaid C, Rice S, Wright K, Jenkins B, Woolacott N (2011) Paracetamol and selective and non-selective non-steroidal anti-inflammatory drugs for the reduction in morphine-related side-effects after major surgery: a systematic review. Br J Anaesth 106(3):292–297
McDonald S, Hetrick S, Green S (2004) Pre-operative education for hip or knee replacement. Cochrane Database Syst Rev (1):CD003526
Memtsoudis SG, Sun X, Chiu YL, Stundner O, Liu SS, Banerjee S, Mazumdar M, Sharrock NE (2013) Perioperative comparative effectiveness of anesthetic technique in orthopedic patients. Anesthesiology 118(5):1046–1058
Meunier A, Aspenberg P, Good L (2009) Celecoxib does not appear to affect prosthesis fixation in total knee replacement: a randomized study using radiostereometry in 50 patients. Acta Orthop 80(1):46–50
Paul JE, Nantha-Aree M, Buckley N, Cheng J, Thabane L, Tidy A, DeBeer J, Winemaker M, Wismer D, Punthakee D, Avram V (2013) Gabapentin does not improve multimodal analgesia outcomes for total knee arthroplasty: a randomized controlled trial. Can J Anaesth 60(5):423–431
Pumberger M, Memtsoudis SG, Stundner O, Herzog R, Boettner F, Gausden E, Hughes AP (2013) An analysis of the safety of epidural and spinal neuraxial anesthesia in more than 100,000 consecutive major lower extremity joint replacements. Reg Anesth Pain Med 38(6):515–519
Schroer WC, Diesfeld PJ, LeMarr AR, Reedy ME (2011) Benefits of prolonged postoperative cyclooxygenase-2 inhibitor administration on total knee arthroplasty recovery: a double-blind, placebo-controlled study. J Arthroplasty 26(6 Suppl):2–7
Silkman Baker C, McKeon JM (2012) Does preoperative rehabilitation improve patient-based outcomes in persons who have undergone total knee arthroplasty? A systematic review. PM R 4(10):756–767
Singh JA, Lewallen DG (2013) Medical and psychological comorbidity predicts poor pain outcomes after total knee arthroplasty. Rheumatology (Oxford) 52(5):916–923
Solovyova O, Lewis CG, Abrams JH, Grady-Benson J, Joyce ME, Schutzer SF, Arumugam S, Caminiti S, Sinha SK (2013) Local infiltration analgesia followed by continuous infusion of local anesthetic solution for total hip arthroplasty: a prospective, randomized, double-blind, placebo-controlled study. J Bone Joint Surg Am 95(21):1935–1941
Tiippana EM, Hamunen K, Kontinen VK, Kalso E (2007) Do surgical patients benefit from perioperative gabapentin/pregabalin? A systematic review of efficacy and safety. Anesth Analg 104(6):1545–1556
Vissers MM, Bussmann JB, Verhaar JA, Busschbach JJ, Bierma-Zeinstra SM, Reijman M (2012) Psychological factors affecting the outcome of total hip and knee arthroplasty: a systematic review. Semin Arthritis Rheum 41(4):576–588
Williams A, Dunning T, Manias E (2007) Continuity of care and general wellbeing of patients with comorbidities requiring joint replacement. J Adv Nurs 57: 244–256

Dealing with Pain Using a "Fast-Track" (Multimodal) Protocol: The Experience from the United States

16

Priscilla K. Cavanaugh, Snir Heller, and Javad Parvizi

Open Questions

- Where is postoperative pain coming from? How should we manage it?
- Is patient-controlled epidural analgesia suitable for a fast-track protocol?
- Which is the best peripheral nerve block for THA and TKA?
- Which drugs should be used for preemptive analgesia before arthroplasty procedures?

16.1 Introduction

Total joint arthroplasty (TJA) is one of the most common and successful operations in orthopedics. By 2030 the demand for both total knee arthroplasty (TKA) and total hip arthroplasty (THA) is estimated to increase by 673 and 174 %, respectively, in the United States (Kurtz et al. 2007). The increasing number of patients undergoing TJA procedures places pressure on the orthopedic community to continue searching for ways to both improve perioperative pain management and obtain better postoperative results. Although these procedures are performed to reduce pain and improve function (Singh 2011), patients may be reluctant to undergo surgery due to the fear of uncontrolled postoperative pain.

Literature has shown that approximately 80 % of patients experience acute postoperative pain and, further, that pain management after joint replacement has commonly been suboptimal (Apfelbaum et al. 2003). Inadequately treated postoperative pain can significantly impact early and late orthopedic surgical outcomes by affecting patient satisfaction, ambulation, and physical therapy compliance (Brokelman et al. 2003). Further, inadequate management of postoperative pain has shown to delay ambulation, slow patient rehabilitation, and prolong hospital stay and cost of care and has been associated with long-term functional impairment (Morrison et al. 2003).

The use of opioids via intravenous patient-controlled analgesia (PCA) has long been the mainstay of pain management after joint reconstruction (Horlocker 2010). Unfortunately, opioids can be associated with significant dose-dependent systemic side effects that include nausea, vomiting, respiratory depression, urinary retention, confusion, sedation, and delirium (Horlocker 2010; Wheeler et al. 2002). As a

P.K. Cavanaugh (✉) • S. Heller
J. Parvizi
Rothman Institute of Orthopaedics at Thomas Jefferson University, 925 Chestnut Street, Philadelphia, PA 19107, USA
e-mail: priscilla.ku@rothmaninstitute.com; snirheller@gmail.com

A. Baldini, P. Caldora (eds.), *Perioperative Medical Management for Total Joint Arthroplasty: How to Control Hemostasis, Pain and Infection*, DOI 10.1007/978-3-319-07203-6_16,

result, orthopedic practitioners may use less than optimal doses of opioids in an effort to decrease the risk of serious adverse effects and enhance rehabilitation.

Inadequate pain management after TJA has led the orthopedic community on a search for more effective strategies. In 1988, Wall (1988) introduced a multimodal approach to pain management that was later refined and popularized by Kehlet and Dahl (1993). Multimodal pain management aims to achieve more effective and safe pain control without heavily relying on opioids.

This chapter reviews multimodal pain management for joint arthroplasty by providing an overview of the approach, discussing its different components, and describing how the approach is implemented at our institution. Components discussed are neuraxial analgesia, nerve blockade, cryotherapy, acetaminophen, nonsteroidal anti-inflammatory drugs (NSAIDS), selective cyclooxygenase (COX)-2 inhibitors, gabapentinoids, tramadol, N-methyl-D-aspartate (NMDA) non-competitive antagonists, and local analgesics.

16.2 Pain Perception

A fundamental understanding of the process of pain generation is necessary to understand the multimodal approach to pain management. Tissue damage triggers the release of inflammatory mediators that include histamine, prostaglandins, bradykinin, substance P, and potassium ions (DeLeo 2006). Pain and temperature stimuli are detected by receptors, which subsequently initiate afferent signals in the peripheral nervous system via myelinated A delta and unmyelinated C fibers (DeLeo 2006). Sensory information reaches the dorsal root ganglion through these fibers and synapse in the dorsal horn of the spinal cord (DeLeo 2006). The dorsal horn is the first integration site of pain pathways where spinal modulation of afferent input can occur through opioids, N-methyl-D-aspartate (NMDA) receptor antagonists, and $\alpha 2$ agonists (Parvizi et al. 2011). These ascending signals are carried by the spinothalamic tracts that carry the information to higher central modulatory areas (DeLeo 2006). The aim of a multimodal pain management regimen is to take advantage of these different steps involved in the common pain pathway, using various analgesics that vary in both their site of action and mechanism of action.

16.3 Multimodal Pain Management

Multimodal pain management refers to a multidisciplinary approach to postoperative pain control. The approach combines different analgesic modalities that act at different steps in the pain pathway, resulting in synergistic analgesia, which can then reduce the overall dose and adverse effects of any individual drug (Kehlet and Dahl 1993). Therefore, multimodal pain management has the potential to provide appropriate postoperative pain relief with less reliance on opioids. The decreased use of perioperative opioids in pain control is a significant component of this approach, as many of the serious adverse effects associated with pain control are opioid related (Horlocker 2010). Decreased opioid consumption and superior pain control have been shown when peripheral or neuraxial regional anesthesia, along with a combination of nonopioid and opioid analgesics, was used after surgery (Hanna et al. 2009; Capdevila et al. 1999; Singelyn et al. 1998; Murphy et al. 2012).

Preemptive analgesia is another aspect of multimodal pain management which refers to the administration of anti-inflammatory agents and analgesics prior to surgery (Wall 1988; Parvizi et al. 2011). The use of preemptive analgesia combined with multimodal pain management after orthopedic surgery reduces postoperative pain and opioid use compared with patients who do not receive this combination (Kang et al. 2013).

16.4 Components of Multimodal Pain Management

16.4.1 Neuraxial Analgesia

Neuraxial analgesia/anesthesia encompasses spinally and epidurally administered anesthetic agents that provide pain relief after joint reconstruction through single-dose or continuous infusion techniques. Intraoperatively, neuraxial anesthesia has been associated with a lower incidence of postoperative venous thromboembolism and reduction in intraoperative blood loss, operative time, and need for transfusion (Hu et al. 2009; Macfarlane et al. 2009). Lower rates of respiratory complications and inpatient mortality after hip fracture surgery have been associated with the use of neuraxial anesthesia compared with general anesthesia (Neuman et al. 2012). Additionally, neuraxial anesthesia has been shown to decrease nausea, vomiting, postoperative pain, risk of postoperative systemic infection, and narcotic consumption following THA (Macfarlane et al. 2009; Liu et al. 2013). Neuraxial analgesia has been widely used following TJA, often yielding both satisfactory postoperative pain control and a reduction of overall narcotic use (Rathmell et al. 2003).

16.4.1.1 Spinal Analgesia

Spinal analgesia refers to the administration of anesthetic agents into the intrathecal space. The addition of intrathecal lipophilic opioids has enhanced the quality of pain relief, the effect lasting longer than local anesthetics alone (Hamber and Viscomi 1999). The onset and duration of neuraxial administered opioids are determined by their lipid solubility (Horlocker 2010). Lipid solubility is determined by octanol-water partitioning, the distribution of a compound between water and octanol, which is then used to calculate a partition coefficient (Hurley and Wu 2009). Lipophilic drugs have high octanol-water partition coefficients, while hydrophilic ones have lower octanol-water partition coefficients (Hurley and Wu 2009). Therefore, lipophilic opioids have a more rapid onset of action accompanied by a shorter duration of action secondary to a more rapid diffusion from the cerebrospinal fluid (CSF) compared with hydrophilic opioids (Hurley and Wu 2009). Conversely, hydrophilic opioids remain in the CSF longer, resulting in a delayed but longer duration of analgesia (Hurley and Wu 2009). The longer duration of opioid-receptor interaction in the latter group generally results in higher prevalence for opioid-related adverse effects (Hurley and Wu 2009). Commonly, spinal analgesia using either fentanyl or morphine is usually used, although in recent years, the recognition of the fact that intrathecal opioids may result in serious gastrointestinal disturbances has led many—including our institution—to abandon the use of intrathecal opioids with spinal anesthesia.

Compared with general anesthesia, the use of regional anesthesia has been shown to decrease morbidity, mortality, requirement for blood transfusion, narcotic usage, and pain after surgery (Rathmell et al. 2003; Rodgers et al. 2000; Guay 2006). A study of patients undergoing joint arthroplasty using either intrathecal ketorolac, intrathecal morphine, a combination of the two, or intrathecal saline postoperatively found that both spinal ketorolac-controlled pain and morphine-controlled pain are longer than that in the control group with no significant adverse effects (Lauretti et al. 2013). Furthermore, the individual use of spinal ketorolac or morphine provided 7 h of analgesia, but the combination of the two resulted in 15 h of postoperative analgesia (Lauretti et al. 2013). The administration of intrathecal opioids occurs at a variety of doses. Rathmell et al. (2003) administered intrathecal opioid doses ranging from 0 to 0.3 mg in patients undergoing hip arthroplasty. Patients that received higher doses were more satisfied with their postoperative pain management, and their use of PCA with morphine was significantly lower (Rathmell et al. 2003). When combined with a regional block, the use of low-dose intrathecal bupivacaine (5 mg) for knee arthroplasty has been associated with earlier discharge from the postanesthesia care unit (PACU) compared with using the standard 10 mg dose (Awad et al. 2013).

In contrast, some studies of patients undergoing joint arthroplasty under either general anesthesia or spinal anesthesia show delayed mobility and recovery, equal or sometimes increased postoperative pain, and a longer hospital stay with the use of the latter (Harsten et al. 2013b). Adverse effects associated with spinal analgesia include postoperative nausea, vomiting, pruritis, and respiratory depression (Rathmell et al. 2003; Harsten et al. 2013a, b).

16.4.1.2 Epidural Analgesia

Epidural anesthesia/analgesia occurs through single-dose or continuous delivery of analgesic agents to the epidural space (Hurley and Wu 2009). The combination of an opioid and epinephrine is typically administered; the latter provides local vasoconstriction resulting in reduced systemic absorption and therefore an increase of both local anesthetic concentration and analgesia (Huang et al. 1993). Postoperative pain can be managed by maintaining the intraoperatively administered epidural anesthesia (American Society of Anesthesiologists Task Force on Acute Pain Management 2012). Overall, epidural analgesia has been a well-established form of postoperative pain management.

When compared with patient-controlled analgesia (PCA), epidural analgesia was found to improve pain control (Block et al. 2003). Casati et al. (2008) evaluated the efficacy of continuous epidural levobupivacaine (0.125 %) infusion given for 72 h after total knee replacement for pain control. All patients received PCA with morphine, and of these patients a group was randomized to receive continuous epidural analgesia. Better pain scores, decreased morphine consumption, and no decrease in motor function were observed in the epidural analgesia group (Casati et al. 2008). The development of extended-release opioids permits long postoperative epidural analgesia via a single injection, without the need for continuous infusion (Kahl et al. 2010). Among a group of patients who underwent TKA, Hartrick et al. (2006) observed decreased opioid consumption and pain in patients who received extended-release epidural morphine and patient-controlled opioids, compared with recipients of sham epidural. Kahl et al. (2010) showed that extended-release epidural morphine provided better pain relief after THA compared with spinal anesthesia on postoperative day 1. However, extended-release epidural morphine was also associated with a higher incidence of pruritis, vomiting, nausea, and even pulmonary embolism (Kahl et al. 2010).

In addition to postoperative pain control, past studies have shown additional benefits to epidural analgesia including decreased pulmonary, cardiovascular, and gastrointestinal morbidity (Ballantyne et al. 1998; Beattie et al. 2001; Jørgensen et al. 2001). Despite these benefits, the use of epidural analgesia carries risks. These risks include nausea, vomiting, pruritis, dizziness, respiratory depression, hypotension, motor weakness, and development of epidural hematoma especially if combined with thromboprophylaxis (Viscusi 2005; Choi et al. 2003).

16.4.2 Peripheral Nerve Block

Lower extremity peripheral nerve blockade is a common modality used for pain control after TJA. The type of block used mainly depends on the surgical site. Patients undergoing THA benefit from psoas compartment blocks targeting the full lumbar plexus (which includes the femoral, obturator, and lateral femoral cutaneous nerves) (Awad and Duggan 2005; Capdevila et al. 2005). For patients treated with TKA, receiving a femoral nerve block with or without a sciatic nerve block can be effective. The latter is sometimes added because femoral nerve blocks (FNB) do not cover the sciatic nerve, a nerve that innervates the area posterior to the knee (Awad and Duggan 2005; Capdevila et al. 2005). The addition of a sciatic nerve block to FNB was investigated by two recent studies. A recent randomized control trial (RCT) showed that continuous sciatic nerve block improved analgesia, decreased morphine consumption, and improved early rehabilitation compared with single-dose sciatic nerve block (Cappelleri et al. 2011). On the other hand, a systematic review by Abdallah and Brull (2011) was unable to define the effect of combining a sciatic nerve block with FNB secondary to inconclusive evidence in the literature.

Peripheral nerve blocks may be administered by a one-time injection or by continuous infusion via an indwelling catheter. When administered in a single dose, blocks have a shorter duration of action usually lasting less than 12 h (Bono et al. 2012). Continuous infusion blockade provides longer postoperative analgesia and involves the placement of an indwelling catheter on the day of surgery, which usually remains in place for approximately 24 h (Bono et al. 2012). An RCT comparing continuous with single-dose femoral blockade after TKA showed significantly better pain control in the former group (Soto Mesa et al. 2012). Another RCT of patients undergoing TKA found that both single-injection and continuous FNB provided superior pain relief in the first 24 h after surgery compared with PCA, with continuous FNB providing better analgesia than single-injection FNB (Chan et al. 2013). Furthermore, nerve preemptive analgesia, an important part of multimodal pain management, specifically refers to the blockade of afferent nerve fibers prior to painful stimuli. An RCT of patients treated with TKA found that both preoperative and postoperative treatments using single-shot FNB with IV PCA resulted in equally successful postoperative pain control (Chan et al. 2012).

Substantial evidence in the literature has established the effectiveness of peripheral nerve blockade for postoperative analgesia. Siddiqui et al. (2007) randomized patients treated with hip arthroplasty to receive either continuous lumbar plexus block with PCA or PCA alone. The group that received a continuous lumbar plexus block combined with PCA had significantly better pain scores and less opioid consumption (Siddiqui et al. 2007). In a meta-analysis of 23 randomized control studies comparing FNB analgesia with or without sciatic nerve block with opioid PCA and epidural analgesia, Paul et al. (2010) found that both single-dosed and continuous FNB (with PCA) were superior to PCA alone for postoperative pain control in knee arthroplasty patients. Ozen et al. (2006) compared the effect of a single-shot preoperative three-in-one femoral nerve block (femoral nerve, obturator nerve, and lateral femoral cutaneous nerve blocks) with the use of no block in patients treated with TKA. Significantly lower visual analog scale (VAS) pain scores ($p<0.05$) and morphine consumption ($p<0.001$) were noted in the three-in-one FNB group. Another study showed faster rehabilitation in TKA patients receiving continuous nerve block versus PCA with morphine (Singelyn et al. 1998). Finally, a meta-analysis by Richmann et al. (2006) investigated the use of continuous peripheral nerve block versus systemic opioids for postoperative pain. When compared with opioid analgesia, continuous peripheral nerve analgesia proved superior in postoperative analgesia and was associated with less opioid-related adverse effects (Richman et al. 2006).

Additional benefits of peripheral nerve blocks can best be appreciated when compared with other available methods of postoperative analgesia. Peripheral nerve blockade provides comparable postoperative pain control to continuous epidural analgesia without the risk of epidural-associated adverse effects, such as hypotension and urinary retention (Fowler et al. 2008). Patients on anticoagulation therapy can safely use nerve blockade, while this same group of patients are at an increased risk for hematoma formation with spinal anesthesia (Dilger 2000).

The complications associated with regional nerve blockade are rare but should be noted. Complications include nerve damage, muscle weakness, and inflammation and/or infection associated with perineural catheters. Regarding nerve damage risk, Barrington et al. (2009) found that from over 6,000 patients who received 8,189 peripheral nerve or plexus blocks, only 0.5 % developed postoperative nerve symptoms, and further, the incidence of symptoms actually related to block-related nerve injury was 0.4 per 1,000 blocks. A meta-analysis of 32 peripheral nerve blockade studies published between 1995 and 2005 found the incidence of symptomatic postoperative neuropathy to be 0.34 % (Brull et al. 2007). However, a recent retrospective series including 1,802 nerve blocks or catheters performed reported a 1.94 % incidence of sensorial neurological symptoms involving the femoral nerve distribution after surgery (Widmer et al. 2013). All patients had full motor function with grade five motor strength and normal deep tendon reflexes. Furthermore, indwelling catheters have been associated with infections rates from 0.2 to 3.2 % (Wiegel et al. 2007; Neuburger et al. 2007).

Peripheral nerve blocks associated with the femoral nerve can result in quadriceps weakness (Bono et al. 2012). This adverse effect is undesirable, as early mobilization after joint arthroplasty can enhance functional recovery and decrease the risk for complications associated with immobility. Additionally, prolonged quadriceps weakness may lead to an increased fall risk postoperatively (Ilfeld et al. 2010). Recently, a meta-analysis of five studies involving patients undergoing lower extremity orthopedic surgery found a significant increase in the risk for falls in patients who received continuous lumbar plexus blockade ($p < 0.005$) compared with those who received noncontinuous blockade or no blockade (Johnson et al. 2013).

In the attempt to reduce quadriceps muscle involvement, the use of saphenous (adductor canal) nerve blocks for knee arthroplasty has been explored. Theoretically, an adductor canal block (ACB) is predominantly a sensory block, unlike femoral nerve blocks (Jæger et al. 2013). The ACB has shown to provide adequate analgesia while better preserving quadriceps muscle strength (Jaeger et al. 2012). Jaeger et al. (2013) randomized total knee arthroplasty patients to receive either continuous ACB or FNB after surgery; quadriceps muscle strength was better preserved in the ACB group without a significant difference in pain control. However, the study was unable to show a significant difference in mobilization ability, regardless of better quadriceps preservation in the ACB group. Yet, another study by Beebe et al. (2013) showed that continuous FNB (with single-shot sciatic block) provided adequate analgesia without preventing early ambulation after TKA.

16.4.3 Cryotherapy

Cryotherapy is a therapeutic procedure that has been commonly used in the postoperative management of edema and pain control after TKA (Dundon et al. 2013). It involves the application of cold to the skin around the surgical site using cooled water, ice, or other devices (Banerjee et al. 2013). The application of cold by these devices penetrates approximately 4 cm in depth (Banerjee et al. 2013). The cold travels through the soft tissue and reduces the internal temperature inside the joint, which subsequently reduces nerve conduction velocity and tissue metabolism and causes vasoconstriction (Martin et al. 2002; Abramson et al. 1966). The reduction in blood flow decreases local edema formation and inflammatory response (Kullenberg et al. 2006). Meanwhile, the slowing of pain signal transmission provides an anesthetic effect (Abramson et al. 1966).

Levy and Marmar (1993) studied the effect of normal versus cold compression dressings in the postoperative management of TKA. The cold compression group demonstrated reduced blood loss and narcotic consumption (Levy and Marmar 1993). In another prospective randomized study of patients treated with TKA, Kullenberg et al. (2006) compared the effects of postoperative management using either cold compression or epidural analgesia. Patients treated with cryotherapy experienced improved range of motion and a shorter hospital stay; however, there were no differences in analgesic consumption and visual analog scores (VAS) in the two groups (Kullenberg et al. 2006). In a recent Cochrane review of 11 randomized trials and one controlled clinical trial of 809 TKA patients, Adie et al. (2012) found evidence from ten trials (666 participants) of patients treated with TKA supporting that postoperative cryotherapy may have a small significant benefit in range of motion and blood loss. However, the authors concluded that these potential benefits of cryotherapy might be too small and not clinically significant. No significant complications from cryotherapy were reported in the review.

The overall safety of cryotherapy is supported by current evidence, with serious adverse effects being rare (Dundon et al. 2013; Banerjee et al. 2013). The potential benefits, ease of use, and low cost of cryotherapy justify its continued use as an adjunct to pharmacologic pain management after joint arthroplasty. However, more adequately powered randomized control trials are needed to more accurately determine the effects of this modality of postoperative treatment.

16.4.4 Acetaminophen

Acetaminophen or paracetamol is a centrally acting analgesic and antipyretic agent. The exact mechanism by which this agent produces analgesia is not fully understood (Pergolizzi et al. 2012). A variety of mechanisms have been suggested which include the inhibition of cyclooxygenase production with subsequent effects on prostaglandin production and effects on the serotonin pathway (Pergolizzi et al. 2012; O'Neal 2013). This agent is often used orally alone or in combination with opioids as part of a multimodal pain control regimen. The intravenous (IV) form of acetaminophen, available in Europe since 2002, was approved in the United States in November 2010 (Anon 2013).

A study by Imasogie et al. (2009) evaluated the use of oral tramadol/acetaminophen combined with opioid analgesia in patients 70 years or older after lower extremity joint replacement. Decreased opioid consumption was found with the postoperative use of oral tramadol/acetaminophen (Imasogie et al. 2009). The efficacy of IV acetaminophen was evaluated by Sinatra et al. (2005) in a randomized, double-blind, placebo-controlled, three-parallel group study comparing IV acetaminophen with its prodrug and placebo for pain control after major orthopedic surgery. Results demonstrated that both treatment groups had significantly improved pain responses and reduced opioid consumption as compared to placebo (Sinatra et al. 2005). Similar rates of adverse effects were reported in the acetaminophen and placebo groups (Sinatra et al. 2005). Later, a subsequent expanded analysis by the same group found significant longer times to opioid rescue dose requirement in the IV acetaminophen group compared to placebo after TKA and THA (2.1 and 3.9 h, respectively, versus 0.8 in placebo cohort) (Sinatra et al. 2012). In a systematic review of randomized, placebo-controlled, clinical trials of perioperative IV acetaminophen for the treatment of postsurgical pain, lower pain scores were found in the IV acetaminophen group in 12 of the 14 studies (Macario and Royal 2011). Moreover, 10 of the 14 trials found lower postoperative opioid consumption with perioperative IV acetaminophen use (Macario and Royal 2011).

Acetaminophen advantageously is not associated with nonsteroidal anti-inflammatory drug (NSAID)-induced gastrointestinal effects and opioid-related respiratory depression (Bertolini et al. 2006). However, just as any drug, acetaminophen may cause adverse effects. Major adverse effects associated with acetaminophen are liver or kidney toxicity (especially in patients with prior liver or kidney disease) (Bono et al. 2012). Further, patients who drink moderate levels of alcohol daily should use acetaminophen with caution, taking care to decrease their intake of acetaminophen appropriately (Bono et al. 2012).

16.4.5 NSAIDs and COX-2 Inhibitors

Prostaglandins, metabolites of arachidonic acid, decrease the threshold for pain at the site of injury, causing primary hyperalgesia. They also cause secondary hyperalgesia by acting on the central nervous system. The production of prostaglandins from arachidonic acid is utilized through the cyclooxygenase (COX) reaction. Several crystal types of NSAIDs are available in the market. They interact with the active site of the COX enzymes and inhibit its action on arachidonic acid. There are two subtypes of NSAIDs: the classical NSAID and the COX-2 inhibitor. Classical NSAIDs (nonselective COX inhibitors) inhibit both COX-1 and COX-2 isozymes, but their affinity to COX-1 is stronger (Smith et al. 2000). COX-2 inhibitors are 100–1,000 times more selective for the COX-2 isozyme (Parvizi et al. 2011). COX-1 enzyme is widespread in most body organs, whereas COX-2 is more prevalent in inflammatory tissue. Roughly 1 % of chronic NSAID users develop gastric ulcers. These ulcers result from inhibition of prostaglandin synthesis by COX-1 in the stomach lining. The use of COX-2 inhibitors provides the same anti-inflammatory response as nonselective NSAIDs with minimal gastrointestinal side effects (Eisen et al. 2005; Moore et al. 2005).

There is abundant data in the literature in support of the use of NSAIDs or COX-2 inhibitors as a part of multimodal pain management of TJAs. Nonselective NSAIDs and selective COX-2 inhibitors have shown to reduce postoperative pain following hip and knee arthroplasty. A meta-analysis by Lin et al. (2013) compared eight randomized controlled trials evaluating COX-2 inhibitors for TKAs. They found that when comparing to placebo, perioperative administration of COX-2 inhibitors significantly reduced VAS during the first 72 h after surgery (0–24 h: $p=.0007$; 24–48 h: $p=.01$; 48–72 h: $p=.0001$). Opioid consumption and side effect rates (itching, nausea, and vomiting) were also reduced in the study group (OR 0.49 [95 % CI 0.31–0.79]; $p=.003$). The COX-2 group also had improved range of motion (ROM) on the third day after surgery (mean difference −7.45 [95 % CI 2.76–12.14]; $p=.002$). Concerns regarding the effects of NSAIDs or selective COX-2 inhibitors on platelet aggregation and bleeding have been raised. However, a recent meta-analysis did not show increased blood loss with the use of COX-2 inhibitors when compared to placebo (Lin et al. 2013).

Renner et al. (2012) studied the influence of preoperative administration of etoricoxib on pain and production of proinflammatory mediators compared to placebo. They showed that the administration of etoricoxib 2 h before surgery reduced the plasma levels of interleukin 6 (IL-6) and wound fluid levels of IL-6 and PGE2 up to 48 h after the surgery (Renner et al. 2012). Another RCT evaluated the influence of intravenous administration of parecoxib before and after surgical incision in patients undergoing THA. The authors showed decreased VAS scores and opioid consumption in the preincisional group. They also reported lower plasma concentrations of IL-6 and IL-8 24 h after the surgery (Bao et al. 2012).

There is inconsistent evidence regarding the association of cardiac morbidity with the use of COX-2 inhibitors. Rofecoxib, a selective COX-2 inhibitor, was withdrawn from the market in 2004 because long-term usage (longer than 18 months) had been associated with increased risk for myocardial infarction. A systematic review and meta-analysis by Caldwell et al. (2006) showed an increased risk for myocardial infarction when comparing celecoxib to placebo (OR 2.26, 95 % CI 1.0–5.1) or to nonselective NSAIDs (OR 1.88, 95 % CI 1.15–3.08). In most of the studies included in that meta-analysis, celecoxib was administered for at least 1 year and the dosage was 800 mg per day. Two studies that were of 6 weeks' duration with celecoxib daily dosage of 200 mg added only two cardiovascular events to the meta-analysis (Caldwell et al. 2006). The Coxib and traditional NSAID Trialists' (CNT) collaboration recently published a meta-analysis comparing vascular and upper GI complications in RCTs comparing coxibs to placebo and to classic NSAIDs. This meta-analysis showed increased risk for cardiovascular events (by about a third) and heart failure in both classic NSAIDs and newer coxibs comparing to placebo. The rates of cardiovascular event were minimal for low-risk patients, whereas 0.7–0.8 % of high-risk patients had major vascular events and 0.2 % had fatal events. Unfortunately, the duration of treatment was not analyzed in that study. As expected, while traditional NSAIDs increased the risk for upper GI bleeding by 2–4-fold, coxibs yielded the lowest risk of such complications (Coxib and traditional NSAID Trialists' (CNT) Collaboration et al. 2013).

There is also a concern regarding the negative effect of NSAIDS on bone healing and osteointegration. An RCT comparing ibuprofen to placebo for the treatment of heterotopic ossification with a 10-year follow-up showed increased failure rates in the study group (Persson et al. 2005). Another RCT examined prosthesis migration with radiostereometric analysis following TKAs. Patients were randomized to either celecoxib 200 mg twice daily or placebo. No difference was found between the groups at the 2-year follow-up (Meunier et al. 2009).

While it is necessary to weigh the benefits and risks of NSAIDs and COX-2 inhibitors in every individual case, these agents should remain an integral part in the armamentarium of multimodal pain management.

16.4.6 Gabapentin/Pregabalin

Gabapentin and pregabalin are analogs of the major inhibitor neurotransmitter GABA (gamma-aminobutyric acid). They were originally developed for treatment of neuropathic pain, epilepsy, and generalized anxiety disorder. They bind to the presynaptic alpha-2-delta subunit of the voltage-sensitive calcium channels along the dorsal horn synapse in the spinal neurons. The result is a reduction in the depolarization-induced calcium influx at nerve terminals and a decrease in the excitatory signal release along the afferent pathway by lowering the release of the neurotransmitters norepinephrine and glutamate (Ben-Menachem 2004; Shneker and McAuley 2005). By reducing the hyperexcitability of the dorsal horn neurons, the gabapentinoids prevent the surgery-induced hyperalgesia that contributes to persistent postoperative pain (Field et al. 1997).

Several prospective trials favor the use of gabapentinoids over placebo after total knee replacements (Mathiesen et al. 2008; Buvanendran et al. 2010; Clarke et al. 2009). Buvanendran et al. (2010) showed in a prospective RCT that the administration of pregabalin (300 mg/day) 1–2 h before surgery and for 14 days after surgery resulted in better pain control than placebo in terms of residual neuropathic pain, decreased opioid consumption, and better ROM over the first month after surgery. A higher risk of side effects was reported in the study group (sedation, confusion, and dry mouth). All adverse events had resolved by the 6-month follow-up visit (Buvanendran et al. 2010).

Two meta-analyses by Engelman and Cateloy (2011) and by Zhang et al. (2011) evaluated the efficacy and safety of pregablin in non-orthopedic patients. Both concluded that pregabalin reduces postoperative pain and reduces opioid consumption during the first 24 h after surgery. It also reduced the incidence of postoperative nausea and vomiting. Its side effects included increased the risk of dizziness, somnolence, and visual disturbances. However, these were limited to the time pregabalin was administered and resolved upon discontinuation (Engelman and Cateloy 2011; Zhang et al. 2011). In another meta-analysis by Clarke et al. (2012), 11 RCTs were evaluated for long-term postoperative pain (more than 2 months). They showed significant reduction in chronic postsurgical pain for patients treated with either pregabalin (OR 0.09; 95 % CI 0.02–0.79; $p = 0.007$) or gabapentin (OR 0.52; 95 % CI 0.27–0.98; $p = 0.04$) (Clarke et al. 2012).

More research is warranted to identify the optimal dosage necessary to maximize efficacy while minimizing adverse effects and to identify the best mode of administration of gabapentinoids following arthroplasty.

16.4.7 Tramadol

Tramadol is a synthetic atypical opioid. It is distinguished from other opioids by its dual mode of action. It is both a weak opioid agonist acting on the central and peripheral μ-opioid receptors and also a weak inhibitor of the monoaminergic receptors (noradrenalin and serotonin) (Scott and Perry 2000). Tramadol has less sedative influence and respiratory depressive effects than other opioids and therefore is more appealing for usage following TJA (Houmes et al. 1992). However, some of the studies that evaluated its efficacy after TJA had disappointing results. Stubhaug et al. (1995) conducted a prospective double-blind RCT that assessed the efficacy of tramadol versus codeine plus paracetamol and placebo after THA. They found that 50 and 100 mg of tramadol administrated per os had no significant analgesic effect compared to placebo (Stubhaug et al. 1995). A study comparing the intravenous administration of tramadol (400 mg/day) to placebo after TKA showed significantly less morphine consumption in the study group with no significant difference in the rates of adverse events (Stiller et al. 2007). Another study compared the effect of tramadol to morphine, both administrated via PCA following TKA. The authors showed that the administration of tramadol at high doses (more than 800 mg/48 h) provided the same analgesic effect as morphine but with higher rates of nausea and vomiting (48 % versus 28 %) (Pang et al. 1999). The paucity of prospective clinical trials makes it difficult to ascertain the role of tramadol in the multimodal pain management after TJA.

16.4.8 Local Analgesia

Local infiltration analgesia (LIA) and local infusion analgesia (LINFA) have rapidly gained popularity during the recent years. Several prospective studies that assessed the influence of LIA and LINFA found these methods to be effective and rejected the concern of toxicity due to systemic absorption. An RCT by Tammachote et al. (2013) found that LIA with multimodal drugs (bupivacaine 0.5 %, epinephrine, morphine sulfate, and ketorolac) is comparable to intrathecal administration of morphine regarding pain level, analgesic drug consumption, and function. However, there were significantly less nausea or pruritus events in the former group (Tammachote et al. 2013). Other studies comparing LIA to either femoral nerve block or to epidural infusion also found LIA to be as effective with lower rates of adverse events (Andersen et al. 2010; Affas et al. 2011; Busch et al. 2006). In a prospective, double-blind, placebo-controlled study by Goyal et al. (2013), patients were randomized to receive either 0.5 % bupivacaine or normal saline at 5 ml/h for 2 days in addition to the standard preemptive analgesia and multimodal pain control after the TKA. The patients in the study group reported lower VAS scores and significantly reduced opioid consumption compared with the control group (Goyal et al. 2013).

On the other hand, a similar double-blind RCT by Williams et al. (2013) failed to show any difference (VAS, opiates consumption, or their side effects) between patients who received 5 % bupivacaine at a rate of 2 ml/h and those who received placebo. In that study the LINFA rate was lower and patients from both groups also received LIA during the surgery (Williams et al. 2013). Another randomized double-blind and placebo-controlled clinical trial evaluating the effect of LINFA was conducted on patients having THA. All patients received standard preemptive analgesia plus LIA. Patients received either LINFA with ropivacaine, ketorolac, and adrenaline or placebo. The authors failed to find evidence for any effect of LIFNA on pain relief or opioid consumption (Specht et al. 2011).

Most of the studies comparing LIA or LINFA to placebo or with other analgesic treatment options advocate the use of local analgesia as part of the multimodal treatment. It is not clear, however, if there is any additive effect when combining LIA and LIFNA. A meta-analysis is warranted in order to establish more conclusive recommendations.

16.4.9 Ketamine

Ketamine, an N-methyl-D-aspartate (NMDA) receptor antagonist, is a potent antihyperalgesic agent that was shown to potentiate opioid analgesic function. The coadministration of low-dose ketamine and morphine reduces the overall morphine consumption (Suzuki 2009). Aveline et al. (2009) compared the effect of low-dose ketamine at 1 μg/kg/min to nefopam (monoamine reuptake inhibitor) and placebo following TKA. Patients treated with ketamine had better pain scores and improved ROM compared with those in the two other groups. Patients from the ketamine group also had up to a 30 % reduction in morphine consumption and lower nausea/vomiting rate compared with those who received placebo (Aveline et al. 2009). Another study evaluated the long-term influence of low-dose ketamine as a part of multimodal analgesia. A total of 154 patients were randomized to receive ketamine at a rate of 2 μg/kg/min or placebo for 24 h after THA. Opioid consumption was reduced by 28 % in the study group. The authors noticed significantly lower rates of reported residual hip pain in the ketamine group up to 6 months after surgery (Remérand et al. 2009).

Common concerns regarding adverse events include hallucinations and vision changes. None of them are reported with low-dose ketamine. The reported adverse events at low doses include nausea and vomiting, with the rates comparable to those associated with morphine (Suzuki 2009; Aveline et al. 2009; Remérand et al. 2009; Himmelseher et al. 2001; Adam et al. 2005; Lamplot et al. 2014).

16.4.10 Author's Preferred Approach

The literature supports the use of multimodal analgesia for patients having TJA. The combination of preemptive analgesia, intraoperative measurements, and postoperative pain medications is preferred over PCA (Lamplot et al. 2014). This multimodal regimen minimizes the use of opioids and therefore facilitates rehabilitation, shortens the length of hospitalization, and prevents

Table 16.1 Multimodal postoperative pain regimen for total joint arthroplasty at our institution

Drug	Preemptive dose	Postoperative dose	Route of administration
Acetaminophen	*975 mg*	*650 mg q6h*	*IV/PO*
Paracetamol	2 g	2 g q4h	IV/PO
Celecoxib	*400 mg*	*200 mg q12h*	*PO*
Naproxen	500 mg	500 mg q12h	PO
Ketorolac	12–30 mg	15–30 mg q6h	IV/PO
Ibuprofen	600 mg	600 mg q6h	PO
Pregabalin	*75 mg*	*75 mg q12h*	*PO*
Gabapentin	300 mg	300 mg q24h	PO
Tramadol	–	50 mg q6h	PO
Oxycodone	–	10 mg q6h	PO

unwanted adverse effects. There is substantial evidence supporting the use of spinal over general anesthesia, acetaminophen, NSAIDS/COX-2 inhibitors, gabapentinoids, local analgesia, and peripheral neural blocks. The treatment regimen at our institute is tailored for each patient individually depending on age, comorbidities, and drug allergies. The mainstay of treatment is summarized in Table 16.1. Preemptive analgesia consists of the TLC (Tylenol/Lyrica/Celebrex) protocol: Acetaminophen (Tylenol) 975 mg is administered within 2 h prior to surgery. If the patient has liver disease, acetaminophen is withheld; pregabalin (Lyrica) 75 mg is given within 2 h preoperatively; celecoxib (Celebrex) 400 mg is administrated within 2 h prior to surgery. In case of sulfa allergy or drug intolerance, naprosyn 500 mg is administrated instead. Spinal anesthesia is now preferred for both TKAs and THAs. We currently do not use local infiltration analgesia. At the end of TKAs, an intraarticular catheter is placed. Bupivacaine 5 % is then administered through an elastomeric pump at a rate of 5 ml/h. The infusion is discontinued and the pump is removed on the second postoperative day. Acetaminophen 650 mg q6h, celecoxib 200 mg q12h, and pregabalin 75 mg q12h are continued until discharge. Ice is provided to all patients and patients are mobilized on the day of surgery as tolerated.

Breakthrough pain is managed with intravenous ketorolac 30 mg (or ibuprofen 600 mg), oral tramadol 50 mg, or oral oxycodone 10 mg. PCA is used only if the patient is not responding to any of the above-mentioned measures. Once PCA is used, fentanyl is the preferred drug and Dilaudid is used as a second line agent.

16.5 Overview

Pain management has significantly contributed to the overall satisfaction of patients undergoing TJA. The main principle of modern pain management in TJA patients is pain prevention rather than pain treatment. It is widely accepted that reducing opioid consumption and their side effects is crucial for successful "fast-track rehabilitation" after TJA. The reduction of opioid consumption is achieved by implementation of the multimodal pain management principles. Preemptive analgesia has a major role in TJA pain management by lowering the initial inflammatory response related to the surgery. The current literature strongly supports the use of NSAIDs, acetaminophen, and gabapentinoids prior to the incision. There is substantial evidence showing that spinal and/or epidural anesthesia is superior to general anesthesia in terms of venous opioid-induced adverse events, thromboembolism, intraoperative blood loss, respiratory complications, and mortality. Local analgesia, either by infiltration of the surrounding tissue or by intraarticular continuous administration, has been shown to reduce opioid consumption and their related side effects, and its usage is rapidly expanding during the recent years. The cumulating effects of other treatment options are not as well studied as the former medications in the setting of multimodal pain management. There is still conflicting and insufficient data regarding the use of tramadol, NMDA receptor antagonists, cryotherapy, and the preferred nerve blockade, and substantial research is warranted before a widely accepted protocol could be proposed.

Key Points

- Modern pain management in TJA patients is pain prevention rather than pain treatment.
- Reducing opioid consumption and their side effects with multimodal pain management is crucial for successful "fast-track rehabilitation" after TJA.
- Spinal and/or epidural anesthesia is preferred rather than general anesthesia.
- Local analgesia, either by infiltration of the surrounding tissue or by intra-articular continuous administration, has been shown to reduce opioid consumption.
- The use of tramadol, NMDA receptor antagonists, cryotherapy, and the preferred nerve blockade is still under scrutiny in order to define their correct application.

References

Abdallah FW, Brull R (2011) Is sciatic nerve block advantageous when combined with femoral nerve block for postoperative analgesia following total knee arthroplasty? A systematic review. Reg Anesth Pain Med 36(5):493–498

Abramson DI et al (1966) Effect of tissue temperatures and blood flow on motor nerve conduction velocity. JAMA 198(10):1082–1088

Adam F et al (2005) Small-dose ketamine infusion improves postoperative analgesia and rehabilitation after total knee arthroplasty. Anesth Analg 100(2):475–480

Adie S et al (2012) Cryotherapy following total knee replacement. Cochrane Database Syst Rev (9): CD007911

Affas F et al (2011) Pain control after total knee arthroplasty: a randomized trial comparing local infiltration anesthesia and continuous femoral block. Acta Orthop 82(4):441–447

American Society of Anesthesiologists Task Force on Acute Pain Management (2012) Practice guidelines for acute pain management in the perioperative setting: an updated report by the American Society of Anesthesiologists Task Force on Acute Pain Management. Anesthesiology 116(2):248–273

Andersen KV et al (2010) A randomized, controlled trial comparing local infiltration analgesia with epidural infusion for total knee arthroplasty. Acta Orthop 81(5):606–610

Anon, Drugs@FDA: FDA Approved Drug Products. Available at: http://www.accessdata.fda.gov/scripts/cder/drugsatfda/index.cfm/fuseaction=Search. Accessed 30 Dec 2013

Apfelbaum JL et al (2003) Postoperative pain experience: results from a national survey suggest postoperative pain continues to be undermanaged. Anesth Analg 97(2):534–540, table of contents

Aveline C et al (2009) Postoperative analgesia and early rehabilitation after total knee replacement: a comparison of continuous low-dose intravenous ketamine versus nefopam. Eur J Pain (London, England) 13(6):613–619

Awad IT, Duggan EM (2005) Posterior lumbar plexus block: anatomy, approaches, and techniques. Reg Anesth Pain Med 30(2):143–149

Awad IT et al (2013) Low-dose spinal bupivacaine for total knee arthroplasty facilitates recovery room discharge: a randomized controlled trial. Can J Anaesth 60(3):259–265

Ballantyne JC et al (1998) The comparative effects of postoperative analgesic therapies on pulmonary outcome: cumulative meta-analyses of randomized, controlled trials. Anesth Analg 86(3):598–612

Banerjee S et al (2013) Postoperative blood loss prevention in total knee arthroplasty. J Knee Surg 26(06): 395–400

Bao Y et al (2012) Comparison of preincisional and postincisional parecoxib administration on postoperative pain control and cytokine response after total hip replacement. J Int Med Res 40(5):1804–1811

Barrington MJ et al (2009) Preliminary results of the Australasian Regional Anaesthesia Collaboration: a prospective audit of more than 7000 peripheral nerve and plexus blocks for neurologic and other complications. Reg Anesth Pain Med 34(6):534–541

Beattie WS, Badner NH, Choi P (2001) Epidural analgesia reduces postoperative myocardial infarction: a meta-analysis. Anesth Analg 93(4):853–858

Beebe MJ et al (2014) Continuous femoral nerve block using 0.125% bupivacaine does not prevent early ambulation after total knee arthroplasty. Clin Orthop Relat Res 472(5):1394–1399

Ben-Menachem E (2004) Pregabalin pharmacology and its relevance to clinical practice. Epilepsia 45(Suppl 6): 13–18

Bertolini A et al (2006) Paracetamol: new vistas of an old drug. CNS Drug Rev 12(3–4):250–275

Block BM et al (2003) Efficacy of postoperative epidural analgesia: a meta-analysis. JAMA 290(18):2455–2463
Bono JV et al (2012) Pharmacologic pain management before and after total joint replacement of the hip and knee. Clin Geriatr Med 28(3):459–470
Brokelman RBG, van Loon CJM, Rijnberg WJ (2003) Patient versus surgeon satisfaction after total hip arthroplasty. J Bone Joint Surg Br 85(4):495–498
Brull R et al (2007) Neurological complications after regional anesthesia: contemporary estimates of risk. Anesth Analg 104(4):965–974
Busch CA et al (2006) Efficacy of periarticular multimodal drug injection in total knee arthroplasty. A randomized trial. J Bone Joint Surg Am 88(5):959–963
Buvanendran A et al (2010) Perioperative oral pregabalin reduces chronic pain after total knee arthroplasty: a prospective, randomized, controlled trial. Anesth Analg 110(1):199–207
Caldwell B et al (2006) Risk of cardiovascular events and celecoxib: a systematic review and meta-analysis. J R Soc Med 99(3):132–140
Capdevila X et al (1999) Effects of perioperative analgesic technique on the surgical outcome and duration of rehabilitation after major knee surgery. Anesthesiology 91(1):8–15
Capdevila X, Coimbra C, Choquet O (2005) Approaches to the lumbar plexus: success, risks, and outcome. Reg Anesth Pain Med 30(2):150–162
Cappelleri G et al (2011) Does continuous sciatic nerve block improve postoperative analgesia and early rehabilitation after total knee arthroplasty? A prospective, randomized, double-blinded study. Reg Anesth Pain Med 36(5):489–492
Casati A et al (2008) 72-hour epidural infusion of 0.125% levobupivacaine following total knee replacement: a prospective, randomized, controlled, multicenter evaluation. Acta Biomed 79(1):28–35
Chan M-H et al (2012) Single-injection femoral nerve block lacks preemptive effect on postoperative pain and morphine consumption in total knee arthroplasty. Acta Anaesthesiol Taiwan 50(2):54–58
Chan E-Y et al (2013) Comparing the analgesia effects of single-injection and continuous femoral nerve blocks with patient controlled analgesia after total knee arthroplasty. J Arthroplasty 28(4):608–613
Choi PT et al (2003) Epidural analgesia for pain relief following hip or knee replacement. Cochrane Database Syst Rev (3):CD003071
Clarke H et al (2009) Gabapentin decreases morphine consumption and improves functional recovery following total knee arthroplasty. Pain Res Manag 14(3):217–222
Clarke H et al (2012) The prevention of chronic postsurgical pain using gabapentin and pregabalin: a combined systematic review and meta-analysis. Anesth Analg 115(2):428–442
Coxib and traditional NSAID Trialists' (CNT) Collaboration et al (2013) Vascular and upper gastrointestinal effects of non-steroidal anti-inflammatory drugs: meta-analyses of individual participant data from randomised trials. Lancet 382(9894):769–779
DeLeo JA (2006) Basic science of pain. J Bone Joint Surg Am 88(Suppl 2):58–62
Dilger JA (2000) Lower extremity nerve blocks. Anesthesiol Clin North America 18(2):319–340
Dundon JM, Rymer MC, Johnson RM (2013) Total patellar skin loss from cryotherapy after total knee arthroplasty. J Arthroplasty 28(2):376.e5–7
Eisen GM et al (2005) Meta-analysis: upper gastrointestinal tolerability of valdecoxib, a cyclooxygenase-2-specific inhibitor, compared with nonspecific nonsteroidal anti-inflammatory drugs among patients with osteoarthritis and rheumatoid arthritis. Aliment Pharmacol Ther 21(5):591–598
Engelman E, Cateloy F (2011) Efficacy and safety of perioperative pregabalin for post-operative pain: a meta-analysis of randomized-controlled trials. Acta Anaesthesiol Scand 55(8):927–943
Field MJ et al (1997) Evaluation of gabapentin and S-(+)-3-isobutylgaba in a rat model of postoperative pain. J Pharmacol Exp Ther 282(3):1242–1246
Fowler SJ et al (2008) Epidural analgesia compared with peripheral nerve blockade after major knee surgery: a systematic review and meta-analysis of randomized trials. Br J Anaesth 100(2):154–164
Goyal N et al (2013) The 2012 Chitranjan Ranawat award: intraarticular analgesia after TKA reduces pain: a randomized, double-blinded, placebo-controlled, prospective study. Clin Orthop Relat Res 471(1):64–75
Guay J (2006) The effect of neuraxial blocks on surgical blood loss and blood transfusion requirements: a meta-analysis. J Clin Anesth 18(2):124–128
Hamber EA, Viscomi CM (1999) Intrathecal lipophilic opioids as adjuncts to surgical spinal anesthesia. Reg Anesth Pain Med 24(3):255–263
Hanna MN et al (2009) Regional techniques and outcome: what is the evidence? Curr Opin Anaesthesiol 22(5):672–677
Harsten A et al (2013a) General anaesthesia with multimodal principles versus intrathecal analgesia with conventional principles in total knee arthroplasty: a consecutive, randomized study. J Clin Med Res 5(1):42–48
Harsten A, Kehlet H, Toksvig-Larsen S (2013b) Recovery after total intravenous general anaesthesia or spinal anaesthesia for total knee arthroplasty: a randomized trial. Br J Anaesth 111(3):391–399
Hartrick CT et al (2006) Evaluation of a single-dose, extended-release epidural morphine formulation for pain after knee arthroplasty. J Bone Joint Surg Am 88(2):273–281
Himmelseher S et al (2001) Small-dose S(+)-ketamine reduces postoperative pain when applied with ropivacaine in epidural anesthesia for total knee arthroplasty. Anesth Analg 92(5):1290–1295
Horlocker TT (2010) Pain management in total joint arthroplasty: a historical review. Orthopedics 33(9 Suppl):14–19
Houmes RJ et al (1992) Efficacy and safety of tramadol versus morphine for moderate and severe postoperative pain with special regard to respiratory depression. Anesth Analg 74(4):510–514

Hu S et al (2009) A comparison of regional and general anaesthesia for total replacement of the hip or knee: a meta-analysis. J Bone Joint Surg Br 91(7):935–942. [Review] [43 refs]

Huang KS et al (1993) Influence of epinephrine as an adjuvant to epidural morphine for postoperative analgesia. Ma Zui Xue Za Zhi 31(4):245–248

Hurley R, Wu C (2009) Chapter 87. Acute postoperative pain. In: Miller's anesthesia. Churchill Livingstone, Philadelphia, pp 2757–2781

Ilfeld BM, Duke KB, Donohue MC (2010) The association between lower extremity continuous peripheral nerve blocks and patient falls after knee and hip arthroplasty. Anesth Analg 111(6):1552–1554

Imasogie NN et al (2009) Ultra low-dose naloxone and tramadol/acetaminophen in elderly patients undergoing joint replacement surgery: a pilot study. Pain Res Manag 14(2):103–108

Jaeger P et al (2012) Effect of adductor-canal-blockade on established, severe post-operative pain after total knee arthroplasty: a randomised study. Acta Anaesthesiol Scand 56(8):1013–1019

Jæger P et al (2013) Adductor canal block versus femoral nerve block for analgesia after total knee arthroplasty: a randomized, double-blind study. Reg Anesth Pain Med 38(6):526–532

Johnson RL et al (2013) Falls and major orthopaedic surgery with peripheral nerve blockade: a systematic review and meta-analysis. Br J Anaesth 110(4):518–528

Jørgensen H et al (2001) Epidural local anaesthetics versus opioid-based analgesic regimens on postoperative gastrointestinal paralysis, PONV and pain after abdominal surgery. Cochrane Database Syst Rev (1):CD001893 doi:10.1002/14651858.CD001893

Kahl L et al (2010) Lessons learned with extended-release epidural morphine after total hip arthroplasty. Clin Orthop Relat Res 468(4):1082–1087

Kang H et al (2013) Effectiveness of multimodal pain management after bipolar hemiarthroplasty for hip fracture: a randomized, controlled study. J Bone Joint Surg Am 95(4):291–296

Kehlet H, Dahl JB (1993) The value of "multimodal" or "balanced analgesia" in postoperative pain treatment. Anesth Analg 77(5):1048–1056

Kullenberg B et al (2006) Postoperative cryotherapy after total knee arthroplasty: a prospective study of 86 patients. J Arthroplasty 21(8):1175–1179

Kurtz S et al (2007) Projections of primary and revision hip and knee arthroplasty in the United States from 2005 to 2030. J Bone Joint Surg Am 89(4):780–785

Lamplot JD, Wagner ER, Manning DW (2014) Multimodal pain management in total knee arthroplasty: a prospective randomized controlled trial. J Arthroplasty 29(2):329–334

Lauretti GR, Righeti CCF, Mattos AL (2013) Intrathecal ketorolac enhances intrathecal morphine analgesia following total knee arthroplasty. J Anaesthesiol Clin Pharmacol 29(4):503–508

Levy AS, Marmar E (1993) The role of cold compression dressings in the postoperative treatment of total knee arthroplasty. Clin Orthop Relat Res 297:174–178

Lin J, Zhang L, Yang H (2013) Perioperative administration of selective cyclooxygenase-2 inhibitors for postoperative pain management in patients after total knee arthroplasty. J Arthroplasty 28(2):207–213.e2

Liu J et al (2013) Neuraxial anesthesia decreases postoperative systemic infection risk compared with general anesthesia in knee arthroplasty. Anesth Analg 117(4): 1010–1016

Macario A, Royal MA (2011) A literature review of randomized clinical trials of intravenous acetaminophen (paracetamol) for acute postoperative pain. Pain Pract 11(3):290–296

Macfarlane AJR et al (2009) Does regional anaesthesia improve outcome after total hip arthroplasty? A systematic review. Br J Anaesth 103(3):335–345

Martin SS et al (2002) Does cryotherapy affect intraarticular temperature after knee arthroscopy? Clin Orthop Relat Res 400:184–189

Mathiesen O et al (2008) Pregabalin and dexamethasone for postoperative pain control: a randomized controlled study in hip arthroplasty. Br J Anaesth 101(4):535–541

Meunier A, Aspenberg P, Good L (2009) Celecoxib does not appear to affect prosthesis fixation in total knee replacement: a randomized study using radiostereometry in 50 patients. Acta Orthop 80(1):46–50

Moore RA et al (2005) Tolerability and adverse events in clinical trials of celecoxib in osteoarthritis and rheumatoid arthritis: systematic review and meta-analysis of information from company clinical trial reports. Arthritis Res Ther 7(3):R644–R665

Morrison RS et al (2003) The impact of post-operative pain on outcomes following hip fracture. Pain 103(3):303–311

Murphy TP et al (2012) Can a periarticular levobupivacaine injection reduce postoperative opiate consumption during primary hip arthroplasty? Clin Orthop Relat Res 470(4):1151–1157

Neuburger M et al (2007) Inflammation and infection complications of 2285 perineural catheters: a prospective study. Acta Anaesthesiol Scand 51(1):108–114

Neuman MD et al (2012) Comparative effectiveness of regional versus general anesthesia for hip fracture surgery in adults. Anesthesiology 117(1):72–92

O'Neal JB (2013) The utility of intravenous acetaminophen in the perioperative period. Front Public Health 1:25

Ozen M et al (2006) The effect of 3-in-1 femoral nerve block with ropivacaine 0.375% on postoperative morphine consumption in elderly patients after total knee replacement surgery. Agri 18(4):44–50

Pang WW et al (1999) Comparison of patient-controlled analgesia (PCA) with tramadol or morphine. Can J Anaesth 46(11):1030–1035

Parvizi J, Miller A, Gandhi K (2011) Multimodal pain management after total joint arthroplasty. J Bone Joint Surg Am 93(11):1075–1084

Paul JE et al (2010) Femoral nerve block improves analgesia outcomes after total knee arthroplasty: a meta-analysis of randomized controlled trials. Anesthesiology 113(5):1144–1162

Pergolizzi JV Jr et al (2012) Continuous multimechanistic postoperative analgesia: a rationale for transitioning from intravenous acetaminophen and opioids to oral formulations. Pain Pract 12(2):159–173

Persson P-E, Nilsson OS, Berggren A-M (2005) Do nonsteroidal anti-inflammatory drugs cause endoprosthetic loosening? A 10-year follow-up of a randomized trial on ibuprofen for prevention of heterotopic ossification after hip arthroplasty. Acta Orthop 76(6): 735–740

Rathmell JP et al (2003) Intrathecal morphine for postoperative analgesia: a randomized, controlled, dose-ranging study after hip and knee arthroplasty. Anesth Analg 97(5):1452–1457

Remérand F et al (2009) The early and delayed analgesic effects of ketamine after total hip arthroplasty: a prospective, randomized, controlled, double-blind study. Anesth Analg 109(6):1963–1971

Renner B et al (2012) Preoperative administration of etoricoxib in patients undergoing hip replacement causes inhibition of inflammatory mediators and pain relief. Eur J Pain (London, England) 16(6):838–848

Richman JM et al (2006) Does continuous peripheral nerve block provide superior pain control to opioids? A meta-analysis. Anesth Analg 102(1):248–257

Rodgers A et al (2000) Reduction of postoperative mortality and morbidity with epidural or spinal anaesthesia: results from overview of randomised trials. BMJ (Clinical research ed) 321(7275):1493

Scott LJ, Perry CM (2000) Tramadol: a review of its use in perioperative pain. Drugs 60(1):139–176

Shneker BF, McAuley JW (2005) Pregabalin: a new neuromodulator with broad therapeutic indications. Ann Pharmacother 39(12):2029–2037

Siddiqui ZI et al (2007) Continuous lumbar plexus block provides improved analgesia with fewer side effects compared with systemic opioids after hip arthroplasty: a randomized controlled trial. Reg Anesth Pain Med 32(5):393–398

Sinatra RS et al (2005) Efficacy and safety of single and repeated administration of 1 gram intravenous acetaminophen injection (paracetamol) for pain management after major orthopedic surgery. Anesthesiology 102(4):822–831

Sinatra RS et al (2012) Intravenous acetaminophen for pain after major orthopedic surgery: an expanded analysis. Pain Pract 12(5):357–365

Singelyn FJ et al (1998) Effects of intravenous patient-controlled analgesia with morphine, continuous epidural analgesia, and continuous three-in-one block on postoperative pain and knee rehabilitation after unilateral total knee arthroplasty. Anesth Analg 87(1): 88–92

Singh JA (2011) Epidemiology of knee and hip arthroplasty: a systematic review. Open Orthop J 5:80–85

Smith WL, DeWitt DL, Garavito RM (2000) Cyclooxygenases: structural, cellular, and molecular biology. Annu Rev Biochem 69:145–182

Soto Mesa D et al (2012) Control of postoperative pain in knee arthroplasty: single dose femoral nerve block versus continuous femoral block. Rev Esp Anestesiol Reanim 59(4):204–209

Specht K et al (2011) No evidence of a clinically important effect of adding local infusion analgesia administrated through a catheter in pain treatment after total hip arthroplasty. Acta Orthop 82(3):315–320

Stiller C-O et al (2007) The addition of tramadol to morphine via patient-controlled analgesia does not lead to better post-operative pain relief after total knee arthroplasty. Acta Anaesthesiol Scand 51(3):322–330

Stubhaug A, Grimstad J, Breivik H (1995) Lack of analgesic effect of 50 and 100 mg oral tramadol after orthopaedic surgery: a randomized, double-blind, placebo and standard active drug comparison. Pain 62(1):111–118

Suzuki M (2009) Role of N-methyl-D-aspartate receptor antagonists in postoperative pain management. Curr Opin Anaesthesiol 22(5):618–622

Tammachote N et al (2013) Is pain after TKA better with periarticular injection or intrathecal morphine? Clin Orthop Relat Res 471(6):1992–1999

Viscusi ER (2005) Emerging techniques in the management of acute pain: epidural analgesia. Anesth Analg 105(1):176–183. Available at: http://ovidsp.ovid.com.ezproxy2.library.drexel.edu/ovidweb.cgi?T=JS&CSC=Y&NEWS=N&PAGE=fulltext&D=ovfth&AN=00000539-200511001-00003. Accessed 6 Jan 2014

Wall PD (1988) The prevention of postoperative pain. Pain 33(3):289–290

Wheeler M et al (2002) Adverse events associated with postoperative opioid analgesia: a systematic review. J Pain 3(3):159–180

Widmer B et al (2013) Incidence and severity of complications due to femoral nerve blocks performed for knee surgery. Knee 20(3):181–185

Wiegel M et al (2007) Complications and adverse effects associated with continuous peripheral nerve blocks in orthopedic patients. Anesth Analg 104(6):1578–1582, table of contents

Williams D et al (2013) Continuous infusion of bupivacaine following total knee arthroplasty: a randomized control trial pilot study. J Arthroplasty 28(3):479–484

Zhang J, Ho K-Y, Wang Y (2011) Efficacy of pregabalin in acute postoperative pain: a meta-analysis. Br J Anaesth 106(4):454–462

Perspectives: Best Techniques for Local Wound Infiltrations

17

Emmanuel Thienpont and Francesco Traverso

Open Questions

- Why is local infiltration analgesia becoming a pillar of multimodal pain management?
- Which drugs, volumes and concentrations makes the ideal "cocktail"?
- Where should the surgeon perform the infiltrations?
- What does "anatomical knee block" mean?
- What are the results of recent prolonged-release local anesthetics for infiltrations?

17.1 The Injection Site Matters

Emmanuel Thienpont

E. Thienpont (✉)
Department of Orthopaedic Surgery, University Hospital Saint Luc, Av. Hippocrate 10 Brussels, 1200, Belgium
e-mail: emmanuel.thienpont@uclouvain.be

F. Traverso (✉)
Hip and Knee Arthroplasty and Arthroscopic Unit, Humanitas Clinical and Research Center, Via Manzoni 56, Rozzano, Milan 20089, Italy
e-mail: francesco.traverso@humanitas.it

17.1.1 Supporting Points

- Total knee arthroplasty (TKA) is a painful procedure that can be associated with severe acute postoperative pain in over one-third of patients
- Severe postoperative pain, which may result from both peripheral and central sensitization, delays rehabilitation, increases hospital stay and is a risk factor for persistent postoperative pain (PPSP)
- Traditional analgesic techniques are associated with known side-effects and potentially debilitating complications which can affect rehabilitation and recovery, sparking interest in multimodal analgesia
- Local infiltration analgesia (LIA) is a simple, safe and inexpensive technique in which the surgical wound is infiltrated with a mixture of local anaesthetics or a mixture of different drugs (cocktail with NSAIDs, adrenaline, steroids and antibiotics)
- Although early studies demonstrated improved pain control and shorter length of stay (LOS), recent meta-analyses have suggested that the evidence for the use of LIA is not currently definitive
- One factor may be the variety in the mixture, concentration and volume of LIA constituents and the wide range of techniques employed, which underscores the need for further, well-designed studies into this promising area to provide a consensus on the optimal technique

A. Baldini, P. Caldora (eds.), *Perioperative Medical Management for Total Joint Arthroplasty: How to Control Hemostasis, Pain and Infection*, DOI 10.1007/978-3-319-07203-6_17,

17.1.2 Introduction

Total knee arthroplasty (TKA) is a common and very successful procedure. However, it can be painful (McCartney and McLeod 2011) or at least has a high risk of severe acute postoperative pain (McCartney and McLeod 2011; Carli et al. 2010) which may become chronic in a substantial proportion of cases (McCartney and McLeod 2011). One study estimated the incidence of persistent pain after primary TKA at 36 %, with the most important predictor of pain being the degree of pain relief in the first week after the operation (Puolakka et al. 2010). Notably, the proportion of TKA patients with severe postoperative pain is higher than for all surgical patients combined, and especially those undergoing total hip arthroplasty (THA) (Thomas et al. 1998; Wylde et al. 2011).

Pain in TKA arises from incisional pain, which is a combination of nociceptive, ischemic and inflammatory mechanisms, in addition to nerve damage (Grosu et al. 2013). Nociceptive pain results from peripheral pain receptor activation resulting from surgical tissue incisions, while inflammatory pain is a response to tissue injury and the release of inflammatory mediators, which lowers the nociceptor threshold (Grosu et al. 2013). The combination of tissue injury and local inflammation causes hyperalgesia to any subsequent noxious stimuli and allodynia to ordinarily innocuous stimuli (Grosu et al. 2013), which contributes to postoperative pain both at the wound site and at a distance (Xu and Brennan 2011). This amplified response is due partly to sensitisation of peripheral nociceptors and to central sensitisation in the spinal cord and further up in the central nervous system (Woolf 2011).

17.1.3 The Consequences of Postoperative Pain

Severe postoperative pain, as well as causing suffering and discomfort for the patient, delays rehabilitation (Kehlet et al. 2006; Carli et al. 2010), increases hospital length of stay (LOS) and is a risk factor for the development of persistent postsurgical pain (PPSP) (Kehlet et al. 2006), which is associated with higher pain intensity (Torrance et al. 2006). For patients embarking on rehabilitation programmes, it is important to distinguish between pain at rest (PAR) and movement-evoked pain (MEP) (Grosu et al. 2013) as MEP is potentially more than twice as intense as PAR in the first three postoperative days (Srikandarajah and Gilron 2011). Moreover, poorly relieved MEP may enhance central sensitisation and further increases the risk of PPSP (Grosu et al. 2013).

Although the majority of patients experience a reduction in pain within 3 months of undergoing TKA (Vilardo and Shah 2011), approximately 20 % endure pain for a long time (Beswick et al. 2012). Perhaps unsurprisingly, almost the same proportion (19 %) of TKA patients are unsatisfied with the outcome of the operation (Bourne et al. 2010), with persistent postsurgical pain (PPSP) being the apparent primary predictor of dissatisfaction (Bourne et al. 2010). There have been few studies on the consequences of PPSP (Grosu et al. 2013), and in particular on the impact of the long-term use of analgesics (Steyaert and Lavand'homme 2013). Nevertheless, 56 % of patients continue to receive analgesics at 30 days postoperatively (Andersen et al. 2009), 40 % are still taking them at 4 months (Puolakka et al. 2010) and approximately 25 % still require analgesics after 2 years (Carroll et al. 2012).

Efforts to improve effective pain relief after TKA are therefore required (Carli et al. 2010) to improve both patient comfort and early postoperative function and provide the optimal conditions for rehabilitation (McCartney and McLeod 2011; Sisak 2013). Early mobilisation, which is associated with adequate pain control, has been identified as paramount for achieving a good clinical outcome (Dillon et al. 2012), with accelerated rehabilitation achieving early functional recovery in the motivated patient (Sisak 2013). A recent study indicated that starting rehabilitation within the first postoperative 24 h is associated with a reduced length of stay and a more rapid return to independent walking (Labraca et al. 2011).

17.1.4 The Evolution of Analgesia in TKA

Over recent decades, advances in implant and instruments design, along with less invasive techniques, have reduced the severity of the surgical impact for the patient (Shen et al. 2009). Improvements in anaesthetic techniques and operative treatment has also led to quicker recovery, improved patient satisfaction and earlier independent walking (Berger et al. 2004; Lombardi et al. 2006).

Innovations in analgesic approaches and techniques have not been so dramatic in recent years. Peri-operative analgesia has traditionally relied on techniques such as general anaesthesia with per- and postoperative intravenous opioids, epidurals with or without catheters, and femoral and/or sciatic regional nerve blocks with or without continuous postoperative infusions (Sisak 2013). All these techniques are still being used, despite known and well-defined failure and complication rates (Sisak 2013).

For example, parenteral opioids may not provide adequate pain relief but are especially affected by adverse events like nausea and vomiting, confusion, constipation, urinary retention, sedation, respiratory depression and pruritus, all of which may prevent rapid rehabilitation and influence the perception of the quality of postoperative care (McCartney and McLeod 2011; Dillon et al. 2012; Grosu et al. 2013). Moreover, opioids may induce hyperalgesia and acute tolerance, and exacerbate postoperative pain (Grosu et al. 2013). Although epidural anaesthesia is used widely and can achieve good pain control (McCartney and McLeod 2011), it could be associated with adverse events such as excessive motor block and the failure rate can be as high as 20 % (McLeod et al. 2001). Moreover, when it is removed the patient experiences pain later on in the postoperative period (Grosu et al. 2013).

In contrast, peripheral nerve blocks, such as continuous femoral nerve block, provides pain control comparable to epidural analgesia, but with fewer adverse effects (Singelyn et al. 1998). Continuous femoral nerve block has therefore become regarded by many as the gold standard for pain relief in TKA (Hadzic et al. 2010). However, it is hampered by being technically demanding, more time consuming and requires acquired skill vs simpler techniques (McCartney and McLeod 2011; Sisak 2013) and it may cause prolonged motor block (Kandasami et al. 2009).

17.1.5 Multimodal Analgesia

One solution to the issue of pain relief in TKA is that of multimodal analgesia, with the aim of minimising the need for opioid analgesia (Kehlet and Dahl 1993). Furthermore, recognition of the role of the incision in the initiation and maintenance of pain sensitisation has meant that intra-wound analgesia has received increasing attention (Grosu et al. 2013).

For example, adding posterior capsule infiltration to femoral nerve block has been shown to reduce pain scores and improves extension of the knee in the first postoperative 12 h (Krenzel et al. 2009). A systematic review also demonstrated that general anaesthesia plus femoral nerve block or spinal anaesthesia in TKA provides intra-operative anaesthesia and improves postoperative pain relief (Fischer et al. 2008). Importantly, severe complications following peripheral nerve block and spinal anaesthesia are rare (Aromaa et al. 1997; Auroy et al. 1997).

However, a note of caution should be observed, as patients receiving multimodal analgesia may remain in significant pain following TKA (Davies et al. 2004), potentially increasing the risk of chronic pain (Perkins and Kehlet 2000). Furthermore, intra-articular analgesia does not, on its own, improve patients' pain, satisfaction or range of motion (Joo et al. 2011).

17.1.6 Local Infiltration Analgesia

The ongoing quest to find the ideal analgesic approach for TKA has led to the relatively novel technique of local infiltration analgesia (LIA). This involves the intra-operative infiltration of anaesthetic agents locally into the surgical wound to provide an additional form of analgesia

(Keijsers et al. 2013; Ibrahim et al. 2013). The term was coined in the late 1990s, when it was developed as part of a multimodal pain management and early mobilisation protocol after joint replacement (Kerr and Kohan 2008; Ibrahim et al. 2013).

LIA is a promising technique which is easy to use, safe and inexpensive, providing simple, effective pain relief with few adverse effects, due to the local administration (Keijsers et al. 2013; Affas et al. 2011; Kerr and Kohan 2008; McCartney and McLeod 2011; Vendittoli et al. 2006). Moreover, it avoids the need for peripheral nerve blocks and/or catheters (Sisak 2013) and may reduce opioid consumption (Kerr and Kohan 2008). Consequently, LIA has become relatively common for several types of surgical procedures (McCartney and McLeod 2011; Keijsers et al. 2013).

Typically, the LIA injection consists of a mixture of an anaesthetic drug and a non-steroidal anti-inflammatory drug (NSAID), to which adrenaline or a corticosteroid may be added (Raeder 2011). This may be followed by small boluses of the same mixture postoperatively using an intra-articular catheter (Ibrahim et al. 2013).

Initially a small randomised controlled trial comparing LIA with placebo established the benefits of local infiltration during TKA (Bianconi et al. 2003). Kerr and Kohan used LIA to manage postoperative pain in 325 patients presenting for THA, elective hip resurfacing or TKA (Kerr and Kohan 2008). They found that two-thirds of patients did not require morphine for postoperative pain control, and few patients experienced limiting adverse effects. The majority of patients were able to walk with assistance 5–6 h after surgery, with independent mobility achieved 13–22 h postoperatively, and 71 % of patients were discharged after a single night in hospital.

17.1.7 Current Evidence for LIA in TKA

Since then there have been a number of studies of LIA in TKA (McCartney and McLeod 2011), several indicating that the technique is associated with lower morphine consumption, reduced pain and shorter LOS (Essving et al. 2011; Andersen et al. 2007). LIA has also achieved favourable outcomes vs epidural analgesia (Andersen et al. 2010; Spreng et al. 2010) and has been advocated as an alternative to femoral nerve block due to the reduced risk of affecting quadriceps function (Chaumeron et al. 2013).

Two meta-analyses have been published recently in an attempt to summarise the evidence so far on the use of LIA in TKA (Gibbs et al. 2012; Keijsers et al. 2013). Gibbs et al. identified 29 randomised controlled trials of LIA following TKA (Gibbs et al., 2012a, b). Thirteen studies compared LIA with control, of which seven concluded that LIA was beneficial in providing analgesia, while six concluded it was of no benefit. LIA was not compared with peripheral nerve block in any of the identified studies; however, it was shown to be beneficial against a background of epidural analgesia in one sufficiently controlled study. Other studies included in the analysis either lacked systematic infiltration or used sub-therapeutic doses. Looking at outcomes for continuous infusion vs multiple analgesic administration, Gibbs et al. identified 11 randomised controlled trials, of which seven used multiple administration and four continuous administration. For multiple administration, five studies reported that local infiltration was effective, as did three continuous infusion studies. However, two studies indicated that local infiltration was less effective than continuous femoral nerve block (Carli et al. 2010; Toftdahl et al. 2007). Interestingly, Andersen et al. and Essving et al. demonstrated that an injection given 24 h postoperatively decreased both PAR and MEP (Andersen et al. 2008b; Essving et al. 2010). Gibbs et al. identified nine studies that examined LOS, in six of which LIA failed to reduce LOS significantly, although two of those reported that the time to be ready for discharge was reduced without affecting LOS.

The meta-analysis by Keijsers et al. involved 7 studies, with a total of 406 TKAs in 374 patients (Keijsers et al. 2013). Postoperative pain visual analogue scales (VAS) scores were in favour of LIA. However, the reductions were modest, at just 12.3 % on the first postoperative day across all studies, with a heterogeneity in scores of 71 %. There were no significant differences in pain scores on postoperative day 2, and no difference in pain scores on activity. Patients in the LIA group used 14.8 % less opioids than those in the placebo group on the first postoperative day. However, there was no difference in opioid usage by 48 h. Keijsers et al. concluded that LIA may be able to reduce pain and opioid use on the first postoperative day, but the effect is small and not clinically relevant (Keijsers et al. 2013).

17.1.8 Differences in LIA Technique May Affect Efficacy

The lack of a definitive body of evidence for LIA in TKA may be due to inconsistencies in the techniques used in the different studies. The basic procedure, as outlined above and originally defined by Kerr and Kohan, is for the surgeon to infiltrate the joint and surrounding tissues with a high volume of anaesthetic, typically including ropivacaine, adrenaline and adjuvant drugs such as NSAIDs, clonidine, corticosteroids or opioids (Kerr and Kohan 2008; Maheshwari et al. 2009a, b). Specifically, 'local infiltration' may be characterised as the systematic injection into all the tissues which are exposed, instrumented or incised during surgery, including the capsule, ligaments and other soft tissues, along with the subcutaneous layers (Andersen et al. 2008b).

A number of different infiltration techniques have been described, involving various agents and methods of administration (Sisak 2013). Agents used in addition to local anaesthetics include steroids (Fu et al. 2010), magnesium sulphate (Chen et al. 2009), morphine (Ritter et al. 1999) and NSAIDS, (Vendittoli et al. 2006a, b), while the methods of administration include intra-articular injection (Badner et al. 1996), infiltration of all traumatised tissues (Andersen et al. 2008a), intra-articular infusion (Ong et al. 2010) or a single shot intra-articular injection (Keijsers et al. 2013).

Due to the lack of consensus over the optimal technique for LIA; with a wide variety in mixture, concentration and volume of analgesics administered but also for the anatomical location where the mixture is infiltrated (Keijsers et al. 2013). In one study, the addition of ketorolac was advocated after it was demonstrated that combining it with ropivacaine reduced morphine consumption, reduced pain intensity and shortened the patients' readiness for discharge (Andersen et al. 2013). Another study of 100 unilateral TKA patients examined the impact of adding 40 mg triamcinolone to the LIA mixture, with recipients recording lower pain scores and better ranges of motion up to 6 months postoperatively vs controls (Bramlett et al. 2012).

Another issue is that the duration of action of an intra-operative bolus of LIA appears to be short (Busch et al. 2006) and it is unclear whether an indwelling catheter should be placed to extend the duration of action through intermittent boluses of local anaesthetic (McCartney and McLeod 2011; Kehlet and Andersen 2011). There are, however, concerns over the risk of infection with an indwelling catheter (McCartney and McLeod 2011; Grosu et al. 2013).

For their meta-analysis, Gibbs et al. examined the different techniques used for LIA in TKA, focusing on five studies that used the same initial infiltration of ropivacaine and adrenaline of all instrumented tissues (Gibbs et al. 2012a, b). Patients received slight variations in the volume and concentration of analgesia, the use of bandaging, catheter site placement, and additional subcutaneous analgesia administration. None of the variations could demonstrate superiority of efficacy.

17.1.8.1 Anatomical Knee Block

Another possible explanation for the observed differences in LIA efficacy in TKA is the anatomical localisation of the infiltration. For LIA to be efficient, it is important to understand the principles of pain and pain control in TKA. The knee joint is highly innervated, with many nerve branches to the joint, where, during TKA, large areas of bone are cut and bone morphogenic proteins are released. If intramedullary alignment is used, the femoral and tibial periosteum is violated and bone marrow release induces inflammatory processes. Finally, hemarthrosis and joint swelling can be an important aspect of the pain experience (Grosu et al. 2013).

With an anatomical knee block, the different structures are infiltrated step-by-step. Due to the progressive nature of the procedure, the risk of local anaesthetic intoxication is extremely limited and allows the surgeon to use an important volume of ropivicaine.

The first infiltration is made during the surgical approach, which is, in our cases, a far medial subvastus approach (Koninckx et al. 2013; Thienpont 2013). The distal aspect of the saphenous nerve is infiltrated as a distal adductor canal blockade. We then address the suprapatellar pouch by infiltrating the anterior surface of the femoral bone under the fat pad. The periosteum of the femur is infiltrated medially and laterally, followed by a para-femoral injection at the supracondylar level.

After making the tibial cut and removing the bone piece, the soft tissues around the tibia are infiltrated under the medial collateral ligament and the lateral periosteum of the tibia. After making the femoral four-in-one cuts and preparing the box, posterior infiltrations should be made both medially and laterally. Staying close to the posterior femoral bone is crucial, alongside infiltration of the posterior capsule. We prefer to infiltrate the area of the lateral genicular artery to obtain chemically controlled blood loss in that area.

After preparing the tibial tray, the periosteum of the tibia is infiltrated. In smaller patients, if some volume of local anaesthetic is available, we prefer to inject intra-articularly after closure of the arthrotomy. A subfascial infiltration of the cutaneous nerves may be performed, although surgeons should be aware that the presence of adrenaline in the LIA solution may cause soft-tissue necrosis of the skin in patients who have undergone multiple operations, are diabetic or have vascular impairment.

17.1.9 Conclusion

LIA is an attractive technique due to its simplicity vs the placing of peri-neural catheters, its safety and the short time required for administration (McCartney and McLeod 2011; Sisak 2013; Grosu et al. 2013), thus potentially reducing anaesthetic time and healthcare costs without affecting patient comfort (Sisak 2013). Consequently, LIA has been adopted by a number of centres worldwide (McCartney and McLeod 2011).

There is nevertheless a lack of definitive evidence on the performance of LIA (Grosu et al. 2013) and it is not yet clear whether the technique offers equivalent analgesia to continuous femoral nerve block or even the same record of safety (Capdevila et al. 2005; McCartney and McLeod 2011). A number of questions remain about LIA, including which components are working, and at what dose (Sisak 2013), whether glucocorticoids should be added (Ikeuchi et al. 2013) and how LIA compares with the alternatives in terms of safety, efficacy and costs (Sisak 2013). There are also concerns as to the potential for local and central toxicity of injecting large volumes of local anaesthetic and other adjuvant drugs around the knee joint (McCartney and McLeod 2011). Finally, it remains to be seen whether LIA actually reduces LOS and the time to achieve recovery goals (Sisak 2013).

Further, well-designed studies will help to determine whether LIA can be recommended as a standalone technique or adjunct to femoral nerve block to improve pain outcomes after TKA, and the required combination, volume and concentration of constituents for the LIA mixture.

17.2 The Drug Matters

Francesco Traverso

The use of peri-articular multimodal drug injection (PMDI) in TKA was proposed 10 years ago with the aim of obtaining a better patient outcome after surgery. Several studies on the use of PMDI showed stable and promising results on pain control, primarily in the first 24 h after surgery, better patient satisfaction, lower morphine consumption during the first 48 post-operative hours, reduction of average length of stay, and improvement of the knee function while minimizing complications (Essving et al. 2010a, b; Husted et al. 2010; Park et al. 2014). However many concerns about this approach need to be elucidated, including the relevance of the drug's choice, the site and timing for wound delivery of local anesthetic agent after TKA.

One of the best topics is about the choice of the drugs used in PMDI. A large consensus in the literature establishes that the most frequently used is a combined mix of local anaesthetic (generally bupivacaine or ropivacaine), magnesium sulphate, morphine, non-steroidal anti-inflammatory drugs (ketorolac), sometimes steroids (depending on the author's preference) and epinephrine. These agents cover all the pathways of the pain as opioid receptors, nociceptors and local inflammatory mediators. Peripheral opioid receptors, covered by morphine, are the first expressed after surgical trauma, sending immediately information to central receptors. NSAID agents such as ketorolac inhibit the production of prostaglandin inflammatory mediators, leading to an anti-inflammatory, antipyretic and analgesic effect. A local anaesthetic such as bupivacaine inhibits the nociceptor and its action is prolonged, with less risk of systemic toxicity, by epinephrine's local vasoconstriction (Lamplot et al. 2014). The use of magnesium sulphate is to "stabilise" the plasma membrane of nociceptors leading to a more difficult transmission of nociceptive stimuli.

Regarding the physiology of pain transmission, the PMDI plays an important role in reducing or avoiding the "early transmission" that leads to the recruitment phenomenon in which painful stimuli induce hyperpolarisation of the neural pathway which makes it difficult to control the subsequent pain.

This pain reduction through its transmission mechanism at peripheral and central levels allows better patient participation in the rehab program and consequently faster discharge from hospital, improving the overall outcome (Maheshwari et al. 2009a, b).

Despite the action of PMDI seldom extending over the first 24–48 h postoperatively, it is helpful, in association with multimodal analgesia program, in assessing the patient's immediate postoperative program, avoiding the experience of "early" pain with lower opioid consumption and faster home readiness, particularly in a "fast track" program (Husted et al. 2010; Lamplot et al. 2014).

Another important issue is the injection site. Randomised studies have reported no differences of analgesic efficacy of intra-capsular vs intra-articular injection, and intra-articular vs extra-articular wound space (Husted et al. 2010; Ruder et al. 2014).

Moreover, local infiltration of the posterior capsule of the knee with a cocktail based on marcaine, morphine, adrenaline antibiotic and corticosteroids before cementing the implants followed by a second infiltration prior to closure did not reduce the morphine consumption and did not improve the recovery of walking capacity, physical activity and knee function vs continuous femoral block (Meftah et al. 2012). Conversely, peri-articular injection of ropivacaine, morphine, non-steroidal anti-inflammatory drug (ketorolac), epinephrine, and cefuroxime after cementation of the prostheses into the sheath of the medial and lateral collateral ligaments and posterior capsule in simultaneous bilateral TKA improved early post-operative pain control, but not patient satisfaction (Koh et al. 2010, 2012). Similar outcomes have been observed after peri-articular injection of bupivacaine, ketorolac after implantation or before wound closure. Overall these data suggest that it is not the injection site which is important (Table 17.1) but the dose and the type of multiple agents used.

Gibbs et al. in a review of literature about the local infiltration in TKA suggested that an infiltration of specific cocktail, made by ropivacaine, adrenaline and ketorolac, inside all the exposed tissues and not just the specific site of the joint

Table 17.1 Multimodal analgesia outcomes achieved by using different cocktails of analgesic and different site of injection

Patients (*n*)	PMDI Cocktail	Administration	Injection	Site of injection	Outcome	Reference
55	200–400 mg Marcaine 0.5 % 0.8 mL Morphine sulphate (8 mg) 0.3 mL Adrenaline (300 μg) 750 mg Antibiotic 40 mg Corticosteroids 22 mL Normal saline	Peri-articular	2	Deep (first injection in three areas: posterior capsule, postero-medial structures and periarticular synovium) Superficial (second injection in six areas: extensor mechanism, pes anserinus, anteromedial capsule, periosteum, iliotibial band and subcutaneous plane)	No differences between PMDI and PCEA/FNB; PCEA/FNB better pain control in deambulation	Meftah et al. (2012)
55	300 mg Ropivacaine (40 mL) 10 mg Morphine sulphate (10 mL) 30 mg Ketorolac (1 mL) 300 μg Epinephrine 1:1,000 (0.3 mL) 750 mg Cefuroxime (10 mL) 38,7 mL Normal saline	Peri-articular after cementation of prostheses in simultaneous bilateral TKAs	1 (100 mL)	20 mL (sheath of the medial and lateral collateral ligaments and posterior capsule) 30 mL before closure (synovium, capsule and quadriceps muscle) 50 mL after closure (subcutaneous tissue, capsule and quadriceps muscle)	Significant reduction of the pain score only during operation night (POD 1)	Koh et al. (2010)
87	300 mg Ropivacaine (40 mL) 10 mg Morphine sulphate (10 mL) 30 mg Ketorolac (1 mL) 300 μg Epinephrine 1:1,000 (0.3 mL) 750 mg Cefuroxime (10 mL) 38.7 mL Normal saline	Peri-articular after cementation of prostheses	1 (100 mL)	20 mL (sheath of the medial and lateral collateral ligaments and posterior capsule) 30 mL before closure (synovium, capsule and quadriceps muscle) 50 mL after closure (subcutaneous tissue, capsule and quadriceps muscle)	PMDI in combination with IV-PCA reduced pain level and opioid consumption over 24 h after surgery	Koh et al. (2012)
36	30 mL Bupivacaine 0.5 % 10 mg $MgSO_4$ 15 mg Ketorolac	Peri-articular before wound closure	1	Posterior capsule in the posteromedial and posterolateral soft tissue, synovium, pes anserinus and iliotibial band at Gerdy's tubercle	PMDI in combination with multimodal analgesics reduced significantly the narcotic consumption, pain score and length of hospital stay	Lamplot et al. (2014)

57	100 mg Bupivacaine (0.5 %) 20 mL 5 mg Morphine sulphate (5 mL) 0.6 mg Epinephrine (1:1,000) 0.6 mL 30 mg Ketorolac trimethamine (1 mL)	Peri-articular before implantation and during the cementation	1 (100 mL)	25 mL (posterior knee capsule, soft tissue around the medial and lateral collateral ligaments before implantation) 75 mL (quadriceps muscle, reticacular tissues, pes anserinus, suprapatellar and infrapatellar fat pat during cementation)	PMDI showed reduction in ketorolac consumption during the 12–16 h after surgery; but higher incidence of nausea and pruritus	Tammachote et al. (2013)
42	275 mg Ropivacaine 30 mg Ketorolac 0.5 mg Adrenaline	Local infiltration	1	Intra-articular via catheter-	Reduced opioid consumption for 48 h after surgery and reduced pain for 48 h	Vendittoli et al. (2006a, b)
67	*ROC (Ranawat Orthopaedic Center) cocktail* *First injection* 200-400 mg Bupivacaine (0.5 %) 24 mL 8 mg Morphine sulphate 0.8 mL 300 µg Epinephrine 1:1,000 0.3 mL 40 mg Methylprednisolone acetate 1 mL 750 mg Cefuroxime 10 mL Sodium chloride (0.9 %) 20 mL *Second injection* Bupivacaine (0.5 %) 20 mL Sodium chloride (0.9 %) 20 mL	Peri-articular	2	All the soft tissues surrounding the hip and knee	Reduction in narcotic consumption, shorter hospital stay, better ASLR	Maheshwari et al. (2009a, b), Aad et al. (2010)
60	100 mL Ropivacaine (0.2 %) with adrenaline 50 mL Ropivacaine (0.2 %)	Intracapsular vs intra-articular	1 (150 mL)	50 mL before insertion in posterior capsule 50 mL after insertion in anterior capsule 50 mL surrounding the joints	No significant differences	Ruder et al. (2014)

is important for more effective pain management (Gibbs et al. 2012a, b).

Although the local infiltration of anaesthetic agents into the surgical wound provides good post-operative pain control, the short lifetime of action of the drugs including bupivacaine remains an important issue to be addressed. Indeed, plasma bupivacaine HCl concentration is sustained within 12 h of local injection and thereafter decreases rapidly (Hu et al. 2013). In order to improve the effects of local analgesia by enhancing its duration of action, a new bupivacaine liposome has recently been designed (EXPAREL, Pacira Pharmaceuticals Parsippany, NJ). A liposome-based delivery system consists of a controlled release of the drug. The liposomes are vesicles formed by an aqueous core surrounded by an outer phospholipid bilayer. They are biodegradable, biocompatible, safe and not immunogenic. Given the capability to facilitate the penetration of poorly absorbed drugs and bind the surface, which leads to increased retention time, the liposome represent a successful carrier for a wide variety of drug and paved the way for new therapeutic strategies including pain management (Hua and Wu 2013).

Bupivacaine liposome is an injectable suspension, approved by the Food Drug Administration (FDA) in 2011 as a new multivesicular formulation designed for rapid absorption and prolonged release of bupivacaine in association with others analgesic (http://investor.pacira.com/phoenix.zhtml?c=220759&p=irol-newsArticle&ID=1623529&highlight=Exparel). In the USA it is available commercially at a concentration of 13.3 mg/mL for a single-dose infiltration (EXPAREL, Pacira Pharmaceuticals Parsippany, NJ). Wound infiltration with liposomal bupivacaine (LB) before site closure is a feasible approach to be performed without the need for specific training for surgeons and nurse, or specific surgical devices. The absorption of LB varies depending on the surgical procedure and size of the incision (Golf et al. 2011; Haas et al. 2012). A single intra-operative administration of LB into the surgical site for up to 72 h resulted in markedly prolonged plasma levels and analgesia with a corresponding reduction in use of opioids. (Gorfine et al. 2011; Bramlett et al. 2012a, b; Cohen 2012; Haas et al. 2012; Smoot et al. 2012; FDA approval of Exparel for postsurgical pain management 2014). Bupivacaine, reducing the influx of sodium ions, prevents the depolarisation of plasma membrane of nerve cells and, thereby, the propagation of impulse along the nerve (Buckenmaier and Bleckner 2005). Once administrated locally as liposome delivery, bupivacaine power seems to increase. In line with this, comparative analysis of the pharmacokinetic profile between liposome bupivacaine and bupivacaine HCl based on data from four phase II and III randomised, active – and placebo-controlled trials in patients undergoing inguinal hernia repair, TKA, haemorrhoidectomy or bunionectomy, revealed extended plasma bupivacaine levels over time in the patients treated with liposome bupivacaine compared those with bupivacaine HCl. Looking at the levels of plasma bupivacaine concentrations vs time, the authors observed bimodal kinetics characterised by an initial peak soon after administration of the LB (probably associated with a small amount (3 %) of extra-liposomal bupivacaine), and by a second later peak (about 12–36 h later) (associated with the liposome-loaded bupivacaine), thus indicating a slow release from the liposomal vesicles (Hu et al. 2013). This new formulation thereby promoted a rapid uptake of bupivacaine during the first few hours after administration, and delayed release within 96 h later. Albeit generally well-tolerated in all four studies (Hu et al. 2013), the high dose of LB (532 mg) was associated with higher adverse effects in the patients and provoked a reduction to the limit of Cmax with a high toxicological risk for the central nervous system and cardiovascular system. In contrast, no signs of neuro- or cardiac toxicity have been observed in other independent studies using a dose ranging from 66 to 532 mg of LB (Bergese et al. 2012a, b; Naseem et al. 2012), even though no statistically significant difference in terms of pain score within 72 h after drug injection has recorded between LB and bupivacaine HCl in TKA.

Taking advantage of the pharmacokinetic properties, LB is administrated in association with other analgesic or NSAIDs with intra-operative local infiltration analgesia during TKA. A recent study of Hawkins RJ (ICJR Symposium at AAOS, Chicago 2013) has analyzed 200 TKA patients, 100 treated with femoral block pain management and 100 treated with EXPAREL multi-module pain management. No significant difference was observed in terms of average resting pain score at 72 h, while improved assisted ambulation and shorter length of stay was found in the EXPAREL group. In addition, a pilot evaluation, conducted by Lombardi V (JIS experience 2012–2013 available on ICJR Webinar) on 229 patients with TJR, 120 treated with intra-articular LB in association with epinephrine, ketorolac and bupivacaine HCl compared to 109 patients with intra-articular injection of ropivacaine, epinephrine and ketorolac, showed a significant reduction in opioid use within 24–48 h in the LB group. However, the average pain rating was better in the first 24 h post-operative with less differences over 36–60 h post-operatively. Furthermore, the hospital length of stay was comparable in the two groups. Although interesting and promising, further studies are still necessary to corroborate the beneficial effects of LB administration in TKA. The approval and free marking of LB, which at the moment is limited only in US, will probably help to attest better its advantages and eventual adverse effects.

References

Aad G, Abbott B et al (2010) Observation of a centrality-dependent dijet asymmetry in lead-lead collisions at sqrt[S(NN)] =2.76 TeV with the ATLAS detector at the LHC. Phys Rev Lett 105(25):252303

Affas F, Nygards EB, Stiller CO et al (2011) Pain control after total knee arthroplasty: a randomized trial comparing local infiltration anesthesia and continuous femoral block. Acta Orthop 82:441–447

Andersen KV, Bak M, Christensen BV et al (2010) A randomized, controlled trial comparing local infiltration analgesia with epidural infusion for total knee arthroplasty. Acta Orthop 81:606–610

Andersen KV, Nikolajsen L, Haraldsted V et al (2013) Local infiltration analgesia for total knee arthroplasty: should ketorolac be added? Br J Anaesth 111:242–248

Andersen KV, Pfeiffer-Jensen M, Haraldsted V et al (2007) Reduced hospital stay and narcotic consumption, and improved mobilization with local and intraarticular infiltration after hip arthroplasty: a randomized clinical trial of an intraarticular technique versus epidural infusion in 80 patients. Acta Orthop 78:180–186

Andersen LO, Gaarn-Larsen L, Kristensen BB et al (2009) Subacute pain and function after fast-track hip and knee arthroplasty. Anaesthesia 64:508–513

Andersen LO, Husted H, Otte KS et al (2008a) A compression bandage improves local infiltration analgesia in total knee arthroplasty. Acta Orthop 79:806–811

Andersen LO, Husted H, Otte KS et al (2008b) High-volume infiltration analgesia in total knee arthroplasty: a randomized, double-blind, placebo-controlled trial. Acta Anaesthesiol Scand 52:1331–1335

Aromaa U, Lahdensuu M, Cozanitis DA (1997) Severe complications associated with epidural and spinal anaesthesias in Finland 1987-1993. A study based on patient insurance claims [see comment]. Acta Anaesthesiol Scand 41:445–452

Auroy Y, Narchi P, Messiah A et al (1997) Serious complications related to regional anesthesia: results of a prospective survey in France. Anesthesiology 87:479–486

Badner NH, Bourne RB, Rorabeck CH et al (1996) Intra-articular injection of bupivacaine in knee-replacement operations. Results of use for analgesia and for preemptive blockade. J Bone Joint Surg Am 78:734–738

Berger RA, Jacobs JJ, Meneghini RM et al (2004) Rapid rehabilitation and recovery with minimally invasive total hip arthroplasty. Clin Orthop Relat Res 429:239–247

Bergese SD, Onel E et al (2012a) Bupivacaine extended-release liposome injection exhibits a favorable cardiac safety profile. Reg Anesth Pain Med 37(2):145–151

Bergese SD, Ramamoorthy S et al (2012b) Efficacy profile of liposome bupivacaine, a novel formulation of bupivacaine for postsurgical analgesia. J Pain Res 5:107–116

Beswick AD, Wylde V, Gooberman-Hill R et al (2012) What proportion of patients report long-term pain after total hip or knee replacement for osteoarthritis? A systematic review of prospective studies in unselected patients. BMJ Open 2:e000435

Bianconi M, Ferraro L, Traina GC et al (2003) Pharmacokinetics and efficacy of ropivacaine continuous wound instillation after joint replacement surgery. Br J Anaesth 91:830–835

Bourne RB, Chesworth BM, Davis AM et al (2010) Patient satisfaction after total knee arthroplasty: who is satisfied and who is not? Clin Orthop Relat Res 468:57–63

Bramlett K, Onel E, Viscusi ER et al (2012) A randomized, double-blind, dose-ranging study comparing wound infiltration of DepoFoam bupivacaine, an extended-release liposomal bupivacaine, to bupivacaine HCl for postsurgical analgesia in total knee arthroplasty. Knee 19:530–536

Buckenmaier CC 3rd, Bleckner LL (2005) Anaesthetic agents for advanced regional anaesthesia: a North American perspective. Drugs 65(6):745–759

Busch CA, Shore BJ, Bhandari R et al (2006) Efficacy of periarticular multimodal drug injection in total knee

arthroplasty. A randomized trial. J Bone Joint Surg Am 88:959–963
Capdevila X, Pirat P, Bringuier S et al (2005) Continuous peripheral nerve blocks in hospital wards after orthopedic surgery: a multicenter prospective analysis of the quality of postoperative analgesia and complications in 1,416 patients. Anesthesiology 103:1035–1045
Carli F, Clemente A, Asenjo JF et al (2010) Analgesia and functional outcome after total knee arthroplasty: periarticular infiltration vs continuous femoral nerve block. Br J Anaesth 105:185–195
Carroll I, Barelka P, Wang CK et al (2012) A pilot cohort study of the determinants of longitudinal opioid use after surgery. Anesth Analg 115:694–702
Chaumeron A, Audy D, Drolet P et al (2013) Periarticular injection in knee arthroplasty improves quadriceps function. Clin Orthop Relat Res 471:2284–2295
Chen Y, Zhang Y, Zhu YL et al (2009) Efficacy and safety of an intra-operative intra-articular magnesium/ropivacaine injection for pain control following total knee arthroplasty. J Int Med Res 37:1733–1741
Cohen SM (2012) Extended pain relief trial utilizing infiltration of Exparel((R)), a long-acting multivesicular liposome formulation of bupivacaine: a Phase IV health economic trial in adult patients undergoing open colectomy. J Pain Res 5:567–572
Davies AF, Segar EP, Murdoch J et al (2004) Epidural infusion or combined femoral and sciatic nerve blocks as perioperative analgesia for knee arthroplasty. Br J Anaesth 93:368–374
Dillon JP, Brennan L, Mitchell D (2012) Local infiltration analgesia in hip and knee arthroplasty: an emerging technique. Acta Orthop Belg 78:158–163
Essving P, Axelsson K, Aberg E et al (2011) Local infiltration analgesia versus intrathecal morphine for postoperative pain management after total knee arthroplasty: a randomized controlled trial. Anesth Analg 113:926–933
Essving P, Axelsson K, Kjellberg J et al (2010) Reduced morphine consumption and pain intensity with local infiltration analgesia (LIA) following total knee arthroplasty. Acta Orthop 81:354–360
FDA approval of Exparel for postsurgical pain management. January 24. http://investor.pacira.com/phoenix.zhtml?c=220759&p=irol-newsArticle&ID=1623529&highlight=Exparel. (Visited on 8 May 2014)
Fischer HB, Simanski CJ, Sharp C et al (2008) A procedure-specific systematic review and consensus recommendations for postoperative analgesia following total knee arthroplasty. Anaesthesia 63:1105–1123
Fu PL, Xiao J, Zhu YL et al (2010) Efficacy of a multimodal analgesia protocol in total knee arthroplasty: a randomized, controlled trial. J Int Med Res 38:1404–1412
Gibbs DM, Green TP, Esler CN (2012) The local infiltration of analgesia following total knee replacement: a review of current literature. J Bone Joint Surg Br 94:1154–1159
Golf M, Daniels SE et al (2011) A phase 3, randomized, placebo-controlled trial of DepoFoam(R) bupivacaine (extended-release bupivacaine local analgesic) in bunionectomy. Adv Ther 28(9):776–788
Gorfine SR, Onel E et al (2011) Bupivacaine extended-release liposome injection for prolonged postsurgical analgesia in patients undergoing hemorrhoidectomy: a multicenter, randomized, double-blind, placebo-controlled trial. Dis Colon Rectum 54(12):1552–1559
Grosu I, Lavand'homme P, Thienpont E (2014) Pain after knee arthroplasty: an unresolved issue. Knee Surg Sports Traumatol Arthrosc 22(8):1744–58
Haas E, Onel E et al (2012) A double-blind, randomized, active-controlled study for post-hemorrhoidectomy pain management with liposome bupivacaine, a novel local analgesic formulation. Am Surg 78(5):574–581
Hadzic A, Houle TT, Capdevila X et al (2010) Femoral nerve block for analgesia in patients having knee arthroplasty. Anesthesiology 113:1014–1015
Hu D, Onel E et al (2013) Pharmacokinetic profile of liposome bupivacaine injection following a single administration at the surgical site. Clin Drug Investig 33(2):109–115
Hua S, Wu SY (2013) The use of lipid-based nanocarriers for targeted pain therapies. Front Pharmacol 4:143. eCollection 2013
Husted H, Solgaard S, Hansen TB, Søballe K, Kehlet H (2010) Care principles at four fast-track arthroplasty departments in Denmark. Dan Med Bull 57(7):A4166
Ibrahim MS, Alazzawi S, Nizam I et al (2013) An evidence-based review of enhanced recovery interventions in knee replacement surgery. Ann R Coll Surg Engl 95:386–389
Ikeuchi M, Kamimoto Y, Izumi M et al. (2014). Effects of dexamethasone on local infiltration analgesia in total knee arthroplasty: a randomized controlled trial. Knee Surg Sports Traumatol Arthrosc 22(7):1638–43
Joo JH, Park JW, Kim JS et al (2011) Is intra-articular multimodal drug injection effective in pain management after total knee arthroplasty? A randomized, double-blinded, prospective study. J Arthroplasty 26:1095–1099
Kandasami M, Kinninmonth AW, Sarungi M et al (2009) Femoral nerve block for total knee replacement – a word of caution. Knee 16:98–100
Kehlet H, Andersen LO (2011) Local infiltration analgesia in joint replacement: the evidence and recommendations for clinical practice. Acta Anaesthesiol Scand 55:778–784
Kehlet H, Dahl JB (1993) The value of "multimodal" or "balanced analgesia" in postoperative pain treatment. Anesth Analg 77:1048–1056
Kehlet H, Jensen TS, Woolf CJ (2006) Persistent postsurgical pain: risk factors and prevention. Lancet 367:1618–1625
Keijsers R, Van Delft R, Van Den Bekerom MP et al. (2013). Local infiltration analgesia following total knee arthroplasty: effect on post-operative pain and opioid consumption-a meta-analysis. Knee Surg Sports Traumatol Arthrosc
Kerr DR, Kohan L (2008) Local infiltration analgesia: a technique for the control of acute postoperative pain

following knee and hip surgery: a case study of 325 patients. Acta Orthop 79:174–183

Koh IJ, Kang YG et al (2010) Additional pain relieving effect of intraoperative periarticular injections after simultaneous bilateral TKA: a randomized, controlled study. Knee Surg Sports Traumatol Arthrosc 18(7):916–922

Koh IJ, Kang YG et al (2012) Does periarticular injection have additional pain relieving effects during contemporary multimodal pain control protocols for TKA?: a randomised, controlled study. Knee 19(4):253–259

Koninckx A, Schwab PE, Deltour A et al. (2014). The minimally invasive far medial subvastus approach for total knee arthroplasty in valgus knees. Knee Surg Sports Traumatol Arthrosc 22(8):1765–70

Krenzel BA, Cook C, Martin GN et al (2009) Posterior capsular injections of ropivacaine during total knee arthroplasty: a randomized, double-blind, placebo-controlled study. J Arthroplasty 24:138–143

Labraca NS, Castro-Sánchez AM, Matarán-Peñarrocha GA et al (2011) Benefits of starting rehabilitation within 24 hours of primary total knee arthroplasty: randomized clinical trial. Clin Rehabil 25:557–566

Lamplot JD, Wagner ER et al (2014) Multimodal pain management in total knee arthroplasty: a prospective randomized controlled trial. J Arthroplasty 29(2):329–334

Lombardi AV Jr, Viacava AJ, Berend KR (2006) Rapid recovery protocols and minimally invasive surgery help achieve high knee flexion. Clin Orthop Relat Res 452:117–122

Maheshwari AV, Blum YC, Shekhar L et al (2009) Multimodal pain management after total hip and knee arthroplasty at the Ranawat Orthopaedic Center. Clin Orthop Relat Res 467:1418–1423

McCartney CJ, McLeod GA (2011) Local infiltration analgesia for total knee arthroplasty. Br J Anaesth 107:487–489

Mcleod G, Davies H, Munnoch N et al (2001) Postoperative pain relief using thoracic epidural analgesia: outstanding success and disappointing failures. Anaesthesia 56:75–81

Meftah M, Wong AC et al (2012) Pain management after total knee arthroplasty using a multimodal approach. Orthopedics 35(5):e660–e664

Naseem A, Harada T et al (2012) Bupivacaine extended release liposome injection does not prolong QTc interval in a thorough QT/QTc study in healthy volunteers. J Clin Pharmacol 52(9):1441–1447

Ong JC, Chin PL, Fook-Chong SM et al (2010) Continuous infiltration of local anaesthetic following total knee arthroplasty. J Orthop Surg (Hong Kong) 18:203–207

Park C, Klatman S et al (2014) Acute host reaction after anterior cruciate ligament reconstruction. Am J Orthop (Belle Mead NJ) 43(2):78–82

Perkins FM, Kehlet H (2000) Chronic pain as an outcome of surgery. A review of predictive factors. Anesthesiology 93:1123–1133

Puolakka PA, Rorarius MG, Roviola M et al (2010) Persistent pain following knee arthroplasty. Eur J Anaesthesiol 27:455–460

Raeder JC (2011) Local infiltration analgesia for pain after total knee replacement surgery: a winner or just a strong runner-up? Anesth Analg 113:684–686

Ritter MA, Koehler M, Keating EM et al (1999) Intra-articular morphine and/or bupivacaine after total knee replacement. J Bone Joint Surg Br 81:301–303

Ruder JA, Magennis E et al (2014) Clinical and morphologic factors associated with suture anchor refixation of labral tears in the hip. HSS J 10(1):18–24

Shen H, Zhang N, Zhang X et al (2009) C-reactive protein levels after 4 types of arthroplasty. Acta Orthop 80:330–333

Singelyn FJ, Deyaert M, Joris D et al (1998) Effects of intravenous patient-controlled analgesia with morphine, continuous epidural analgesia, and continuous three-in-one block on postoperative pain and knee rehabilitation after unilateral total knee arthroplasty. Anesth Analg 87:88–92

Sisak K (2013) Local infiltration analgesia for total knee replacement: is it the answer? Available: http://www.boneandjoint.org.uk/content/local-infiltration-analgesia-total-knee-replacement-it-answer. Accessed 9 Jan 2014

Smoot JD, Bergese SD et al (2012) The efficacy and safety of DepoFoam bupivacaine in patients undergoing bilateral, cosmetic, submuscular augmentation mammaplasty: a randomized, double-blind, active-control study. Aesthet Surg J 32(1):69–76

Spreng UJ, Dahl V, Hjall A et al (2010) High-volume local infiltration analgesia combined with intravenous or local ketorolac+morphine compared with epidural analgesia after total knee arthroplasty. Br J Anaesth 105:675–682

Srikandarajah S, Gilron I (2011) Systematic review of movement-evoked pain versus pain at rest in postsurgical clinical trials and meta-analyses: a fundamental distinction requiring standardized measurement. Pain 152:1734–1739

Steyaert A, Lavand'homme P (2013) Postoperative opioids: let us take responsibility for the possible consequences. Eur J Anaesthesiol 30:50–52

Tammachote N, Kanitnate S et al (2013) Is pain after TKA better with periarticular injection or intrathecal morphine? Clin Orthop Relat Res 471(6):1992–1999

Thienpont E (2013) Faster quadriceps recovery with the far medial subvastus approach in minimally invasive total knee arthroplasty. Knee Surg Sports Traumatol Arthrosc 21:2370–2374

Thomas T, Robinson C, Champion D et al (1998) Prediction and assessment of the severity of post-operative pain and of satisfaction with management. Pain 75:177–185

Toftdahl K, Nikolajsen L, Haraldsted V et al (2007) Comparison of peri- and intraarticular analgesia with femoral nerve block after total knee arthroplasty: a randomized clinical trial. Acta Orthop 78:172–179

Torrance N, Smith BH, Bennett MI et al (2006) The epidemiology of chronic pain of predominantly neuropathic origin. Results from a general population survey. J Pain 7:281–289

Vendittoli PA, Makinen P, Drolet P et al (2006) A multimodal analgesia protocol for total knee arthroplasty. A randomized, controlled study. J Bone Joint Surg Am 88:282–289

Vilardo L, Shah M (2011) Chronic pain after hip and knee replacement. Tech Reg Anesth Pain Manag 15:110–115

Woolf CJ (2011) Central sensitization: implications for the diagnosis and treatment of pain. Pain 152:S2–S15

Wylde V, Gooberman-Hill R, Horwood J et al (2011) The effect of local anaesthetic wound infiltration on chronic pain after lower limb joint replacement: a protocol for a double-blind randomised controlled trial. BMC Musculoskelet Disord 12:53

Xu J, Brennan TJ (2011) The pathophysiology of acute pain: animal models. Curr Opin Anaesthesiol 24:508–514

Part III

Infection Control

18 Prevention of Infection: The Host Factors

Matteo Carlo Ferrari and Guido Grappiolo

Open Questions

- How important are the host risk factors in prosthetic joint infections?
- What is the role of obesity in periprosthetic joint infections?
- Is it cost-effective to identify preoperatively all the medical risk factors and try to correct them before surgery?
- Multidisciplinary preoperative approach to detect and to correct the major host risk factors: is it advisable?
- Should we change the standard antibiotic prophylaxis for patients with multiple comorbidities?

18.1 Prosthetic Joint Infections: Classification, Incidence, Causes, and Microorganism Factors

Orthopedic device-related infections are relatively uncommon (0.6–2.5 % for primary and up to 10–20 % for revision) (Jamsen et al. 2010; Urquhart et al. 2010; Cataldo et al. 2010; Moran et al. 2010; Peel et al. 2011; Shuman et al. 2012). They cause significant morbidity and mortality and an elevated health care expenditure (three times more than first implants).

Surgical risk factors include simultaneous bilateral arthroplasty, a long operative time (more than 2.5 h), and allogenic blood transfusion.

Post-operative risk factors include wound-healing complications such as superficial infection, delayed healing, necrosis, dehiscence, hematoma, bacteremia, prolonged wound drainage, permanence of a urinary catheter, and prolonged hospital stay.

The frequency of infection increases as the number of primary and revision arthroplasties increases (Trampuz and Zimmerli 2006a; Kurd et al. 2010; Laudermilch et al. 2010; Ghanem et al. 2009; Mittal et al. 2007; Estes et al. 2010; Jafari et al. 2010; Mortazavi et al. 2010; Atkins et al. 1998; Zimmerli et al. 2004; Trampuz and Zimmerli 2005).

Almost any microorganism can cause prosthetic joint infections, such as Gram-positive bacteria (accounting for about two-thirds of total), Gram-negative bacteria and polymicrobic flora (accounting for about 10–15 % each), and fungi (rare).

Many classification systems of periprosthetic joint infections have been proposed in the literature. The Centers for Disease Control and Prevention (CDC) defined Surgical Site Infection as an infection of or near the operative site within

M.C. Ferrari (✉) • G. Grappiolo
Hip Orthopedics and Prosthesis,
Humanitas Clinical and Research Center,
Via Manzoni 56, Rozzano, Milan 20089, Italy
e-mail: matteo_carlo.ferrari@humanitas.it

A. Baldini, P. Caldora (eds.), *Perioperative Medical Management for Total Joint Arthroplasty: How to Control Hemostasis, Pain and Infection*, DOI 10.1007/978-3-319-07203-6_18,

the first 30 days of surgical procedure or within 1 year with an implant in place (Hidron et al. 2008). Tsukayama's classification attempted to correlate the time of infection onset with the therapeutic strategy (Tsukayama et al. 1996). His classification, adopted by the Musculoskeletal Infection Society, has been used as a guide for selection of surgical treatment. It defines an early infection as one that occurs within 1 month of index arthroplasty and any infection beyond this point as late. Acute hematogenous infection is also included in this classification system. The Zimmerli/Trampuz classification considers an early infection as one that occurs within 3 months of index surgery. Infections with onset between 3 and 24 months are delayed infections and those occurring >24 months after index arthroplasty are classified as late (Zimmerli et al. 2004; Trampuz and Zimmerli 2005). These classification systems are useful since they provide a description for pathogenesis. It is admitted that early infections may be the result of seeding during surgery, whereas late infections are likely acquired by hematogenous spread. Another classification proposed by Senneville et al. (2009) relies mostly on duration of symptoms and places less emphasis on the timing of index arthroplasty. Based on this classification, acute infection is one with less than 1 month of symptoms and any infection with greater than 1 month of symptoms is considered late. The classification proposed by McPherson considers criteria other than timing, such as host factors and microorganism factors, and looks at periods shorter than 3 weeks (McPherson et al. 2002). Considering the host factors, the McPherson classification quantifies the infection risk factors, making a systemic host grading and a local extremity grading. From the McPherson classification the Musculoskeletal Infection Society scoring system was derived, taking into account the infection type, the systemic host grade and the local extremity grade. The scoring system produces prognostic and therapeutic suggestions regarding the functional results, risks of reimplantation, and risks of limb amputation (McPherson et al. 2002).

Early infections are usually associated with acute onset of pain, effusion, erythema, warmth at the implant site, fever, and increase of inflammatory markers, such as white blood cells, platelet count, C-reactive protein, erythrocyte sedimentation rate, fibrinogen, pro-calcitonin, IL-1, and IL-6 (Greidanus et al. 2007); the formation of a sinus tract with purulent discharge may also occur. Acute infections are usually caused by virulent microorganisms, such as *Staphylococcus aureus* or, less frequently, Gram-negative bacteria.

Delayed or low-grade infections are most frequently observed and present with insidious signs and symptoms such as implant loosening, persistent joint pain, and non-specific low-grade increase of inflammatory markers. These signs are usually difficult to distinguish from aseptic failure modes. Delayed infections are caused by less aggressive microorganisms such as coagulase-negative staphylococci (CoNS) or streptococci/enterococci. Early and delayed infections are considered acquired from index surgery.

Late infections are predominantly acquired by hematogenous seeding from the skin, respiratory tract, dental apparatus, and urinary or gastrointestinal tract (Trampuz and Widmer 2006).

Other classifications (Coventry 1975) divide the acute postoperative infections into superficial and deep, depending on the infection site.

Superficial infection is limited to the superficial wound layers, above the fascia or capsular layer, and can be treated in most cases by soft tissue debridement with prosthesis retention.

Deep infections below the fascia involving the periprosthetic space are more difficult to treat. In the case of early acute infection starting in the first 3–4 weeks after surgery, an aggressive debridement changing the modular components of the prosthesis may be attempted. In all late chronic deep periprosthetic joint infections, prosthesis removal and exchange (in one or, more commonly, two stages) represents the gold standard.

The key point of all the surgical procedures for fighting periprosthetic joint infection – irrigation and debridement, one stage exchange, or two stage procedures – is the bacteria slime production. Biofilm is the most important factor conditioning the result from irrigation and debridement in acute postoperative infection. Bacterial biofilm production probably starts a few hours after bacterial colonization and prosthesis adhesion but a postoperative period of 3–4 weeks after surgery is allowed for choosing between irrigation and debridement in the case of deep acute periprosthetic infection (Costerton et al. 1999). Further investigations on biofilm are advisable to identify other factors influencing the outcome of the surgical strategies adopted for periprosthetic joint infections.

The management of infections is not completely standardized and the outcome is frequently poor or at least unsatisfactory because of the increasing number of highly virulent and antibiotic-resistant bacteria (Trampuz and Zimmerli 2006b; Gould et al. 2009; Prokuski 2008).

18.2 Prosthetic Joint Infections: The Host Factors

Considering host factors, patients with infected prostheses usually present with many pre-existing risk factors: obesity, diabetes mellitus, rheumatoid arthritis, other autoimmune diseases, and immunosuppression related to a number of causes (such as previous or active neoplasm, HIV, etc.), tobacco use, previous multiple procedures, and previous infection associated with a prosthetic joint at the same site.

Overweight patients should be counseled to lose weight before surgery. Patients receiving immunosuppressive therapies must be advised to suspend them 2 weeks before surgery and not to resume them for approximately 3 weeks after surgery. Only HIV positive patients should not stop their antiretroviral therapy.

Considering other aspects related to the prevention of prosthetic infections, we must take into account the skin aspects: skin preparation (hair removal), type of skin disinfection, previous scars, adequate blood supply (previous flaps, vein and capillary refilling, arterial local conditions), and presence of pressure sores. The presence of postoperative hematoma is another risk factor because of the more frequent bacterial colonization and the absence of an adequate leukocyte blood supply.

Another aspect which has to be considered is strict glycemic blood level control in diabetic patients. As is well known, high glucose levels worsen leukocyte chemotaxis and blood circulation, reducing the host defenses at the surgical site; moreover, peripheral neuropathy could reduce patient awareness as well as suspicion of infection because of lack of the pain. Furthermore, typical diabetic arterial damage could complicate the postoperative period with acute ischemic limb disease, especially for tourniquet-related knee procedures and for intraoperative leg torsions related to hip procedures. Diabetic patients have a significant increase of ischemic heart and brain events in the postoperative period due to anemia.

Smoking should be strongly discouraged because it increases the infection risk fourfold, probably due to vascular damage. Another possible complication in heavy smokers is COPD exacerbation and an increase in the risk of hospital-acquired pneumonia.

Patients with renal function impairment (especially those on dialysis) and major liver diseases have higher infection risks and drug-related and postoperative side effects, such as allergies, thrombocytopenia and coagulation problems (preexisting and acquired) with the risk of bleeding from the surgical site and hematoma, kidney and liver failure.

Before surgery, the medical team should investigate and take into account the possible treatment of any ongoing source of infection from the teeth and gums, skin, soft tissue, urinary tract, respiratory tract, and gastrointestinal tract.

Prosthetic joint infections are classified by several authors including McPherson et al. (2002), Cierny and DiPasquale (2002), and Cierny et al. (2003).

McPherson developed a staging system for periprosthetic infections, taking into consideration the timing of infection, the overall medical and immune health status of the patient, and the local wound condition.

This staging system considers and integrates three aspects: infection timing type (early <4 postoperative weeks; haematogenous <4 weeks duration; late chronic >4 weeks duration), systemic host grade (A: uncompromised; B: compromised with —one or two compromising factors; C: significantly compromised with more than two compromising factors), and local extremity wound grade (1: uncompromised; 2: compromised with —one or two compromising factors; 3: significantly compromised with more than two compromising factors).

Cierny et al. integrated the classification system for osteomyelitis in adult patients with the classification of periprosthetic total joint infections.

In these classifications, prosthetic joint infections are entered as anatomic types of the disease: early and superficial osteomyelitis (the old Type II osteomyelitis staging system), late and chronic refractory osteomyelitis (Type IV of the previous osteomyelitis staging system).

In addition, these authors added local and systemic host factors which may influence treatment and prognosis, dividing patients into three categories: A-, B-, and C-hosts. A-hosts are healthy and without healing deficiencies; B-hosts are compromised by one or more local and/or systemic parameters; C-hosts are patients in whom the severity of the underlying pre-existing diseases exceeds their ability to undergo the necessary aggressive treatment, and are therefore directed to more conservative therapies.

18.3 Our Approach for Infection Prevention in Arthroplasty

Many different protocols are published in the literature (national and international guidelines, SNICh in Italy, acronym for National Surgical Site Infections Surveillance System) using first- or second-class cephalosporin or vancomycin/clindamycin in beta-lactamic-allergic patients as well as in high methicillin-resistant *Staphylococcus aureus* incidence hospitals. The importance of short duration and proper timing of prophylaxis is well demonstrated. In primary and revision total hip and knee arthroplasty, the duration of the procedure is often unpredictable.

Our department is a high-volume arthroplasty unit with approximately 1,500 hip and knee prosthetic joint replacement procedures per year. We prospectively collected data on prosthetic joint infection from 2009 and observed an infection incidence of 0.68 % on that year. This rate increased to 1.19 % in 2010 using a 48-h prophylaxis with cefazolin in repeated rigid time scheduled shots of antibiotics.

In 2011 we decided to shorten the prophylaxis time to 24 h (as recommended by the most important recent international guidelines) starting 20–60 min before surgery (depending on the antibiotic class) and, at the same time, to introduce continuous intravenous antibiotic use. Specifically, we use cefazolin 2 g i.v. 20 min before surgical incision, followed by cefazolin 4 g in 250 cc normal saline over 24 h starting immediately after surgical incision (20 mL/h). In beta-lactamic-allergic patients we use vancomycin 1 g 60 min before surgical incision, followed by 2 g in 500 cc normal saline over 24 h (20 mL/h).

The idea of using continuous intravenous beta-lactams infusion arises from the time-dependent antimicrobial activity, which depends on the maintenance of antibiotic concentrations permanently above the minimal inhibiting concentration (MIC) of pathogens. To our knowledge, this is the first antibiotic continuous intravenous prophylaxis protocol described in the literature. In 2011, with the new prophylaxis, there was a significant decrease in infections to 0.39 % ($p=0.012$), and confirmed in 2012 with 0.38 % ($p=0.01$).

In the 36 infections analyzed out of 5,631 total arthroplasty procedures (primary and revision cases), 13 patients were affected by diabetes mellitus or increased fasting glucose (36.1 %), 11 patients were obese (30.5 %), 5 patients had autoimmune pre-existing conditions (13.9 %), 6 patients had previous neoplasm (16.7 %), 8 patients had cardiovascular diseases (22.2 %) (especially atrial fibrillation) and/or diffuse atherosclerosis, and 8 patients were active smokers (22.2 %). All of these comorbidities except obesity were significantly more frequent in infected patients compared to our controls.

In 31 cases the infection site was the hip and in the remaining 5 was the knee. The majority (72.2 %) of them were revisions (74.2 % of hips and 60 % of knees).

Considering the infected patients without predisposing risk factors, the majority had delayed infection. The involved bacteria were mainly not very aggressive microorganisms such as CoNS, and in two cases polymicrobic (one with *Enterococcus faecalis* and one with Corynebacterium spp), *Enterococcus faecalis* in one case, *Streptococcus agalactiae* in two cases, whereas MSSA caused two early and one delayed infection.

More aggressive bacteria, such as MRSA, *Enterococcus faecium* and Gram-negative bacteria are almost exclusively isolated in patients carrying one or more risk factors.

Our switch to the continuous infusion prophylaxis regimen found a number of possible topics which deserve further investigation. First, continuous antibiotic prophylaxis seems able to reduce CoNS and MRSA infections. Second, the new approach to antibiotic prophylaxis does not have any impact on costs.

Third, the orthopedic surgeon is able to minimize concern because the antibiotic concentration remains stable during surgery independent of the duration.

18.4 How to Manage Patients at Risk

First of all, we should be aware that the vast majority of the prosthetic joint infections are acquired in the operating room and/or during hospital stay. Thus, each patient is at risk of infection if physicians act with superficiality.

In any case, as described above, it is possible and necessary to identify more sensitive patients and therefore those more at risk of infection.

Before surgery:

- All overweight patients should be encouraged to lose weight
- Patients receiving immunosuppressive therapies must be advised to suspend them 2 weeks before surgery and not to resume until at least 2 weeks after surgery, with the exception of HIV positive subjects
- Good glycemic and blood pressure control must be achieved
- Smoking habits should be strongly discouraged
- Any possible ongoing source of infection at any level should be found and successfully treated
- The best possible liver and kidney metabolism should be achieved in patients with renal and hepatic function impairments
- In patients with infected prosthesis and one or more general risk factors, the correct preoperative bacterial identification (synovial fluid aspiration and culture, WBC and neutrophil count) is mandatory to start the correct antibiotic treatment immediately (any previous antibiotic therapy must be stopped at least 2 weeks before surgery)

During surgery:

- The best available antibiotic prophylaxis must be used, in terms of drug choice, dosage, proper timing, and correct duration
- The quickest possible surgery must be encouraged, with the best hemostasis control
- The least invasive anesthetic technique possible should be used
- In infected patients many samples in different tissues must be collected to improve the microbiological chance of correct bacterial identification (if available the removed prosthesis sonication could be useful)

After surgery:

- Good glycemic control must be maintained
- Good blood pressure level must be maintained to ensure heart and brain perfusion, as well as good surgical site blood supply
- Good liver and kidney perfusion must be maintained
- Good pain control must be achieved
- Strict control on blood tests must be stressed (hemoglobin level, white blood cells and platelet count, liver and kidney function, sodium, potassium, and calcium levels, coagulation parameters)

- Careful monitoring of vital signs (body temperature and arterial peripheral blood O_2 saturation, heart rate to identify eventual atrial fibrillation correctly) must be done
- Quick and correct diagnosis and treatment of any postoperative general complications must be kept in mind
- In infected patients a good cooperation with microbiologists and infectious disease specialists is a milestone for giving them the best available treatment in terms of best choice of the antibiotic type, dosage, interval between doses, route of administration, and duration of therapy
- In infected patients the type of follow-up in terms of blood test control, treatment, and clinical monitoring should be shared, informing them about possible side effects and the time needed for healing and reoperation

Key Points

- Prosthetic joint infections are rare but they are a devastating complication.
- Almost any microorganism may cause prosthetic joint infections.
- The management of infections is difficult and the outcome is frequently unsatisfactory because of the increasing number of highly virulent and antibiotic-resistant bacteria.
- The best available antibiotic prophylaxis must be used, in terms of drug choice, proper timing, and correct duration.
- We suggest, based on our experience, that continuous i.v. 24-h antibiotic prophylaxis should be considered.
- There are many host factors predisposing to prosthetic joint infections, most of which are known or at least predictable, and correctable or improvable.
- Human and environmental variables must be taken into account and improved as much as possible.
- Any possible ongoing source of infection must be found and treated before surgery.
- Good cooperation between hospitalist, orthopedic surgeon, microbiologists, and infectious disease specialist is very desirable to ensure the best available treatment and the best cure rate for the patients.
- Good clinical practice and good clinical experience makes the difference in overall outcome.

References

Atkins BL, Athanasou N, Deeks JJ, Crook DW, Simpson H, Peto TE, McLardy-Smith P, Berendt AR (1998) Prospective evaluation of criteria for microbiological diagnosis of prosthetic-joint infection at revision arthroplasty. The OSIRIS Collaborative Study Group. J Clin Microbiol 36(10):2932–2939

Cataldo MA, Petrosillo N, Cipriani M, Cauda R, Tacconelli E (2010) Prosthetic joint infection: recent developments in diagnosis and management. J Infect 61:443–448

Cierny G 3rd, DiPasquale D (2002) Periprosthetic total joint infections. Staging, treatment, and outcomes. Clin Orthop Relat Res 403:23–28

Cierny G 3rd, Mader JT, Penninck JJ (2003) A clinical staging system for adult osteomyelitis. Clin Orthop Relat Res 414:7–24

Costerton JW, Stewart PS, Greenberg EP (1999) Bacterial biofilms: a common cause of persistent infections. Science 284(5418):1318–1322

Coventry MB (1975) Treatment of infection occurring in total hip surgery. Orthop Clin North Am 6: 991–1003

Estes CS, Beauchamp CP, Clarke HD, Spangehl MJ (2010) A two-stage retention debridement protocol for acute periprosthetic joint infections. Clin Orthop Relat Res 468:2029–2038

Ghanem E, Azzam K, Seeley M, Joshi A, Parvizi J (2009) Staged revision for knee arthroplasty infection: what is the role of serologic tests before reimplantation? Clin Orthop Relat Res 467:1699–1705

Gould KF, Brindle R, Chadwick PR, Fraise AP, Hill S, Nathwani D, Ridgway GL, Spry MJ, Warren RE (2009) Guidelines (2008) for the prophylaxis and treatment of methicillin-resistant Staphylococcus aureus (MRSA) infections in the United Kingdom. J Antimicrob Chemother 63(5):849–861

Greidanus NV, Masri BA, Garbuz DS, Wilson SD, McAlinden MG, Xu M, Duncan CP (2007) Use of erythrocyte sedimentation rate and C-reactive protein level to diagnose infection before revision total knee arthroplasty. J Bone Joint Surg Am 89:1409–1416

Hidron AI, Edwards JR, Patel J et al (2008) NHSN annual update: antimicrobial-resistant pathogens associated with healthcare-associated infections: annual summary of data reported to the National Healthcare Safety Network at the Center for Disease Control and Prevention, 2006–2007. Infect Control Hosp Epidemiol 29(11):996–1011

Jafari SM, Coyle C, Mortazavi SM, Sharkey PF, Parvizi J (2010) Revision hip arthroplasty. Infection in the most common cause of failure. Clin Orthop Relat Res 468:2046–2051

Jamsen E, Varonen M, Huhtala H, Letho MU, Lumio J, Konttinen YT, Moilanen T (2010) Incidence of prosthetic joint infections after primary knee arthroplasty. J Arthroplasty 25:87–92

Kurd MF, Ghanem E, Steinbrecher J, Parvizi J (2010) Two-stage exchange knee arthroplasty: does resistance of the infected organism influence the outcome? Clin Orthop Relat Res 468:2060–2066

Laudermilch DJ, Fedorka CJ, Heyl A, Rao N, McGough RL (2010) Outcomes of revision of total knee arthroplasty after methicillin-resistant staphylococcus aureus infection. Clin Orthop Relat Res 468:2067–2073

McPherson EJ, Woodson C, Holtom P, Roidis N, Shufelt C, Patzakis M (2002) Periprosthetic total hip infection. Outcomes using a staging system. Clin Orthop Relat Res 403:8–15

Mittal Y, Fehring TK, Hanssen A, Marculescu C, Odum SM, Osmon D (2007) Two-stage reimplantation for periprosthetic knee infection involving resistant organisms. J Bone Joint Surg Am 89:1227–1231

Moran E, Byren I, Atkins BL (2010) The diagnosis and management of prosthetic joint infections. J Antimicrob Chemother 65(suppl 3):45–54

Mortazavi SM, Schwartzenberger J, Austin MS, Purtill JJ, Parvizi J (2010) Revision total knee arthroplasty infection. Incidence and predictors. Clin Orthop Relat Res 468:2052–2059

Peel TN, Buising KL, Choong PF (2011) Prosthetic joint infection: challenges of diagnosis and treatment. ANZ J Surg 81:32–39

Prokuski L (2008) Prophylactic antibiotics in orthopaedic surgery. J Am Acad Orthop Surg 16:283–293

Senneville E, Joulie D, Legout L et al (2009) Outcome and predictors of treatment failure in total hip/knee prosthetic joint infections due to Staphylococcus aureus. Clin Infect Dis 53(4):334–340

Shuman EK, Urquhart A, Malani PN (2012) Management and prevention of prosthetic joint infection. Infect Dis Clin North Am 26:29–39

Trampuz A, Widmer AF (2006) Infections associated with orthopedic implants. Curr Opin Infect Dis 19: 349–356

Trampuz A, Zimmerli W (2005) Prosthetic joint infections: update in diagnosis and treatment. Swiss Med Wkly 135:243–251

Trampuz A, Zimmerli W (2006a) Antimicrobial agents in orthopaedic surgery: prophylaxis and treatment. Drugs 66:1089–1105

Trampuz A, Zimmerli W (2006b) Diagnosis and treatment of infections associated with fracture-fixation devices. Injury 37(Suppl 2):59–66

Tsukayama DT, Estrada R, Gustilo RB (1996) Infection after total hip arthroplasty. A study of the treatment of one hundred and six infections. J Bone Joint Surg Am 78(4):512–523

Urquhart DM, Hanna FS, Brennan SL, Wluka AE, Leder K, Cameron PA, Graves SE, Cicuttini FM (2010) Incidence and risk factors for deep surgical site infection after primary total hip arthroplasty: a systematic review. J Arthroplasty 25:1216–1222

Zimmerli W, Trampuz A, Ochsner PE (2004) Prosthetic-joint infections. N Engl J Med 351:1645–1654

19 Prevention of Infection: The Wound Factors

Pouya Alijanipour and Javad Parvizi

Open Questions on Debated or Unanswered Issues

- What are the risk factors that can influence the normal process of surgical wound healing?
- What wound-related problems are serious and require early intervention?
- What evidence is available regarding surgery-related factors and details of perioperative management in relationship with surgical wound healing and complications?
- What are the best available strategies to approach wound-related complications such as dehiscence, hematoma, necrosis, or persistent drainage?

19.1 Introduction

In recent years and with the recognition of the importance of wound-related complications, more attention has been paid to surgical management of wound-related problems following total joint arthroplasty. The surgical wound, besides its importance to the patient as a reflection of what has occurred inside, plays an important role in eventual outcome of any surgical procedure. Wound-related problems can occur with a relative frequency. Most of these complications are usually minor and rarely require surgical intervention. However, serious problems of surgical wound can lead to catastrophic situations, which will influence adversely the final outcome of the surgery. Complications such as wound dehiscence, skin-edge necrosis, superficial infection, and delayed healing are associated with deep wound infection (Berbari et al. 1998) and increase the risk of periprosthetic joint infection (PJI) up to 4 times over 5 years after total knee replacement (Mortazavi et al. 2010). Furthermore, patient with successful treatment of superficial surgical wound infection should be closely followed up for any possibility of PJI in the future (Saleh et al. 2002).

Two models were proposed to explain the relationship between superficial surgical site infection (SSI) and PJI (Saleh et al. 2002). The first model suggests that there are common risk factors that predispose the patients to both superficial wound and deep periprosthetic joint infections. In the second model, the relationship between superficial SSI and PJI is causal in which superficial SSI creates a source of quiescent residual infection until an unknown factor triggers a process that finally leads to deep infection. While these models are not mutually opposing, both

P. Alijanipour • J. Parvizi (✉)
Department of Adult Reconstruction, Rothman Institute of Orthopaedics at Thomas Jefferson University, 925 Chestnut Street, Philadelphia, PA 19107, USA
e-mail: pouya@alijanipour.com; parvj@aol.com

A. Baldini, P. Caldora (eds.), *Perioperative Medical Management for Total Joint Arthroplasty: How to Control Hemostasis, Pain and Infection*, DOI 10.1007/978-3-319-07203-6_19,

emphasize the fact that any tactic that improves the process of wound healing and decreases the incidence of superficial SSI confers double benefit to the patients. The main focus in this chapter is on the factors that influence surgical wounds that are to heal by primary intention. Wounds that need to be closed by secondary intention should be considered in a different context.

19.2 Prevention of Surgical Wound Complications

Prevention, elimination, or mitigation of risk factors that can potentially influence the normal process of wound healing is probably the most efficient method for avoiding infection. These factors can be related to the host or to the surgical intervention. However, if any complication related to surgical wound occurred, an appropriate and timely management strategy would be of utmost importance for decreasing the risk of more serious complications particularly superficial and deep wound infection.

19.3 Patient Optimization

Many risk factors for PJI may have direct or indirect influence on the process of wound healing and local defense mechanisms against invading bacteria at the site of the surgical field. The preoperative evaluation is an opportunity to identify high-risk patients. Recognition and optimization of risk factors can considerably reduce risk of PJI and promote the possibility of optimal patient recovery after surgery.

19.3.1 Malnutrition

Poor nutritional status has been shown to delay wound healing through its negative influence on collagen and proteoglycan synthesis and subsequent wound remodeling (Greene et al. 1991). Malnutrition also interferes with immune system function. Malnutrition does not necessarily happen independently and can be associated with other comorbidities. It has been defined using several indices, the most common of which are serum albumin less that 3.5 g/dL, serum transferrin less than 200 mg/dL, and total lymphocyte count less than 1,500 per mm^3. These indices in general are good indicators of protein deficiency but do not indicate the state of calorie and vitamin deficiency that can potentially be present in patients who are to undergo total joint arthroplasty (Nawabi et al. 2010). An increased rate of surgical wound complications has been observed in patients with perioperative nutritional depletion. Adequate nutritional reserve can lessen the adverse effects of catabolic state following a major surgery such as total joint arthroplasty (Lavernia et al. 1999). Malnutrition has been associated with increased surgical and anesthesia time and longer postoperative in-hospital stay (Lavernia et al. 1999; Gherini et al. 1993; Marín et al. 2002). Moreover, malnutrition was reported as a risk factor for failure of irrigation and debridement in the setting of persistent wound drainage following total joint replacement (Jaberi et al. 2008).

19.3.2 Hyperglycemia and Diabetes

Hyperglycemia with or without diabetes mellitus is a recognized risk factor for suboptimal perioperative outcomes in nearly all surgical interventions, and improving glycemic levels has lowered the rate of perioperative complications (Umpierrez et al. 2012; Pomposelli et al. 1998). The link between hyperglycemia and the susceptibility to infection has been well established (Pozzilli and Leslie 1994). Uncontrolled glycemia impairs local innate immune system mechanisms through decreasing vascular permeability, oxygen delivery and redox reactions, neutrophil adherence, chemotaxis, phagocytosis, efficacy of antibodies, function of complement components, and intracellular bactericidal activity (Dronge et al. 2006). Furthermore, surgical wound healing is a concern among diabetic patients as hyperglycemia delays collagen synthesis, and rates between 1.2 and 12 % have been reported for surgical wound-related complications in diabetic patients undergoing TKA (England et al. 1990;

Papagelopoulos et al. 1996; Serna et al. 1994; Yang et al. 2001). Debates exist regarding the best indicator of controlled glycemia. Fasting glucose level more than 200 mg/dL (10 mmol/L) and hemoglobin A1C >7 % have been most commonly used, but the former is just a real-time indicator of glucose levels and with the latter has not been consistently shown to be of value in the identification of high-risk patients (Iorio et al. 2012; Adams et al. 2013).

19.3.3 Smoking

Smoking is a general risk factor for complications following elective total joint replacement. Coexistence of chronic obstructive pulmonary disease, atherosclerosis, and other systematic comorbidities confounds the relationship between smoking and postoperative complications. Evidence shows smoking intervenes with wound healing (Galat et al. 2009) probably through impeding collagen synthesis and maturation in subcutaneous tissue surrounding surgical wounds (Jorgensen et al. 1998). Adequate oxygen supply is essential for healing of surgical wound and local defense against microorganisms (Sørensen et al. 2009). Hypoxia negatively affects oxygen-dependent defense mechanisms in neutrophils (Hopf et al. 1997). Smoking can induce hypoxia through nicotine-induced release of catecholamines that leads to microvascular vasospasm and subcutaneous hypoperfusion. The same mechanism can cause platelet aggregation and formation of microthrombi. Moreover, inhaled carbon monoxide shifts the oxyhemoglobin dissociation curve to the left (via formation of carboxyhemoglobin) and significantly decreases oxygen delivery to the peripheral tissues. Interestingly, smoking cessation programs 6–8 weeks before elective hip or knee surgery have been effective in decreasing postoperative wound-related complications, especially infection (Thomsen et al. 2010; Møller et al. 2002). Although unfavorable influence of smoking on early postoperative complications seems to be evident, there are two long-term studies on smokers who underwent total hip or knee replacement in which no association between smoking and PJI was found (Dowsey and Choong 2009; Khan et al. 2009).

19.3.4 Alcohol Consumption

Frequent alcohol use may increase the risk for postoperative complications after arthroplasty (Harris et al. 2011), and excessive alcohol consumption was associated with SSI and other postoperative infectious complications in patients who underwent major noncardiac surgery (Bradley et al. 2011). Similar to smoking, it seems that many detrimental effects of alcohol consumption on the outcome of surgery happen during the perioperative period. However, the optimal period of cessation of alcohol consumption has not been defined yet, and at least 4 weeks of abstinence has been proposed for recovery of physiologic abnormalities that place patients at increased risk of postoperative complications (Tonnesen et al. 1999). Patients should be encouraged to decrease their level of alcohol consumption during preoperative evaluation. Alcohol-dependent patients should be counseled for consideration of cessation programs before undergoing their elective surgery.

19.3.5 Organ Insufficiency (Renal Disease, Liver Disease, and Immune System Dysfunction)

End-stage organ insufficiency can seriously influence postoperative recovery of patients following elective major surgery. Studies reported occurrence of significant morbidity and mortality, including infectious complications, in patients with end-stage kidney or liver disease (Hsieh et al. 2003; Sunday et al. 2002; Lieberman et al. 1995). On the other hand, the immune system can also be considered as an organ that has significant contribution to the outcome of surgery both locally at the level of surgical wound or systematically. Many situations that cause immune system dysfunction have been shown to impair surgical wound healing and increase the risk of surgical site infection. These include malignancy (Berbari et al. 1998), chronic inflammatory disorders such as rheumatoid arthritis (White et al. 1990), use of immunosuppressive medications (Wicke et al. 2000), and acquired immune deficiency syndrome (AIDS) (Luck et al. 1996). The abovementioned associations can happen through multiple complex pathophysiologic mechanisms. The presence of any organ failure can affect the function of other systems including repair mechanisms and local and systemic immune function. Nevertheless, they indicate the fact that maximum effort should be placed prior to the surgery to optimize patients with organ insufficiencies that per se do not contraindicate total joint replacement or anesthesia.

19.3.6 Obesity

Retrospective studies reported that body mass index (BMI) over 35 kg/m^2 increased the risk of infection up to 4 and 7 times following Total Hip Arthroplasty (THA) and Total Knee Arthroplasty (TKA), respectively (Namba et al. 2005). Obese patients are at increased risk of postoperative surgical wound complications. Poorly vascularized bulky subcutaneous fat tissue leads to lower oxygen tension in the peri-incisional zone, which is not favorable for wound healing (Hopf et al. 1997). Wound dehiscence can occur due to increased surface tension (Winiarsky et al. 1998; Guss and Bhattacharyya 2006). Moreover, due to extensive dissection required during surgery, prolonged wound drainage and formation of hematoma and seroma are more likely to occur (Patel et al. 2007). Also, local immune response in the surgical field may be diminished in obese patients because of metabolic derangement. Prolonged surgical time due to intraoperative technical challenges can also increase the risk of PJI independently. Weight reduction strategies including modification of diet and activity or even bariatric surgery along with correcting nutritional deficiencies should be considered as part of patient optimization (Parvizi et al. 2000). However, excessive weight loss in a short period of time may induce a catabolic state that is unfavorable for perioperative recovery.

19.3.7 Anticoagulation

Excessive anticoagulation can be an underlying factor for persistent surgical wound drainage, hematoma formation, and susceptibility for infection (Parvizi et al. 2007). Chronic anticoagulation was found to be an independent risk factor for mortality after total joint replacement in a case-control study in which 38 patients who were reoperated because of hematoma after THA or TKA were matched with 117 patients without hematoma formation (Mortazavi et al. 2013). Higher rates of clinically important hemorrhagic complications were reported among patients taking injectable forms of low molecular weight heparin compared to oral warfarin (Colwell et al. 1999; Fitzgerald et al. 2001). Low molecular weight heparin was reported to significantly prolong the time required for the surgical wound to become dry in comparison with a group of patients who received aspirin and mechanical foot compression and another group of patients who received warfarin. This difference existed until postoperative day 5 (Patel et al. 2007). Prophylactic warfarin was associated with greater likelihood of both superficial and deep surgical wound infections in one study comparing patients who received warfarin as preoperative thromboprophylaxis for total joint arthroplasty with those who did not receive any form of thromboprophylaxis (Sachs et al. 2003). In those patients who receive warfarin as anticoagulant, an international normalized ratio (INR) of 2–3 is usually the optimal range of anticoagulation. INR greater than 3 was significantly associated with wound-related complications (such as bleeding, hematoma formation, persistent drainage) as well as deep PJI in two studies (Minnema et al. 2004; Parvizi et al. 2007). However, the optimal level of anticoagulation should probably be individualized to diminish the likelihood of hemorrhagic, wound healing, and infectious complications.

19.3.8 Active Cutaneous Lesions

The condition of the skin at the site of surgical incision is undoubtedly of utmost importance.

Elective total joint replacement should not be performed in the presence of active cutaneous lesions such as psoriasis and eczema. Previous studies have reported increased risk of surgical site infection in patients with psoriasis or eczema (Menon and Wroblewski 1983; Stern et al. 1989).

19.4 Intraoperative Care

A considerable variety exists in the details of protocols that are routinely used in different institutions. Similarly, substantial heterogeneity is found in the available evidence. While it might be difficult, if not impossible, to make definite conclusions due to this diversity, in some instances, significant difference does not seem to exist among different methods or strategies that are already in common practice.

19.4.1 Preoperative Skin Cleansing with Antiseptic Solutions

Although preoperative whole-body showering and skin cleansing with chlorhexidine gluconate on the night prior to surgery has been recommended by Centers for Disease Control (CDC) (Mangram et al. 1999), strong evidence to prove the benefit of this strategy in the prevention of surgical site infection does not exist (Webster et al. 2012b; Johnson et al. 2010; Zywiel et al. 2011). Moreover, the available evidence does not clearly support the use of non-rinse skin decontamination with chlorhexidine gluconate to decolonize methicillin-resistant *S. aureus* (MRSA) (Karki and Cheng 2012). The methods for skin cleansing proposed in different studies vary considerably which makes it difficult to reach a conclusion for an evidence-based protocol. However, excessive preoperative washing is discouraged as it can cause skin irritation.

19.4.2 Skin Preparation

Different methods exist for preparation of the skin, and in the lack of a methodologically sound prospective investigation, it is impossible to recommend one solution over the other (Mangram et al. 1999). Both chlorhexidine gluconate and Betadine and other iodine-based antiseptics have been effective in the reduction of surgical site infection (Dumville et al. 2013), and literature is inconsistent in terms of one being better than the other (Darouiche et al. 2010; Swenson et al. 2009). Anyhow, alcohol should be considered as part of the antiseptic solution since it is an effective rapidly acting (yet of short duration) antiseptic solution. Hair removal should be performed only if the hair at the site of incision site interferes with the surgery (Mangram et al. 1999). If hair removal is necessary, it should be done in the hospital, yet out of the operating room and as close to the time of surgery as possible since early hair removal has been correlated with increased risk of infection (Alexander et al. 1983). Clippers are preferred because they have been more effective in randomized prospective studies in reducing surgical site infection compared to razors (Tanner et al. 2011).

19.4.3 Draping

There is wide variation in clinical practice for draping. The use of sticky U-drapes to isolate the perineum has been in practice for decades, but there is no evidence regarding their influence on and cost-efficiency for the prevention of SSI or PJI. Evidence regarding comparison of disposable or reusable drapes is only experimental, using models that do not resemble real-life conditions. Passage of bacteria through dry drapes does happen. However, it will be enhanced when wetted by normal saline or blood and diminished when wetted by antiseptic solutions. Moreover, other factors such as pressure, friction, and contact time with the contaminated material should also be taken into consideration (Blom et al. 2002; Laufman et al. 1979). Disposable drapes considerably decrease the load of passing bacteria and therefore resist better than woven drapes to bacterial penetration (Blom et al. 2000), but they are not completely impermeable (Blom et al. 2007). Two randomized trials compared the incidence of

SSI as their main outcome with use of reusable or disposable draping in elective abdominal surgery and coronary artery bypass graft surgery and did not find any significant difference (Bellchambers et al. 1999; Garibaldi et al. 1986).

Incise draping can be clear or impregnated with iodine-based antiseptic solutions. They are utilized on already prepped surgical sites to provide additional protection and address the concern about recolonization of the skin with the normal flora (Jacobson et al. 2005; Johnston et al. 1987). The use of incise drapes alone as a substitute for conventional skin preparation is not recommended since bactericidal action of iodine-containing incise drapes was inferior to conventional skin preparation solutions such as Betadine (Lewis et al. 1984). The use of non-impregnated drapes was questioned in a recent study for facilitating recolonization of skin flora in one study (Falk-Brynhildsen et al. 2013), in contrast to another similar older study that reported no multiplication or migration of bacteria beneath the plastic drape (French et al. 1976). While it has been shown that impregnated incise drapes decrease the recolonization rate of skin flora in clean and clean-contaminated surgeries measured by colony-forming units (Fairclough et al. 1986; Chiu et al. 1993), clinical studies of adequate size and quality are missing, leading to confusing conclusions on the prevention of SSI (Webster and Alghamdi 2013). Another important issue is the influence of method of skin preparation on drape adhesion. Separation of incise drapes from the skin has been associated with 6-fold increase in skin contamination (Alexander et al. 1985). A prospective RCT on patients with TJA confirmed that DuraPrep solution was associated with better drape adhesion than povidone-iodine scrub and paint. However, there was no difference in skin contamination between the two groups, although DuraPrep was associated with slightly lower rate of contamination (Jacobson et al. 2005).

19.4.3.1 Surgical Wound Management

Undermining of the skin should be avoided. Tissues should be handled gently during surgery and the procedure should be performed expeditiously.

19.4.3.2 Intraoperative Irrigation

Irrigation has the advantage of diluting and physically removing the contaminants and non-viable tissues from the surgical site (Bratzler et al. 2013). There are several different methods for irrigation including the type of solution, volume of irrigation delivering systems, and finally type of surgical procedure being done, with each being able to influence other factors, making definition of an ideal irrigation protocol difficult. As an example, increasing the volume of the irrigation solution removes more bacteria and particulate matter, but this effect plateaus depending on the delivery system (Niki et al. 2007). Furthermore, the conclusions of studies regarding irrigations in clean-contaminated gastrointestinal surgeries or interventions for open fractures are not totally expandable to a clean surgical field like arthroplasty. In one study in which pulsatile lavage with normal saline was used after cemented TKA, the authors collected all particles larger than 1 μm (most of bacteria) after each liter of irrigation and found that irrigation beyond four liters did not remove further particles (Niki et al. 2007). Generally irrigation with pressures below 15 psi (103.4 kPa) and over 35 psi (241.3 kPa) are considered low- and high-pressure lavage, respectively, although the definition of high- and low-pressure irrigation has not been standardized yet (Hassinger et al. 2005). An appropriate cutoff point for high-pressure lavage is yet to be defined, and interestingly studies suggest that even lavage pressures that were considered to be too low to have macroscopic influence may still have an effect on bone marrow mesenchymal cells and direct them to differentiate into adipocyte tissues, thus declining the content of osteoblasts in the marrow (Bhandari et al. 1999). High-pressure pulsatile lavage may have potential benefits of being time-saving and effective in removal of necrotic tissue and debris and offering better mechanical stability of cemented arthroplasty by allowing better cement penetration in cancellous bone tissue (Seeger et al. 2013; Kalteis et al. 2007). However, concerns exist regarding its mechanical damage to the tissues, propagation of bacteria into the deeper layers, and negative influence on healing and new bone formation (Hassinger et al. 2005; Polzin et al. 2006; Dirschl et al. 1998). Strong clinical evidence is lacking. However, a prospective RCT showed pulsatile lavage in comparison with normal lavage by syringe or jug was associated with a lower incidence of PJI after cemented hemiarthroplasty for hip fracture (3/164 versus 10/192 for pulsatile and syringe lavage groups, respectively) (Hargrove et al. 2006). In another study, the use of high-pressure pulsatile lavage during open debridement for the treatment of acute orthopedic implant infections (mainly TKA, THA, and hip hemiarthroplasty) was associated with a similar success rate compared with the conventional manual low-pressure lavage ($n = 79$) (Muñoz-Mahamud et al. 2011). High-pressure pulsatile lavage should perhaps be reserved for severely contaminated wounds. Low-pressure irrigation should probably be sufficient if contamination is minimal (Bhandari et al. 1999). Detergents such as castile soap or benzalkonium chloride are effective decontaminators because of their surface-active properties which act by disrupting hydrophobic and electrostatic forces and limit the ability of bacteria to bind to soft tissue and bone (Anglen et al. 2003). Weak evidence is available for the benefit of irrigation with diluted Betadine solution before closure of the surgical wound. However, no deleterious influence on wound healing or any other major adverse effects have been associated with their use. Concerns for its potential chondrocytotoxicity are only supported by experimental evidence. Lower concentrations (0.35–0.5 %) with a short time of lavage might avoid potential chondrocytotoxic effects in partial knee arthroplasty. Evidence regarding wound irrigation with antibiotic solutions mainly comes from non-orthopedic surgical specialties with clean-contaminated surgeries. Most of the RCTs found that adding antibiotics to irrigation solutions did not decrease the incidence of SSI significantly in comparison with irrigation with normal saline solution (Greig et al. 1987; Rambo 1972; Schein et al. 1990; Sherman et al. 1976) and their findings have also been supported by experimental studies (Conroy et al. 1999). Further high-level evidence with SSI or PJI as endpoints is required to evaluate the efficacy and potential adverse effects of local irrigation with antibiotic solutions on the surgical site.

19.4.4 Optimal Closure

Optimal closure consists of minimizing bacterial contamination and dead space while maximizing blood flow. One investigation measured blood flow on either sides of abdominal incisions of uninjured skin with different suturing techniques and found higher blood flow in wounds closed with subcuticular sutures (Zografos et al. 1992). However, there is no strong evidence demonstrating clear superiority of one method of closure over the others. Layered closure with monofilament suture is recommended consisting of separate closure of the fascia along with subcuticular closure. Topical skin adhesive can also be applied at the end of the closure. Most of the studies comparing methods of closure are underpowered, have used inadequate definitions for surgical site infection, and have not taken into consideration the host factors for wound healing. A meta-analysis comparing clinical outcomes of staples versus sutures in orthopedic surgery found a significantly higher risk of developing wound infection in the wounds closed with staples in comparison with sutures (17/350 versus 3/333 superficial or deep infections for staples and sutures, respectively). In this study, six small-sized RCTs were included, five of which were conducted on patients undergoing hip surgery, and unfortunately, their definition of superficial and deep infections was not distinguishable. Anyhow, it should be considered that staples can potentiate wound complications in the presence of necrotic tissue, hematoma, and dead space. Moreover, surgical wounds in arthroplasty particularly in TKA require a method of closure with adequate strength to overcome mechanical tension. Tissue adhesives such as (2-octyl or n-butyl-2 or OCA) have also been added to wounds closed with sutures. One trial including 90 patients with TKA found that patients with staple had longer hospital stay in comparison with sutures alone or sutures combined with OCA (Eggers et al. 2011). Another RCT in patients with TKA and THA found that although wound drainage was less in patients with OCT compared with staples or sutures alone, the use of OCT was associated with prolonged wound drainage in the TKA subgroup (Khan et al. 2006). A Cochrane meta-analysis regarding the effects of various tissue adhesives and conventional skin closure techniques (staples, sutures, and tapes) on the healing of surgical wounds concluded there is inadequate evidence to support or disprove the use of tissue adhesive for the purpose of obtaining better outcome in terms of dehiscence, satisfaction with cosmetic appearance, patients' and surgeons' general satisfaction, or infection (Coulthard et al. 2010).

Autologous blood-derived products such as platelet gel and fibrin sealant have recently been proposed for application at the end of surgery. However, there is not adequate evidence for making a confident conclusion regarding their effectiveness. Small-sized randomized clinical trials showed their use in TKA (Everts et al. 2006) and in THA (Lassen et al. 2006) was associated with lower incidence of wound leakage, wound healing disturbance, surgical site infection, and blood transfusion. One review included six trials that studied the use of fibrin sealants in orthopedic surgery (Carless et al. 2003) and found that the use of fibrin sealant was associated with a reduced postoperative blood loss on average around 223 mL per patient and reduced the risk of exposure to allogeneic red blood cell transfusion by 32 % without any influence on wound infection or hematoma formation.

19.4.5 Drains

There is no evidence to demonstrate that use of closed drains increases the risk of SSI/PJI following TJA. There is no conclusive evidence for the optimal timing of drain removal. Based on a Cochrane meta-analysis and systematic review encompassing various orthopedic procedures including total joint replacement, use of drains was not associated with any difference in hematoma formation or incidence of SSI. However, their use was associated with higher blood loss and transfusion rate (Parker et al. 2007). Most of the drainage of the surgical site occurs in the first 24 h after the surgery. Leaving drains for more prolonged time will be of no benefit and only increases the risk of bacterial colonization (Zamora-Navas et al. 1999) which can be a potential risk factor for surgical site infection (Felippe et al. 2007).

19.4.6 Optimal Dressing Characteristics

An ideal dressing is expected to have the following characteristics: it should be *permeable* since moist wound environment promotes healing. Nevertheless, excessive moisture predisposes wounds to maceration and blister formation; it should provide an adequate *physical barrier* to prevent microbial ingress into the wound. It should also be waterproof from outside to allow showering early after the surgery; it should be *occlusive* because hypoxic environment accelerates angiogenesis and promotes repair and non-occlusive dressings would not be able to maintain such an environment for wound healing; it should also be *nonadherent to the wound bed* for patient's comfort and ease of removal so it can eliminate the need for analgesics during dressing change. Moreover, an optimal dressing should be adequately *thick* in order to decrease the need for frequent changes and risk of exposure of the wound. Finally, the design of the dressing should be *simple* enough for the ease of family members or caretakers.

19.4.7 Modern Dressings Versus Traditional Gauze Dressings

Hydrofiber dressing (such as Aquacel) absorbs the exudate and swell. A fibrin layer is formed between the dressing and the wound, acting as an extra physical barrier for the surgical wound. Based on a rat model, it seems that hydrofiber dressings provide a selective barrier for inflammatory cells (Hoekstra et al. 2002). Polymorphonuclear (PMN) cells that are mainly responsible for defense could infiltrate hydrofiber dressing and remain active even when they were captured, resulting in a reduced number of PMN cells in the wounds in comparison with traditional dressings (adhesive dressing with an integral absorbent pad). However, although macrophages (which have a more reparative role) infiltrated in the wound bed, they could not be found in the dressing. Two prospective studies including one randomized clinical trial (Burke et al. 2012) and a prospective clinical audit (Clarke et al. 2009) showed that occlusive dressings secured with hydrocolloid have a lower incidence of blister formation, leakage, dressing changes, delayed discharge, and SSI rate while providing longer wear time in comparison to traditional gauze dressings. A trend for shorter hospital stay was also reported for hydrocolloid occlusive dressings. The addition of silver has been suggested to better control the infection and promote wound healing mainly in diabetic ulcers, venous insufficiency ulcers, and other contaminated types of wounds including complicated surgical wounds, but its role in noncomplicated surgical wounds that are to be healed by primary intention is less clear.

19.5 Postoperative Care of Surgical Wound

19.5.1 Frequency of Dressing Change

Frequent changing of dressing exposes the wound to exogenous bacteria and is a risk factor for surgical site infection. Mitotic cell division and leukocyte activity are critical for wound healing and increase with the use of occlusive dressing. After dressing changes, it takes 3–4 h for these activities to resume. With increasing risk of nosocomial infection (particularly MRSA infection), uncomplicated wounds may be better served with limited wound exposure in high-risk environments such as hospitals, rehabilitation facilities, and skilled nursing facilities. We recommend the first dressing be changed at 7 days after surgery, and during this time, the wound should not be exposed to the environment. Moreover, pain and discomfort associated with dressing change can be avoided. The patient can shower immediately after surgery with modern occlusive dressings, and unless strikethrough happened, dressing change would not be required. The importance of patient education should also be considered. This is especially important in patients undergoing TKA, whose dressings are continuously under their vision. Patients may become concerned and assume the dressing should be changed just because it appears to be soaked.

19.6 Wound-Related Complications

19.6.1 Hematoma

Several factors can contribute to hematoma formation including inadequate hemostasis during surgery, underlying coagulopathy, and administration of anticoagulants. Hematomas usually resorb without any associated adverse event (Fitzgerald et al. 2001), but when large enough, they should be considered as serious complication which can lead to surgical wound problems such as skin necrosis and persistent wound drainage (Stern et al. 2000). Furthermore, they can limit the access of antibiotics to surgical field. A study reported that hematoma, despite adequate treatment, was an independent risk factor for adverse outcomes and increasing morbidity and mortality (Mortazavi et al. 2013). The same study defined perioperative anticoagulation, blood loss, administration of fresh frozen plasma and vitamin K, and hormonal therapy as independent predictors for hematoma formation. Other investigations showed it increases the risk of PJI with 2-year cumulative probability of 10.8 % in comparison with 0.8 % in patients without hematomas requiring surgery (Galat et al. 2008). The surgeon should have low threshold for irrigation and debridement if hematoma is large, active, and associated with drainage.

19.6.2 Persistent Drainage of Surgical Wound

Persistent postoperative wound drainage has been shown to be associated with deep infection after total joint arthroplasty (Saleh et al. 2002; Parvizi et al. 2007). It has been reported that if the surgical wound continues to drain more than 5–7 days, it is 12.5 times more likely to develop infection (Saleh et al. 2002). A retrospective study found that with every additional day of prolonged drainage, the probability for infection is substantially increased by 42 % in hips and 29 % in knees (Patel et al. 2007). As the surgical wound continues to drain, the hospital stay is also extended which is another risk factor for nosocomial infections and overall adverse outcome (Dennis 1997; Patel et al. 2007). A clear definition for persistent postoperative wound drainage does not exist, and different definitions in terms of volume of the drainage exudate and its duration have been described. Expressions such as "discharge from the wound", "strikethrough of dressing of the surgical wound" (Jaberi et al. 2008), and "area of soaking the covering dressing greater than of 2×2 cm^{2}" (Patel et al. 2007) have been utilized to describe the warning limit for the volume of surgical wound drainage. A duration of 48 hr (Saleh et al. 2002) up to 1 week (Dennis 1997). However, continuous drainage for more than 72 h seems to be a reasonable and practical definition as it allows for early intervention to limit adverse consequences. Risk factors associated with prolonged wound drainage are numerous. Higher volume of drain output is an independent factor (Patel et al. 2007). Conditions that intervene with wound healing (i.e., diabetes mellitus, rheumatoid arthritis, malnutrition, immune-modifying medications, smoking, advanced age, and obesity) can potentially predispose the patients to worrisome wound drainage (Galat et al. 2009). Postoperative antithrombotic prophylaxis with low molecular weight heparin has been associated with longer drainage in comparison with aspirin and warfarin (Patel et al. 2007).

Swab sampling is not recommended. It is an inexpensive and easy-to-use method but has high risk of contamination (false positives). Moreover, microorganism growth inhibition, poor specimen volume, and bacterial adherence can occur with swab sampling and result in false-negative results.

If persistent drainage happens, observation is not an appropriate strategy. As stated before, lengthier drainage is associated with higher risk of PJI. Blind use of antibiotics should be avoided because they can mask the symptoms and signs of an underlying infection. Moreover, they may reduce the chance of isolation of the causative bacteria via microbiologic culture of synovial fluid samples.

19.6.3 Negative-Pressure Wound Therapy (NPWT)

Although high-quality and adequately powered evidence regarding NPWT is still lacking, there is no evidence for the effectiveness of NPWT on the complete healing of wounds that are expected to heal by primary intention (Webster et al. 2012a). A prospective RCT has shown that NPWT decreases the size of seroma when used for patients with large surgical wounds after THA (Pachowsky et al. 2012). Another retrospective study on patients who received NPWT due to persistent wound drainage after THA reported 76 % of patients required no further intervention (Hansen et al. 2013). The same study also found that international normalized ratio level greater than 2, greater than one prior to hip surgery, and device application greater than 48 h were risk factors for failure of NPWT application. It seems that NPWT can be a reasonable option for patients at high risk for postoperative drainage such as obese patients with large incisions or wounds of revision surgery. We usually use 75–100 mmHg of suction pressure on continuous mode for 48 h.

Cutoff point for the best time for surgical intervention is difficult to define, particularly because various factors should be taken into consideration to indicate surgery. Patient-related factors are general health status, the underlying comorbid conditions (especially malnutrition), and patient's preference. Other factors to be considered are amount of blood loss and anticoagulation status of the patient. If persistent drainage seems to be more concerning, lower threshold for performing irrigation and debridement is recommended and it has been suggested to be treated as infection (Vince and Abdeen 2006). Early surgical intervention at 5–7 days after the index arthroplasty has been demonstrated to have better outcome than later surgery (Jaberi et al. 2008; Saleh et al. 2002). Adequate samples for microbiologic culture should be taken. If complete closure of the wound is not possible, NPWT can be utilized during immediate postoperative period followed by later plastic surgery intervention for definitive closure of the wound. According to a registry-based study of TKA patients, patients who undergo early surgical intervention due to wound complication of their index arthroplasty procedure have 6 % chance for developing deep infection and 5.3 % chance for undergoing another major surgery (component removal, plastic surgery for wound coverage, or amputation) within 2 years (Galat et al. 2009).

Our recommendation in the situation of persistent wound drainage consists of maintaining range of motion exercises (particularly in TKA), application of compressive wrap if no signs or symptoms of infection exist, and local wound care. If available, NPWT can also be considered. Anyhow, the threshold for reoperation of a continuously draining wound should be low, and if the drainage persists for more than 5 days, the patient should be taken to the OR for surgical inspection of the wound. The procedure should include opening the fascia, taking adequate samples for microbiologic culture, irrigation and debridement, exchange of modular components, and meticulous closure. Parenteral prophylactic antibiotics should be administered as usual. However, they should be extended for 6 weeks if there is adequate evidence for infection. NPWR can be considered if adequate closure is impossible with considering further surgery of skin coverage when drainage is controlled and infection is excluded or controlled. Early intervention was shown to be successful in 76 % of the cases, though in 24 % patients required further surgical interventions (Jaberi et al. 2008). Moreover, irrigation and debridement with polyethylene exchange has considerably high failure rate in acute PJI, with one study reporting failure in 57 % of cases in which further surgeries or lifelong suppressive antibiotic therapy was required (Gardner et al. 2011).

19.6.4 Skin Blistering

Blistering can be attributed to movement between the skin and dressing over time. Its formation depends on the dressing type and technique and soft tissue edema. Some patients may be more susceptible to blister formation due to underlying dermatological, vascular, or allergic disorders. Although blister exudate is sterile, it can rapidly become contaminated with skin flora after rupture (Varela et al. 1993). Blisters precipitate the breakdown of the epithelial barrier layer of the skin and increase the risk of developing local infection. Also, blisters are a source of discomfort for the patients and may require dressing changes, extra nursing care, and sometimes prolonged hospital stay (Abuzakuk et al. 2006). Small blisters (less than 5 mm) should be observed. Adequate protection might be the only strategy required for small blisters. Larger blisters should be drained in a sterile fashion, but it is recommended to leave the blister roof intact to function as barrier. After draining, the skin should be cleansed using an antibacterial solution and hydrocolloid dressing, or antibacterial ointment should be applied to cover the skin particularly if the blister has become unroofed (Knapik et al. 1995). There is no evidence to support the use of systemic antibiotic for apparently uninfected blisters. If the blister fluid seems to be purulent or surrounding cellulitis exists, the blister should be unroofed and drained completely and then cleansed with an antibacterial solution followed by a short course of systemic antibiotics with frequent examination of the skin (Brennan 2002).

19.6.5 Skin Necrosis

Superficial soft tissue necrosis requires debridement. If less than 3 cm, consider local care versus delayed closure; if more than 3 cm, soft tissue coverage is required which can be split thickness skin grafts or fascio-cutaneous flaps. For full-thickness necrosis, immediate debridement should be performed. Unfortunately, secondary closure often fails and vascular tissue transfer should be considered to cover the defect.

Key Points

- Patients should be optimized prior to total joint arthroplasty to minimize the risk of postoperative complications and improve the final outcome.
- Recognition and treatment of potential risk factors for surgical wound complications is of utmost importance. However, debates regarding the definition of some of these risk factors and their most efficient management strategies still exist.
- A number of perioperative details can influence wound healing. While debate exists regarding which strategy is most efficient, surgeons should adapt their routine care based on the most updated evidence and available resources.
- Surgical wound-related complications should not be underestimated, and the surgeon should adopt a reasonable evidence-based approach in case of their occurrence. More evidence is required to develop a balanced strategy to avoid excessively aggressive or negligent attitude.

References

Abuzakuk TM et al (2006) The management of wounds following primary lower limb arthroplasty: a prospective, randomised study comparing hydrofibre and central pad dressings. Int Wound J 3(2):133–137

Adams AL et al (2013) Surgical outcomes of total knee replacement according to diabetes status and glycemic control. J bone Joint Surg Am 95(6):481–487

Alexander JW et al (1983) The influence of hair-removal methods on wound infections. Arch Surg (Chicago, Ill: 1960) 118(3):347–352

Alexander JW, Aerni S, Plettner JP (1985) Development of a safe and effective one-minute preoperative skin preparation. Arch Surg (Chicago, Ill: 1960) 120(12): 1357–1361

Anglen JO et al (2003) The use of detergent irrigation for musculoskeletal wounds. Int Orthop 27(1):40–46

Bellchambers J et al (1999) A prospective study of wound infection in coronary artery surgery. Eur J Cardiothoracic Surg 15(1):45–50

Berbari EF et al (1998) Risk factors for prosthetic joint infection: case-control study. Clin Infect Dis 27(5): 1247–1254

Bhandari M et al (1999) High and low pressure pulsatile lavage of contaminated tibial fractures: an in vitro study of bacterial adherence and bone damage. J Orthop Trauma 13(8):526–533

Blom A et al (2000) The passage of bacteria through surgical drapes. Ann R Coll Surg Engl 82(6):405–407

Blom AW et al (2002) Bacterial strike-through of re-usable surgical drapes: the effect of different wetting agents. J Hosp Infect 52(1):52–55

Blom AW et al (2007) Resistance of disposable drapes to bacterial penetration. J Orthop Surg (Hong Kong) 15(3):267–269

Bradley KA et al (2011) Alcohol screening and risk of postoperative complications in male VA patients undergoing major non-cardiac surgery. J Gen Intern Med 26(2):162–169

Bratzler DW et al (2013) Clinical practice guidelines for antimicrobial prophylaxis in surgery. Am J Health Syst Pharm 70(3):195–283

Brennan FH Jr (2002) Managing blisters in competitive athletes. Curr Sports Med Rep 1(6):319–322

Burke NG et al (2012) A prospective randomised study comparing the jubilee dressing method to a standard adhesive dressing for total hip and knee replacements. J Tissue Viability 21(3):84–87

Carless PA, Henry DA, Anthony DM (2003) Fibrin sealant use for minimising peri-operative allogeneic blood transfusion. Cochrane Database Syst Rev (Online) (2):CD004171

Chiu KY et al (1993) Plastic adhesive drapes and wound infection after hip fracture surgery. Aust N Z J Surg 63(10):798–801

Clarke JV et al (2009) A prospective clinical audit of a new dressing design for lower limb arthroplasty wounds. J Wound Care 18(1):5–8, 10–11

Colwell CW Jr et al (1999) Comparison of enoxaparin and warfarin for the prevention of venous thromboembolic disease after total hip arthroplasty. Evaluation during hospitalization and three months after discharge. J Bone Joint Surg Am 81(7): 932–940

Conroy BP et al (1999) Comparison of castile soap, benzalkonium chloride, and bacitracin as irrigation solutions for complex contaminated orthopaedic wounds. J Orthop Trauma 13(5):332–337

Coulthard P et al (2010) Tissue adhesives for closure of surgical incisions. Cochrane Database Syst Rev (Online) (5):CD004287

Darouiche RO et al (2010) Chlorhexidine-alcohol versus povidone-iodine for surgical-site antisepsis. N Engl J Med 362(1):18–26

Dennis DA (1997) Wound complications in total knee arthroplasty. Instr Course Lect 46:165–169

Dirschl DR et al (1998) High pressure pulsatile lavage irrigation of intraarticular fractures: effects on fracture healing. J Orthop Trauma 12(7):460–463

Dowsey MM, Choong PFM (2009) Obese diabetic patients are at substantial risk for deep infection after primary TKA. Clin Orthop Relat Res 467(6): 1577–1581

Dronge AS et al (2006) Long-term glycemic control and postoperative infectious complications. Arch Surg (Chicago, Ill: 1960) 141(4):375–380; discussion 380

Dumville JC et al (2013) Preoperative skin antiseptics for preventing surgical wound infections after clean surgery. Cochrane Database Syst Rev (3):CD003949

Eggers MD, Fang L, Lionberger DR (2011) A comparison of wound closure techniques for total knee arthroplasty. J Arthroplasty 26(8):1251–1258.e1–4

England SP et al (1990) Total knee arthroplasty in diabetes mellitus. Clin Orthop Relat Res 260:130–134

Everts PM et al (2006) Platelet gel and fibrin sealant reduce allogeneic blood transfusions in total knee arthroplasty. Acta Anaesthesiol Scand 50(5):593–599

Fairclough JA, Johnson D, Mackie I (1986) The prevention of wound contamination by skin organisms by the pre-operative application of an iodophor impregnated plastic adhesive drape. J Int Med Res 14(2): 105–109

Falk-Brynhildsen K et al (2013) Bacterial colonization of the skin following aseptic preoperative preparation and impact of the use of plastic adhesive drapes. Biol Res Nurs 15(2):242–248

Felippe WAB, Werneck GL, Santoro-Lopes G (2007) Surgical site infection among women discharged with a drain in situ after breast cancer surgery. World J Surg 31(12):2293–2299; discussion 2300–2301

Fitzgerald RH et al (2001) Prevention of venous thromboembolic disease following primary total knee arthroplasty. A randomized, multicenter, open-label, parallel-group comparison of enoxaparin and warfarin. J Bone Joint Surg Am 83-A(6):900–906

French ML, Eitzen HE, Ritter MA (1976) The plastic surgical adhesive drape: an evaluation of its efficacy as a microbial barrier. Ann Surg 184(1):46–50

Galat DD et al (2008) Early return to surgery for evacuation of a postoperative hematoma after primary total knee arthroplasty. J Bone Joint Surg Am 90(11): 2331–2336

Galat DD et al (2009) Surgical treatment of early wound complications following primary total knee arthroplasty. J Bone Joint Surg Am 91(1):48–54

Gardner J, Gioe TJ, Tatman P (2011) Can this prosthesis be saved?: implant salvage attempts in infected primary TKA. Clin Orthop Relat Res 469(4):970–976

Garibaldi RA et al (1986) Comparison of nonwoven and woven gown and drape fabric to prevent intraoperative wound contamination and postoperative infection. Am J Surg 152(5):505–509

Gherini S et al (1993) Delayed wound healing and nutritional deficiencies after total hip arthroplasty. Clin Orthop Relat Res 293:188–195

Greene KA, Wilde AH, Stulberg BN (1991) Preoperative nutritional status of total joint patients. Relationship to postoperative wound complications. J Arthroplasty 6(4):321–325

Greig J et al (1987) Wound sepsis after colorectal surgery: the effect of cefotetan lavage. Chemioter Int J Mediterr Soc Chemother 6(2 Suppl):595–596

Guss D, Bhattacharyya T (2006) Perioperative management of the obese orthopaedic patient. J Am Acad Orthop Surg 14(7):425–432

Hansen E et al (2013) Negative pressure wound therapy is associated with resolution of incisional drainage in most wounds after hip arthroplasty. Clin Orthop Relat Res 471(10):3230–3236

Hargrove R et al (2006) Does pulse lavage reduce hip hemiarthroplasty infection rates? J Hosp Infect 62(4):446–449

Harris AHS et al (2011) Preoperative alcohol screening scores: association with complications in men undergoing total joint arthroplasty. J Bone Joint Surg Am 93(4):321–327

Hassinger SM, Harding G, Wongworawat MD (2005) High-pressure pulsatile lavage propagates bacteria into soft tissue. Clin Orthop Relat Res 439:27–31

Hoekstra MJ et al (2002) A histological comparison of acute inflammatory responses with a hydrofibre or tulle gauze dressing. J Wound Care 11(3):113–117

Hopf HW et al (1997) Wound tissue oxygen tension predicts the risk of wound infection in surgical patients. Arch Surg (Chicago, Ill: 1960) 132(9):997–1004; discussion 1005

Hsieh PH et al (2003) Hip arthroplasty in patients with cirrhosis of the liver. J Bone Joint Surg Br 85(6): 818–821

Iorio R et al (2012) Diabetes mellitus, hemoglobin A1C, and the incidence of total joint arthroplasty infection. J Arthroplasty 27(5):726–729.e1

Jaberi FM et al (2008) Procrastination of wound drainage and malnutrition affect the outcome of joint arthroplasty. Clin Orthop Relat Res 466(6):1368–1371

Jacobson C et al (2005) Prevention of wound contamination using DuraPrep solution plus Ioban 2 drapes. Clin Orthop Relat Res 439:32–37

Johnson AJ et al (2010) Preoperative chlorhexidine preparation and the incidence of surgical site infections after hip arthroplasty. J Arthroplasty 25(6 Suppl):98–102

Johnston DH et al (1987) Rate of bacterial recolonization of the skin after preparation: four methods compared. Br J Surg 74(1):64

Jorgensen LN et al (1998) Less collagen production in smokers. Surgery 123(4):450–455

Kalteis T et al (2007) An experimental comparison of different devices for pulsatile high-pressure lavage and

their relevance to cement intrusion into cancellous bone. Arch Orthop Trauma Surg 127(10):873–877
Karki S, Cheng AC (2012) Impact of non-rinse skin cleansing with chlorhexidine gluconate on prevention of healthcare-associated infections and colonization with multi-resistant organisms: a systematic review. J Hosp Infect 82(2):71–84
Khan LAK et al (2009) The complication rate and medium-term functional outcome after total hip replacement in smokers. Hip Int J Clin Exp Res Hip Pathol Ther 19(1):47–51
Khan RJK et al (2006) A comparison of three methods of wound closure following arthroplasty: a prospective, randomised, controlled trial. J Bone Joint Surg 88(2):238–242
Knapik JJ et al (1995) Friction blisters. Pathophysiology, prevention and treatment. Sports Med (Auckland, NZ) 20(3):136–147
Lassen MR et al (2006) A pilot study of the effects of Vivostat patient-derived fibrin sealant in reducing blood loss in primary hip arthroplasty. Clin Appl Thromb Hemost 12(3):352–357
Laufman H, Siegal JD, Edberg SC (1979) Moist bacterial strike-through of surgical materials: confirmatory tests. Ann Surg 189(1):68
Lavernia CJ, Sierra RJ, Baerga L (1999) Nutritional parameters and short term outcome in arthroplasty. J Am Coll Nutr 18(3):274–278
Lewis DA, Leaper DJ, Speller DC (1984) Prevention of bacterial colonization of wounds at operation: comparison of iodine-impregnated ('Ioban') drapes with conventional methods. J Hosp Infect 5(4):431–437
Lieberman JR et al (1995) Hip arthroplasty in patients with chronic renal failure. J Arthroplasty 10(2):191–195
Luck JV et al (1996) Human immunodeficiency virus infection: complications and outcome of orthopaedic surgery. J Am Acad Orthop Surg 4(6):297–304
Mangram AJ et al (1999) Guideline for prevention of surgical site infection, Hospital Infection Control Practices Advisory Committee. Infect Control Hosp Epidemiol 20(4):250–278; quiz 279–280
Marín LA et al (2002) Preoperative nutritional evaluation as a prognostic tool for wound healing. Acta Orthop Scand 73(1):2–5
Menon TJ, Wroblewski BM (1983) Charnley low-friction arthroplasty in patients with psoriasis. Clin Orthop Relat Res 176:127–128
Minnema B et al (2004) Risk factors for surgical-site infection following primary total knee arthroplasty. Infect Control Hosp Epidemiol 25(6):477–480
Møller AM et al (2002) Effect of preoperative smoking intervention on postoperative complications: a randomised clinical trial. Lancet 359(9301):114–117
Mortazavi SMJ et al (2013) Hematoma following primary total hip arthroplasty: a grave complication. J Arthroplasty 28(3):498–503
Mortazavi SMJ et al (2010) Revision total knee arthroplasty infection: incidence and predictors. Clin Orthop Relat Res 468(8):2052–2059
Muñoz-Mahamud E et al (2011) Comparison of a low-pressure and a high-pressure pulsatile lavage during débridement for orthopaedic implant infection. Arch Orthop Trauma Surg 131(9):1233–1238
Namba RS et al (2005) Obesity and perioperative morbidity in total hip and total knee arthroplasty patients. J Arthroplasty 20(Supplement 3):46–50
Nawabi DH et al (2010) Vitamin D deficiency in patients with osteoarthritis undergoing total hip replacement: a cause for concern? J Bone Joint Surg Br 92(4):496–499
Niki Y et al (2007) How much sterile saline should be used for efficient lavage during total knee arthroplasty? Effects of pulse lavage irrigation on removal of bone and cement debris. J Arthroplasty 22(1):95–99
Pachowsky M et al (2012) Negative pressure wound therapy to prevent seromas and treat surgical incisions after total hip arthroplasty. Int Orthop 36(4):719–722
Papagelopoulos PJ et al (1996) Long term outcome and survivorship analysis of primary total knee arthroplasty in patients with diabetes mellitus. Clin Orthop Relat Res 330:124–132
Parker MJ et al (2007) Closed suction surgical wound drainage after orthopaedic surgery. Cochrane Database Syst Rev (3):CD001825
Parvizi J et al (2007) Does "excessive" anticoagulation predispose to periprosthetic infection? J Arthroplasty 22(6 Suppl 2):24–28
Parvizi J, Trousdale RT, Sarr MG (2000) Total joint arthroplasty in patients surgically treated for morbid obesity. J Arthroplasty 15(8):1003–1008
Patel VP et al (2007) Factors associated with prolonged wound drainage after primary total hip and knee arthroplasty. J Bone Joint Surg Am 89(1):33–38
Polzin B, Ellis T, Dirschl DR (2006) Effects of varying pulsatile lavage pressure on cancellous bone structure and fracture healing. J Orthop Trauma 20(4):261–266
Pomposelli JJ et al (1998) Early postoperative glucose control predicts nosocomial infection rate in diabetic patients. JPEN J Parenter Enteral Nutr 22(2):77–81
Pozzilli P, Leslie RD (1994) Infections and diabetes: mechanisms and prospects for prevention. Diabet Medicine 11(10):935–941
Rambo WM (1972) Irrigation of the peritoneal cavity with cephalothin. Am J Surg 123(2):192–195
Sachs RA et al (2003) Does anticoagulation do more harm than good?: a comparison of patients treated without prophylaxis and patients treated with low-dose warfarin after total knee arthroplasty. J Arthroplasty 18(4):389–395
Saleh K et al (2002) Predictors of wound infection in hip and knee joint replacement: results from a 20 year surveillance program. J Orthop Res 20(3):506–515
Schein M et al (1990) Peritoneal lavage in abdominal sepsis. A controlled clinical study. Arch Surg (Chicago, Ill: 1960) 125(9):1132–1135
Seeger JB et al (2013) The effect of bone lavage on femoral cement penetration and interface temperature during Oxford unicompartmental knee arthroplasty with cement. J Bone Joint Surg 95(1):48–53

Serna F et al (1994) Total knee arthroplasty in diabetic patients. Comparison to a matched control group. J Arthroplasty 9(4):375–379

Sherman JO, Luck SR, Borger JA (1976) Irrigation of the peritoneal cavity for appendicitis in children: a double-blind study. J Pediatr Surg 11(3):371–374

Sørensen LT et al (2009) Acute effects of nicotine and smoking on blood flow, tissue oxygen, and aerobe metabolism of the skin and subcutis. J Surg Res 152(2):224–230

Stern SH et al (1989) Total knee arthroplasty in patients with psoriasis. Clin Orthop Relat Res 248:108–110; discussion 111

Stern SH, Wixson RL, O'Connor D (2000) Evaluation of the safety and efficacy of enoxaparin and warfarin for prevention of deep vein thrombosis after total knee arthroplasty. J Arthroplasty 15(2):153–158

Sunday JM, Guille JT, Torg JS (2002) Complications of joint arthroplasty in patients with end-stage renal disease on hemodialysis. Clin Orthop Relat Res 397:350–355

Swenson BR et al (2009) Effects of preoperative skin preparation on postoperative wound infection rates: a prospective study of 3 skin preparation protocols. Infect Control Hosp Epidemiol 30(10):964–971

Tanner J, Norrie P, Melen K (2011) Preoperative hair removal to reduce surgical site infection. Cochrane Database Syst Rev (11):CD004122

Thomsen T, Villebro N, Møller AM (2010) Interventions for preoperative smoking cessation. Cochrane Database Syst Rev (Online) (7):CD002294

Tonnesen H et al (1999) Effect of preoperative abstinence on poor postoperative outcome in alcohol misusers: randomised controlled trial. BMJ (Clinical research ed) 318(7194):1311–1316

Umpierrez GE et al (2012) Management of hyperglycemia in hospitalized patients in non-critical care setting: an endocrine society clinical practice guideline. J Clin Endocrinol Metab 97(1):16–38

Varela CD et al (1993) Fracture blisters: clinical and pathological aspects. J Orthop Trauma 7(5):417–427

Vince KG, Abdeen A (2006) Wound problems in total knee arthroplasty. Clin Orthop Relat Res 452:88–90

Webster J et al (2012) Negative pressure wound therapy for skin grafts and surgical wounds healing by primary intention. Cochrane Database Syst Rev (4):CD009261

Webster J et al (2012b) Preoperative bathing or showering with skin antiseptics to prevent surgical site infection. In: The Cochrane library. Wiley. Available at: http://onlinelibrary.wiley.com/doi/10.1002/14651858.CD004985.pub3/abstract. Accessed 12 March 2012

Webster J, Alghamdi A (2013) Use of plastic adhesive drapes during surgery for preventing surgical site infection. Cochrane Database Syst Rev (Online) (1):CD006353

White RH, McCurdy SA, Marder RA (1990) Early morbidity after total hip replacement: rheumatoid arthritis versus osteoarthritis. J Gen Intern Med 5(4):304–309

Wicke C et al (2000) Effects of steroids and retinoids on wound healing. Arch Surg (Chicago, Ill: 1960) 135(11):1265–1270

Winiarsky R, Barth P, Lotke P (1998) Total knee arthroplasty in morbidly obese patients. J Bone Joint Surg Am 80(12):1770–1774

Yang K et al (2001) Total knee arthroplasty in diabetic patients: a study of 109 consecutive cases. J Arthroplasty 16(1):102–106

Zamora-Navas P, Collado-Torres F, de la Torre-Solís F (1999) Closed suction drainage after knee arthroplasty. A prospective study of the effectiveness of the operation and of bacterial contamination. Acta Orthop Belg 65(1):44–47

Zografos GC, Martis K, Morris DL (1992) Laser Doppler flowmetry in evaluation of cutaneous wound blood flow using various suturing techniques. Ann Surg 215(3):266–268

Zywiel MG et al (2011) Advance pre-operative chlorhexidine reduces the incidence of surgical site infections in knee arthroplasty. Int Orthop 35(7):1001–1006

20 Environmental Factors and Infection in Total Joint Replacement Surgery

Erik Schnaser and Alejandro Gonzalez Della Valle

Open Questions

- What is the major source of environmental contamination in the operating room?
- Is the intraoperative bacterial contamination of the surgical field the major source of prosthetic joint infection?
- What is the role of laminar airflow in reducing the rate of prosthetic joint infection?
- Has routine use of ultraviolet light been associated with a reduction of wound contamination?
- Does the use of disposable impervious drapes decrease surgical contamination rate?
- Can the used of close suction drainage be avoided without increasing the risk of wound hematomas and infection?
- Should we screen and decolonize all patients carrying nasal staphylococci?
- Does the use of body exhaust suits reduce periprosthetic joint infections or improve surgical team safety?

20.1 Background

Intraoperative bacterial contamination of the surgical wound is a major source of periprosthetic joint infection (PJI). In order to reduce wound contamination and surgical site infections (SSI), several strategies have been developed, tested, and implemented. These strategies include those which address specific operating room variables (such as improvements in operating room ventilation systems), surgical factors (draping materials, irrigation, wound closure, etc.), patient factors such as improving the patient's immune response or diminishing the bacterial load present on the patient's skin (patient's temperature, MRSA contamination), and factors controlled by the surgical team (hand cleansing, use of face masks, etc.) (Salvati et al. 2003). This chapter will discuss the different sources of bacterial contamination in the operating room, the approaches to reduce them, and their effect in diminishing the rates of SSI with particular emphasis in joint replacement (JR) surgery.

20.2 Operating Room Factors

20.2.1 Bacterial Load in the Operating Room

Sir John Charnley realized that one of the main sources of wound contamination and PJI was the air in the operating room (Evans 2011). Particulate

E. Schnaser • A. Gonzalez Della Valle (✉)
Department of Orthopaedic Surgery,
Hospital for Special Surgery, Weill Medical College of Cornell University, 535 East 70th Street,
New York, NY 10021, USA
e-mail: gonzaleza@hss.edu

A. Baldini, P. Caldora (eds.), *Perioperative Medical Management for Total Joint Arthroplasty: How to Control Hemostasis, Pain and Infection*, DOI 10.1007/978-3-319-07203-6_20,

size greater than 10 μm is considered to be a surrogate for viable bacteria capable of contaminating the surgical field. The number of airborne particulate near the surgical site has been correlated with the incidence of PJI. They originate from the operating room personnel, the patient, the equipment present or introduced in the theater during the procedure, and the circulating air. Particulate is spread throughout the operating room via air currents created by the air ventilation system, the movement of people, structures and equipment, and/or by opening and closing the operating room doors. It is reasonable to believe that reducing the bacterial load and the particulate count in the surgical field will likely lead to a reduction in SSI. This theory has led to the development of strategies and technologies to reduce the number of airborne particulates in the operating room.

20.2.2 Clean Air Technology

In order to reduce the particle load and minimize turbulence, air filtration and laminar air flow (LAF) units are increasingly being used in operating rooms devoted to orthopedic procedures.

High efficiency particulate arrest (HEPA) filters remove from the air that circulates into the operating room 99.9 % of particles with a diameter equal to or greater than 0.3 um. This means that bacteria are virtually eliminated from the delivered air (Salvati et al. 1982). Horizontal LAF operating rooms have units that push a HEPA-filtered positive pressure plane of air or "plenum" in a horizontal direction over the surgical site (wall to wall). Vertical LAF units push the plenum from the ceiling to the floor.

Vertical LAF units are considered to be superior to horizontal LAF as the filtered air is directed without obstacles toward the surgical site. In our own institution devoted to the care of patients with diverse orthopedic conditions, Eduardo Salvati et al. studied the effect of ventilation systems in the operating room on the infection rates following 3,175 unilateral total hip (THR) and total knee replacements (TKR). All surgeries were performed with prophylactic antibiotics and in operating rooms equipped with a horizontal, unidirectional, LAF system. Although the infection rate of THRs diminished from 1.4 to 0.9 %, that of TKRs increased from 1.4 to 3.9 %. The changes in the infection rates were likely the cause of the position of the operating team during surgery: during TKR surgery, the surgical team was positioned between the air source and the wound, whereas during THR surgery, the patient was positioned between the air source and the surgical team. Consequently, during TKR surgery, bacteria shed by the team were carried to the wound by laminar airflow (Salvati et al. 1982). All our operating rooms devoted to JR surgery are currently equipped with vertical LAF. Outside the canopy area, the downward flow of air is brought up and recirculated along with the new air (Evans 2011). HEPA filtration can also be used in operating theaters that are not equipped with LAF units.

In spite of the previously mentioned theoretical advantages, the clinical benefit of using operating rooms equipped with LAF units remains controversial. The initial studies supporting the use of LAF technology were conducted in the 1970s and 1980s. Charnley reported an initial infection rate of 9.5 % for his series of primary THR patients. Using a combination of clean air systems and occlusive operating gowns, he reported a reduction in PJI nearly 20-fold to 0.5 % (Charnley and Eftekhar 1969; Charnley 1972). Lidwell et al. authored a multicenter study of over 8,136 joint replacements performed in 19 hospitals in England, Scotland, and Sweden. The infection rate was reduced from 1.6 to 0.6 % when surgeries were performed in operating rooms equipped with ultra-clean air technology (Lidwell et al. 1982). In the early era of THR surgery at Hospital for Special Surgery, Paolo Aglietti, Eduardo Salvati, and coworkers demonstrated that THR surgeries performed in conventional operating rooms had a higher risk of persistent wound drained than those performed in rooms equipped with LAF (Aglietti et al. 1974).

Other investigators have suggested that the use of LAF technology by itself is unlikely to reduce infection rates (Breier et al. 2011; Hooper et al. 2011).

draping and minimizing environmental exposure of the instruments to open air likely reduce instrumentation contamination, and attempting to adhere to such principle is likely important, but no study shows that these practices are associated with lower infection rates in JR surgery.

We have studied the effect of exposure of instruments to the air in the operating room at Hospital for Special Surgery on the development of SSI following bilateral sequential THR surgery performed in ideal aseptic conditions (vertical LAF operating rooms, full body exhaust suits, preoperative antibiotics, and devoted specialized surgical team) (González Della Valle et al. 2006). Two hundred and seventy-one consecutive patients underwent surgery with different sterile setups for each side (a complete sterile setup was used for the second side), and 289 patients were operated using the same instruments (instruments and sterile setup were not changed for the second side). There was one deep infection in the first group and one superficial wound infection in the second group during the first year ($p \sim 1.0$). We concluded that given the very low prevalence of deep infection of the first and second side in each group (0.2 and 0 %, respectively), it would be necessary to analyze more than 2,300 patients in each group to achieve statistical significance. Based on this experience, the use of the same set of instruments for the second side in the ideal operating room conditions described in this study appears safe.

Several surgeons employ the practice of changing knife blades after initial incision and frequent changing electrocautery tips as well as sucker tips. Changing knife blades after initial incision and using a fresh blade on deep tissue for the sole reason of avoiding bacterial contamination is controversial (Schindler et al. 2006; Davis et al. 1999) (Ritter et al. 1975b; Fairclough et al. 1983; Grabe et al. 1985). Little data exists that would recommend for or against regular changing of the electrocautery tip; however, due to the extreme temperatures created at the tip, it is unlikely that microorganisms can survive (Bennett and Kraffert 1990).

On the other hand, there is ample evidence to suggest changing the sucker tip reduces bacterial contamination. Contamination rates of sucker tips in JR surgery have been reported to be between 37 and 78 % (Greenough 1986; Robinson et al. 1993; Strange-Vognsen and Klareskov 1988; Givissis et al. 2008), and there is at least one case in the literature where the organism in a surgical site infection was the same organism isolated on the sucker tip at the time of surgery (Givissis et al. 2008). It is believed that the increased flow of air through the narrow suction tip is responsible for the high contamination rates. Givissis et al. showed that there was a 9 % rate of sucker tip contamination if the procedure lasted less than an hour and a 67 % rate of contamination if the procedure lasted more than an hour. They recommend changing the sucker tip every hour (Givissis et al. 2008). Given the data above, it is reasonable to recommend that the suction tip be changed every hour during prolonged JR procedures.

The role of patient specific instrumentation used for TKR in reducing infection rates is speculative (Barrack et al. 2012). Mont et al. did show a decrease in instrument contamination rates when using disposable cutting blocks and trials (Mont et al. 2013).

20.3.6 Irrigation and Antiseptic Irrigation

Irrigation with normal saline during surgery has been shown to be beneficial in reducing bacterial counts and SSIs (Bratzler et al. 2013; Cervantes-Sánchez et al. 2000; Eklund and Tunevall 1987). Moreover, the first four liters of pulsatile lavage with saline solution has been shown to reduce the number of particles in wound after TKR surgery (Niki et al. 2007). An additional advantage of pulsatile high-pressure lavage in combination with dry suction is that it appears to increase the strength of the cement-bone interface by allowing enhanced cement penetration into clean, blood-free, and dry cancellous bone (Kalteis et al. 2007; Maistrelli et al. 1995; Miskovsky et al. 1992; Seeger et al. 2013).

The solution used for lavage during surgery may contain soap, antibiotics, iodine, or normal saline. The data is conflicting when it comes to recommending one solution over the other. The surgeon should rely on their own clinic experience, patient factors (such as allergies or history of contact dermatitis), as sufficient evidence to recommend one particular solution is lacking. Detergents/soaps may be effective in decreasing the bacterial wound burden by acting as a surfactant that disrupts the hydrophobic and electrostatic properties that allow bacteria to bind to hardware and tissue (Anglen et al. 2003). Some detergents such as castile soap may be more efficacious than other solutions, such as normal saline, in removing bacteria from surgical wounds, but a clear reduction in infections has yet to have been shown (Anon 2011; Anglen et al. 2003; Howell et al. 1993a, b). The FLOW (fluid lavage of open wounds) consortium publish their multicenter, blinded, randomized controlled trial looking at castile soap vs. low pressure saline in 111 open contaminated orthopedic trauma cases (Gustilo type I–IIIb) (Anon 2011). Eighty-nine of the 111 patients were followed for at least 1 year and failed to show a significant difference in wound infection between castile soap (23 %) and low-pressure saline lavage (24 %). The investigators acknowledged that this study was underpowered and called for a larger series. Randomized controlled trials in non-orthopedic literature and experimental evidence suggests that adding antibiotic irrigation to clean-contaminated wounds does not significantly decrease the incidence of SSIs in comparison to irrigation with normal saline (Brown et al. 1978; Farnell et al. 1986; Greig et al. 1987; Rambo 1972; Schein et al. 1990; Sherman et al. 1976; Anglen et al. 2003; Conroy et al. 1999).

In a systematic review of different surgical specialties, it was suggested that povidone-iodine irrigation was significantly more effective at preventing SSIs than the comparative interventions of saline, water, or no irrigation (Chundamala and Wright 2007). It should be noted that povidone-iodine solution should not be used in patients with iodine sensitivity, renal disease, burns, or patients with thyroid disease. Taken together, these conditions may be somewhat prevalent in the population undergoing JR.

If the surgeon chooses to irrigate with an antibiotic containing solution, the ideal antibiotic is one, which has high efficacy, low systemic absorption, is inexpensive, and has a low potential to harm the patient. Though toxic if given systemically, bacitracin and polymyxin B can be added to irrigation solutions, are bactericidal, and are commonly used in orthopedic procedures. The antibiotics have low absorption rate during wound irrigation and are relatively safe when used topically. Other commonly used topical antibiotics are cephalosporins, aminoglycosides (neomycin), and chloramphenicol (McHugh et al. 2011). Topical antibiotics like bacitracin, polymyxin, and neomycin can cause contact dermatitis, anaphylaxis, deafness, and renal failure (Eedy et al. 1990; Bratzler et al. 2013; Antevil et al. 2003; Dirschl and Wilson 1991; Gelman et al. 1979). Even though no evidence exists that directly connects the use of topical antibiotic irrigation to a lower risk of infection (Dimick et al. 2000; McHugh et al. 2011), we use bacitracin in the irrigation solution during surgeries on patients who are considered to be at a high risk of infection.

Fluid-filled basins to be used for irrigation of surgical wounds or to clean surgical instruments kept in the back table have a high level of contamination (Andersson et al. 1984; Baird et al. 1984; Anto et al. 2006; Glait et al. 2011), and consequently, their use should be avoided.

20.3.7 Wound Closure/Closed Suction Drainage

Obtaining appropriate tension-free tissue apposition of the surgical wound is important in minimizing wound complications, and several methods including superficial suture, subcuticular closure, and staples exist. There is insufficient evidence that one type of closure method over the other reduces the rate of SSI (Smith et al. 2010; Eggers et al. 2011). Tissue adhesives such as 2-octylcyanoacrylate (OCA) should be viewed as a biologic dressing with insufficient mechanical strength to be used by itself for closure (Khan et al. 2006). OCA may be effective in reducing early wound discharge when combined with other closure methods which may indirectly reduce postoperative infection; however, no clear reduction in infection has been observed (El-Gazzar et al. 2013; Khan et al. 2006).

The use of closed suction drainage after JR is controversial. Closed suction drainage theoretically provides a route for bacteria to travel in a retrograde fashion to the surgical site; on the other hand, drains may provide a route for wound decompression, lower wound-related complications, and joint stiffness. Several prospective studies including randomized controlled trials and meta-analysis have failed to show a benefit of closed suction drainage in JR and have not definitively shown an effect in wound infection rates (Walmsley et al. 2005; Parker et al. 2004; Chen et al. 2013; Zhou et al. 2013; González Della Valle et al. 2004). In our own prospective randomized trial, we assessed the use of close suction drainage in 104 elective primary THRs (González Della Valle et al. 2004). We observed no difference in the early infection rates between the two groups. Similarly, Walmsley et al., in a study of 577 THAs in 552 patients, concluded that drains provided little benefit while increasing surgical cost as well as increasing transfusion rates (Walmsley et al. 2005). There is a vast body of literature suggesting that the use of closed suction drainage in an elective, primary, uncomplicated JR can be avoided without an increase in the infection rate.

20.4 Patient Factors

20.4.1 Patient Temperature and the Use of Forced Air Warming Blankets

Mild hypothermia may promote SSI by triggering vasoconstriction, which leads to a decrease in oxygen tension. Reduced oxygen tension impairs the oxidative mechanisms that allow neutrophils to attack bacteria. In a general surgery study, Kurz et al. analyzed 200 patients who underwent colorectal surgery. Patients were assigned to either the "routine" care group (hypothermia group) or to the warmed, "normothermia," group. Not only did the authors see a significant increase in the SSIs in the hypothermia group, hypothermic patients tended to have longer hospital lengths of stay and their sutures stayed in longer (Kurz et al. 1996). Other studies from the general surgery literature support patient warming in clean surgeries to reduce infection rates (Melling et al. 2001). Currently, the literature regarding intraoperative patient temperature and SSI in JR surgery is lacking.

Patients generally are kept warm in the operating rooms by the use of conventional or forced-air warming blankets (FAW). Concern has been raised about the possibility of bacterial contamination by the air circulating out of air warming blankets. Such airflow could disrupt laminar airflow in operating rooms and increase bacterial counts over the surgical field. McGovern et al. conducted an experimental study utilizing soap bubbles to analyze airflow in the operating room and found more bubbles migrated over the surgical site when a FAW device was used compared to a conventional warming blanket (McGovern et al. 2011). In another experimental study that simulated a TKR, Legg et al. compared a torso FAW device (Bair Hugger; Arizant UK Limited, Wakefield, UK) to a radiant warming blanket (Hot-Dog, Eden Prairie, Minnesota) in an enclosed laminar flow operating room (ExFlow 90 Howorth enclosure) and found an increase in air particles (0.3–5 μm) and temperature over the surgical field when a FAW device was used (Legg et al. 2012). The authors concluded further work is required to confirm that unidirectional airflow produced by LAF is disrupted by FAW devices as they did not study airflow over the surgical site. On the other hand, several studies on this subject have failed to link FAW systems to a direct increase in bacterial air counts and/or SSI (Moretti et al. 2009; Tumia and Ashcroft 2002; Zink and Iaizzo 1993). Moretti et al. studied the risk of surgical site contamination by Bair Hugger blankets in 30 THR surgeries. The authors quantified the level of bacterial contamination of the air in the operating room with and without the use of the FAW device (Moretti et al. 2009). They concluded that the Bair Hugger system does not pose a real risk for nosocomial infection and offers the advantage of potentially preventing hypothermia.

Currently, the benefits of keeping the patient in normothermia, as outlined above, outweigh the theoretical risks of wound bacterial air contamination. We routinely use forced air warming (FAW) blankets at our hospital and have not attributed a higher infection rate to their use. As long as the surgical field is appropriately sealed off from the rest of the patients' body, the benefits of keeping the patient normothermic likely outweigh the risks. We use a combination of multilayered surgical drapes, incise drapes (Ioban), and vertical laminar flow which may prevent contaminated air from that FAW to cross over the surgical field.

20.4.2 MSSA/MRSA Colonization

A strong link has been establish between patients who carry *Staphylococcus aureus* (methicillin sensitive (MSSA) and methicillin resistant (MRSA)) in their nares and surgical site infection (Perl and Golub 1998). Kalmeijer et al. studied risk factors for the development of infection in patients undergoing orthopedic surgery that received implants. They determined that high levels of nasal *S. aureus* were not only the most important but the only independent risk factor for the development of an SSI (Kalmeijer et al. 2000).

Though the link to patient colonization and infection has been made, much debate exists regarding methods of decolonization. Mupirocin nasal ointment has been widely adopted for reducing nasal colonization of MRSA, but concern over the development of bacterial resistance exists. However, Fawley et al. were not able to identify an increasing prevalence in mupirocin resistance over a 4-year study period when mupirocin was combined with topical triclosan (Fawley et al. 2006). Other forms of decolonization include preoperative photo disinfection, total body chlorhexidine gluconate showers and wipes, and iodine-based solutions. Due to several controversies on the subject, our institution does not have standard policy on this subject, but we feel that patients with a history of MRSA or MSSA colonization should probably be rescreened prior to additional surgical procedures. If a patient is screened, cultures are taken from the nares, oropharynx, axilla, and groin. If positive for MRSA, we recommend the use of a chlorhexidine total body wash, nasal mupirocin, and IV vancomycin as the perioperative antibiotic of choice.

Recommendations for screening healthcare workers to assess if they are carriers of MSSA and MRSA vary by country. The Dutch Working Party for infection recommends screening workers who have been exposed to MRSA-positive patients (Kluymans-Vandenbergh et al. 2005). The advantages of a screening policy include the determination of the full extent of MRSA colonization and work exclusion; the disadvantages include detection of transient nasal carriage, disruption of staff routine, and stigmatization. Screening of heathcare workers can be a valuable tool in the control of MRSA outbreaks, but it should be used selectively (Lessing et al. 1996).

20.5 Operating Room Personnel

20.5.1 Hand Cleansing

Hand washing has been identified as one of the most important gestures to avoid the spread of community and hospital infections. It is a basic gesture that is performed by all personnel before dressing with surgical scrubs. A number of regulatory bodies like the Centers of Disease Control (CDC) and the Association of Perioperative Registered Nurses recommend washing hands for a period of 2–5 min (Mangram et al. 1999; Association of periOperative Registered Nurses Recommended Practices Committee 2004). There is evidence to suggest that shorter hand cleansing procedures are as effective as the conventional hand washing alone at reducing operating room staff bacterial counts (Kappstein et al. 1993).

20.5.2 Operating Room Masks

Surgical face masks were originally developed to contain and filter droplets containing microorganisms expelled from the mouth and nasopharynx of healthcare workers during surgery, thereby providing protection for the patient. Operating room masks should be worn by all operating room personnel as they are cost effective, produce little, if any, morbidity for the personnel, and, at minimum, provide a barrier between the OR personnel's bacterial-laden mouth and the surgical wound. However, to the best of our knowledge, there is no study showing that use of a mask in TJA reduces surgical site infections (Tunevall and Jörbeck 1992; Tunevall 1991; Lipp and Edwards 2005; Webster et al. 2010).

20.5.3 Body Exhaust Suits

Body exhaust suits or "space suits" may offer a level of protection and comfort for the surgeon, but their role in SSIs in TJA is somewhat controversial. It is reasonable to believe that they are beneficial in reducing infection in a laminar airflow setting (Salvati et al. 1982; Taylor and Bannister 1993). On the other hand, studies have also linked them to an increase in SSI rates (Hooper et al. 2011; Miner et al. 2007). If the surgical team utilizes body exhaust suits, it is important to remember that the rules of meticulous surgical sterility do not change.

It is also important to recognize that the properly worn, conventional sterile gown can be a source of contamination. Bible et al. recently determined that despite proper use of surgical gown and sterile technique, all 50 gowns tested after spinal operations were contaminated with bacteria. The least contaminated areas were between the chest and the level of the surgical field, whereas the most contaminated were the areas below the waist, the neck, and the elbow creases (Bible et al. 2009).

20.5.4 Garments

Wearing clean operating room attire including scrubs, head covering, and masks is important. Surgical attire should be clean and made of tightly woven material (McHugh et al. 2013). Scrubs that are worn outside of the hospital as well as scrubs that have been worn in the presence of a patient with a bacterial infection should probably not be worn during a subsequent, elective JR surgery. Ensuring mechanical barriers such as masks, head coverings, and scrubs are clean and regularly changed add no risk to the patient. Its practice should be a regular habit for the operating room personnel.

20.5.5 Portable Electronic Devices

Mobile phones improve the efficiency of clinical communication and are increasingly involved in all areas of healthcare. Personal electronic devices (PEDs) such as cell phones and smartphones are frequently used in the OR, and their utility in the OR may be increased with time (Peters et al. 2012). The surgeon and OR personnel should use PEDs with caution as many studies have shown there is a high contamination rate in PEDs used in hospitals by healthcare workers (Brady et al. 2012; Ulger et al. 2009; Lee et al. 2013; Jeske et al. 2007; Sadat-Ali et al. 2010; Ustun and Cihangiroglu 2012; Singh and Purohit 2012). Ulger et al. noted that 52 % of the *Staphylococcus aureus* strains isolated from cell phones were methicillin-resistant (Ulger et al. 2009). Lee et al. showed a higher rate of contamination in "smart" cell phone compared to "non-smart" cell phones (Lee et al. 2013). If personal electronic devices must be used, then they should be wiped down with an alcohol-based solution as this can significantly reduce contamination (Singh et al. 2002; Brady et al. 2012). The operating room personnel should be aware of this potential source of contamination, and PED use should be limited. If their utility in JR surgery grows, it may be beneficial for hospitals to acquire their own devices or develop sterile cases or bags that seal them off from the operating room environment.

20.5.6 Operating Room Traffic and Intraoperative Radiology

Operating room traffic, the number of people in the operating room, and the number of times the operating room door is opened should be kept to a minimum. Anderson et al. showed a positive correlation between operating room traffic flow rates as well as the number of personnel in the operating room to increased bacterial counts in orthopedic procedures (Andersson et al. 1984). Ritter also showed that bacterial counts increased from 13 CFUs/ft2/h to 24 CFUs/ft2/h when doors were left open in the operating room; however, when 5 people were introduced into the operating room, the bacterial counts soared comparatively (447 CFUs/ft2/h) (Ritter et al. 1975a). They concluded that people are the major source of environmental contamination in the operating room and unnecessary personnel should be minimized. Quraishi further confirmed that increased activity with OR personnel led to a higher rate of surgical field contamination during clean procedures (Quraishi et al. 1983). Not surprisingly, circulating nurses and implant technicians/sales representatives have been implicated to be the major source of traffic (Panahi et al. 2012).

Opening the door in an operating room also creates turbulence which may contribute to air contamination (Lynch et al. 2009). In rooms equipped with LAF, opening the door leads to a drop in the pressure gradient which, in turn, requires more air to be pumped in through the laminar flow system. Anticipation to the needs and steps of surgery plays a major role in minimizing door openings during surgery. Preoperative templating (Gonzalez Della Valle et al. 2005) and having appropriate implants and instruments available in the room at the start of the case are plausible ways to reduce operating room traffic. With the growing popularity of THR performed through an anterior approach, the use of intraoperative fluoroscopy has increased. Theoretically, having a C-arm over the field could increase contamination risk, but no studies exist on this topic. Kaska et al. points out that unstandardized, inefficient, and wasteful techniques that violate AORN standards of keeping sterile fields are currently used during intraoperative fluoroscopy (Kaska 2010). They point out that rotation of the C-arm into the horizontal position introduces a non-sterile object (x-ray tube) and/or contaminated drape(s) into the sterile field. This rotation is often required multiple times throughout a surgical case. This increases the potential for contamination. By preoperative templating and minimizing the rotational use of the fluoroscopic arm, surgeons can reduce the chance of C-arm-related contamination.

20.6 Summary

Wound contamination during JR surgery is a multifactorial phenomenon. A number of factors involving the operating room environment, conduct and gestures of operating room personnel, and patient-related factors are involved. Though the majority of the factors discussed in this chapter may not individually contribute to a significant reduction in PJI, it is very likely that when used together, they result in a drastic reduction in the rate of acute postoperative infection (Parvizi and Gehrke 2013). In the experience of the senior author, when all the previously mentioned factors and gestures are taken into account, the rate of deep, acute infection of elective primary THR and TKR has been negligible with only three cases observed in the span of 9 years (approximate rate: 0.1 %).

Key Points

- Unnecessary personnel should not be present in the operating room.
- Intraoperative bacterial contamination of the surgical wound is a major source of surgical site infections and periprosthetic joint infections.
- It is reasonable to believe that the use of vertical LAF technology together with other important factors such as the administration of preoperative antibiotics and attention to following a sterile surgical technique has a beneficial effect in reducing the infection rates following joint replacement surgery.
- The use of UVL technology has shown to be effective in reducing the rate of SSI.
- Despite the perceived advantage, two randomized controlled trials have shown no difference in contamination rates when comparing reusable drapes to disposable ones. Experimental evidence suggests that disposable drapes have better resistance to bacterial penetration.
- There is strong evidence in literature suggesting that the use of closed suction drainage in an elective, primary, uncomplicated JR can be avoided without an increase in the infection rate.
- Since a strong link has been established between patients who carry *Staphylococcus aureus* (MSSA and MRSA) in their nares and surgical site infection, patients with a history of MRSA or MSSA colonization should probably be rescreened and eventually treated prior to undergoing elective surgery.
- Body exhaust suits may offer more protection, comfort, and safety for the surgeon, but their role in SSIs and in PJI is somewhat controversial.

Acknowledgement This work was partially funded by the generous donation of Mr. Glenn Bergenfield and The Sidney Milton and Leoma Simon Foundation.

References

Abolghasemian M et al (2013) Is arthroplasty immediately after an infected case a risk factor for infection? Clin Orthop Relat Res 471(7):2253–2258

Aglietti P et al (1974) Effect of a surgical horizontal unidirectional filtered air flow unit on wound bacterial contamination and wound healing. Clin Orthop Relat Res 101:99–104

Al-Maiyah M et al (2005) Glove perforation and contamination in primary total hip arthroplasty. J Bone Joint Surg Br 87(4):556–559

Andersson BM et al (1984) Contamination of irrigation solutions in an operating theatre. Infect Control 5(7):339–341

Anglen JO et al (2003) The use of detergent irrigation for musculoskeletal wounds. Int Orthop 27(1):40–46

Anon (2011) Fluid lavage of open wounds (FLOW): a multicenter, blinded, factorial pilot trial comparing alternative irrigating solutions and pressures in patients with open fractures. J Trauma 71(3):596–606

Antevil JL et al (2003) Intraoperative anaphylactic shock associated with bacitracin irrigation during revision total knee arthroplasty. A case report. J Bone Joint Surg Am 85-A(2):339–342

Anto B et al (2006) Splash basin bacterial contamination during elective arthroplasty. J Infect 52(3):231–232

AORN Recommended Practices Committee (2006) Recommended practices for maintaining a sterile field. AORN J 83(2):402–404, 407–410, 413–416

Association of periOperative Registered Nurses Recommended Practices Committee (2004) Recommended practices for surgical hand antisepsis/hand scrubs. AORN J 79(2):416–418, 421–416, 429–431

Baird RA et al (1984) Splash basin contamination in orthopaedic surgery. Clin Orthop Relat Res 187:129–133

Barrack RL et al (2012) Patient specific cutting blocks are currently of no proven value. J Bone Joint Surg Br 94(11 Suppl A):95–99

Bellchambers J et al (1999) A prospective study of wound infection in coronary artery surgery. Eur J Cardiothorac Surg 15(1):45–50

Bennett RG, Kraffert CA (1990) Bacterial transference during electrodesiccation and electrocoagulation. Arch Dermatol 126(6):751–755

Berg M, Bergman BR, Hoborn J (1989) Shortwave ultraviolet radiation in operating rooms. J Bone Joint Surg Br 71(3):483–485

Berg M, Bergman BR, Hoborn J (1991) Ultraviolet radiation compared to an ultra-clean air enclosure. Comparison of air bacteria counts in operating rooms. J Bone Joint Surg Br 73(5):811–815

Bible JE et al (2009) Which regions of the operating gown should be considered most sterile? Clin Orthop Relat Res 467(3):825–830

Blom A et al (2000) The passage of bacteria through surgical drapes. Ann R Coll Surg Engl 82(6):405–407

Blom AW et al (2002) Bacterial strike-through of re-usable surgical drapes: the effect of different wetting agents. J Hosp Infect 52(1):52–55

Blom AW et al (2007) Resistance of disposable drapes to bacterial penetration. J Orthop Surg (Hong Kong) 15(3):267–269

Brady RRW et al (2012) NHS connecting for health: healthcare professionals, mobile technology, and infection control. Telemed J E Health 18(4):289–291

Bratzler DW et al (2013) Clinical practice guidelines for antimicrobial prophylaxis in surgery. Surg Infect (Larchmt) 14(1):73–156

Breier A-C et al (2011) Laminar airflow ceiling size: no impact on infection rates following hip and knee prosthesis. Infect Control Hosp Epidemiol 32(11): 1097–1102

Brown LL et al (1978) Evaluation of wound irrigation by pulsatile jet and conventional methods. Ann Surg 187(2):170–173

Brown AR, Taylor GJ, Gregg PJ (1996) Air contamination during skin preparation and draping in joint replacement surgery. J Bone Joint Surg Br 78(1):92–94

Carlsson AS et al (1986) Ultraviolet radiation and air contamination during total hip replacement. J Hosp Infect 7(2):176–184

Carroll K et al (2014) Risk factors for superficial wound complications in hip and knee arthroplasty. Clin Microbiol Infect 20(2):130–135

Carter AH et al (2012) A prospective analysis of glove perforation in primary and revision total hip and total knee arthroplasty. J Arthroplasty 27(7):1271–1275

Cervantes-Sánchez CR et al (2000) Syringe pressure irrigation of subdermic tissue after appendectomy to decrease the incidence of postoperative wound infection. World J Surg 24(1):38–41; discussion 41–42

Charnley J (1972) Postoperative infection after total hip replacement with special reference to air contamination in the operating room. Clin Orthop Relat Res 87:167–187

Charnley J, Eftekhar N (1969) Postoperative infection in total prosthetic replacement arthroplasty of the hip-joint. With special reference to the bacterial content of the air of the operating room. Br J Surg 56(9):641–649

Chen ZY Gao Y, Chen W, Li X, Zhang YZ (2013) Is wound drainage necessary in hip arthroplasty? A meta-analysis of randomized controlled trials. Eur J Orthop Surg Traumatol (Epub ahead of print)

Chiu KY et al (1993) Plastic adhesive drapes and wound infection after hip fracture surgery. Aust N Z J Surg 63(10):798–801

Chosky SA, Modha D, Taylor GJ (1996) Optimisation of ultraclean air. The role of instrument preparation. J Bone Joint Surg Br 78(5):835–837

Chundamala J, Wright JG (2007) The efficacy and risks of using povidone-iodine irrigation to prevent surgical site infection: an evidence-based review. Can J Surg 50(6):473–481

Conroy BP et al (1999) Comparison of castile soap, benzalkonium chloride, and bacitracin as irrigation solu-

tions for complex contaminated orthopaedic wounds. J Orthop Trauma 13(5):332–337
Cordero-Ampuero J, de Dios M (2010) What are the risk factors for infection in hemiarthroplasties and total hip arthroplasties? Clin Orthop Relat Res 468(12): 3268–3277
Dalstrom DJ et al (2008) Time-dependent contamination of opened sterile operating-room trays. J Bone Joint Surg Am 90(5):1022–1025
Davis N et al (1999) Intraoperative bacterial contamination in operations for joint replacement. J Bone Joint Surg Br 81(5):886–889
de Boer AS et al (2001) Risk assessment for surgical site infections following total hip and total knee prostheses. J Chemother (Florence, Italy) 13 Spec No 1(1): 42–47
Demircay E et al (2010) Glove perforation in hip and knee arthroplasty. J Orthop Sci 15(6):790–794
Dewan PA et al (1987) The use of an iodophor-impregnated plastic incise drape in abdominal surgery–a controlled clinical trial. Aust N Z J Surg 57(11):859–863
Dimick JB, Lipsett PA, Kostuik JP (2000) Spine update: antimicrobial prophylaxis in spine surgery: basic principles and recent advances. Spine 25(19): 2544–2548
Dirschl DR, Wilson FC (1991) Topical antibiotic irrigation in the prophylaxis of operative wound infections in orthopedic surgery. Orthop Clin North Am 22(3): 419–426
Edwards JP et al (2012) Wound protectors reduce surgical site infection: a meta-analysis of randomized controlled trials. Ann Surg 256(1):53–59
Eedy DJ, McMillan JC, Bingham EA (1990) Anaphylactic reactions to topical antibiotic combinations. Postgrad Med J 66(780):858–859
Eggers MD, Fang L, Lionberger DR (2011) A comparison of wound closure techniques for total knee arthroplasty. J Arthroplasty 26(8):1251–1258.e1–4
Eklund AE, Tunevall TG (1987) Prevention of postoperative wound infection after appendectomy by local application of tinidazole: a double-blind study. World J Surg 11(2):263–266
El-Gazzar Y et al (2013) The use of dermabond® as an adjunct to wound closure after total knee arthroplasty: examining immediate post-operative wound drainage. J Arthroplasty 28(4):553–556
Erdmann S, Hertl M, Merk HF (1999) Allergic contact dermatitis from povidone-iodine. Contact Dermatitis 40(6):331–332
Evans RP (2011) Current concepts for clean air and total joint arthroplasty: laminar airflow and ultraviolet radiation: a systematic review. Clin Orthop Relat Res 469(4):945–953
Fairclough JA et al (1983) The contaminated skin-knife. A surgical myth. J Bone Joint Surg Br 65(2):210
Fairclough JA, Johnson D, Mackie I (1986) The prevention of wound contamination by skin organisms by the pre-operative application of an iodophor impregnated plastic adhesive drape. J Int Med Res 14(2): 105–109
Falk-Brynhildsen K et al (2013) Bacterial colonization of the skin following aseptic preoperative preparation and impact of the use of plastic adhesive drapes. Biol Res Nurs 15(2):242–248
Farnell MB et al (1986) Closure of abdominal incisions with subcutaneous catheters. A prospective randomized trial. Arch Surg 121(6):641–648
Fawley WN et al (2006) Surveillance for mupirocin resistance following introduction of routine peri-operative prophylaxis with nasal mupirocin. J Hosp Infect 62(3):327–332
Garibaldi RA et al (1986) Comparison of nonwoven and woven gown and drape fabric to prevent intraoperative wound contamination and postoperative infection. Am J Surg 152(5):505–509
Garibaldi RA, Cushing D, Lerer T (1991a) Predictors of intraoperative-acquired surgical wound infections. J Hosp Infect 18(Suppl A):289–298
Garibaldi RA, Cushing D, Lerer T (1991b) Risk factors for postoperative infection. Am J Med 91(3B): 158S–163S
Gelman ML, Frazier CH, Chandler HP (1979) Acute renal failure after total hip replacement. J Bone Joint Surg Am 61(5):657–660
Gheorghe A et al (2012) Systematic review of the clinical effectiveness of wound-edge protection devices in reducing surgical site infection in patients undergoing open abdominal surgery. Ann Surg 255(6): 1017–1029
Gilliam DL, Nelson CL (1990) Comparison of a one-step iodophor skin preparation versus traditional preparation in total joint surgery. Clin Orthop Relat Res 250:258–260
Givissis P et al (2008) Suction during orthopaedic surgery. How safe is the suction tip? Acta Orthop Belg 74(4):531–533
Glait SA et al (2011) Is repetitive intraoperative splash basin use a source of bacterial contamination in total joint replacement? Orthopedics 34(9):e546–e549
González Della Valle A et al (2004) No need for routine closed suction drainage in elective arthroplasty of the hip: a prospective randomized trial in 104 operations. Acta Orthop Scand 75(1):30–33
González Della Valle A, Padgett DE, Salvati EA (2005) Preoperative planning for primary total hip arthroplasty. J Am Acad Orthop Surg 13(7):455–462
González Della Valle A et al (2006) Prevalence of infection in bilateral total hip arthroplasty: a comparison of single-stage 565 bilateral procedures performed with 1 or 2 sets of instruments. J Arthroplasty 21(2): 157–160
Grabe N et al (1985) The contaminated skin-knife–fact or fiction. J Hosp Infect 6(3):252–256
Greenough CG (1986) An investigation into contamination of operative suction. J Bone Joint Surg Br 68(1):151–153
Greig J et al (1987) Wound sepsis after colorectal surgery: the effect of cefotetan lavage. Chemioterapia 6(2 Suppl):595–596
Han CD et al (2013) A randomized prospective study of glove perforation in orthopaedic surgery: is a thick glove more effective? J Arthroplasty 28(10):1878–1881

Hart D (1960) Bactericidal ultraviolet radiation in the operating room. Twenty-nine-year study for control of infections. J Am Med Assoc 172:1019–1028
Hester RA, Nelson CL, Harrison S (1992) Control of contamination of the operative team in total joint arthroplasty. J Arthroplasty 7(3):267–269
Hooper GJ et al (2011) Does the use of laminar flow and space suits reduce early deep infection after total hip and knee replacement?: the ten-year results of the New Zealand Joint Registry. J Bone Joint Surg Br 93(1): 85–90
Howell JM, Dhindsa HS et al (1993a) Effect of scrubbing and irrigation on staphylococcal and streptococcal counts in contaminated lacerations. Antimicrob Agents Chemother 37(12):2754–2755
Howell JM, Stair TO et al (1993b) The effect of scrubbing and irrigation with normal saline, povidone iodine, and cefazolin on wound bacterial counts in a guinea pig model. Am J Emerg Med 11(2):134–138
Hussein JR et al (2001) Use of light handles in the laminar flow operating theatre–is it a cause of bacterial concern? Ann R Coll Surg Engl 83(5):353–354
Jacobson C et al (2005) Prevention of wound contamination using DuraPrep solution plus Ioban 2 drapes. Clin Orthop Relat Res 439:32–37
Jeske H-C et al (2007) Bacterial contamination of anaesthetists' hands by personal mobile phone and fixed phone use in the operating theatre. Anaesthesia 62(9):904–906
Kalmeijer MD et al (2000) Nasal carriage of staphylococcus aureus is a major risk factor for surgical-site infections in orthopedic surgery. Infect Control Hosp Epidemiol 21(5):319–323
Kalteis T et al (2007) An experimental comparison of different devices for pulsatile high-pressure lavage and their relevance to cement intrusion into cancellous bone. Arch Orthop Trauma Surg 127(10):873–877
Kappstein I et al (1993) Microbiological and economic studies of abbreviated procedures for surgical hand disinfection. Chirurg 64(5):400–405
Kaska SC (2010) A standardized and safe method of sterile field maintenance during intra-operative horizontal plane fluoroscopy. Patient Saf Surg 4(1):20
Kaya I et al (2012) Glove perforation time and frequency in total hip arthroplasty procedures. Acta Orthop Traumatol Turc 46(1):57–60
Khan RJK et al (2006) A comparison of three methods of wound closure following arthroplasty: a prospective, randomised, controlled trial. J Bone Joint Surg Br 88(2):238–242
Kluytmans-Vandenbergh MF, Kluytmans JA, Voss A (2005) Dutch guideline for preventing nosocomial transmission of highly resistant microorganisms. Infection 33(5-6):309–13
Kurz A, Sessler DI, Lenhardt R (1996) Perioperative normothermia to reduce the incidence of surgical-wound infection and shorten hospitalization. Study of Wound Infection and Temperature Group. N Engl J Med 334(19):1209–1215
Lee YJ et al (2013) Contamination rates between smart cell phones and non-smart cell phones of healthcare workers. J Hosp Med 8(3):144–147
Legg AJ, Cannon T, Hamer AJ (2012) Do forced air patient-warming devices disrupt unidirectional downward airflow? J Bone Joint Surg Br 94(2):254–256
Lessing MP, Jordens JZ, Bowler IC (1996) When should healthcare workers be screened for methicillin-resistant Staphylococcus aureus? J Hosp Infect 34(3):205–210
Lewis DA, Leaper DJ, Speller DC (1984) Prevention of bacterial colonization of wounds at operation: comparison of iodine-impregnated ("Ioban") drapes with conventional methods. J Hosp Infect 5(4):431–437
Lidwell OM (1994) Ultraviolet radiation and the control of airborne contamination in the operating room. J Hosp Infect 28(4):245–248
Lidwell OM et al (1982) Effect of ultraclean air in operating rooms on deep sepsis in the joint after total hip or knee replacement: a randomised study. Br Med J (Clin Res Ed) 285(6334):10–14
Lipp A, Edwards P (2005) Disposable surgical face masks: a systematic review. Can Oper Room Nurs J 23(3):20–21, 24–25, 33–38
Lowell JD et al (1980) Ultraviolet radiation and reduction of deep wound infection following hip and knee arthroplasty. Ann N Y Acad Sci 353:285–293
Lynch RJ et al (2009) Measurement of foot traffic in the operating room: implications for infection control. Am J Med Qual 24(1):45–52
Mackintosh CA, Lidwell OM (1980) The evaluation of fabrics in relation to their use as protective garments in nursing and surgery. III. Wet penetration and contact transfer of particles through clothing. J Hyg 85(3):393–403
Maistrelli GL et al (1995) Cement penetration with pulsed lavage versus syringe irrigation in total knee arthroplasty. Clin Orthop Relat Res 312:261–265
Mangram AJ et al (1999) Guideline for Prevention of Surgical Site Infection, 1999. Centers for Disease Control and Prevention (CDC) Hospital Infection Control Practices Advisory Committee. Am J Infect Control 27(2): 97–132; quiz 133–134, discussion 96
McGovern PD et al (2011) Forced-air warming and ultraclean ventilation do not mix: an investigation of theatre ventilation, patient warming and joint replacement infection in orthopaedics. J Bone Joint Surg Br 93(11): 1537–1544
McHugh SM et al (2011) The role of topical antibiotics used as prophylaxis in surgical site infection prevention. J Antimicrob Chemother 66(4):693–701
McHugh SM et al (2014) Surgical attire, practices and their perception in the prevention of surgical site infection. Surgeon 12(1):47–52
Melling AC et al (2001) Effects of preoperative warming on the incidence of wound infection after clean surgery: a randomised controlled trial. Lancet 358(9285):876–880
Miner AL et al (2007) Deep infection after total knee replacement: impact of laminar airflow systems and body exhaust suits in the modern operating room. Infect Control Hosp Epidemiol 28(2):222–226
Miskovsky C, Whiteside LA, White SE (1992) The cemented unicondylar knee arthroplasty. An in vitro comparison of three cement techniques. Clin Orthop Relat Res 284:215–220

Moggio M et al (1979) Wound infections in patients undergoing total hip arthroplasty. Ultraviolet light for the control of airborne bacteria. Arch Surg 114(7):815–823
Mont MA et al (2013) Single-use instrumentation, cutting blocks, and trials decrease contamination during total knee arthroplasty: a prospective comparison of navigated and nonnavigated cases. J Knee Surg 26(4):285–290
Moretti B et al (2009) Active warming systems to maintain perioperative normothermia in hip replacement surgery: a therapeutic aid or a vector of infection? J Hosp Infect 73(1):58–63
Niki Y et al (2007) How much sterile saline should be used for efficient lavage during total knee arthroplasty? Effects of pulse lavage irrigation on removal of bone and cement debris. J Arthroplasty 22(1): 95–99
Panahi P et al (2012) Operating room traffic is a major concern during total joint arthroplasty. Clin Orthop Relat Res 470(10):2690–2694
Parker MJ, Roberts CP, Hay D (2004) Closed suction drainage for hip and knee arthroplasty. A meta-analysis. J Bone Joint Surg Am 86-A(6):1146–1152
Parvizi J, Gehrke T (eds) (2013) Proceedings of the international consensus meeting on periprosthetic joint infection. Data Trace Publishing Company, Brooklandville, Maryland
Pedersen AB et al (2010) Risk factors for revision due to infection after primary total hip arthroplasty. A population-based study of 80,756 primary procedures in the Danish Hip Arthroplasty Registry. Acta Orthop 81(5):542–547
Peersman G et al (2006) Prolonged operative time correlates with increased infection rate after total knee arthroplasty. HSS J 2(1):70–72
Perl TM, Golub JE (1998) New approaches to reduce staphylococcus aureus nosocomial infection rates: treating S. aureus nasal carriage. Ann Pharmacother 32(1):S7–S16
Peters FM et al (2012) Improving acetabular cup orientation in total hip arthroplasty by using smartphone technology. J Arthroplasty 27(7):1324–1330
Quraishi ZA et al (1983) Movement of personnel and wound contamination. AORN J 38(1):146–147, 150–156
Rambo WM (1972) Irrigation of the peritoneal cavity with cephalothin. Am J Surg 123(2):192–195
Ridgeway S et al (2005) Infection of the surgical site after arthroplasty of the hip. J Bone Joint Surg Br 87(6): 844–850
Ritter MA, Eitzen H et al (1975a) The operating room environment as affected by people and the surgical face mask. Clin Orthop Relat Res 111:147–150
Ritter MA, French ML, Eitzen HE (1975b) Bacterial contamination of the surgical knife. Clin Orthop Relat Res 108:158–160
Ritter MA, Olberding EM, Malinzak RA (2007) Ultraviolet lighting during orthopaedic surgery and the rate of infection. J Bone Joint Surg Am 89(9):1935–1940
Robinson AH et al (1993) Suction tip contamination in the ultraclean-air operating theatre. Ann R Coll Surg Engl 75(4):254–256
Sadat-Ali M et al (2010) Bacterial flora on cell phones of health care providers in a teaching institution. Am J Infect Control 38(5):404–405
Salvati EA et al (1982) Infection rates after 3175 total hip and total knee replacements performed with and without a horizontal unidirectional filtered air-flow system. J Bone Joint Surg Am 64(4):525–535
Salvati EA et al (2003) The infected total hip arthroplasty. Instr Course Lect 52:223–245
Savitz SI et al (1994) Investigations of the bacteriological factors in clean neurosurgical wounds. Neurosurgery 34(3):417–420; discussion 420–421
Schein M et al (1990) Peritoneal lavage in abdominal sepsis. A controlled clinical study. Arch Surg 125(9): 1132–1135
Schindler OS, Spencer RF, Smith MD (2006) Should we use a separate knife for the skin? J Bone Joint Surg Br 88(3):382–385
Seeger JB et al (2013) The effect of bone lavage on femoral cement penetration and interface temperature during Oxford unicompartmental knee arthroplasty with cement. J Bone Joint Surg Am 95(1):48–53
Sherman JO, Luck SR, Borger JA (1976) Irrigation of the peritoneal cavity for appendicitis in children: a double-blind study. J Pediatr Surg 11(3):371–374
Siegel JD et al (2007) 2007 guideline for isolation precautions: preventing transmission of infectious agents in health care settings. Am J Infect Control 35(10 Suppl 2):S65–S164
Singh A, Purohit B (2012) Mobile phones in hospital settings: a serious threat to infection. Occup Health Saf 81(3):42–44
Singh D et al (2002) Bacterial contamination of hospital pagers. Infect Control Hosp Epidemiol 23(5): 274–276
Skråmm I, Saltytė Benth J, Bukholm G (2012) Decreasing time trend in SSI incidence for orthopaedic procedures: surveillance matters! J Hosp Infect 82(4):243–247
Småbrekke A et al (2004) Operating time and survival of primary total hip replacements: an analysis of 31,745 primary cemented and uncemented total hip replacements from local hospitals reported to the Norwegian Arthroplasty Register 1987–2001. Acta Orthop Scand 75(5):524–532
Smith TO et al (2010) Sutures versus staples for skin closure in orthopaedic surgery: meta-analysis. BMJ 340:c1199
Strange-Vognsen HH, Klareskov B (1988) Bacteriologic contamination of suction tips during hip arthroplasty. Acta Orthop Scand 59(4):410–411
Sutton PM, Greene T, Howell FR (1998) The protective effect of a cut-resistant glove liner. A prospective, randomised trial. J Bone Joint Surg Br 80(3):411–413
Taylor GJ, Bannister GC (1993) Infection and interposition between ultraclean air source and wound. J Bone Joint Surg Br 75(3):503–504
Taylor GJ, Bannister GC, Leeming JP (1995) Wound disinfection with ultraviolet radiation. J Hosp Infect 30(2):85–93
Tumia N, Ashcroft GP (2002) Convection warmers–a possible source of contamination in laminar airflow operating theatres? J Hosp Infect 52(3):171–174

Tunevall TG (1991) Postoperative wound infections and surgical face masks: a controlled study. World J Surg 15(3):383–387; discussion 387–388

Tunevall TG, Jörbeck H (1992) Influence of wearing masks on the density of airborne bacteria in the vicinity of the surgical wound. Eur J Surg 158(5):263–266

Ulger F et al (2009) Are we aware how contaminated our mobile phones with nosocomial pathogens? Ann Clin Microbiol Antimicrob 8(1):7

Ustun C, Cihangiroglu M (2012) Health care workers' mobile phones: a potential cause of microbial cross-contamination between hospitals and community. J Occup Environ Hyg 9(9):538–542

Walmsley PJ et al (2005) A prospective, randomised, controlled trial of the use of drains in total hip arthroplasty. J Bone Joint Surg Br 87(10):1397–1401

Webster J, Alghamdi AA (2007) Use of plastic adhesive drapes during surgery for preventing surgical site infection. Cochrane Database Syst Rev (4):CD006353

Webster J et al (2010) Use of face masks by non-scrubbed operating room staff: a randomized controlled trial. ANZ J Surg 80(3):169–173

Willis-Owen CA, Konyves A, Martin DK (2010) Factors affecting the incidence of infection in hip and knee replacement: an analysis of 5277 cases. J Bone Joint Surg Br 92(8):1128–1133

Wilson SE (2008) Microbial sealing: a new approach to reducing contamination. J Hosp Infect 70(Suppl 2): 11–14

Wymenga AB et al (1992) Perioperative factors associated with septic arthritis after arthroplasty. Prospective multicenter study of 362 knee and 2,651 hip operations. Acta Orthop Scand 63(6):665–671

Zhou X-D et al (2013) Do we really need closed-suction drainage in total hip arthroplasty? A meta-analysis. Int Orthop 37(11):2109–2118

Zink RS, Iaizzo PA (1993) Convective warming therapy does not increase the risk of wound contamination in the operating room. Anesth Analg 76(1):50–53

Zokaie S, White IR, McFadden JD (2011) Allergic contact dermatitis caused by iodophor-impregnated surgical incise drape. Contact Dermatitis 65(5):309

The Fight Against the Slime: Can We Ever Win?

21

Michele Lisanti, Nicola Piolanti, Enrico Tagliaferri, Lorenzo Andreani, Paolo Parchi, and Francesco Menichetti

Open Questions

- Which are the phases of slime production?
- Which are the biofilm-related mechanisms of virulence?
- Prevention and treatment of biofilm implant-related infection in hip and knee arthroplasty: what should be done in the clinical practice?
- How do antiadhension and antimatrix agents work?

21.1 Introduction

It has been shown that joint replacement is among the most successful surgical procedures performed in terms of consistent improvement of the patient's quality of life (Rorabeck et al. 1994; Wiklund and Romanus 1991).

M. Lisanti • N. Piolanti (✉) • L. Andreani • P. Parchi
Ortopedia e Traumatologia I, Azienda Ospedaliera Universitaria Pisana, Via Paradisa 2, Pisa 56124, Italy
e-mail: lisanti@med.unipi.it; nicpio@hotmail.it; l.andreani@hotmail.it; parchip@tiscali.it

E. Tagliaferri • F. Menichetti
U.O. Malattie Infettive, Azienda Ospedaliera Universitaria Pisana, Via Paradisa 2, Pisa 56124, Italy
e-mail: tagliaferrienrico@alice.it; menichettifrancesco@gmail.com

Aside from the life-threatening complications of total hip replacement, no postoperative complication can be more devastating than infection. The use of perioperative antimicrobial prophylaxis and laminar airflow surgical environment and further reduction of other risk factors have diminished the infection's rate to less than one prcent for hip prosthesis and 2 % for other prostheses. Unfortunately these percentage are probably underestimated because of unrecognized infections, and considering the US annual infection rate for orthopedic implants, this raised to 4.3 % (Zimmerli et al. 2004; Trampuz and Zimmerli 2005; Hetrick and Schoenfisch 2006).

Such infections may lead to implant failure, revision surgery, and even though in very selective cases to limb amputation. All these procedures are associated with extremely high medical costs and long-lasting suffering status of the patients (Fig. 21.1).

Schamalzried, in order to better characterize the cause of prosthetic joint infection (PJI), described four different modes of infection: mode 1, intraoperative surgical contaminations; mode 2, hematogenous spread; mode 3, a recurrence of sepsis in a previously infected hip; and mode 4, contiguous spread of infection from local source (Schamalzried et al. 1992).

Another useful way to classify the periprosthetic joint infections (PJIs) is according to Coventry's classification that distinguishes three categories: acute postoperative infections

A. Baldini, P. Caldora (eds.), *Perioperative Medical Management for Total Joint Arthroplasty: How to Control Hemostasis, Pain and Infection*, DOI 10.1007/978-3-319-07203-6_21,

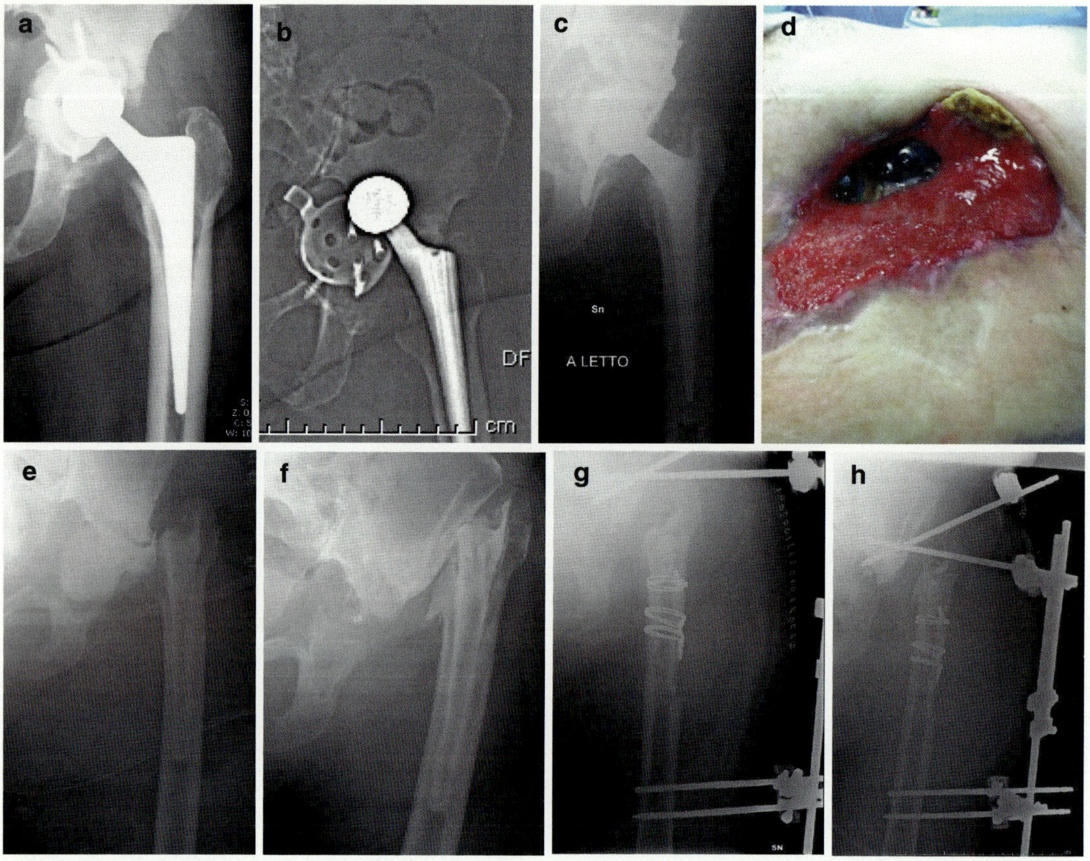

Fig. 21.1 (**a**, **b**) Progressive acetabular component mobilization; (**c**) X-ray after revision with an anti-protrusion cage; (**d**) catastrophic clinical aspect with exposure of the bone of the implant due to infection; (**e–h**) resection arthroplasty still in treatment 1 year after the outset of the infection

(infection is caused by contamination at the time of the operation), delayed infections (usually at least 8 weeks after operation in the form of an indolent, chronic, low-grade infection), and late hematogenous infections (it can happen at any time with a presentation similar to that of acute infection) (Coventry 1975).

From an etiological point of view, PJIs are mainly caused by staphylococci (45–55 %), particularly *Staphylococcus aureus* (33–43 %), and coagulase-negative staphylococci (17–21 %). However, other microorganisms can be involved such as streptococci (11–12 %) and more rarely Gram-negative bacteria (5–14 %), enterococci, and anaerobes. In 5–13 % of cases, mixed flora is found, while in 5 % of infections no microorganism is isolated (Giulieri et al. 2004; Laffer et al. 2006; Rao et al. 2008; Fulkerson et al. 2006).

Adhesion and fixation of bacteria onto biomaterial surfaces represent the first fundamental step in the development of PJI (Arciola et al. 2002).

Among various mechanisms involved in bacterial adhesion, the production of extracellular substance of polysaccharidic nature termed slime appears to play a relevant role; this phenomenon is now regularly referred to as biofilm formation (An and Friedmann 1998; Foster and McDevit 1994; Mack et al. 2000; Montanaro and Arciola 2000; Cristhensen et al. 1982).

It is well accepted that bacteria growing in a biofilm are more recalcitrant to the action of antibiotics than cells growing in a planktonic state and are associated with chronic inflammation and resistance to the innate immune system (Stewart and Costerton 2001).

More than 65 % and the majority of PJIs treated by clinicians in the developed world are now known to be caused by organisms growing in biofilm (Stoodley et al. 2011; Costerton et al. 1999).

The aim of this overview is to analyze the development of the biofilm and examine the most recent literature on this topic in particular about the efficiency of new and old treatments and possible perspectives for the future.

21.2 Bacterial Adhesion and Development of Biofilm

To understand the diagnostic principles and treatment models of PJI, it is imperative to understand the development and functions of biofilm. The transition from planktonic growth to biofilm occurs in response to environmental changes, such as the presence of a prosthetic device, and involves multiple regulatory networks. This communication termed "quorum sensing" (QS) is analogous to the paracrine signaling in multicellular organisms and enables the bacteria to regulate their gene synthesis (Gristina and Costerton 2009).

At the end, biofilm formation enables single-cell organisms to assume a temporary multicellular lifestyle, in which "group behavior" facilitates survival in adverse environments. What was once defined as the formation of a community of microorganisms attached to a surface has come to be recognized as a complex developmental process that is multifaceted and dynamic in nature (Kostakioti et al. 2013).

This cellular reprogramming alters the expression of surface molecules, nutrient utilization, and virulence factors and equips bacteria with an arsenal of properties that enable their survival in unfavorable conditions (Whiteley et al. 2001; Stanley et al. 2003; Vuong et al. 2004; Lenz et al. 2008).

As soon as a new device gets implanted in a surgical site, a process notoriously called "race for the surface" begins (Gristina et al. 1995).

According to this concept, there is a competition for colonizing the surface between extracellular matrix proteins (fibrinogen, fibronectin, vitronectin, thrombospondin, bone sialoprotein) and eukaryotic cells (fibroblasts, osteoblasts, endothelial cells) on one hand and prokaryotic bacterial cells on the other. Matrix proteins are known to cover foreign material as soon as it appears in the human body. In the next step, fibroblasts interact with a layer of matrix proteins using specific receptors called integrins. In such a way, the implant becomes covered by a viable barrier, capable of defense functions against bacteria. In case there are bacteria present at the time of implantation, they enter the competition for the surface, and the outcome largely depends on their number and features.

Bacterial adhesion to biomaterial surfaces and development of biofilm are thought to consist of four separate stages regulated through different mechanisms among which the best studied is QS (Lazar 2011; Costerton et al. 2007) (Fig. 21.2).

Stage I can be subdivided in to two phases. In the first, bacteria inoculated in planktonic form diffuse through fluids propelled by nonspecific physical factors like gravity, Brownian motion, surface tension, and van der Waals bonds. While this process for the majority of pathogen is at least in part stochastic, motile bacteria such as *Pseudomonas aeruginosa* have a competitive advantage. When bacteria come into proximity of an implant at distances smaller than 3 nm, they start interacting with biomaterial by means of hydrogen, ionic, and hydrophobic bonds. Energy needed for disruption of these bonds is small; therefore, initial attachment is dynamic and reversible (Donlan 2002; Krekeler et al. 1989; Kostakioti et al. 2013).

The second phase, mediated by multiple macromolecules able to bond with the implant surface and in general called adhesins, is less reversible. Microorganisms appear to have different adhesins for different surface materials (Hasty et al. 1992).

Pseudomonas aeruginosa, *Escherichia coli*, and others, mainly Gram-negative bacteria, connect to implant surface using flagella (Darouiche 2001). Flagella are protein hooks sized 20 nm used for grabbing the surroundings (An and Friedman 1998). Some bacterial species adhere to implant surface using specific means, e.g., *Staphylococcus aureus* uses MSCRAMM adhesive molecule (microbial

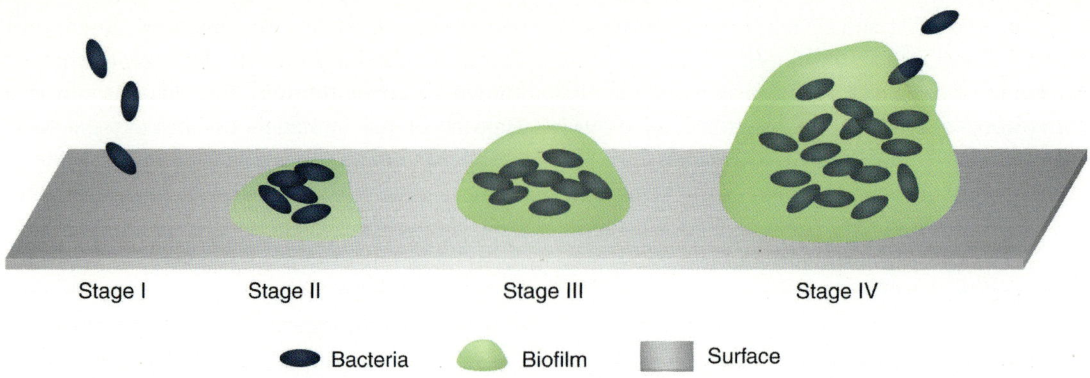

Fig. 21.2 Four stages of biofilm formation. (*Stage I*) bacteria inoculated in planktonic form diffuse through fluids, initial adherence to the foreign body; (*stage II*) accumulation phase, irreversible binding to the surface the now sessile (or fixed) organisms begin to multiply and forming; (*stage III*) maturation, in this stage biofilms reach their ultimate thickness, generally greater than 100 μm with mushroom-shaped or tower-like microcolonies. At that stage the biofilm shows maximum resistance to antibiotics. (*Stage IV*) focal areas of the biofilm dissolve, so some of the bacteria develop the planktonic phenotype and leave the biofilm; such event may cause expansion of the infection and a reactivation of clinical manifestation

surface components recognizing adhesive matrix molecules) to connect with extracellular matrix proteins covering the implant (Patti et al. 1994). Adhesion to a surface leads to important changes in many aspects of bacterial metabolism. Genes needed for biofilm development become activated. There are also other prerequisites for induction of this process like availability of nutrients, temperature, pH, osmolality, availability of iron, and presence of different signal molecules from other bacteria. During this stage, bacterial cells form a monolayer and exhibit a logarithmic grow rate.

Stage II, also called accumulation phase, is characterized by the irreversible binding to the surface and begins from minutes to hours after the first stage. Once adherence has taken place, the now sessile (or fixed) organisms begin to multiply and forming microcolonies while emitting chemical signals that "intercommunicate" between bacterial cells (Høiby et al. 2010a).

When the signal intensity exceeds a certain threshold level, the genetic mechanisms underlying extracellular polymeric substances (EPSs) production are activated. EPSs consist primarily of polysaccharides and contribute 50–90 % of the organic matter in biofilms. This matrix is highly hydrated (98 % water), and apart from water and microbial cells, it is a very complex material. Biofilm in fact is not only tenaciously bounded to the underlying surface but also has a propensity to act almost as filters to entrap particles of various kinds, including minerals and host components such as fibrin, RBCs, platelets, and planktonic bacteria (Costerton et al. 1999).

Therefore, all major classes of macromolecules (proteins, polysaccharides, and nucleic acids) are present in addition to peptidoglycan, lipids, phospholipids, and other cell components (Taraszkiewicz et al. 2013).

In case of *Staphylococcal* infection, this second stage is mediated by multiple molecules including polysaccharide intercellular adhesin (PIA)/poly-N-acetyl glucosamine (PNAG); proteins such as biofilm-associated protein (Bap), accumulation-associated protein (Aap), or fibronectin-binding protein (FnBp); and eDNA (Rohde et al. 2010).

Stage III is also known as maturation; it is characterized by the synthesis of tower-like structures containing, in part, eDNA from lysed bacteria and the generation of multiple metabolic niches that include bacteria growing under aerobic conditions, microaerobic-anaerobic conditions, dormant, and dead cells.

The production of QS signals bacterial surface components such as exopolysaccharides (EPSs) is required for the formation of a mature biofilm.

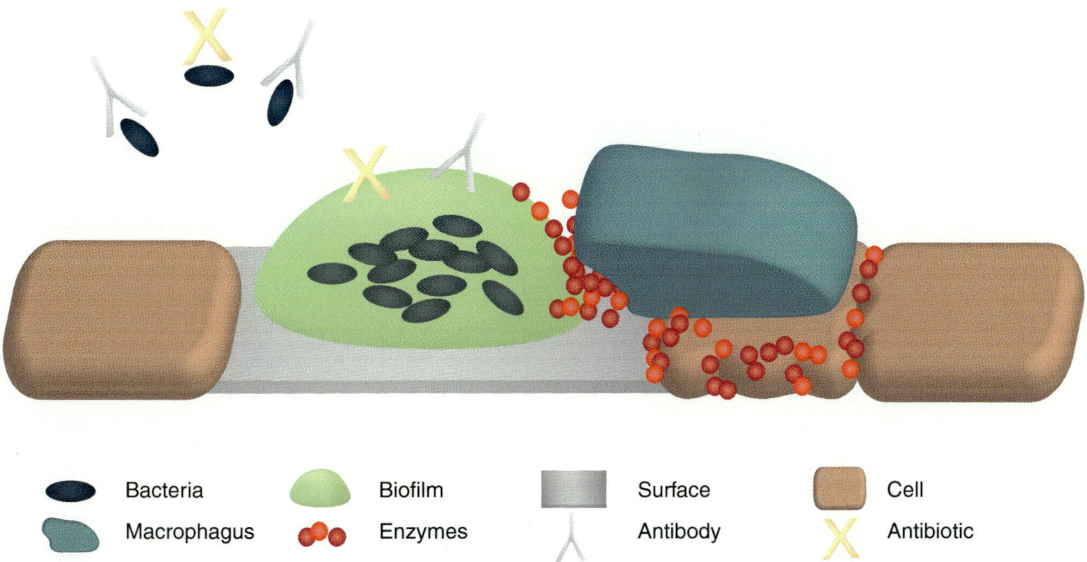

Fig. 21.3 While bacteria in planktonic can be cleaned by host defense mechanisms and antibiotic, sessile forms are protected. Enzymes and other host defense mechanisms that enable to destroy biofilm and enzymes and other inflammatory molecules released may cause damage to the host cells. Such damage could be responsible of implant mobilization

In this stage biofilms reach their ultimate thickness, generally greater than 100 μm with mushroom-shaped or tower-like microcolonies (Zoubos et al. 2012).

At this stage the biofilm shows maximum resistance to antibiotics (Høiby et al. 2010b).

Stage IV, during this stage, maybe due to bacteriophage activity within the biofilm, focal areas of the biofilm dissolve, so that some of the bacteria develop the planktonic phenotype and leave the biofilm, such event may cause metastatic expansion of the infection and a reactivation of clinical features (Webb et al. 2003; Gristina et al. 1987) (Figs. 21.3 and 21.4).

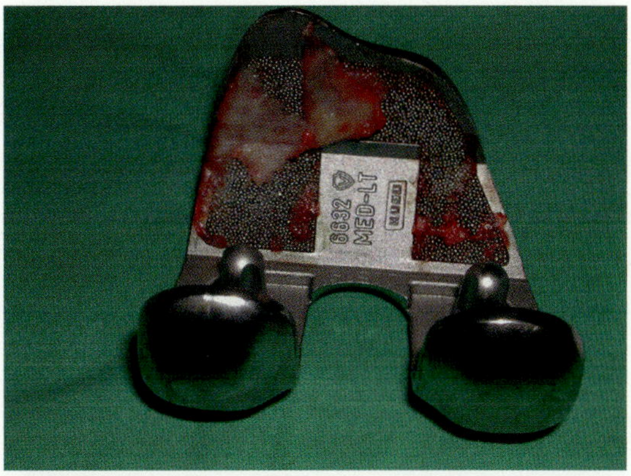

Fig. 21.4 Macroscopic aspect of a biofilm colony on a femoral knee prosthesis component explanted due to infection

21.3 Biofilm, a "Survival" or "Virulence" Mechanism for Bacteria

Using QS, biofilm bacteria behave very intelligently, adjusting the growth of colonies in response to various challenges; the complexity of biofilm structure and metabolism has led to the analogy of biofilms to tissues of more complex organisms (Costerton et al. 1995).

Living in biofilms, the bacteria are protected from deleterious conditions; this structure and its physiological attributes confer an inherent resistance to antimicrobial agents, whether these antimicrobial agents are antibiotics, disinfectants, or germicides. Cells in different regions of a biofilm exhibit different patterns of gene expression; likewise, growth, protein synthesis, and metabolic activity are stratified in biofilms (Davies et al. 1993).

Even if the structures that form biofilms contain channels in which nutrients can circulate (An YH and Friedmann RJ 1998), inspection of environmental as well as in vitro biofilms has revealed that the oxygen as well as nutrition concentration may be different in different areas of the matrix (Beer et al. 1994; Costerton et al. 1995).

Because of these nutritional and oxygen gradient, bacteria within a biofilm exist in different metabolic zones (Stewart and Franklin 2008). Nutrient-depleted zones can result in a stationary phase – like dormancy within the biofilm – which may be responsible for the general resistance of biofilms forming bacteria to antibiotics. Therefore, limited penetration of nutrients, rather than restricted antibiotic diffusion, may contribute to a generalized resistance or tolerance to antibiotics (Stoodley and Stoodley 2009).

Example of such metabolic heterogeneity is as described by Rani et al. (Rani et al. 2007) that *S. epidermidis* growing in a biofilm existed in four metabolic states: aerobic, fermentative growth, dead, and dormant.

Due to increased production of endogenous reactive oxygen species and a deficient antioxidant system, the mutation frequency of biofilm-growing bacteria is significantly increased compared with planktonically growing isogenic bacteria, and there is increased horizontal gene transmission in biofilms. Plasmid interchange is largely facilitated inside biofilm. The reason is the close proximity of bacteria; reduction of shear forces by the slime also eases conjugating process (Ehlers and Bouwer 1999).

These physiological conditions may explain why biofilm-growing bacteria easily become multidrug resistant by means of traditional resistance mechanisms against β-lactam antibiotics, aminoglycosides, and fluoroquinolones, which are detected by routine susceptibility testing in the clinical microbiology laboratory where planktonic bacterial growth is investigated. Thus, bacterial cells in biofilms may simultaneously produce enzymes that degrade antibiotics, have antibiotic targets of low affinity, and over-express efflux pumps that have a broad range of substrates (Driffield et al. 2008; Molin and Tolker-Nielsen 2003).

The matrix can provide bacteria with protection also from host defense mechanisms. Bacterial cells inside the biofilm are well protected from complement system, neutrophilic granulocytes, killer cells, antibiotic peptides, antibodies, and phagocytosis. This impairment of host defense mechanisms has been demonstrated in a number of in vitro models.

Staphylococcus epidermidis is the paradigmatic example of virulence due to biofilm. Such a bacterium is generally not considered pathogenic, and its presence on normal skin and mucosal surface is not normally associated with any signs of inflammatory or immune reactions. However, the host-staphylococcal balance becomes disrupted if the bacterium gains entry into the tissues and especially if it reaches an orthopedic implant. After adhering to the implant surface, *Staphylococcus epidermidis* secretes a layer of slime that can inhibit the phagocytic activity of neutrophils (Shiau and Wu 1998) and decreases its antibiotic susceptibility significantly making this infection very hard to treat (Sousa 2011; Shiau and Wu 1998).

21.4 The Fight Against the Slime

As Roman's said "divide et impera," the better way to fight against biofilm forming bacteria is before the bacterial adherence to the foreign material has taken place, therefore before bacteria assume multicellular lifestyle. In such a "war," the host, the wound, and all the environmental factors are involved. In the next pages, we will focus on antimicrobial prophylaxis, the role of the antimicrobial therapy in the treatment of PJI, and perspectives for the future possible new molecules and target.

21.4.1 Antimicrobial Prophylaxis

Perioperative antibiotic prophylaxis in orthopedic surgery is a broadly accepted practice, especially in prosthetic surgery (Borens et al. 2013).

It must be emphasized that perioperative antibiotic prophylaxis is not intended to sterilize tissues but to reduce the microbial burden of intraoperative contamination to a level that cannot overwhelm host defenses (Mangram et al. 1999). The goal is to achieve serum and tissue drug levels that exceed, for the duration of the operation, the minimum inhibitory concentration (MIC) for the organisms likely to be encountered during the operation (Bratzler and Houck 2004).

Important questions related to antibiotics before surgery are: *which antibiotics to give, when to give, and for how long.*

21.4.1.1 Which Antibiotics in Prophylaxis

In general, the selection of prophylactic antibiotic should be based on its spectrum of action, pharmacokinetics and safety profile, local hospital infections epidemiology and resistance patterns, antibiotics availability, and their relative cost. For practical reasons and due to better biodisponibility, prophylaxis is routinely given intravenously (i.v.).

In particular, in orthopedic prosthetic surgery, the agent must have a half-life that covers the decisive interval (the first 2 h after incision or contamination) with therapeutic tissue concentrations from the time of incision to wound closure and must be active against *Staphylococcus aureus* and *Staphylococcus epidermidis* which cause the majority of the implant-related infections (Rao 2008; Fulkerson 2006).

According to the present state of knowledge, cefazolin, the first-generation cephalosporin, is the most commonly studied and used for perioperative antibiotic prophylaxis in primary total joint replacement with a recommended dose of 1–2 g IV.

Cefazolin is preferred because of its activity against methicillin-sensitive *Staphylococcus aureus* (MSSA) and streptococci, for its safety profile, excellent distribution in the bone, muscle, and synovia, and low cost. Cefuroxime is a second-generation cephalosporin and has broader activity against Gram-negative bacteria than the first generation [61].

Recently cefuroxime at a dosage of 1.5 g i.v. has been recommended for total hip arthroplasty (Prokuski 2008; Bratzler and Hunt 2006; Kalman and Barriere 1990).

In case of a serious allergy or adverse reaction to β-lactams, although there are few data supporting its use for routine prophylaxis, clindamycin (600–900 mg) currently is the preferred alternative (Bratzler and Houck 2004; Gradl et al. 2011; Matar et al. 2010).

Patients with previous history of methicillin-resistant *Staphylococcus aureus* (MRSA) infection, institutions with high rate of MRSA (>10 %) and methicillin-resistant *Staphylococcus epidermidis* (MRSE) (>20 %) orthopedic surgical site infections (SSIs), and patients colonized with MRSA should undergo to perioperative prophylaxis with vancomycin (American Society of Health-System Pharmacists 2011).

Vancomycin has adequate activity against the most common high-resistant pathogens involved in orthopedic procedures, and it reaches high concentrations in the bone, synovia, and muscle within minutes after administration (Eshkenazi et al. 2001). It is important to keep in mind that the recommended dose should be adjusted to patient's weight. A routine use of vancomycin should be discouraged since its routinely prophylactic use is associated with vancomycin-resistant *Enterococcus* colonization and infection (French 1998).

21.4.1.2 When to Give Antibiotics

The importance of antibiotic delivery timing is known since the 1970s when Miles and Burke established that the efficacy of antibiotics in reducing the dermal lesions after subcutaneous bacterial inoculation in a guinea pig model was associated with its administration during surgery or a few hours after wound closing. By delaying the administration of antibiotics by only 3 or 4 h, the resulting lesions were identical in size to those of animals not receiving antibiotic prophylaxis. This concept was confirmed in 1992 by Classen in a large study including surgical procedures performed in 2.847 patients in which 313 (11 %) were arthroplasty.

The authors found that the rate of infection was lower for patients who had received an antibiotic from zero to 2 h before the incision (Classen et al. 1992).

A study from Switzerland performed further investigations about the timing of prophylactic

Table 21.1 Prophylaxis recommendations during prosthetic surgery

	Institution with <10 % SSIs MRSA <20 % SSIs MRSE	Institution with >10 % SSIs MRSA >20 % SSIs MRSE
Cefazolin 1–2 g IV or Cefuroxime 1.5 g IV	X	X
Vancomycin 1 g IV	_	X
Patients with adverse reaction to β-lactams clindamycin 600–900 mg iv	X	X

antibiotics. That study shows that administration of cefuroxime 59–30 min before incision is more effective than during the last half hour (Weber et al. 2008).

Hence, the American Academy of Orthopedic Surgeons (AAOS) recommends prophylactic antibiotics to be completely infused within 1 h before the surgical incision (American Academy of Orthopaedic Surgeons http://www.aaos.org/about/papers/ advistmt/1027.asp).

Other issues of antibiotic prophylaxis may be pointed out as follows:

1. Dose amount should be proportional to patient weight; for patients >80 kg, the doses of cefazolin should be doubled.
2. Vancomycin due to an extended infusion time, (10 mg/min or less to avoid infusion related events, i.e., "red man" syndrome) should be started within 2 h prior to incision. It is imperative to completely infuse antibiotic solution before surgical incision.
3. Additional intraoperative doses of antibiotic are advised if:
   - The duration of the procedure exceeds one to two times the antibiotic's half-life. As prophylaxis, cefazolin can be re-dosed every 2–5 h, cefuroxime every 3–4 h, clindamycin ever 3–6 h, and vancomycin every 6–12 h (American Society of Health-System Pharmacists 1999).
   - There is significant blood loss during the procedure (more than 1.5 l).

21.4.1.3 For How Long Antibiotics Must Be Administrated?

The duration of antibiotic prophylaxis in total joint arthroplasty is still controversial, and there is still insufficient evidence to support single-dose regimens. Mauerhan et al. compared the efficacy of a 1-day regimen of cefuroxime with a 3-day regimen in a prospective, double-blind, multicenter study of 1,354 patients treated with an arthroplasty and concluded that there was no significant difference in the prevalence of wound infections between the two groups (Mauerhan et al. 1994).

The current recommendation of the AAOS is that prophylactic antibiotics should be discontinued within 24 h of the end of surgery (Table 21.1) (American Academy of Orthopaedic Surgeons http://www.aaos.org/about/papers/ advistmt/1027.asp).

21.4.2 The Role of Antibiotic Therapy After PJI

The management of PJI generally relies on a combination of antimicrobial therapy and surgery. Two-stage reimplantation is considered the standard surgical procedure (Fig. 21.5) while other surgical strategies include: one-stage exchange procedures, resection arthroplasty, amputation, and debridement and retention. The latter can be considered in patients with a short duration of symptoms (patients diagnosed with a PJI within approximately 30 days from prosthesis implantation or <3 weeks of onset of infectious) in the absence of implant loosening and soft tissue damage. Finally, whenever surgical procedures cannot be performed and infected prosthesis is retained, a chronic suppressive antibiotic treatment is advisable (Laffer, et al. 2006; Matthews et al. 2009; Trampuz and

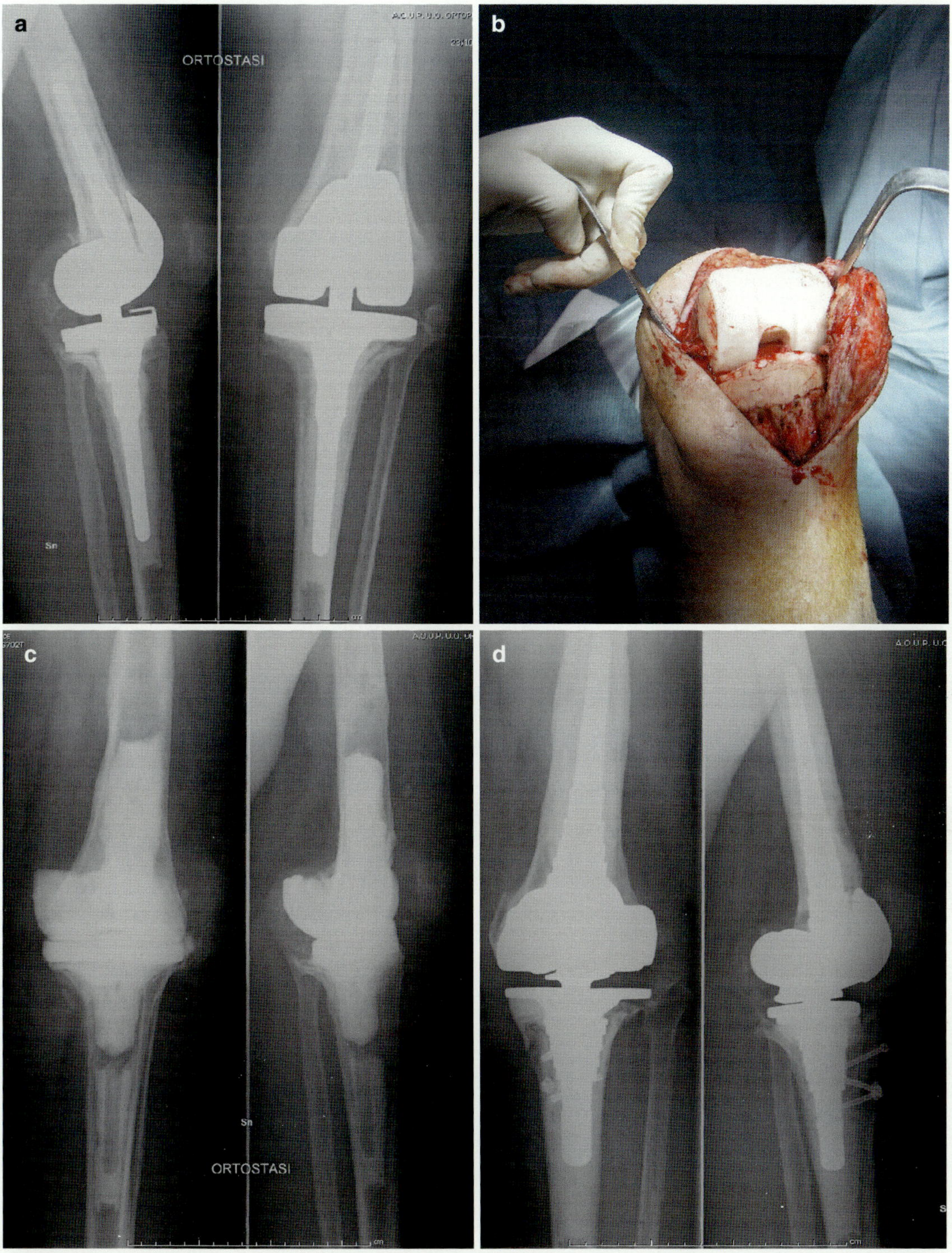

Fig. 21.5 (**a**) X-ray showing a mobilization of a revision knee prosthesis due to infection, (**b**) intraoperative picture of the cement spacer used during two-stage exchange, (**c**) X-ray of the cement spacer, (**d**) X-ray 1 year after the spacer removal

Table 21.2 Adapted and simplified IDSA guidelines on the management of prosthetic joint infections

Microorganism	Preferred treatment	Alternative treatment
Staphylococci, methicillin susceptible	Nafcillin sodium 1.5–2 g i.v. q4-6 h or Cefazolin 1–2 g i.v. q8 h or Ceftriaxone 1–2 g i.v. q24 h	Vancomycin 15–20 mg/kg i.v. q12h or Daptomycin 6 mg/kg i.v. q24 h or Linezolid 600 mg po/i.v. q12 h
Staphylococci, methicillin resistant	Vancomycin 15–20 mg/kg i.v. q12 h	Daptomycin 6 mg/kg i.v. q24 h or Linezolid 600 mg po/i.v. q12 h
Enterococcus spp., penicillin susceptible	Penicillin G 20–24 million units q24 h i.v. or Ampicillin sodium 12 g i.v. q24 h	Vancomycin 15–20 mg/kg i.v. q12 h or Daptomycin 6 mg/kg q24 h or Linezolid 600 mg po/i.v. q12 h
Enterococcus spp, penicillin resistant	Vancomycin 15–20 mg/kg i.v. q12 h	Linezolid 600 mg po/i.v. q12 h or Daptomycin 6 mg i.v. q24 h
Pseudomonas aeruginosa	Cefepime 2 g i.v. q12 h or Meropenem 1 g i.v. q8 h	Ciprofloxacin 500–750 mg po q12 h Ceftazidime 2 g i.v. q8 h

Reproduced with permission from Osmon et al. (2013), Oxford University Press
Abbreviations: *i.v.* intravenous, *q* every, *po* per oral, *h* hours

Zimmerli 2008; Zimmerli, et al. 2004, 1998; Stewart and Costerton 2001).

In any case, it is of paramount importance the use of pathogen-targeted and biofilm-active antibiotics, particularly in case of retention of the prosthesis.

Guidelines on the management of prosthetic joint infections have been issued in 2013 by the Infectious Diseases Society of America (IDSA), and pathogen-targeted options are reported in Table 21.2 (Osmon et al. 2013).

In addition to that, there are several published studies both in vivo and in vitro performed to evaluate antibiotics activity against sessile bacteria. Widmer et al. analyzed the efficacy of different antibiotics on animal infection models in which prosthetic infection was caused by *Staphylococcus epidermidis*. It was noted that fluoroquinolones monotherapy (like ciprofloxacin) has a low efficacy, but this rises to 90 % if combined with rifampicin (Widmer et al. 1990). Among the antibiotics indicated for implant-related staphylococcal infections, rifampicin not only has a good bioavailability and an excellent anti-staphylococcal activity, but it also has an excellent penetration in soft tissues, bone, abscesses, and polymorphonucleates. It also succeeds in eradicating organisms that adhere to prosthetic surfaces during a steady growth stage. However, the use of rifampicin is limited by rapid development of resistance (therefore, it must always be combined with another antibiotic), toxic effects (such as nausea, hepatic disorder), and drugs interactions (Darley and MacGowan 2004).

Last-generation fluoroquinolones (such as moxifloxacin and levofloxacin) present lower MICs in vitro than ciprofloxacin in the presence of Gram-positive microorganisms. However, data regarding their penetration and efficacy in bone infections are still not available. Furthermore, the resistance of nosocomial staphylococci to quinolones has dramatically increased. At the moment, 90 % of nosocomial MRSA are also resistant to quinolones (Darley and MacGowan 2004; Stein et al. 1998).

Clinical studies show that the use of rifampicin and fluoroquinolones as a monotherapy in the cure of orthopedic implant infections associated with staphylococci results in the emergence of antibiotic-resistant isolates in most cases. The association of fluoroquinolones and rifampicin is highly effective in eradicating implant-associated staphylococci and in preventing the emergence of ciprofloxacin-resistant strains. This association has also the advantage of an excellent oral bioavailability of both active principles, which reach serum concentrations comparable to those obtained during intravenous therapy. High levels of intracellular penetration and activity against intracellular staphylococci are also obtained (Bernard et al. 2004; Zimmerli et al. 1998).

Daptomycin has been demonstrated to be more effective than vancomycin for the treatment of experimental foreign body and systemic infections by biofilm-producing methicillin-resistant *S. epidermidis* [1]. However, better results were obtained by the combination of daptomycin and netilmicin, as opposed to daptomycin monotherapy. Similarly, better results were obtained with vancomycin in combination with netilmicin compared to vancomycin monotherapy (Domínguez-Herrera et al. 2012; Widmer et al. 1990).

Linezolid, a relatively recently introduced oxazolidinone compound, is also active against beta-lactam and vancomycin-resistant Gram-positive bacteria, and it has been used in the treatment of PJI with encouraging results (Bassetti et al. 2005). A combination of linezolid and high-dose daptomycin was more effective than each agent alone in an in vitro model of biofilm-producing *Staphylococcus aureus* infection (Parra-Ruiz et al. 2012).

In an in vitro biofilm model of *S. aureus* infection, fosfomycin enhanced the activity of linezolid, minocycline, vancomycin, and teicoplanin, and these combinatorial treatments were even better than rifampicin combination regimens (Tang et al. 2012).

Indeed the properties of the biofilm change with time; with age, many biofilms become increasingly resistant to antibiotics. Monzon et al. demonstrated the efficacy of vancomycin against *Staphylococcus epidermidis* decreased as a biofilm aged. This phenomenon was not demonstrated for all antibiotics; the activity of rifampicin and tetracyclines was not altered (Monzon, et al. 2002).

In conclusion, evidence suggests that combination regimens can be more effective in treatment of biofilm-associated infections, with respect to monotherapy. Particularly, rifampicin seems to represent an ideal partner drug in most cases.

The duration of antibiotic after debridement and retention varies in reported clinical studies ranging from 6 months to greater than 4 years. In a study by Laffer et al., there was no difference in outcome in patients receiving 3–6 months of antibiotics compared with greater than 6 months (91 % vs. 87 % success). Recent IDSA guidelines recommend, in case of debridement and retention of the prosthesis, 2–6 weeks of pathogen-specific intravenous antimicrobial therapy in combination with oral rifampicin followed by rifampicin plus a companion oral drug for a total of 3 months for a hip prosthesis infection and 6 months for a knee prosthesis infection (Laffer et al. 2006; Osmon et al. 2013).

21.4.3 Future Perspectives: New Molecules and Target

The increasing scientific knowledge on the molecular mechanisms of adhesion and development of bacterial biofilm has opened the way to find new therapeutical targets and a number of molecules and new strategies to "fight" against any stage of biofilm formation (Kostakioti et al. 2013).

Anti-adhesion agents such as mannosides and pilicides have been developed to contrast bacterial attachment to the foreign body (stage I). Cusumano et al. demonstrated in vitro that mannosides prevented uropathogenic *Escherichia coli* (UPEC) biofilm formation in vitro and were shown to disrupt preformed biofilms (Cusumano et al. 2011).

Pilicides which are compounds rationally designed to interfere with export of the corresponding pilin subunits were shown to inhibit UPEC biofilm formation in vitro by 50 %, at concentrations as low as 3 mM (Chorell et al. 2010).

"Antimatrix" agents such as enzymes and chelating agents. These molecules are able to interfere with stage II of the biofilm formation disrupting components of the extracellular matrix. Burton et al. (2006) tested the effect of inhibitors of the N-acetil-D-glucosamine-1-phosphate acetyltransferase (GlmU) which is implicated in the LPS synthesis. Such inhibitors showed antibiofilm activity against clinical isolates of *E. coli, P. aeruginosa, K. pneumoniae, S. epidermidis, and E. faecalis* (Burton et al. 2006).

Similar results were shown with other enzymes with different targets such as DNase I and dispersin B engineered into a phage (Guiton et al. 2009; Lu and Collins 2007).

Other possible antibiofilm molecules are *QS inhibitors*, able to interfere with bacterial signaling cascades which is, as mentioned above of paramount importance, during colony formation and maturation (Bearson and Bearson 2008; Wang et al. 2011).

For instance, QS inhibitors injected systemically into rats have been found to have strong activity in preventing methicillin-resistant *Staphylococcus aureus* graft infections (Balaban et al. 2007).

Various other agents have been reported to have a possible activity on bacterial biofilms, including corticosteroids (Goggin et al. 2013), nonsteroidal anti-inflammatory drugs (Bink et al. 2012), ginseng extracts (Wu et al. 2011), and electrical current (Del Pozo et al. 2009). However, more studies are needed to assess their efficacy and clinical applicability.

Conclusions

Biofilm development is an essential step in the establishment of a PJI, conferring to bacteria a biological advantage against antibiotics; thus surgery becomes necessary.

Currently, prevention with adequate pharmacological prophylaxis is mandatory. The surgical treatment of an established PJI in conjunction with pathogen-specific antibiotics, biofilm-specific antibiotics, and combined antimicrobial regimens results of paramount importance.

The knowledge on the mechanisms of biofilm formation has greatly deepened, possibly leading in the next future to the development of new weapons and strategies in the armamentarium of physicians for fighting against PJI.

Key Points

- Aside from the life-threatening complications of total hip replacement, no postoperative complication could be more devastating than infection.
- Bacteria growing in a biofilm are more recalcitrant to the action of antibiotics and host defenses than cells growing in a planktonic state.
- Perioperative antibiotic prophylaxis is the standard prevention of infection for all patients undergoing total joint replacement.
- In the near future a better knowledge of the biofilm biology may lead to the developement of new antibiotic molecules and new antimicrobial targets.

Acknowledgments The authors thank Alessia Diaco for the support given in building figures and the editors for the excellent opportunity of writing a chapter of this book.

References

American Academy of Orthopaedic Surgeons. Information statement: recommendations for the use of intravenous antibiotic prophylaxis in primary total joint arthroplasty. http://www.aaos.org/about/papers/advistmt/1027.asp

American Society of Health-System Pharmacists (1999) ASHP therapeutic guidelines on antimicrobial prophylaxis in surgery. Am J Health Syst Pharm 56:1839–1888

American Society of Health-System Pharmacists (2011) Draft therapeutic guidelines on antimicrobial prophylaxis in surgery. 2011. http://www.ashp.org/DocLibrary/BestPractices/TGSurgery.aspx

An YH, Friedmann RJ (1998) Concise review of mechanisms of bacterial adhesion to biomaterial surfaces. J Biomed Mater Res 43:338–348

Arciola CR, Campoccia D, Montanaro L (2002) Effects of antibiotic resistance of Staphylococcus epidermidis following adhesion to polymethylmethacrylate and to silicone surfaces. Biomaterials 23:1495–1502

Balaban N, Cirioni O, Giacometti A et al (2007) Treatment of Staphylococcus aureus biofilm infection by the quorum-sensing inhibitor RIP. Antimicrob Agents Chemother 51(6):2226–2229

Bassetti M, Vitale F, Melica G et al (2005) Linezolid in the treatment of Gram-positive prosthetic joint infections. J Antimicrob Chemother 55:387–390. doi:10.1093/jac/dki016

Bearson BL, Bearson SM (2008) The role of the QseC quorum- sensing sensor kinase in colonization and norepinephrine- enhanced motility of Salmonella enterica serovar Typhimurium. Microb Pathog 44:271–278

Beer D, Stoodley P, Lewandowski Z (1994) Liquid flow in heterogeneous biofilm. Biotechnol Bioeng 44:636–641

Bernard L, Hoffmeyer P, Assal M et al (2004) Trends in the treatment of orthopaedic prosthetic infections. J Antimicrob Chemother 53(2):127–129, Review

Bink A, Kucharíková S, Neirinck B et al (2012) The nonsteroidal antiinflammatory drug diclofenac potentiates the in vivo activity of caspofungin against Candida albicans biofilms. J Infect Dis 206(11):1790–1797

Borens O, Yusuf E, Trampuz A (2013) Surgical Site Infections (SSIs): risk factors and prevention strategies. Eur Instr Lect 13:15–25

Bratzler DW, Houck PM (2004) Antimicrobial prophylaxis for surgery: an advisory statement from the National Surgical Infection Prevention Project. Clin Infect Dis 38:1706–1715

Bratzler DW, Hunt DR (2006) The surgical infection prevention and surgical care improvement projects: national initiatives to improve outcomes for patients having surgery. Clin Infect Dis 43(3):322

Burton E, Gawande PV, Yakandawala N et al (2006) Antibiofilm activity of GlmU enzyme inhibitors against catheter-associated uropathogens. Antimicrob Agents Chemother 50:1835–1840

Chorell E, Pinkner JS, Phan G et al (2010) Design and synthesis of C-2 substituted thiazolo and dihydrothiazolo ring-fused 2-pyridones: pilicides with increased antivirulence activity. J Med Chem 53:5690–5695

Classen DC, Evans RS, Pestotnik SL et al (1992) The timing of prophylactic administration of antibiotics and the risk of surgical-wound infection. N Engl J Med 326(5):281–286

Costerton JW, Lewandowski Z, Caldwell DE et al (1995) Microbial biofilms. Annu Rev Microbiol 49:711–745

Costerton JW, Stewart PS, Greenberg EP (1999) Bacterial biofilms: a common cause of persistent infections. Science 284:1318–1322

Costerton JW, Montanaro L, Arciola CR (2007) Bacterial communications in implant infections: a target for an intelligence war. Int J Artif Organs 30(9):757–763

Coventry MB (1975) Treatment of infections occurring in total hip surgery. Orthop Clin North Am 6(4):991–1003

Cristhensen GD, Simpson WA, Bisno AL et al (1982) Adherence of slime-producing Staphylococcus epidermidis to smooth surfaces. Infect Immun 37(1):318–326

Cusumano CK, Pinkner J, Han Z et al (2011) Treatment and prevention of UTI with orally active mannoside FimH inhibitors. Sci Transl Med 3:109ra115

Darley ES, MacGowan AP (2004) Antibiotic treatment of gram-positive bone and joint infections. J Antimicrob Chemother 53(6):928–935

Darouiche RO (2001) Device-associated infections: a macroproblem that starts with microadherence. Clin Infect Dis 33:1567–1572

Davies DG, Chakrabarty AM, Geesey GG (1993) Exopolysaccharide production in biofilms: substratum activation of alginate gene expression by Pseudomonas aeruginosa. Appl Environ Microbiol 59:1181–1886

Del Pozo JL, Rouse MS, Mandrekar JN et al (2009) Effect of electrical current on the activities of antimicrobial agents against Pseudomonas aeruginosa, Staphylococcus aureus, and Staphylococcus epidermidis biofilms. Antimicrob Agents Chemother 53(1):35–40

Domínguez-Herrera J, Docobo-Pérez F, López-Rojas R et al (2012) Efficacy of daptomycin versus vancomycin in an experimental model of foreign-body and systemic infection caused by biofilm producers and methicillin-resistant Staphylococcus epidermidis. Antimicrob Agents Chemother 56(2):613–617

Donlan RM (2002) Biofilms: microbial life on surfaces. Emerg Infect Dis 8:881–890

Driffield K, Miller K, Bostock M et al (2008) Increased mutability of Pseudomonas aeruginosa in biofilms. J Antimicrob Chemother 61:1053–1056

Ehlers LJ, Bouwer EJ (1999) RP4 plasmid transfer among species of Pseudomonas in a bio fi lm reactor. Water Sci Technol 7:163–171

Eshkenazi AU, Garti A, Tamir L et al (2001) Serum and synovial vancomycin concentrations following prophylactic administration in knee arthroplasty. Am J Knee Surg 14(4):221–223

Foster TJ, McDevit TD (1994) Molecular basis of adherence of staphylococci to biomaterials. In: Bisno AL, Waldvo gel FA (eds) Infection associated with indwelling medical devices. American Society for Microbiology, Washington, pp 31–43

French GL (1998) Enterococci and vancomycin resistance. Clin Infect Dis 27(Suppl 1):S75–S83

Fulkerson E, Valle CJ, Wise B et al (2006) Antibiotic susceptibility of bacteria infecting total joint arthroplasty sites. J Bone Joint Surg Am 88:1231–1237

Giulieri SG, Graber P, Ochsner PE et al (2004) Management of infection associated with total hip arthroplasty according to a treatment algorithm. Infection 32(4):222–228

Goggin R, Jardeleza C, Wormald PJ et al (2013) Corticosteroids directly reduce Staphylococcus aureus biofilm growth: an in vitro study. Laryngoscope(Jul 23)

Gradl G, Horn C, Postl LK et al (2011) Antibiotic prophylaxis in primary and revision hip arthroplasty: what is the evidence? Orthopade 40(6):520–527

Gristina AG, Costerton JW (2009) Bacterial adherence to biomaterials and tissue. The significance of its role in clinical sepsis to biomaterials. J Bone Joint Surg Am 67-A:264–273

Gristina AG, Hobgood CD, Webb LX (1987) Adhesive colonisation of biomaterials and antibiotic resistance. Biomaterials 8:423–426

Gristina AG, Oga M, Webb LX et al (1995) Adherent bacterial colonization in the pathogenesis of osteomyelitis. Science 228:990–993

Guiton PS, Hung CS, Kline KA et al (2009) Contribution of autolysin and Sortase A during Enterococcus faecalis DNA-dependent biofilm development. Infect Immun 77:3626–3638

Hall-Stoodley L, Stoodley P (2009) Evolving concepts in biofilm infections. Cell Microbiol 11(7):1034–1043. doi:10.1111/j.1462-5822.2009.01323

Hasty DL, Ofek I, Courtney HS et al (1992) Multiple adhesins for streptococci. Infect Immun 60:2147–2152

Hetrick EM, Schoenfisch MH (2006) Reducing implant-related infections: active release strategies. Chem Soc Rev 35:780–789

Høiby N, Bjarnsholt T, Givskov M et al (2010a) Antibiotic resistance of bacterial biofilms. Int J Antimicrob Agents 35:322–332

Høiby N, Ciofu O, Bjarnsholt T (2010b) Pseudomonas aeruginosa biofilms in cystic fibrosis. Future Microbiol 5(11):1663–1674
Kalman D, Barriere SL (1990) Review of the pharmacology, pharmacokinetics, and clinical use of cephalosporins. Tex Heart Inst J 17:203–215
Kostakioti M, Hadjifrangiskou M, Hultgren SJ (2013) Bacterial biofilms: development, dispersal, and therapeutic strategies in the dawn of the postantibiotic era. Cold Spring Harb Perspect Med. doi:10.1101/cshperspect.a010306
Krekeler C, Ziehr H, Klein J (1989) Physical methods for characterization of microbial cell surfaces. Experientia 45:1047–1054
Laffer RR, Graber P, Ochsner PE et al (2006) Outcome of prosthetic knee-associated infection: evaluation of 40 consecutive episodes at a single centre. Clin Microbiol Infect 12(5):433–439
Lazar V (2011) Quorum sensing in bioflms—how to destroy the bacterial citadels or their cohesion/power? Anaerobe 17(6):280–285
Lenz AP, Williamson KS, Pitts B et al (2008) Localized gene expression in Pseudomonas aeruginosa biofilms. Appl Environ Microbiol 74:4463–4471
Lu TK, Collins JJ (2007) Dispersing biofilms with engineered enzymatic bacteriophage. Proc Natl Acad Sci 104:11197–11202
Mack KD, Bartscht S, Dobinsky MA et al (2000) Staphylococcal factors involved in adhesion and biofilm formation on biomaterials. In: An YH, Friedmann RJ (eds) Handbook of bacterial adhesion. Principles, principles, methods, and applications. Humana Press Inc, Totowa, pp 307–330
Mangram AJ, Horan TC, Pearson ML et al (1999) The Hospital Infection Control Practices Advisory Committee. Guideline for the prevention of surgical site infection. Infect Control Hosp Epidemiol 20:247–280
Matar WY, Jafari SM, Restrepo C et al (2010) Preventing infection in total joint arthroplasty. J Bone Joint Surg Am 92(Suppl 2):36–46
Matthews PC, Berendt AR, McNally MA et al (2009) Diagnosis and management of prosthetic joint infection. British Medical Journal 338, b1773–b1773
Mauerhan DR, Nelson CL, Smith DL et al (1994) Prophylaxis against infection in total joint arthroplasty. One day of cefuroxime compared with three days of cefazolin. J Bone Joint Surg Am 76:39–45
Molin S, Tolker-Nielsen T (2003) Gene transfer occurs with enhanced efficiency in biofilms and induces enhanced stabilisation of the biofilm structure. Curr Opin Biotechnol 14:255–261
Montanaro L, Arciola CR (2000) Studying bacterial adhesion to irregular or porous surfaces. In: An YH, Friedmann RJ (eds) Handbook of bacterial adhesion. Principles, methods and applications. Humana Press Inc, Totowa, pp 331–343
Monzon M, Oteiza C, Leiva J et al (2002) Biofilm testing of Staphylococcus epidermidis clinical isolates: low performance of vancomycin in relation to other antibiotics. Diagn Microbiol Infect Dis 44:319–324
Osmon DR, Berbari EF, Berendt AR et al (2013) Diagnosis and management of prosthetic joint infection: clinical practice guidelines by the Infectious Diseases Society of America. Clin Infect Dis 56(1):e1–e25
Parra-Ruiz J, Bravo-Molina A, Peña-Monje A et al (2012) Activity of linezolid and high-dose daptomycin, alone or in combination, in an in vitro model of Staphylococcus aureus biofilm. J Antimicrob Chemother 67(11):2682–2685
Patti JM, Allen BL, McGavin MJ et al (1994) MSCRAMM-mediated adherence of microorganisms to host tissues. Annu Rev Microbiol 48:585–617
Prokuski L (2008) Prophylactic antibiotics in orthopaedic surgery. J Am Acad Orthop Surg 16:283–293
Rani SA, Pitts B, Beyenal H et al (2007) Spatial patterns of DNA replication, protein synthesis, and oxygen concentration within bacterial biofilms reveal diverse physiological states. J Bacteriol 189:4223–4233
Rao N, Cannella B, Crossett LS et al (2008) A preoperative decolonization protocol for Staphylococcus aureus prevents orthopaedic infections. Clin Orthop Relat Res 466:1343–1348
Rohde H, Frankenberger S, Z¨ahringer U et al (2010) Structure, function and contribution of polysaccharide intercellular adhesin (PIA) to Staphylococcus epidermidis biofilm formation and pathogenesis of biomaterial-associated infections. Eur J Cell Biol 89:103–111
Rorabeck CH, Bourne RB, Laupacis A et al (1994) A double-blind study of 250 cases comparing cemented with cementless total hip arthroplasty. Cost-effectiveness and its impact on health-related quality of life. Clin Orthop Relat Res 298:156–164
Schamalzried TP, Amstutz HC, Au MK (1992) Etiology of deep sepsis in total hip arthroplasty: the significance of hematogenous and recurrent infections. Clin Orthop Relat Res 280:200–207
Shiau AL, Wu CL (1998) The inhibitory effect of Staphylococcus epidermidis slime on the phagocytosis of murine peritoneal macrophages is interferon-independent. Microbiol Immunol 42:33–40
Sousa C (2011) Staphylococcus epidermidis: adhesion and biofilm formation onto biomaterials. LAP LAMBERT Academic Publishing, Saarbrü cken
Stanley NR, Britton RA, Grossman AD et al (2003) Identification of catabolite repression as a physiological regulator of biofilm formation by Bacillus subtilis by use of DNA microarrays. J Bacteriol 185: 1951–1957
Stein A, Bataille JF, Drancourt M et al (1998) Ambulatory treatment of multidrug-resistant Staphylococcus-infected orthopedic implants with high-dose oral co-trimoxazole (trimethoprim-sulfamethoxazole). Antimicrob Agents Chemother 42(12):3086–3091
Stewart PS, Costerton JW (2001) Antibiotic resistance of bacteria in biofilms. Lancet 358:135–138

Stewart PS, Franklin MJ (2008) Physiological heterogeneity in biofilms. Nat Rev Microbiol 6:199–210

Stoodley P, Ehrlich GD, Sedghizadeh PP et al (2011) Orthopaedic biofilm infections. Curr Orthop Pract 22(6):558–563. doi:10.1097/BCO.0b013e318230efcf

Tang HJ, Chen CC, Cheng KC et al (2012) In vitro efficacy of fosfomycin-containing regimens against methicillin-resistant Staphylococcus aureus in biofilms. J Antimicrob Chemother 67(4):944–950

Taraszkiewicz A, Fila A, Grinholc M et al (2013) Innovative strategies to overcome biofilm resistance. BioMed Res Int 2013, Article ID 150653, 13 pages. http://dx.doi.org/10.1155/2013/150653

Trampuz A, Zimmerli W (2005) New strategies for the treatment of infections associated with prosthetic joints. Curr Opin Investig Drugs 6(2):185–190

Trampuz A, Zimmerli W (2008) Diagnosis and treatment of implant-associated septic arthritis and osteomyelitis. Current Infectious Disease Reports 10, 394–403

Vuong C, Voyich JM, Fischer ER et al (2004) Polysaccharide intercellular adhesin (PIA) protects Staphylococcus epidermidis against major components of the human innate immune system. Cell Microbiol 6:269–275

Wang X, Wang Q, Yang M et al (2011) QseBC controls flagellar motility, fimbrial hemagglutination and intracellular virulence in fish pathogen Edwardsiella tarda. Fish Shellfish Immunol 30:944–953

Webb JS, Thompson LS, James S et al (2003) Cell death in Pseudomonas aeruginosa biofilm development. J Bacteriol 185:4585–4592

Weber WP, Marti WR, Zwahlen M et al (2008) The timing of surgical antimicrobial prophylaxis. Ann Surg 247:918–926

Whiteley M, Bangera MG, Bumgarner RE et al (2001) Gene expression in Pseudomonas aeruginosa biofilms. Nature 413:860–864

Widmer AF, Frei R, Rajacic Z et al (1990) Correlation between in vivo and in vitro efficacy of antimicrobial agents against foreign body infections. J Infect Dis 162(1):96–102

Wiklund I, Romanus B (1991) A comparison of quality of life before and after arthroplasty in patients who had arthrosis of the hip joint. J Bone Joint Surg Am 73(5):765–769

Wu H, Lee B, Yang L et al (2011) Effects of ginseng on Pseudomonas aeruginosa motility and biofilm formation. FEMS Immunol Med Microbiol 62(1):49–56

Zimmerli W, Widmer AF, Blatter M et al (1998) Role of rifampin for treatment of orthopedic implant-related staphylococcal infections: a randomized controlled trial. Foreign-Body Infection (FBI) Study Group. JAMA 279(19):1537–1541

Zimmerli W, Trampuz A, Ochsner PE (2004) Prosthetic-joint infections. N Engl J Med 351(16):1701–1703

Zoubos AB, Galanakos SP, Soucacos PN (2012) Orthopedics and biofilm – what do we know? A review. Med Sci Monit 18(6):RA89–RA96, PMID: 22648264

Antibiofilm Strategies in Orthopedics: Where Are We?

22

Carlo Luca Romanò, Nicola Logoluso, and Lorenzo Drago

Open Questions

- How relevant is biofilm formation for implant-related infections in orthopedics ?
- Is it possible to prevent/treat biofilm formation with specific agents?
- How should we classify antibiofilm agents?
- Is there any example of a clinical application of antibiofilm strategies in orthopedics?
- What is the possible future?

C.L. Romanò (✉) • N. Logoluso
Center for Reconstructive Surgery and Osteoarticular Infections (Centro di Chirurgia Ricostruttiva e delle Infezioni Osteo-articolari – C.R.I.O.),
Istituto Ortopedico IRCCS Galeazzi,
via R. Galeazzi, 4, Milan 20161, Italy
e-mail: carlo.romano@grupposandonato.it; nicola.logoluso@gmail.com

L. Drago
Clinical-Chemistry and Microbiology Lab, Istituto Ortopedico IRCCS Galeazzi,
via R. Galeazzi, 4, Milan 20161, Italy
e-mail: lorenzo.drago@unimi.it

22.1 Introduction

Antimicrobials unquestionably represent the main outcome of medical research of the twentieth century, and they have been widely implemented in medical practices. Still, their application in the treatment of implant-related infections has not been as successful, since periprosthetic infections represent to date the first and third source of US knee and hip infections, respectively, according to Bozic et al. (2010) and Kurtz et al. (2007). In this particular field, in fact, microorganisms can be either suspended/free floating (planktonic) or they can stick to the surface of the biomaterial itself (sessile), and the two types can coexist. This twofold characterization of microorganisms consequently gives rise to a first major concern: the correct identification of pathogen. Cultures for acute infections were usually aimed at the identification of planktonic germs, but sessile bacteria, like those in periprosthetic infections, often fail to be detected through routine cultural techniques. To spot them, further and more advanced techniques, overcoming the failure of standard sampling and culture procedure, are in fact needed (Drago et al. 2012; Romanò et al. 2009; Chen et al. 2011; Stoodley et al. 2011; Arciola et al. 2011; Palmer et al. 2011; Hill et al. 2010; Zameer and Gopal 2010).

Furthermore, the combination of biofilm and sessile microorganisms can undermine the successfulness of the infection treatment itself, if the

A. Baldini, P. Caldora (eds.), *Perioperative Medical Management for Total Joint Arthroplasty: How to Control Hemostasis, Pain and Infection*, DOI 10.1007/978-3-319-07203-6_22,

biomaterial is not removed; sessile bacteria are in fact significantly more resistant to antimicrobial treatment than other, unprotected, microorganisms (Zameer and Gopal 2010), and chronic septic process, together with long-term infection recurrence, cannot be ruled out (Costerton et al. 1999). Microorganisms living in biofilms are reported to be not only more resistant to antibiotic therapies but also more resilient to the host's immune system. Moreover, it has been assessed that the communication between microorganisms living in biofilms is responsible for controlling several physiological processes, among which is the insurgence of antimicrobial resistance (Shih and Huang 2002; Costerton et al. 2005).

The correct treatment of biofilm-related infections thus starts from the correct targeting for both sessile and planktonic bacteria, by interfering with biofilm production and/or detaching/disaggregating mature biofilms. To this purpose, using antibiofilm agents might reduce the incurrence of resiliency and can also target a wide range of bacteria, though with a lower spectrum specificity and a mainly topical or local delivery systems (Fernebro 2011).

Antibiofilms could be potentially applied to a variety of other infections, such as catheter-related, chronic osteomyelitis, otitis media, chronic wounds, etc. Still, due to their high economical and social impact, implant-related infections in orthopedics and trauma appear to be one of the most straightforward applications (Romero and Kolter 2011; Poultsides et al. 2010).

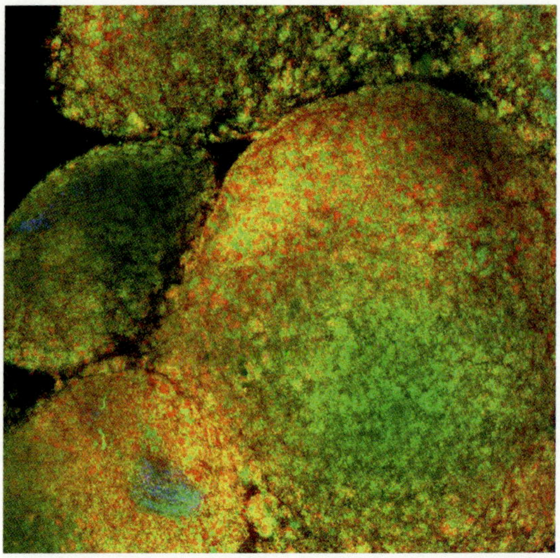

Fig. 22.1 Biofilm production examined by Confocal Laser Microscopy. In red: biofilm; in *green*: bacteria; in *yellow*: bacteria and biofilm mixture

22.2 Classification of Antibiofilm Agents

Biofilms are surface bacterial aggregates encased in a synthesized matrix (Costerton et al. 1999) (Fig. 22.1). The formation of biofilms requires two distinguished steps: the adhesion stage between a substrate surface and bacteria and the maturation stage, during which the adhered bacteria grow and differentiate. Surface adhesins and cell-to-cell communication signaling pathways are specific controls set up for each phase. Microorganisms can spread all over the human body according to the multiple adhesins of bacteria. These adhesins are made of a set of proteins that are able to identify receptors located in the host's tissues and controlled by several inputs (Tojo et al. 1988; Zhang et al. 2003; Nobbs et al. 2009). Biofilms are structurally made of polysaccharides that are in turn produced by bacteria.

The two stages behind the biofilm formation can potentially be affected by antibiofilm compounds. To this purpose, research efforts are not only aimed at the eradication of already formed biofilm but also at impeding its development. Considerable social and economic benefits would in fact be associated with the implementation of a clinical technique that impedes the formation of biofilm on orthopedic implants.

In this chapter, we report some of the most promising antibiofilm agents sorted into classes according to their working mechanism (cf. Table 22.1), providing an overview of the respective in vitro and in vivo studies. When considering the results, attention should be paid to not generalize data, since different bacteria and substrates may make biofilms differ substantially in terms of formation, life cycle, and composition, thus also influencing the potential antibiofilm activity of each compound.

Table 22.1 Antibiofilm therapeutic strategies sorted by their mechanism of action and quick review of the current research

Class	Agent	Molecules	Mode of action/target	Microorganism/model/implanted biomaterial	Reference
BPAs	Anti-adhesins	(Z)-Diarylacrylonitriles Diazoketone Chloromethylketone	Adhesins/sortase inhibition	Gram-positive bacteria In vitro	Maresso et al. (2008)
	Quorum-sensing inhibitors	Furanone derivatives	Interfere with AHSL regulatory system in Gram-negative bacteria and AI-2 signaling system in Gram-positive and Gram-negative bacteria	*Staphylococcus epidermidis* In vitro and in vivo (sheep/polymer) *Pseudomonas aeruginosa* In vitro and in vivo (mouse/lung infection—no implant)	Hume et al. (2004) Hentzer et al. (2003) Wu et al. (2004)
		RIP, hamamelitannin	RNAIII system	*Staphylococcus aureus* In vitro and in vivo (rat/polymer)	Balaban et al. (1998) Kiran et al. (2008)
		Baicalin hydrate, cinnamaldehyde	Acyl-homoserine lactones system	*Pseudomonas aeruginosa*	Geske et al. (2005)
	Nonsteroidal anti-inflammatory drugs	Aspirin, etodolac, diclofenac, celecoxib, nimesulide, ibuprofen, meloxicam	Cyclooxygenase inhibition	*Candida albicans* In vitro *Streptococcus pneumoniae*, *Escherichia coli* In vitro	Alem et al. (2004) del Prado et al. (2010)
	Antimicrobial peptides	Melimine	Membrane disruption Protein functional inhibition	*Staphylococcus aureus*, *Pseudomonas aeruginosa* In vitro and in vivo (rat, guinea pig, rabbit/polymer)	Willcox et al. (2008) Cole et al. (2010)
		Citropin 1.1	DNA binding Polysaccharides detoxification	*Staphylococcus aureus* In vivo (rat) *Streptococcus mutans* In vitro	Cirioni et al. (2006) Li et al. (2010)

(continued)

Table 22.1 (continued)

Class	Agent	Molecules	Mode of action/target	Microorganism/model/implanted biomaterial	Reference
BDAs	Enzymes	Serratiopeptidase	Proteolytic	*Staphylococcus aureus* In vitro and in vivo (rat/metal) *Staphylococcus epidermidis* In vitro and in vivo (rat/metal)	Artini et al. (2011b) Mecikoglu et al. (2006)
		DNase I	Degrades extracellular DNA	*Staphylococcus aureus*, *Staphylococcus epidermidis* In vitro	Kaplan (2009)
		DspB	Hydrolyzes the poly-(beta-1,6)-N-acetylglucosamine exopolysaccharide	*Staphylococcus aureus*, *Staphylococcus epidermidis*, *Escherichia coli* In vitro and in vivo (rabbit/polymer)	Darouiche et al. (2008)
		Maggot *Lucilia sericata* excretions/secretions	Unknown	*Staphylococcus epidermidis*, In vitro *Staphylococcus aureus*, *Staphylococcus epidermidis*, *Klebsiella oxytoca*, *Enterococcus faecalis*, *Enterobacter cloacae* In vitro	Harris et al. (2009) Cazander et al. (2010)
	N-Acetylcysteine	N-Acetylcysteine	Reduces extracellular polysaccharides production and changes the texture of the biofilm formed	*Staphylococcus epidermidis* In vitro Gram-positive and Gram-negative bacteria In vitro *Pseudomonas aeruginosa* In vitro *Escherichia coli* In vitro	Perez-Giraldo et al. (1997) Olofsson et al. (2003) Zhao and Liu (2010) Marchese et al. (2003)

BBPAs	Antibiotics	Daptomycin Minocycline Tigecycline	More effective in decreasing viable biofilm-embedded methicillin-resistant *S. aureus* than rifampin, vancomycin, or linezolid	MRSA In vitro	Raad et al. (2007a, b)
	Photodynamic treatment	Photosensitizers	Photosensitizer penetrates into the bacterial membranes and generate free radicals or singlet oxygen bactericidal to microorganisms	*Staphylococcus aureus*, *Staphylococcus epidermidis* In vitro	Sharma et al. (2008)
	Nanotechnology delivery systems	Nanopolymer-embedded antibiotics	Controlled and prolonged release of antibiotics may be more effective in preventing biofilm formation	*Pseudomonas aeruginosa* In vitro and in vivo (mouse/peritoneal infection—no implant)	Vukomanovic' et al. (2011); Abdelghany et al. (2012)
	Nanoparticles	Nanomeric metals and composites	Direct antibacterial activity	*Staphylococcus aureus*, *Staphylococcus epidermidis* In vitro	Taylor and Webster (2011)
ABV	Vaccine	Quadrivalent vaccine Anti-quorum-sensing vaccine	Membrane-associated proteins Quorum-sensing (AIP)-4 peptide	*Staphylococcus aureus* In vivo (mouse/abscess, no implant) (rabbit/osteomyelitis, no implant)	Park (2007) Brady et al. (2011)

Remarks: *BPA* biofilm prevention agent, *BDA* biofilm-disrupting agent, *BBPA* biofilm-bypassing agent, *ABV* antibiofilm vaccine, *RIP* RNAIII-inhibiting peptides, *DNase I* deoxyribonuclease I, *DspB* dispersin B, *AIP* autoinducing peptide, *MRSA* methicillin-resistant *S. aureus*

22.2.1 Agents Interfering with Biofilm Production (Biofilm Preventing Agents)

22.2.1.1 Anti-adhesins

The process of new biofilm formation can be traced back to the adhesion stage of planktonic cells to specific surfaces or tissues. This essential step is under investigation by many researches; several microbial species and their related surface proteins may in fact represent a potential target of anti-adhesion compounds. The main obstacle for the adhesin characterization is the interaction of multiple adhesion receptors with various affinities.

Sortases are membrane enzymes, commonly found in Gram-positive bacteria, that allow the covalent anchoring of surface proteins to peptidoglycan (Marraffini et al. 2006; Mazmanian et al. 1999; Montanaro et al. 2011). This dynamic surface structure permits several interactions between bacteria and their environment and is fundamental to the biofilm development. Projects on the bacteria genome report that sortase is an enzyme with wide substrates. For each analyzed family, 20 potential sortase substrates have been identified in *S. aureus*, including protein A (Spa), fibronectin-binding proteins (FnbpA, FnbpB), clumping factor (ClfA, ClfB), collagen adhesion protein (CnA), heme-binding proteins (IsdC, IsdB, IsdA), and other surface proteins. These results have been confirmed in other Gram-positive microorganisms, as, for instance, *S. epidermidis* and *S. mutans*. Sortase A (srtA) mutants instead did not show all the surface proteins (Marraffini et al. 2006). Paving the way for future research, tests for sepsis, abscess, septic arthritis, and endocarditis on animal models show that the srtA mutant type is less aggressive than wild-type kinds (Marraffini et al. 2006; Jonsson et al. 2003; Weiss et al. 2004; Gianfaldoni et al. 2009). These outcomes have encouraged researchers to think that sortase could work well as a good drug target for anti-adhesion activities. Up to now, researchers have looked for sortase inhibitors through natural and synthetic compounds (Maresso and Schneewind 2008). Aggregates extracted from *Cocculus trilobus* and *Coptis chinensis* did manage to stop the attachment of microorganisms to fibronectin (Kim et al. 2002), while synthetic compounds, like (Z)-diarylacrylonitriles, successfully passed the researchers' screens.

22.2.1.2 Quorum-Sensing Inhibitors

As mentioned earlier, the second stage of biofilm formation is the maturation stage, when cell-to-cell communication is exploited by microorganisms to control the expressions of the genes that are needed and/or that might be directly involved in the development of the biofilm itself. The lack or failure of cell-to-cell communication may make cells preserve their planktonic state.

Quorum sensing (QS) is a specific microbial type of cell-to-cell communication specific for cell density as well as cell population. Bacteria can detect the presence of other microorganisms nearby by using small molecules secreted by these microorganisms themselves. This observation reveals that bacteria don't act as independent individuals; instead, they behave as a population. In light of this coordination, interferences with the quorum sensing might thus impede bacteria's colonization of an implant (Njoroge and Sperandio 2009; Kaufmann et al. 2008). QS was first described in the 1960s by Tomasz (1965); since then, research efforts have identified and described alternative types of QS, among which are N-acyl homoserine lactone (AHL) system and 4-quinolone system from Gram-negative bacteria, AgrD peptide systems for Gram-positive bacteria, AI2/LuxS systems for both Gram-negative and Gram-positive bacteria, and farnesol systems for fungi.

This identification process has come up with many different quorum-sensing inhibitors (QSI); there are two classes that could be potential leading candidates: the furanones and RNAIII-inhibiting peptide (RIP) ones. There are some superior and inferior plants that are producing QSI, as the algae *Delisea pulchra*, which is an endemic type of algae from Southeastern Australia, producing halogenated furanones that impede the bacterial colonization and the formation of biofilm (Manefield et al. 1999). Furanones prevent the bacteria's settlement and the formation of biofilm by interfering with a fundamental bacteria QS pathway, the AHSL regulatory system in Gram-negative microorganisms. Furanones also interfere with the AI-2 signaling system, generally related to both Gram-negative and Gram-positive bacteria. So far, synthetic programs have proposed a library consisting of up to 200 furanones and furanone analogues, including surface-attached furanone, with its strong in vitro and in vivo antipathogenic characteristics (Lazar 2011). When tested on models of animal disease, furanones did help the host immune system to effectively tackle infections (Wu et al. 2004; Hentzer et al. 2003), and they also did control *S. epidermidis* biofilm formation in vitro, as well as in a sheep model when covalently bound to catheters (Hume et al. 2004). Preliminary results are appealing, but furanones have not been applied to animal models of orthopedic implant-related infections yet.

In vitro applications also identified N-acyl homoserine lactone-based QS system as a predictable target preventing *Pseudomonas* biofilm formation (Geske et al. 2005; Kaufmann et al. 2006). Animal models with polymeric joint-related infections also proved the effectiveness of QS inhibitors in augmenting the vulnerability of bacterial biofilms when subjected to standard antimicrobial agents, such as antibiotics and detergents (Musk and Hergenrother 2006; Pan and Ren 2009; Brackman et al. 2011). Christensen et al. (2012) recently reported intraperitoneal or subcutaneous injection of the QS inhibitor furanone C-30, ajoene, or horseradish juice extract in combination with tobramycin in a mice model of infection. In this model, they inserted silicone tube implants, previously colonized with wild-type *P. aeruginosa*, into the mice's peritoneal cavity. For each QS inhibitor tested, the treated group experienced a significant reduction in the formation of colony compared to placebo.

On the other side, the RNAIII-inhibiting peptide (RIP), in amide form, has effectively inhibited virulence, the onset of biofilm, as well as antibiotic resistance of staphylococci. Kiran et al. (2008) not only proved the effectiveness of RIP against some strains of methicillin-resistant *S. aureus* (MRSA); they also found another RIP, hamamelitannin, which is analogue to the nonpeptide RIP and can impede implant-related MRSA infections in a concentration-dependent manner. This proved to be successful on some animal models, but in vitro studies revealed that the stability and toxicity of the product could be of major concern (Balaban et al. 1998; Giacometti et al. 2003; Anguita-Alonso et al. 1998; Lovetri and Madhyastha 2010; Cirioni et al. 2007).

22.2.1.3 Nonsteroidal Anti-inflammatory Drugs (NSAIDs)

NSAIDs are cyclooxygenase inhibitors able to significantly slow down the in vitro formation of biofilm both in fungi and in bacteria. This cyclooxygenase-dependent synthesis of fungal and bacterial prostaglandin(s) might in fact be relevant in terms of biofilm formation and morphogenesis, and, last but not least, it might also contribute to the regulation phase of these two physiological processes. Approximately 10 years ago, the study carried out by Faber and coworkers revealed that NSAIDs were able to impede the attachment of *Staphylococcus epidermidis* to medical polymers (Farber and Wolff 1992). An analogous effect has been confirmed in more recent studies on aspirin, etodolac, and diclofenac: among these, aspirin has even implied a 95 % inhibition of *Candida albicans* biofilm development. Celecoxib, nimesulide, ibuprofen, and meloxicam did prove able to impede biofilm formation, but with a less dramatic effect than aspirin. Aspirin also turned out to be effective in the treatment of already formed and growing biofilms. To this extent, the efficacy of aspirin was related to the dose applied, and it proved its inhibitor property at pharmacological concentration. Still, this inhibition effect was canceled out when prostaglandin E2 was simultaneously added. At 1 mM, aspirin reduced the viability of biofilm organisms to 1.9 % of that of controls (Alem and Douglas 2004). Also ibuprofen displayed some inhibition properties when tested on the *S. pneumoniae* and *E. coli* strain biofilm formation (del Prado et al. 2010; Naves et al. 2010); some effects also emerged with respect to the attachment of *Escherichia coli* to epithelial cells (Drago et al. 2002). Despite these promising results, these inhibition effects emerged only in in vitro studies: further research on animal models is thus needed to confirm the predicted therapeutic efficacy of NSAIDs on biofilm formation on implanted biomaterials.

22.2.1.4 Antimicrobial Peptides (AMPs)

Antimicrobial peptides are widely diffused molecules in living organisms, whose extensive host defense property makes them fundamental as part of innate immunity. These large molecules, with a net positive charge, contain approximately 50 % hydrophobic residues. Their working mechanism binds the structural molecules that are negatively charged to the microbial membrane. AMPs target a wide range of microbial activity, rarely able to resist them, and they have been described as able to prevent the onset of biofilm on stainless steel surface. Héquet et al. (2011) proved in fact that antibacterial peptides magainin I and misin, with their covalent bound to stainless steel surfaces, were able to reduce in a significant way the attachment of Gram-positive *Listeria ivanovii*. Melamine, a nonhemolytic hybrid peptide between melittin and protamine, decreased the adhesion of bacteria to the contact lenses, to which it was covalently bound, and did not lead to any resistance against *S. aureus* or *P. aeruginosa* during the repeated passage in subminimal inhibitory concentrations (Willcox et al. 2008). Moreover, *P. aeruginosa* guinea pig models revealed that silicone hydrogel lenses with melamine led to a reduction in contact lens-induced acute red eye, and *S. aureus* rabbit models suggested that they also hindered contact lens-induced peripheral ulcers. Citropin 1.1, extracted from *Litoria citropa*, the green tree frog, is powerful to the detriment of biofilm activity and is even more powerful against *S. aureus* biofilm when provided together with rifampin and minocycline (Cirioni et al. 2006). A relevant reduction in the bacterial counts of biofilm emerged in a model of *S. aureus* infection, where rats were treated with central venous catheters previously treated with citropin 1.1 peptides and/or antibiotics (Høiby et al. 2010). The working principle of AMPs include membrane-disrupting action, functional inhibition of proteins, binding with DNA, and detoxification of polysaccharides (lipopolysaccharide and lipoteichoic acid) (Park et al. 2011). The pitfalls related to AMPs treatments are many, as their large-scale production is costly and complicated. Moreover, they are also sensitive to protease digestion. Modified versions of AMPs led to the formation of synthetic antimicrobial peptides, known as SAMPs (second generation of AMPs). Their working mechanism is similar to the AMPs', but SAMPs have better pharmacokinetic properties. This second generation is thus an improvement over the former version, but they are still broad spectrum. As a response, recent studies came up with STAMPs, that is, selectively targeted antimicrobial peptides, to target species-specific biofilm control. In other words, STAMPs are the third generation of AMPs, as they are their modified recombinant version (Eckert et al. 2006; He et al. 2009). The in vivo activity of these compounds has still to be evaluated (Li et al. 2010).

22.2.2 Agents Interfering with Established Biofilm (Biofilm Disruption Agents)

22.2.2.1 Enzymes

To tackle staphylococcal biofilm disruption, many different agents have been considered. Among them, the encouraging results are related to those enzymes capable of attacking biofilm components. Initially, Selan and her coworkers recommended the use of proteolytic enzyme serratiopeptidase for the treatment of biofilm-related infections (Selan et al. 1993; Artini et al. 2011b). Almost 20 years later, in a rat model of joint-related infection due to *S. epidermidis* strain, with a high slime production capacity, serratiopeptidase was injected in the knee affected: the subsequent antibiotic therapy reported a 94.4 % infection healing rate, higher than the 62.5 % cure rate emerged from groups subjected to the antibiotic treatment only. The resulting difference was confirmed to be statistically significant (Mecikoglu et al. 2006). In addition to this enzyme, research has also investigated the biofilm-dispersing property of deoxyribonuclease

I (DNase I) and dispersin B (DspB). Whereas the former degrades extracellular DNA, which is a new structural component contributing to the biofilm steadiness, the latter hydrolyzes the biofilm poly-(beta-1,6)-N-acetylglucosamine exopolysaccharide, also called polysaccharide intercellular adhesin. DNase I also inhibits the formation of biofilm, when present in the culture medium, right at the stage of bacteria onset, but DNase I fails to separate biofilm once it has already formed. More specifically, DNase I is mainly associated to an increase in the biofilm bacteria sensibility to killing by several biocides and to the detachment by anionic detergents and not to the inhibition or detachment of biofilm formation or already formed biofilm. Thus, following Kaplan (2009), biofilm detachment might occur rapidly with DNase I and at a clinically achievable concentration of the enzyme (Kaplan et al. 2012).

Darouiche et al. (2008, 2009) discovered that DspB, combined with antiseptics (triclosan or chlorhexidine), boasted the broad-spectrum antibiofilm and antimicrobial activity against *S. aureus*, *S. epidermidis*, and *Escherichia coli* to coated vascular catheters; moreover, catheters coated with triclosan and DspB effectively showed an in vivo antibacterial activity by subcutaneous implantation of segments in a model with *S. aureus*-infected rabbits.

An ancient approach that considered maggot or larvae therapy can be brushed up and applied in nowadays context: to this purpose, a living and disinfected fly larva is introduced into a nonhealing skin or into soft tissue wounds of animals or humans. This cleans out the necrotic tissues and disinfects and debrides the wound. The *Lucilia sericata* excretions and secretions inhibited the biofilm formation up to 92 %, and this effect has been confirmed by several in vitro applications on various microorganisms (*Staphylococcus aureus*, *Staphylococcus epidermidis*, *Klebsiella oxytoca*, *Enterococcus faecalis*, and *Enterobacter cloacae*) and on several biomaterials, such as polyethylene, titanium, and stainless steel, all currently used in orthopedic practices (Harris et al. 2009; Cazander et al. 2010).

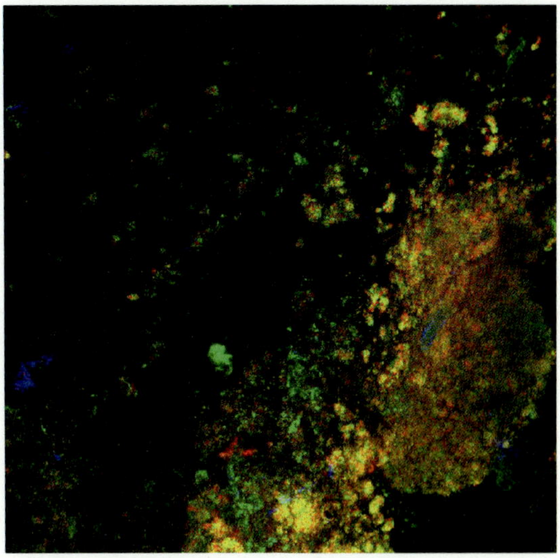

Fig. 22.2 Residual biofilm and bacteria, partially disrupted and removed after antibiofilm treatment with N-acetylcisteine of a titanium disk surface. Confocal Laser Microscopy. In *red*: biofilm; in *green*: bacteria; in *yellow*: bacteria and biofilm mixture

22.2.2.2 N-Acetylcysteine (NAC)

NAC is a mucolytic agent with antibacterial properties. This molecule is an antioxidant containing thiol and breaks disulfide chemical ties in mucus (Sheffner 1963) and competitively impedes amino acid (cysteine) use (Zygmunt and Martin 1968). NAC also diminishes the attachment of staphylococci, as well as the adhesion of some Gram-negative bacilli, to some abiotic materials (Perez-Giraldo et al. 1997; Olofsson et al. 2003; Mansouri and Darouiche 2007; Schwandt et al. 2004). In addition to this, NAC slows down the formation on an extracellular polysaccharide matrix, and, in the meanwhile, it enhances the rupture of mature biofilms. According to our data (Drago et al. 2013), NAC, when dissolved at a final concentration of 100 mg/ml, successfully disrupted *S. aureus*- and *P. aeruginosa*-related biofilm, on disks of polyethylene and titanium, already 3 h after incubation (Fig. 22.2). Still, some differences in the biofilm eradication emerged when targeting already formed *P. aeruginosa* biofilm, according to the type of disk tested: polyethylene displayed a 50 % rate, whereas eradication was successful only on 20 out of 100 titanium disks. The disaggregation of biofilm was monitored for the following 18 h. Figure 22.2 displays the confocal laser scanning microscopy analysis of biofilms untreated and treated with NAC, 18 h after incubation. Live cells, with their intact cell membranes, were stained with Syto9 and were identifiable by their green fluorescence. Furthermore, SYPRO® Ruby stain identifies the extracellular polysaccharide matrix and comes with a red fluorescence. Untreated biofilms were mainly red, but they also contained a green cell that revealed the presence of bacteria in the extracellular polysaccharide matrix. When treated with NAC, after 18 h from incubation, the same analysis revealed a reversed scenario, with more greens and less reds, thus suggesting the successful disruption of biofilm bacteria carried out by NAC agents. Disrupted bacteria returned to their planktonic phenotype. NAC also displays some bactericidal properties, against bacteria clinically relevant and resistant to drugs. Recent studies have tested NAC on organism viability during the planktonic and biofilm stages; the microorganisms tested were, for instance, the methicillin-sensitive and methicillin-resistant *S. aureus* and *S. epidermidis*, the vancomycin-resistant *Enterococcus faecalis*, *Pseudomonas aeruginosa*, *Enterobacter cloacae*, *Klebsiella pneumonia*, *Candida albicans*, and *C. krusei*. At the 80 mg/ml concentration, NAC proved to be bactericidal (with a more than 99.9 % reduction) with respect to all the tested bacteria. On top of that, there were no recoverable organisms only 30 min after incubation and NAC proved to be fungistatic against *Candida* species. In the interval 5–10 mg/ml, NAC displayed the lowest inhibition and bactericidal concentration. The thickness of biofilms treated with NAC decreased significantly on all organisms but vancomycin-resistant enterococci (Aslam and Darouiche 2011).

Agents disrupting biofilms may be exploited in a number of ways, but the pretreatment aimed at the removal of biofilm residues deserves further attention. An analysis carried out by the water industry has revealed that different surfaces homogenously attract planktonic cells, and, when contaminated by organic materials, especially residual biofilm matrices, this attraction process occurs at a speed at least ten times higher. Biofilm formation can occur already at the orthopedic implant manufacturing stage, more specifically when it involves machining techniques using a wet interface between the tool assembly and the implant. To this purpose, sterilization, for instance, ethylene oxide, kills the bacteria on the biofilm but is not enough to totally remove the residues from their matrices. These should be eliminated, applying the available enzyme treatments, before the joint implantation (Olofsson et al. 2003).

When combined with various antibiotics, some synergies emerge. For instance, the combination of NAC and fosfomycin and tigecycline is able to reduce *S. aureus*, *S. epidermidis,* as well as some Gram-negative bacteria (Marchese et al. 2003; Aslam et al. 2007). El-Feky et al. (2009) obtained analogous results in their analysis of nosocomial staphylococci and Gram-negative bacilli retrieved from removed ureteral stents, using NAC (2 and 4 mg/ml) with ciprofloxacin. When comparing the treated and control groups, they obtained is a 94–100 % biofilm formation inhibition rate and a 86–100 % disruption of preformed biofilms. Zhao and Liu (2010) proved that the minimum inhibitory concentrations (MICs) of NAC for most *P. aeruginosa* were achieved at 10–40 mg/ml, whereas at a 0.5 mg/ml concentration NAC would be able to disrupt already formed *P. aeruginosa* biofilms. In their study, the level of biofilm disruption was proportional to the level of NAC concentration, and total disruption was achieved at the 10 mg/ml concentration. Already at 2.5 mg/ml and at >2 MIC, NAC and ciprofloxacin respectively displayed successful *P. aeruginosa* biofilm killing properties. Different combinations of NAC and ciprofloxacin reduced, with respect to the control group, viable biofilm-related bacteria. The most synergic result was obtained at a 0.5 mg/ml NAC concentration, combined with a ½ MIC of CIP. Moreover, the production of extracellular *P. aeruginosa* polysaccharides dropped by 27.64 and 44.59 % at 0.5 and 1 mg/ml NAC concentration, respectively. The studies so far mentioned all report in vitro results, and, over time, clinical experience has made big improvements in the treatment of respiratory tract infections. All these elements make NAC as an ideal antibiofilm agent when dealing with implant-related infections. Still, further animal models are needed to confirm its successful application.

22.2.3 Biofilm-Bypassing Agents

22.2.3.1 Antibiotics

Systemic antibiotics succeed in the elimination of planktonic organisms, but they often fail to clear organisms embedded in the biofilm. Research has proposed alternative explanations for this heterogeneous performance: for instance, limitations to the penetration of the agent (Stewart et al. 2000), presence of dormant cells or alterations in the bacterial metabolism (Brown et al. 1988; Kim 2007; Lewis 2001), and phenotypic variations (Drenkard and Ausubel 2002). The resistance of biofilm depends on many different factors, and it is also organism related. Darouiche et al. (1994) proved that vancomycin was able to penetrate *S. epidermidis* biofilm, but it was not able to completely disrupt the biofilm-embedded bacteria. Gattringer et al. (2010) investigated the time-dependent effects of rifampicin on *S. epidermidis* insediated in biofilm, extracted from patients suffering from cardiac implant infections. Hansen et al. (2010) studied, instead, antibiotic-delivering apparatus and their ability to decrease the development of bacterial biofilm on implanted pacing devices. Both these studies proved that antibiotic doses and delivery times are crucial factors to take into account, as they could effectively act against biofilm-centered infections, especially when surgical treatment cannot be applied. Thus, there are some antibiotics that could emerge as being more effective than others against biofilm-embedded bacteria. According to one study, daptomycin, minocycline, and tigecycline did better than linezolid and vancomycin in the reduction of viable biofilm-embedded MRSA after a 24 h exposure (Raad et al. 2007a). Another study reported that the combination of minocycline, EDTA, and 25 % ethanol was able to disrupt MRSA biofilm after a 15 min exposure (Raad et al. 2007b). Also daptomycin and rifampin, when combined, reported efficacies higher than when applied alone in the prevention of staphylococcal biofilm infections in a rat model (Cirioni et al. 2010). As reported above, adding NAC to tigecycline revealed other synergies to the detriment of several biofilm-embedded organisms and it was also able to eradicate *S. epidermidis* and MRSA from catheter surfaces after 4 h of exposure (Aslam et al. 2007). It is worth mentioning that all these studies might share a common constraint relative to the activity of antibiotics against biofilm bacteria, as there is no standardized laboratory model for testing antimicrobials in biofilms. Coenye and Nelis (2010) provide a complete survey of in vitro and in vivo model systems for the study of microbial biofilm development.

22.2.3.2 Photodynamic Treatment

An alternative approach might eventually be implemented in the treatment of orthopedic chronic wounds: this solution combines the action of a photodynamic treatment with antibiotics, at a lower concentration than other antibiotics working as biofilm inhibitors. Photodynamic treatment (PDT) initially treats bacteria with photosensitizer drug, and then they are consequently treated with a low-intensity visible light of an appropriate wavelength (Jori 2006). Usually, the photodynamic inactivation of bacteria is related to the effect of a photosensitizer dye, aiming at bacterial structures and avoiding eukaryotic tissue cells structures, and these are eventually activated with low doses of visible light, so that free radicals or singlet oxygen bactericidal to microorganisms is generated. PDT has successfully disrupted bacterial biofilm forming in dental plaques and in other oral implants, but it has also turned out successful on *S. epidermidis* and *S. aureus* biofilms (Di Poto et al. 2009; Sharma et al. 2008; Vilela et al. 2011) and on in vitro studies of *E. coli* biofilm (Saino et al. 2010). Saino et al. (2010) proved that PDT is also efficient in the inactivation of staphylococcal biofilms in a variety of implant-related infections accessible to visible light. Still, the real impact of PDT on staphylococcal biofilm eradication is affected by the photosensitizer molecule chosen. The greater effect in terms of photo-efficiency related to bacteria killing is achieved when this photosensitizer molecule can deeply penetrate into the bacterial membranes, thus reaching a higher endocellular concentration. When the bacteria are less resistant to antibiotics, antimicrobial PDT can be an additional clinical therapy, depending on the photosensitizer's pharmacokinetics, on the suitability of the wavelength, on the irradiation time, and, lastly, on the accessibility of the implant site (Maisch 2007; Poggio 2001).

22.2.3.3 Nanotechnologies

At the frontier, research is considering nanotechnologies as the ultimate solution against biofilm formation. Antibacterial nanotherapeutics include nanomaterials that either display antibacterial activity or improve the way other antimicrobials are administered, thus increasing their overall effectiveness and safety. These research efforts can be distinguished into two mainstreams: the development of nanosized carriers from already existing antibiotics as a platform to improve their delivery and creation of new antimicrobial nanoparticles.

The first approach deals with controlled drug delivery. Nanoparticles tend to capture a drug and deliver it directly to the place it is meant to work and/or to release it in a controlled way, thus acting as an innovative drug carrier. There are many benefits related to the implementation of this controlled drug delivery with respect to standard antibiotics administration: (1) more efficient medication, (2) reduction in the required doses, and (3) less side effects related to the drug target and/or localized action. The controlled release of gentamicin formulation using poly(lactide-co-glycolide) nanoparticles is a suitable exemplification of this approach. Entrapping this hydrophilic drug into a hydrophobic poly(lactide-co-glycolide) polymer obtained a controlled gentamicin release for up to 16 days (Abdelghany et al. 2012). An additional example refers to the application of the same approach in the development of core/shell nanoparticles formed from polymeric shell and bioceramic core that were loaded, at the same time, by two forms of available antibiotics. Further analysis proved that these particles were indeed able to provide controlled drug release during the period of at least 30 days. This approach may contribute to the local and controlled delivery of antibiotics already introduced in dental practices as well as for the prevention of bone infections, such as clindamycin base and clindamycin phosphate (Vukomanovic et al. 2011). The main features of these systems of nanotechnological local drug delivery are (1) the dependence of the drug release on the kinetics of polymer degradation, that is, a slow release with no initial burst effect, and (2) the antibacterial mechanism, defined by the activity of the released drug. Both these features help in contrasting the offset of antibiotic side effects, related to the local action; nonetheless, they might theoretically contribute to the development of resistant strains.

The development of antibacterial nanotherapeutics also relies on a second strategy, namely, the synthesis of novel antibacterial nanomaterials. Using inorganic nanoparticles as active agents can in fact positively contribute to the development of these drugs. To this purpose, research is combining materials with natural antimicrobiotics with materials with potential for synthetic activation. The main approaches adopted so far are (1) the formation of composites and hybrids, (2) photoactivation, and (3) functionalized surfaces. The last one provides ability for the attachment of a variety of molecular species on metallic nanoparticles. The special benefit is in development of the route of administration of medicament when it can be led exactly to the predefined place of its action (target drug delivery). This study could be alternatively adopted for the design of the solubility, surface charge, wettability, and other properties that can all provide new behavior of material. Nanoparticles made of gold or platinum, and of other noble metals, with the exception of silver, are all nontoxic particles: as a consequence, their antibacterial ability has to be configured and functionalization might be a suitable approach. Antibacterial activity of vancomycin has been considerably improved once bound to colloidal gold, and it has also proved to be efficient against vancomycin-resistant bacteria. Nanoshell Au-ciprofloxacin performed in a similar way (Burygin et al. 2009; Taylor and Webster 2011).

22.2.4 Antibiofilm Vaccines

As far as the diagnosis of orthopedic biofilm-related infections are concerned, the immunoenzymatic detection of serum IgM levels against staphylococcal slime polysaccharide antigens has proved to be fairly effective (Artini et al. 2011a). Still, all the attempts to the design of an anti-staphylococcal vaccine have failed. In fact, all the whole live or killed *S. aureus* vaccines on animal models have been largely unsuccessful (Watson 1987). Analysis has focused on purified forms of either polysaccharide or protein from the bacterial surface, especially for the capsular polysaccharide types 5 and 8. The StaphVAX vaccine displayed some protective efficacy in infection animal model. Despite this promising result, protection slowly decreased over time down to <30 % 1 year after vaccination (Shinefield et al. 2002). Recently, recombinant forms of four cell walls have been combined with membrane-associated proteins, immunogenic during *S. aureus* biofilm infection, in a quadrivalent vaccine framework: this combination has been tested against *S. aureus* biofilm infection, generally resistant to antimicrobials (Brady et al. 2011). The antigenic proteins included in this study, although not disclosed, were selected among other proteins the same author had previously identified (Brady et al. 2006). One antibiotic, with no effect in terms of eradication of biofilm communities, was used also in the combination with vaccine for the elimination of any trace of planktonic staphylococci. This quadrivalent vaccination, together with antibiotic therapy, was more efficient in terms of infection clearing than either treatment alone. An alternative immunopharmacotherapeutic approach suggests to target the quorum-sensing mechanism of *S. aureus*. An anti-autoinducer monoclonal antibody, AP4-24 H11, successfully inhibited QS in vitro by sequestrating the autoinducing peptide-4 generated by *S. aureus* RN4850. It is worth mentioning that AP4-24H11 eradicated *S. aureus* pathogenicity in a mouse model with abscess formation and also provided total coverage against a lethal *S. aureus* challenge. These results pave the way for further research implementing immunopharmacotherapy on the prevention and treatment of bacterial infections in which QS controls the expression of virulence factors (Park 2011).

22.3 Antibacterial-Loaded Hydrogel Coating and Biofilm Prevention

In the lack of clinically safe and effective antibiofilm agents for systemic administration, current clinical research is more focused on various strategies of local delivery, to protect implanted biomaterials from bacterial colonization and biofilm formation (Romanò et al. 2013; Arciola 2009; Kiedrowski and Horswill 2011) To this aim, various antibacterial coatings have been proposed, but current technologies are far from large-scale application in orthopedics, due to several limitations, including questionable long-term effect on bacterial resistance and on bone ingrowth, regulatory issues, and costs.

Until recently, most of the authors have looked for prolonged or permanent antibacterial coatings (Hickok and Shapiro 2012). Contrary to this common vision, it has been proposed that a fast-resorbable antibacterial-loaded hydrogel coating may offer (1) efficacy toward early bacterial colonization, providing complete protection of the implant for the time needed to win the "run to the surface" (Costerton 2005), i.e., in the first hours after surgery. According to this approach, local antibacterial protection is provided in the very first hours after surgery, much similarly as systemic prophylaxis, that has been shown to be necessary only in the short term perioperatively; (2) safety, as high local concentration and fast and complete

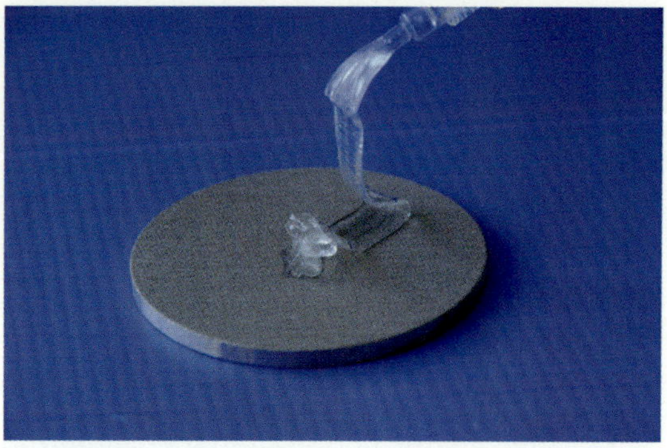

Fig. 22.3 Antibacterial-loaded, fast-resorbable, hydrogel coating (DAC®, Novagenit®, Mezzolombardo, Italy) spread on a sanded titanium disk. The coating, that has received the CE mark and is available for clinical use in Europe, has been proved effective to inhibit biofilm formation on different substrates in vitro and to prevent implant-related infection in an rabbit model of implant-related infection

release of the antibacterial may avoid induction of antibiotic resistance and possible risks of long-term effects on bone healing; (3) versatility, through intraoperative mixing with a choice of different antibacterial agents; (4) ease of handling; and (5) reduced costs for large-scale application.

Studies have demonstrated that this novel approach, using a fast-resorbable hydrogel, composed of covalently linked hyaluronan and poly-D,L-lactide (DAC®, Novagenit®, Mezzolombardo, Italy) (Fig. 22.3), is in fact able to inhibit biofilm formation on different substrates in vitro and to prevent implant-related infection in an animal model of implant-related infection (Giavaresi et al. 2013; Drago et al. 2014).

22.4 Conclusions and New Perspectives

Biofilm-embedded sessile bacteria are overwhelming issues in the treatment of biofilm-related infections in orthopedics and not only. In fact, as publicly announced by US National Institutes of Health, "Biofilms are medically important, accounting for over 80 % of microbial infections in the body" (McLean et al. 2012). Efforts to improve our treatment strategies of biofilm-related infection should take into account the communal, rather than individual, nature of microorganisms, and some attention should be devoted to the understanding of the formation of biofilm communities that are also able to preserve diversity.

Many different targets for antibiofilm agents have been identified. However, despite the worrying recurrence of implant-related infections in orthopedic surgery, their high rate of complications, and social and economic costs, only limited information on antibiofilm strategies and bone- and orthopedic implant-related infections is currently available.

Orthopedic research in this field appears at only a preliminary stage, and some critical points should be better addressed in the future, like biofilm structure and function of different microorganisms; biofilm relationships with different substrates, including bone and cartilage and common biomaterials (both metallic and polymeric); tolerability of antibiofilm agents; etc.

Key Points

- Biofilm formation is probably the main reason for bacteria persistence and treatment failure of implant-related infections in orthopedics.
- Various antibiofilm strategies have been proven in vitro and in vivo to be able to prevent or reduce biofilm formation and to disrupt an established biofilm.
- Antibiofilm agents may be classified according to their mechanism of action, although some may show different activities at the same time.
- Local application of antibacterial and antibiofilm agents, like implant coating, is a feasible and promising approach, while systemic antibiofilm treatment is still restricted to animal models.
- Given the paucity of new antibiotics and their inability to control adequately biofilm-related infections, antibiofilm strategies appear a promising research field to improve clinical results in these challenging conditions.

References

Abdelghany SM, Quinn DJ, Ingram RJ, Gilmore BF, Donnelly RF, Taggart CC, Scott CJ (2012) Gentamicin-loaded nanoparticles show improved antimicrobial effects towards Pseudomonas aeruginosa infection. Int J Nanomedicine 7:4053–4063

Alem MA, Douglas J (2004) Effects of aspirin and other nonsteroidal anti-inflammatory drugs on biofilms and planktonic cells of *Candida albicans*. Antimicrob Agents Chemother 1:41–47

Anguita-Alonso P, Giacometti A, Cirioni O, Ghiselli R, Orlando F, Saba V (1998) RNAIII-inhibiting-peptide loaded polymethylmethacrylate prevents in vivo Staphylococcus aureus biofilm formation. Antimicrob Agents Chemother 51:2594–2596

Arciola CR (2009) New concepts and new weapons in implant infections. Int J Artif Organs 32:533–536

Arciola CR, Montanaro L, Costerton JW (2011) New trends in diagnosis and control strategies for implant infections. Int J Artif Organs 34:727–736

Artini M, Romanò CL, Manzoli L, Scoarughi GL, Papa R, Meani E (2011a) Staphylococcal IgM enzyme-linked immunosorbent assay for diagnosis of periprosthetic joint infections. J Clin Microbiol 49(1):423–425

Artini M, Scoarughi GL, Papa R, Cellini A, Carpentieri A, Pucci P (2011b) A new anti-infective strategy to reduce adhesion-mediated virulence in Staphylococcus aureus affecting surface proteins. Int J Immunopathol Pharmacol 24:661–672

Aslam S, Darouiche RO (2011) Role of antibiofilm-antimicrobial agents in controlling device-related infections. Int J Artif Organs 34:752–758

Aslam S, Trautner BW, Ramanathan V, Darouiche RO (2007) Combination of tigecycline and N-acetylcysteine reduces biofilm-embedded bacteria on vascular catheters. Antimicrob Agents Chemother 51:1556–1558

Balaban N, Goldkorn T, Nhan RT, Dang LB, Scott S, Ridgley RM (1998) Autoinducer of virulence as a target for vaccine and therapy against Staphylococcus aureus. Science 280:438–440

Bozic KJ, Kurtz SM, Lau E, Ong K, Chiu V, Vail TP (2010) The epidemiology of revision total knee arthroplasty in the United States. Clin Orthop Relat Res 468:45–51

Brackman G, Cos P, Maes L, Nelis HJ, Coenye T (2011) Quorum sensing inhibitors increase the susceptibility of bacterial biofilms to antibiotics in vitro and in vivo. Antimicrob Agents Chemother 55:2655–2661

Brady RA, Leid JG, Camper AK, Costerton JW, Shirtliff ME (2006) Identification of Staphylococcus aureus proteins recognized by the antibody-mediated immune response to a biofilm infection. Infect Immun 74: 3415–3426

Brady RA, O'May GA, Leid JG, Prior ML, Costerton JW, Shirtliff ME (2011) Resolution of Staphylococcus aureus biofilm infection using vaccination and antibiotic treatment. Infect Immun 79:1797–1803

Brown MR, Allison DG, Gilbert P (1988) Resistance of bacterial biofilms to antibiotics: a growth-rate related effect? J Antimicrob Chemother 22:777–780

Burygin GL, Khlebtsov BN, Shantrokha AN, Dykman LA, Bogatyrev VA, Khlebtsov NG (2009) On the enhanced antibacterial activity of antibiotics mixed with gold nanoparticles. Nanoscale Res Lett 4(8): 794–801

Cazander G, van de Veerdonk MC, Vandenbroucke-Grauls CM, Schreurs MW, Jukema GN (2010) Maggot excretions inhibit biofilm formation on biomaterials. Clin Orthop Relat Res 468(10):2789–2796

Chen WH, Jiang LS, Dai LY (2011) Influence of bacteria on spinal implant-centered infection: an in vitro and in vivo experimental comparison between Staphylococcus aureus and mycobacterium tuberculosis. Spine 36:103–108

Christensen LD, van Gennip M, Jakobsen TH, Alhede M, Hougen HP, Høiby N, Bjarnsholt T, Givskov M (2012) Synergistic antibacterial efficacy of early combination treatment with tobramycin and quorum-sensing inhibitors against Pseudomonas aeruginosa in an intraperitoneal foreign-body infection mouse model. J Antimicrob Chemother 67(5):1198–1206

Cirioni O, Giacometti A, Ghiselli R, Kamysz W, Orlando F, Mocchegiani F et al (2006) Citropin 1.1-treated central venous catheters improve the efficacy of hydrophobic antibiotics in the treatment of experimental staphylococcal catheter-related infection. Peptides 27:1210–1216

Cirioni O, Ghiselli R, Minardi D, Orlando F, Mocchegiani F, Silvestri C (2007) RNAIII-inhibiting peptide affects biofilm formation in a rat model of staphylococcal ureteral stent infection. Antimicrob Agents Chemother 51:4518–4520

Cirioni O, Mocchegiani F, Ghiselli R, Silvestri C, Gabrielli E, Marchionni E (2010) Daptomycin and rifampin alone and in combination prevent vascular graft biofilm formation and emergence of antibiotic resistance in a subcutaneous rat pouch model of Staphylococcal infection. Eur J Vasc Endovasc Surg 40:817–822

Coenye T, Nelis HJ (2010) In vitro and in vivo model systems to study microbial biofilm formation. J Microbiol Methods 83:89–105

Cole N, Hume EB, Vijay AK, Sankaridurg P, Kumar N, Willcox MD (2010) In vivo performance of melimine as an antimicrobial coating for contact lenses in models of CLARE and CLPU. Invest Ophthalmol Vis Sci 51:390–395

Costerton JW (2005) Biofilm theory can guide the treatment of device-related orthopaedic infections. Clin Orthop Relat Res 437:7–11

Costerton JW, Stewart PS, Greenberg EP (1999) Bacterial biofilms: a common cause of persistent infections. Science 284:1318–1322

Costerton JW, Montanaro L, Arciola CR (2005) Biofilm in implant infections: its production and regulation. Int J Artif Organs 28:1062–1068

Darouiche RO, Dhir A, Miller AJ, Landon GC, Raad II, Musher DM (1994) Vancomycin penetration into

biofilm covering infected prostheses and effect on bacteria. J Infect Dis 170:720–723
Darouiche RO, Mansouri MD, Gawande PV, Madhyastha S (2008) Efficacy of combination of chlorhexidine and protamine sulphate against device-associated pathogens. J Antimicrob Chemother 61:651–657
Darouiche RO, Mansouri MD, Gawande PV, Madhyastha S (2009) Antimicrobial and antibiofilm efficacy of triclosan and DispersinB combination. J Antimicrob Chemother 64:88–93
del Prado G, Ruiz V, Naves P, Rodrı'guez-Cerrato V, Soriano F, del Carmen Ponte M (2010) Biofilm formation by Streptococcus pneumoniae strains and effects of human serum albumin, ibuprofen, N-acetyl-L-cysteine, amoxicillin, erythromycin, and levofloxacin. Diagn Microbiol Infect Dis 67:311–318
Di Poto A, Sbarra MS, Provenza G, Visai L, Speziale P (2009) The effect of photodynamic treatment combined with antibiotic action or host defence mechanisms on Staphylococcus aureus biofilms. Biomaterials 30:3158–3166
Drago L, de Vecchi E, Nicola L, Valli M, Gismondo MR (2002) Effects of subinhibitory concentrations of ibuprofen isobuthanolammonium on virulence factors of uropathogenic *Escherichia coli*. J Chemother 14: 314–315
Drago L, Romanò CL, Mattina R, Signori V, de Vecchi E (2012) Does dithiothreitol improve bacterial detection from infected prosthesis ? A pilot study. Clin Orthop Relat Res. doi:10.1007/s11999-012-2415-3
Drago L, Mattina R, Signori V, De Vecchi E, Romanò CL (2013) Activity of N-acetyl-L-cysteine against biofilm of Staphylococcus aureus and Pseudomonas aeruginosa on orthopaedic prosthetic materials. Int J Artif Organs. doi:10.5301/ijao.5000135
Drago L, Boot W, Dimas K, Malizos K, Hänsch GM, Stuick J, Gawlitta D, Romanò CL (2014) Does implant coating with antibacterial-loaded hydrogel reduce bacterial colonization and biofilm formation in vitro? Clin Orthop Relat Res. doi: 10.1007/s11999-014-3558-1
Drenkard E, Ausubel FM (2002) Pseudomonas biofilm formation and antibiotic resistance are linked to phenotypic variation. Nature 416:740–743
Eckert R, Qi F, Yarbrough DK, He J, Anderson MH, Shi W (2006) Adding selectivity to antimicrobial peptides: rational design of a multidomain peptide against Pseudomonas spp. Antimicrob Agents Chemother 50:1480–1488
El-Feky MA, El-Rehewy MS, Hassan MA, Abolella HA, Abd El-Baky RM, Gad GF (2009) Effect of ciprofloxacin and N-acetylcysteine on bacterial adherence and biofilm formation on ureteral stent surfaces. Pol J Microbiol 58:261–267
Farber BF, Wolff AG (1992) The use of nonsteroidal anti-inflammatory drugs to prevent adherence of Staphylococcus epidermidis to medical polymers. J Infect Dis 166:861–865
Fernebro J (2011) Fighting bacterial infections — future treatment options. Drug Resist Updat 14:125–139
Gattringer KB, Suchomel M, Eder M, Lassnigg AM, Graninger W, Presterl E (2010) Time-dependent effects of rifampicin on staphylococcal biofilms. Int J Artif Organs 33:621–626
Geske GD, Wezeman RJ, Siegel AP, Blackwell HE (2005) Small molecule inhibitors of bacterial quorum sensing and biofilm formation. J Am Chem Soc 127: 12762–12763
Giacometti A, Cirioni O, Gov Y, Ghiselli R, Del Prete MS, Mocchegiani F (2003) RNAIII inhibiting peptide inhibits in vivo biofilm formation by drug-resistant Staphylococcus aureus. Antimicrob Agents Chemother 47:1979–1983
Gianfaldoni C, Maccari S, Pancotto L, Rossi G, Hilleringmann M, Pansegrau W (2009) Sortase A confers protection against Streptococcus pneumoniae in mice. Infect Immun 77:2957–2961
Giavaresi G, Meani E, Sartori M, Ferrari A, Bellini D, Sacchetta AC, Meraner J, Sambri A, Vocale C, Sambri V, Fini M, Romanò CL (2013) Efficacy of antibacterial-loaded coating in an in vivo model of acutely highly contaminated implant. Int Orthop. doi:10.1007/s00264-013-2237-2
Hansen LK, Berg K, Johnson D, Sanders M, Citron M (2010) Efficacy of local rifampin/minocycline delivery (AIGIS(RX)R) to eliminate biofilm formation on implanted pacing devices in a rabbit model. Int J Artif Organs 33:627–635
Harris LG, Bexfield A, Nigam Y, Rohde H, Ratcliffe NA, Mack D (2009) Disruption of Staphylococcus epidermidis biofilms by medicinal maggot Lucilia sericata excretions/secretions. Int J Artif Organs 32:555–564
He J, Anderson MH, Shi W, Eckert R (2009) Design and activity of a 'dual-targeted' antimicrobial peptide. Int J Antimicrob Agents 33:532–537
Hentzer M, Wu H, Andersen JB, Riedel L, Rasmussen TB, Bagge N (2003) Attenuation of Pseudomonas aeruginosa virulence by quorum sensing inhibitors. EMBO J 22:3803–3815
Héquet A, Humblot V, Berjeaud JM, Pradier CM (2011) Optimized grafting of antimicrobial peptides on stainless steel surface and biofilm resistance tests. Colloids Surf B Biointerfaces 84:301–309
Hickok NJ, Shapiro IM (2012) Immobilized antibiotics to prevent orthopaedic implant infections. Adv Drug Deliv Rev 64(12):1165–1176
Hill KE, Malic S, McKee R, Rennison T, Harding KG, Williams DW (2010) An in vitro model of chronic wound biofilms to test wound dressings and assess antimicrobial susceptibilities. J Antimicrob Chemother 65:1195–1206
Høiby N, Bjarnsholt T, Givskov M, Molin S, Ciofu O (2010) Antibiotic resistance of bacterial biofilms. Int J Antimicrob Agents 35:322–332
Hume EBH, Baveja J, Muir B, Schubert TL, Kumar N, Kjelleberg S et al (2004) The control of Staphylococcus epidermidis biofilm formation and in vivo infection rates by covalently bound furanones. Biomaterials 25:5023–5030
Jonsson IM, Mazmanian SK, Schneewind O, Bremell T, Tarkowski A (2003) The role of Staphylococcus aureus sortase A and sortase B in murine arthritis. Microbes Infect 5:775–780

Jori G (2006) Photodynamic therapy of microbial infections: state of the art and perspectives. J Environ Pathol Toxicol Oncol 25:505–519
Kaplan JB (2009) Therapeutic potential of biofilm-dispersing enzymes. Int J Artif Organs 32:545–554
Kaplan JB, Lovetri K, Cardona ST, Madhyastha S, Sadovskaya I, Jabbouri S (2012) Recombinant human DNase I decreases biofilm and increases antimicrobial susceptibility in staphylococci. J Antibiot 65(2):73–77
Kaufmann GF, Sartorio R, Lee SH, Mee JM, Altobell LJ 3rd, Kujawa DP (2006) Antibody interference with N-acyl homoserine lactone-mediated bacterial quorum sensing. J Am Chem Soc 128:2802–2803
Kaufmann GF, Park J, Janda KD (2008) Bacterial quorum sensing: a new target for anti-infective immunotherapy. Expert Opin Biol Ther 8:719–724
Kiedrowski MR, Horswill AR (2011) New approaches for treating staphylococcal biofilm infections. Ann N Y Acad Sci 1241:104–121
Kim L (2007) Persistent cells, dormancy and infectious disease. Nat Rev Microbiol 5:48–56
Kim SW, Chang IM, Oh KB (2002) Inhibition of the bacterial surface protein anchoring transpeptidase sortase by medicinal plants. Biosci Biotechnol Biochem 66:2751–2754
Kiran MD, Giacometti A, Cirioni O, Balaban N (2008) Suppression of biofilm related, device-associated infections by staphylococcal quorum sensing inhibitors. Int J Artif Organs 31:761–770
Kurtz S, Ong K, Lau E, Mowat F, Halpern M (2007) Projections of primary and revision hip and knee arthroplasty in the United States from 2005 to 2030. J Bone Joint Surg Am 89:780–785
Lazar V (2011) Quorum sensing in biofilms — how to destroy the bacterial citadels or their cohesion/power? Anaerobe 17:280–285
Lewis K (2001) Riddle of biofilm resistance. Antimicrob Agents Chemother 45:999–1007
Li YH, Huang S, Du M, Bian Z, Chen Z, Fan MW (2010) Immunogenic characterization and protection against Streptococcus mutans infection induced by intranasal DNA prime-protein boost immunization. Vaccine 28:5370–5376
Lovetri K, Madhyastha S (2010) Antimicrobial and antibiofilm activity of quorum sensing peptides and Peptide analogues against oral biofilm bacteria. Methods Mol Biol 618:383–392
Maisch T (2007) Anti-microbial photodynamic therapy: useful in the future? Lasers Med Sci 22:83–91
Manefield M, de Nys R, Kumar N, Read R, Givskov M, Steinberg P (1999) Evidence that halogenated furanones from Delisea pulchra inhibit acylated homoserine lactone (AHL)- mediated gene expression by displacing the AHL signal from its receptor protein. Microbiology 145:283–291
Mansouri MD, Darouiche RO (2007) In vitro antimicrobial activity of N-acetylcysteine against bacteria colonising central venous catheters. Int J Antimicrob Agents 29:474–476
Marchese A, Bozzolasco M, Gualco L, Debbia EA, Schito GC, Schito AM (2003) Effect of fosfomycin alone and in combination with N-acetylcysteine on *E. coli* biofilms. Int J Antimicrob Agent 22:S95–S100
Maresso AW, Schneewind O (2008) Sortase as a target of antiinfective therapy. Pharmacol Rev 60:128–141
Marraffini LA, Dedent AC, Schneewind O (2006) Sortases and the art of anchoring proteins to the envelopes of gram-positive bacteria. Microbiol Mol Biol Rev 70:192–221
Mazmanian SK, Liu G, Ton-That H, Schneewind O (1999) Staphylococcus aureus sortase, an enzyme that anchors surface proteins to the cell wall. Science 285:760–763
McLean RJC, Lam JS, Graham LL (2012) Training the biofilm generation – a tribute to JW Costerton. J Bacteriol. doi:10.1128/JB.01252-12
Mecikoglu M, Saygi B, Yildirim Y, Karadag-Saygi E, Ramadan SS, Esemenli T (2006) The effect of proteolytic enzyme serratiopeptidase in the treatment of experimental implant-related infection. J Bone Joint Surg Am 88:1208–1214
Montanaro L, Speziale P, Campoccia D, Ravaioli S, Cangini I, Pietrocola G (2011) Scenery of Staphylococcus implant infections in orthopedics. Future Microbiol 6:1329–1349
Musk DJ Jr, Hergenrother PJ (2006) Chemical countermeasures for the control of bacterial biofilms: effective compounds and promising targets. Curr Med Chem 13:2163–2177
Naves P, del Prado G, Huelves L, Rodrı'guez-Cerrato V, Ruiz V, Ponte MC (2010) Effects of human serum albumin, ibuprofen and N-acetyl-L-cysteine against biofilm formation by pathogenic *Escherichia coli* strains. J Hosp Infect 76:165–170
Njoroge J, Sperandio V (2009) Jamming bacterial communication: new approaches for the treatment of infectious diseases. EMBO Mol Med 1:201–210
Nobbs AH, Lamount RJ, Jenkinson H (2009) Streptococcus adherence and colonization. Microbiol Mol Biol Rev 73:407–505
Olofsson AC, Hermansson M, Elwing H (2003) N-acetyl-L-cysteine affects growth, extracellular polysaccharide production, and bacterial biofilm formation on solid surfaces. Appl Environ Microbiol 69: 4814–4822
Palmer M, Costerton W, Sewecke J, Altman D (2011) Molecular techniques to detect biofilm bacteria in long bone nonunion: a case report. Clin Orthop Relat Res 469:3037–3042
Pan JC, Ren DC (2009) Quorum sensing inhibitors: a patent review. Expert Opin Ther Pat 19:1581–1601
Park J (2007) Infection control by antibody disruption of bacterial quorum sensing signaling. Chem Biol 14(10):1119–1127
Park SC, Park Y, Hahm KS (2011) The role of antimicrobial peptides in preventing multidrug-resistant bacterial infections and biofilm formation. Int J Mol Sci 12:5971–5992
Perez-Giraldo C, Rodriguez-Benito A, Moran FJ, Hurtado C, Blanco MT, Gomez-Garcìa AC (1997) Influence of N-acetylcysteine on the formation of biofilm by Staphylococcus epidermidis. J Antimicrob Chemother 39:643–646

Poggio C, Arciola CR, Dagna A, Floridi F, Chiesa M, Saino E (2011) Photoactivated disinfection (PAD) in endodontics: an in vitro microbiological evaluation. Int J Artif Organs 34:889–897

Poultsides LA, Liaropoulos LL, Malizos KN (2010) The socioeconomic impact of musculoskeletal infections. J Bone Joint Surg Am 92:e13

Raad I, Hanna H, Jiang Y, Dvorak T, Reitzel R, Chaiban G (2007a) Comparative activities of daptomycin, linezolid, and tigecycline against catheter related methicillin-resistant Staphylococcus bacteremic isolates embedded in biofilm. Antimicrob Agents Chemother 51:1656–1660

Raad I, Hanna H, Dvorak T, Chaiban G, Hachem R (2007b) Optimal antimicrobial catheter lock solution, using different combinations of minocycline, EDTA, and 25-percent ethanol, rapidly eradicates organisms embedded in biofilm. Antimicrob Agents Chemother 51:78–83

Romanò CL, Romanò D, Bonora C, Degrate A, Mineo G (2009) 'Combined Diagnostic Tool' for joint prosthesis infection. Infez Med 17:141–150

Romanò CL, Toscano M, Romanò D, Drago L (2013) Antibiofilm agents and implant-related infections in orthopaedics: where are we ? J Chemother 25(2):67–80

Romero D, Kolter R (2011) Will biofilm disassembly agents make it to market? Trends Microbiol 19:304–306

Saino E, Sbarra MS, Arciola CR, Scalone M, Bloise N, Nikolov P (2010) Photodynamic action of Tri-meso (N-methyl-pyridyl), meso (N-tetradecyl-pyridyl) porphine on Staphylococcus epidermidis biofilms grown on Ti6Al4V alloy. Int J Artif Organs 33:636–645

Schwandt LQ, van Weissenbruch R, Stokroos I, van der Mei HC, Busscher HJ, Albers FW (2004) Prevention of biofilm formation by dairy products and N-acetylcysteine on voice prostheses in an artificial throat. Acta Otolaryngol 124:726–731

Selan L, Berlutti F, Passariello C, Comodi-Ballanti MR, Thaller MC (1993) Proteolytic enzymes: a new treatment strategy for prosthetic infections? Antimicrob Agents Chemother 37:2618–2621

Sharma M, Visai L, Bragheri F, Cristiani I, Gupta PK, Speziale P (2008) Toluidine blue-mediated photodynamic effects on staphylococcal biofilms. Antimicrob Agents Chemother 52:299–305

Sheffner AL (1963) The reduction in vitro in viscosity of mucoprotein solutions by a new mucolytic agent, N acetyl-L-cysteine. Ann N Y Acad Sci 106:298–310

Shih PC, Huang CT (2002) Effects of quorum-sensing deficiency on Pseudomonas aeruginosa biofilm formation and antibiotic resistance. J Antimicrob Chemother 49:309–314

Shinefield H, Black S, Fattom A, Horwith G, Rasgon S, Ordonez J (2002) Use of a Staphylococcus aureus conjugate vaccine in patients receiving hemodialysis. N Engl J Med 346:491–496

Stewart PS, McFeters GA, Huang CT (2000) Biofilm control by antimicrobial agents. In: Bryers JD (ed) Biofilm: process analysis and applications. Wiley-Liss, New York, pp 373–405

Stoodley P, Conti SF, DeMeo PJ, Nistico L, Melton-Kreft R, Johnson S (2011) Characterization of a mixed MRSA/MRSE biofilm in an explanted total ankle arthroplasty. FEMS Immunol Med Microbiol 62:66–74

Taylor E, Webster TJ (2011) Reducing infections through nanotechnology and nanoparticles. Int J Nanomedicine 6:1463–1473

Tojo M, Yamashita N, Goldmann DA, Pier GB (1988) Isolation and characterization of a capsular polysaccharide adhesin from Staphylococcus epidermidis. J Infect Dis 157:713–722

Tomasz A (1965) Control of the competent state in Pneumococcus by a hormone-like cell product: an example for a new type of regulatory mechanisms in bacteria. Nature 208:155–159

Vilela SF, Junqueira JC, Barbosa JO, Majewski M, Munin E, Jorge AO (2011) Photodynamic inactivation of Staphylococcus aureus and *Escherichia coli* biofilms by malachite green and phenothiazine dyes: an in vitro study. Arch Oral Biol 57:704–710

Vukomanovic M, Skapin SD, Poljansek I, Zagar E, Kralj B, Ignjatovic N, Uskokovic D (2011) Poly(D, L-lactide-co-glycolide)/hydroxyapatite core-shell nanosphere. Part 2: simultaneous release of a drug and a prodrug (clindamycin and clindamycin phosphate). Colloids Surf B Biointerfaces 82(2):414–421

Watson DL (1987) Serological response of sheep to live and killed Staphylococcus aureus vaccines. Vaccine 5:275–278

Weiss WJ, Lenoy E, Murphy T, Tardio L, Burgio O, Projan SJ (2004) Effect of srtA and srtB gene expression on the virulence of Staphylococcus aureus in animal models of infection. J Antimicrob Chemother 53:480–486

Willcox MD, Hume EB, Aliwarga Y, Kumar N, Cole N (2008) A novel cationic-peptide coating for the prevention of microbial colonization on contact lenses. J Appl Microbiol 105:1817–1825

Wu H, Song Z, Hentzer M, Andresen JB, Molin S, Givskov M (2004) Synthetic furanones inhibit quorum-sensing and enhance bacterial clearance in Pseudomonas aeruginosa lung infection in mice. J Antimicrob Chemother 53:1054–1061

Zameer F, Gopal S (2010) Evaluation of antibiotic susceptibility in mixed culture biofilms. Int J Biotech Biochem 6:93–99

Zhang YQ, Ren SX, Li HL, Wang YX, Fu G, Yang J (2003) Genome-based analysis of virulence genes in a non-biofilm-forming Staphylococcus epidermidis strain (ATCC 12228). Mol Microbiol 49:1577–1593

Zhao T, Liu YR (2010) N-acetylcysteine inhibit biofilms produced by *Pseudomonas aeruginosa*. BMC Microbiol 10:140–148

Zygmunt WA, Martin TA (1968) Cysteine analogs as potential amino acid antagonists in bacteria. J Med Chem 11:623–625

Perspectives: The Best Prophylaxis for Primary Arthroplasty

23

Massimo Innocenti, Giovanni Riccio,
Christian Carulli, Gabriele Ristori, Fabrizio Matassi,
and Roberto Civinini

Open Questions

- Is the antibiotic prophylaxis in joint replacement the most important procedure in reducing the infection rate?
- What is the most cost-effective antibiotic family advisable as first choice in prosthetic surgery prophylaxis?
- What are the clinical and environmental conditions justifying the use of glycopeptides for prophylaxis in joint replacement?
- Is there usefulness in combining two antibiotics in a prophylactic regimen?

M. Innocenti • C. Carulli (✉) • G. Ristori
F. Matassi • R. Civinini
Orthopaedic Clinic, University of Florence,
Largo P. Palagi 1, Florence 50139, Italy
e-mail: christian.carulli@unifi.it

G. Riccio (✉)
Regional Center for Infectious Diseases and Septic Orthopedics (Centro Specialistico Regionale Malattie Infettive e Ortopedia Settica, MIOS),
Local Healthcare Unit ASL 2 Savonese,
Ospedale Santa Maria di Misericordia,
Via Martiri della Foce,
Albenga 17031, Italy
e-mail: g.riccio@asl2.liguria.it

23.1 The Infectivologist's Point of View

Giovanni Riccio

Several studies have demonstrated that antibiotic prophylaxis reduces the incidence of infection after orthopaedic surgery, and their use is considered routine for primary and revision joint arthroplasty (AAOS Recommendations 2004).

Three main questions should be answered in discussing about antibiotic prophylaxis:

- Which antibiotic should we choose?
- When do we start its infusion?
- How long do we continue its administration?

Regarding the first point, the characteristics of a good candidate for prophylaxis are as follows:

- To be bactericidal, with a good spectrum against the microorganisms most commonly involved in periprosthetic joint infection.
- It should not be used as in therapeutic regimen.
- It should gain a good tissue penetration and a rapid bioavailability.
- It should have, at the same level of efficacy, lower cost and less adverse effects (Linee Guida ISS 2011).

In order to gain a good tissue concentration of antibiotic during the surgical procedure, the

A. Baldini, P. Caldora (eds.), *Perioperative Medical Management for Total Joint Arthroplasty: How to Control Hemostasis, Pain and Infection*, DOI 10.1007/978-3-319-07203-6_23,

infusion should start between 30 and 60 min before the skin incision, and this range of time seems to be universally accepted. Other reports from the literature have suggested to give the antibiotic within 30 min before the incision or prior the tourniquet inflation in case of knee reconstruction (Van Kasteren et al. 2007a, b). However, the timing of infusion might differ depending on specific drug pharmacokinetics or whether or not a tourniquet is going to be used.

By using vancomycin, for example, that needs a prolonged infusion over 1 h, the infusion should be started, at least, 2 h before skin incision, and this is, of course, more time consuming. In case of the use of a tourniquet, it is important to remember that the whole dose of antibiotic must be infused before the inflation of the tourniquet (Parvizi 2013).

Regarding the third question "how long the prophylaxis has to be continued?", the administration duration time has been well defined from many prospective randomized studies that suggest to stop antibiotic prophylaxis within 24 h after surgery. Medical literature does not demonstrate evidence of benefit when antibiotic prophylaxis is prolonged over this period. Furthermore, giving antibiotic beyond 24 h might lead to the emergence of bacterial resistance and increase the risk of *C. difficile* enteritis (Southorn et al. 1986).

Another aspect often missed by surgeons is the necessity of an intraoperative supplementary dose of antibiotic in case of prolonged operation with surgical time exposure exceeding two times the half-life of the delivered antibiotic or in case of massive blood loss occurring during the procedure (Bratzler et al. 2004). These two situations, indeed, are rare in primary total joint arthroplasties.

Several antibiotics have been suggested for their use as prophylaxis in elective orthopaedic surgery. The main categories are:

- First- and second-generation cephalosporins
- Penicillins
- Glycopeptides (vancomycin and teicoplanin)
- Quinolones
- Clindamycin
- Aminoglycosides

First- and second-generation cephalosporins are the most used as prophylaxis. Their use offers some advantages like an excellent tolerability, the possibility of a more rapid infusion, a good bioavailability and a very low cost.

They are active against oxa-sensitive staphylococci and several Gram-negative microorganisms.

On the other hand, they are not active against oxacillin-resistant staphylococci, enterococci, anaerobes and difficult-to-treat Gram-negative microorganisms (Page et al. 1993).

Penicillins showed, in some studies, results comparable to cefazolin.

Third- and fourth-generation cephalosporins and quinolones should not be chosen as prophylaxis because their use does not ensure better results since they are very useful in the therapeutic regimen and at least more expensive. Like vancomycin, pefloxacin needs a prolonged infusion time (over 1 h).

Glycopeptides seem to be an attractive alternative to second-generation cephalosporins because of their activity against oxacillin-resistant staphylococci, enterococci and anaerobes.

Despite their higher cost, toxicity and management (prolonged infusion time for vancomycin), their cost-effectiveness has been studied by many researchers. Most of these studies showed an equivalent efficacy in preventing SSI, also in centers where oxacillin-resistant staphylococci incidence was higher.

Only one recent study demonstrates a superiority of teicoplanin plus cefuroxime versus cefuroxime alone (Soriano et al. 2006). In other studies, first- and second-generation cephalosporins and glycopeptides showed a similar efficacy in preventing SSI (Vardakas et al. 2005).

Therefore, cefazolin and cefuroxime should be preferred for patients with a standard risk of infection undergoing elective orthopaedic procedures. Clindamycin and vancomycin may be an alternative in the penicillin-allergic patients.

Vancomycin should be used, probably better if in combination with cephalosporin, as first choice in nasal carriers of MRSA or patients coming from communities with a known outbreak of MRSA infection.

Key Points

- The prophylactic infusion time of cephalosporins is 30–60 min before skin incision or tourniquet inflation although one study has suggested that 30 min before incision is admitted.
- In the case of vancomycin, infusion should be started 2 h before skin incision.
- The prophylactic regimen should not be prolonged more than 24 h after surgery.
- Data from the Norwegian Arthroplasty Register showed that four doses/24 h of cefazolin have been more effective than fewer doses, whereas another study showed no differences between one single dose/24 h versus a four-dose regimen.
- In our institution, according to the Italian National Guideline, we recommend one single dose in primary arthroplasty (eventually four doses in particular cases like patients with an ASA score >3) and four doses for prophylaxis in revision surgery.

23.2 The Orthopaedic's Point of View

Massimo Innocenti, Christian Carulli, Gabriele Ristori, Fabrizio Matassi, Roberto Civinini

23.2.1 Introduction

An orthopaedic surgery is a "clean" and successful surgery, as widely demonstrated by several long-term series particularly for hip and knee procedures (Sharkey et al. 2002; Ritter 2009; Corbett et al. 2010; Carulli et al. 2012; Toossi et al. 2013). However, the annual worldwide increasing of the number of hip and knee arthroplasties is leading to a proportional rise of the complications: among these, infections to date represent one of the major risks of failure, reaching up to 15 and 25 % of the indications to revision in hip and knee surgery, respectively (Babkin et al. 2007). The implant of a prosthetic knee or hip induces a susceptibility condition of the host to infections. This situation may be very hard to manage, both for patients and surgeons: moreover, these clinical issues are related to high healthcare and social costs, given the necessity of several medical and surgical procedures. This complication may occur with different clinical patterns: an acute infection, within a few days or weeks from surgery, insidious pain, swelling, rash and possibly with a sinus tract or fistula generally present; a chronic postoperative infection, that realizes from months to years after the implant. In this clinical setting, symptoms are usually nonspecific: it is often difficult to distinguish an infection from an aseptic loosening or a case of hypersensitivity to metals or cement (Carulli et al. 2011; Villano et al. 2011; Innocenti et al. 2014). Finally, the hematogenous seeding type of infection of knee and hip implants usually show as a late infection from index surgery, although as acute clinical presentation: this is not directly correlated to the orthopaedic procedure and may also occur decades after surgery. Fortunately, the infection rates in joint arthroplasties are relatively low and decreasing with respect to the last 30 years: the estimated current incidence is 0.5–1.5 % and 1 % for hip and knee implants, respectively (Engesaeter et al. 2003; Blom et al. 2004; Hamilton and Jamieson 2008; Willis-Owen et al. 2010). These improvements have been achieved by advanced prophylactic perioperative strategies and modern antibiotic therapies. Particularly, the advantages of specific antibiotics has been proved by meticulous randomized trials and demonstrated by important reviews comparing antibiotics with placebo (Heath 1991; Al-Buhairan et al. 2008). Despite this evidence, there is still debate on what should be the best antibiotic to be used as prophylaxis in arthroplasty. Recently, two interesting surveys on the clinical practice of large groups of American and Canadian orthopaedic surgeons have shown a significant variability in the choice of the specific antibiotic, timing and duration of the prophylaxis (Berry and Bozic 2010; de Beer et al. 2009). However, there is no possibility to confirm the superiority of a drug over the others. Given the small percentages of infected implants over the million procedures yearly performed, no randomized trial or head-to-head clinical study may reach a statistical power to assign the greater efficacy of an antibiotic with respect to others. The unique reliability is related to date to the results obtained by the best available evidence in the orthopaedic practice (Parvizi and Gehrke 2013).

23.2.2 Analysis of the Literature and Critical Discussion

The basic requirement to reduce the risk of infection in orthopaedic surgery is to perform the procedures in complete respect of a rigorous sterility: several pre- and intraoperative strategies have been proposed, but only few are supported by scientific evidence (Matar et al. 2010). Preoperative hair removal; the use of a double pair of gloves, surgical gowns and body exhaust suits; laminar flow in the operating room; sterile field by a bacteriostatic and/or bactericidal disinfectant; the use of antibiotic-loaded cement; and antibiotic prophylaxis are now established (Jamsen et al. 2010). Other procedures, such as preoperative shower with antiseptic agents and the use of disposable impervious drapes instead of reusable cotton ones, are still now debated (Merollini et al. 2013).

The main established basic strategy is however the antibiotic prophylaxis. The first choice to be addressed is the specific drug, selected on the basis of the potential agents of infection. In orthopaedic surgery, generally the most involved bacteria are represented by *Staphylococci* (*Staphylococcus aureus* and *epidermidis*), followed by *Streptococci* (Al-Buhairan et al. 2008): specifically, their antibiotic-resistant variants seem to be involved in the septic failures. Several case studies of infected hip and knee implants have been reported in the literature confirming the high rates of bacterial resistance. Phillips et al. reported 4 % of methicillin-resistant *Staphylococcus aureus* (MRSA) and 25 % of methicillin-sensitive *Staphylococcus aureus* (MSSA) in his series (Phillips et al. 2006). Pulido et al. (2001) reported a percentage of MRSA and MSSA of 20 % (Pulido et al. 2008), as similar results have been recently reported (Stefánsdóttir et al. 2013).

Carrega et al. (2008) proposed a hypothesis regarding the type of microbial agent and the timing of occurrence of the infections: early infections are usually induced by non-resistant species of *Staphylococcus aureus* (<3 months), while late infections (>1 year) seem to be correlated to low-virulence bacteria, such as coagulase-negative staphylococci (CoNS). However, the increased number of infections in the interval between 3 months and 1 year is related to resistant species:

- Methicillin-resistant CoNS were identified in 30 % of early infections, in 24 % of delayed infections and in 17 % of late infections.
- MRSA were isolated in 13 % of early infections, in 22 % of delayed infections and in 15 % of late infections.

Therefore, the antibiotic prophylaxis must be essentially focused on *Staphylococci*.

As mentioned, given the current low rates of infection (nowadays decreasing with respect to the 1970s), it is not feasible to conduct a randomized controlled trial that may directly compare the efficacy of two or more antibiotics: thus, there is no evidence of a superiority of an antibiotic over another (Glenny and Song 1999; Al-Buhairan et al. 2008).

The most commonly used and studied antibiotics are first- and second-generation cephalosporins (cefazolin and cefonicid, respectively). They belong to the group of β-lactam molecules with a time-dependent bactericidal action, acting by an irreversible inhibition of the enzyme responsible of the bacterial cell wall integrity. Their pharmacokinetic features as the high water solubility, the elevated tissue penetration, the renal elimination, the absent or negligible toxicity and the half-life (0.5–1.5 h) allow a flexible use in this type of surgery. On the other hand, they have a narrow spectrum of action, mainly active on Gram-positive bacteria (except enterococcus), and in the case of the second-generation cephalosporin, some Gram-negative bacteria (*Escherichia coli*,

Klebsiella pneumoniae, *Proteus mirabilis*). Recent studies revealed a significant increase of antibiotic resistance particularly MRSA but also *Staphylococcus epidermidis* and other methicillin-resistant CoNS (Al-Maiyah et al. 2005; Fulkerson et al. 2006). For these reasons, the use of drugs with a broader spectrum of action as the third-generation cephalosporins (ceftriaxone), extending an action on difficult Gram-negative bacteria, such as *Enterobacter* and *Pseudomonas* species, has been proposed. Similarly, the fourth-generation cephalosporins (Cefepima) showed an enhanced activity on Gram-negative bacteria, maintaining their action on Gram-positive species. These drugs have comparable pharmacokinetic features, but present a longest half-life (ceftriaxone, 4 h; Cefepima, 2 h) with respect to first generation. However, they present an increased risk of colitis by *Clostridium difficile*, associated with a higher mortality risk (from 3.5 to 15.3 %) with respect to the past (Crabtree et al. 1999). For this reason, it is mandatory to reasonably administer the antibiotic prophylaxis in hip and knee surgery to avoid this dangerous complication (Jenkins et al. 2010).

The other major class of antibiotics proposed for the orthopaedic prophylaxis is represented by glycopeptides (vancomycin and teicoplanin). The management of these drugs is absolutely more complex, given the high risk of adverse reactions and limitations. They are almost completely eliminated by the kidneys, and this explains the high rate of (reversible) nephrotoxicity (5 %), and the contraindications in patients with renal insufficiency or in combination with other nephrotoxic drugs. Moreover, vancomycin (but not teicoplanin) may induce a non-immune-mediated release of histamine (5–10 %) in cases of too quick intravenous administration: tachycardia, flushing, tingling, itching, erythema, deafness, tinnitus and in exceptional cases severe arterial hypotension up to shock are reported. Despite these limitations, they are characterized by good pharmacokinetic properties, with long half-life (about 6 h for vancomycin, even more for teicoplanin) and good tissue penetration. Their action is held on all Gram-positive bacteria (except teicoplanin that is not active on enterococcus), and Gram-negative bacteria, acting by an irreversible block of the synthesis of bacterial cell wall. Their spectrum of activity also includes MRSA and methicillin-resistant CoNS, so they are considered "second-line" drugs, reserved for cases of β-lactam resistance or β-lactam allergy. In local ecosystems with specific risks for MRSA infections, it is reasonable to adopt an antibiotic prophylaxis with vancomycin (teicoplanin is more expensive) as "first-line" drugs (Meehan et al. 2009 Smith et al. 2012) with very satisfactory results. Some authors found a recent rise of MRSA and CoNS species with a reduced susceptibility to vancomycin, especially vancomycin-resistant enterococci (VRE) with potential serious consequences (Nixon et al. 2006; Gemmel et al. 2006; Kock et al. 2010). A recent review has concluded that there is insufficient evidence to identify a threshold beyond which it is advisable to switch to routine prophylaxis with glycopeptides (Cranny et al. 2008). The reasonable conclusion is that the analysis of the environmental risks and the patients' features are the main factors to be considered in the choice of the type of drug (Furuno et al. 2006). To date, it has to be considered an increased risk of:

- A previous MRSA infection
- Local environments with a high risk of contamination (elderly communities, hospitalizations in the previous 6–12 months)
- Antibiotic therapy in the previous 30 days, in particular oral fluoroquinolones
- Diabetes mellitus
- Haemodialysis
- Ulcers or unhealed surgical wounds
- Healthcare workers

The first topic (MRSA healthy carriers or shedders) has been the subject of many studies and investigations: in particular, the presence of *Staphylococcus aureus* in nasal colonies in patients undergoing a knee or hip arthroplasty has been evaluated in several papers. It is estimated that 95 million people in the USA are carriers of bacterial colonies inside their nostrils, and in particular, 2.5 million are represented by MRSA species. In these patients, a risk of infection of 2–9 times higher compared to patients without this contamination has been calculated. A dedicated study showed that a prophylaxis with nasal

Table 23.1 International guidelines for the antibiotic prophylaxis in orthopaedics

	AAOS	SIGN	SIOT
1° choice	Cefazolin Cefuroxime	Ceftriaxone (or a low-cost equivalent antibiotic)	Cefazolin
2° choice	Vancomycin Clindamycin (in case of allergy to cephalosporin or of risk for MRSA infection)	Glycopeptides (in case of MRSA infections)	Vancomycin (in case of allergy to cephalosporin or of high risk for MRSA infection)

AAOS American Academy of Orthopaedic Surgeons. Recommendations for the use of intravenous antibiotic prophylaxis in primary total joint arthroplasty (2004)
SIGN Scottish Intercollegiate Guidelines Network. Antibiotic prophylaxis in surgery: a national clinical guideline (2008)
SIOT Società Italiana di Ortopedia e Traumatologia. Profilassi antibiotica perioperatoria nella chirurgia protesica di anca e ginocchio (2011)

mupirocin 5 days prior the intervention in patients with a positive nasal swab was not correlated to a reduction of postoperative infections (Kalmeijer et al. 2002). On the other hand, two papers showed that this type of prophylaxis in association with a preoperative intravenous prophylaxis showed a reduction of infection rate (Rao et al. 2008; Hacek et al. 2008). Currently, nasal decontamination in patients with positive nasal swabs is considered as a good practice (Goyal et al. 2013).

Another debate is on the usefulness of a second antibiotic in the prophylaxis (Sewick et al. 2012). reported on the efficacy of the association of vancomycin and cefazolin: the result was a reduction of the rates of infection by MRSA, while the overall incidence of infections was similar to the single-antibiotic protocol. However, given the large number of patients to be treated to prevent a single case of infection, it is not recommended to extend the indications of a double-antibiotic prophylaxis.

The current trend is to provide the ordinary administration of a first- or second-generation cephalosporin. In selected cases of high risk of MRSA infection as provided by the international guidelines, the choice of a glycopeptide is indicated, as demonstrated by a recent comparative study with cefuroxime, fusidic acid and vancomycin: no superiority of an antibiotic over the others was found, except for vancomycin and MRSA infection (Tyllianakis et al. 2010) (Table 23.1).

Regarding the timing of administration, it is well known that it is fundamental to reach the maximum blood concentration before surgery. Provided that the intravenous administration is the most efficient and useful, the ideal concentration should be achieved before the incision or inflation of the tourniquet, depending on the specific pharmacokinetics of the chosen antibiotic. There is a universal agreement on the fact that it is a crucial step of the procedure (Table 23.2), given the evidence that an inadequate timing of administration is correlated to a rise of the risk for infections (Classen et al. 1992; van Kasteren et al. 2007a, b).

Table 23.2 International guidelines for the timing of the antibiotic prophylaxis in orthopaedics

AAOS	SIGN	SIOT
1 h before incision To be completed before tourniquet Inflation in case of use of vancomycin: 2 h before incision	30 min before incision	30–60 min before incision 5–10 min before tourniquet inflation

AAOS American Academy of Orthopaedic Surgeons. Recommendations for the use of intravenous antibiotic prophylaxis in primary total joint arthroplasty (2004)
SIGN Scottish Intercollegiate Guidelines Network. Antibiotic prophylaxis in surgery: a national clinical guideline (2008)
SIOT Società Italiana di Ortopedia e Traumatologia. Profilassi antibiotica perioperatoria nella chirurgia protesica di anca e ginocchio (2011)

Usually, the preoperative dose corresponds to the therapeutic dose. The following issue is to ensure a stable concentration of antibiotics during the procedure, also by an additional intraoperative dose based on the kinetics of the antibiotic. Indications for a further intraoperative administration are the cases of prolongation of the surgical procedure (timing over twofold the half-life of the antibiotic), an intraoperative non-expected blood loss >1,500 mL or a haemodilution of >15 mL/kg.

Many surgeons are becoming more sensitive to the correct timing of antibiotic administration given the several problems related to the operating rooms (Tan et al. 2006).

The duration time of the prophylaxis is another matter of discussion. The uselessness of the long-term administration is ascertained for two main reasons: firstly, it has been demonstrated that a maintenance of the administration is not correlated to an efficacy in the prevention of an infection (Glenny and Song 1999). On the other hand, a prolonged antibiotic therapy may induce several clinical risks, as adverse reaction, gastric intolerances and possibly a bacterial resistance on the patient and in the community.

Consequently, there is still debate on the opportunity to provide a single versus a multiple (24 h) administration in non-complicated cases: however, there is not enough evidence emerging from the literature. Some authors are in favour of a single shot (Tang et al. 2003; Fonseca et al. 2006), while others support a short-term prophylaxis over the first 24 h after surgery (Wymenga et al. 1992; Engesaeter et al. 2003), considered more efficient in the prevention of an infection.

Many international or national guidelines (AAOS, SIGN, SIOT) indicate that a short-term administration with multiple doses with intervals based on the specific pharmacokinetics of the chosen antibiotic seems to have better results in the control of infection.

Conclusions

As mentioned, it is hard to define a unique protocol of antibiotic prophylaxis in orthopaedic surgery. However, the best available evidence in orthopaedic literature has suggested some specific guidelines worldwide accepted. Antibiotic prophylaxis in orthopaedic surgery should be based on the patients' medical history and health status and set on the local hospital conditions or risk factors; moreover, the duration of the prophylaxis should be varied in cases of prolonged surgical time or intraoperative complications.

The antibiotic of first choice should be a first- or second-generation cephalosporin or, in cases of actual specific risks, a glycopeptide, both by intravenous administration. The first dose of antibiotic should be administered 30–60 min before skin incision and always 30–60 min before the tourniquet is inflated. Finally, considering the duration of the antibiotic prophylaxis, a postoperative period of 24 h is suggested.

Key Points

- So far the preoperative antibiotic prophylaxis represents the most important clinical practice in reducing the infection rate in joint replacement.
- Given the staphylococci are the most frequent contaminants responsible of periprosthetic joint infections, the prophylactic antibiotics most commonly used are first- and second-generation cephalosporins. In the routine practice, for patients and local conditions of standard risks, they are the most cost-effective antibiotic group considered the first choice in prosthetic surgery prophylaxis.
- There is insufficient evidence to identify a threshold beyond which it is advisable to switch from routine prophylaxis to prophylaxis with glycopeptides. It is reasonable that the analysis of the environmental risks (local percentage of MRSA) and the patients' features are the main factors to be considered for switching to a second line of prophylaxis by using glycopeptides. The second reason for using glycopeptides (vancomycin or teicoplanin) in prophylaxis may be a demonstration of a patient's allergy to β-lactamase antibiotics.
- With the exception of selective cases at very high risk of infection or in the presence of concomitant infections (urinary tract) or in patients with an immunodeficiency, it is not recommended to extend the indications of a double-antibiotic prophylaxis.

References

AAOS recommendations for the use of intravenous antibiotic prophylaxis in primary total joint arthroplasty (2004) www.aaos.org

Al-Buhairan B, Hind H, Hutchinson A (2008) Antibiotic prophylaxis for wound infections in total joint arthroplasty: a systematic review. J Bone Joint Surg Br 90:915–919

Al-Maiyah M, Hill D, Bajwa A et al (2005) Bacterial contaminants and antibiotic prophylaxis in total hip arthroplasty. J Bone Joint Surg Br 87:1256–1258

Babkin Y, Raveh D et al (2007) Incidence and risk factors for surgical infection after total knee replacement. Scand J Infect Dis 10:890–895

Berry DJ, Bozic K (2010) Current practice patterns in primary hip and knee arthroplasty among members of the American Association of Hip and Knee Surgeons. J Arthroplasty 25(6 Suppl):2–4

Blom AW, Brown J, Taylor AH et al (2004) Infection after total knee replacement. J Bone Joint Surg Br 86B:688–691

Bratzler DW et al (2004) Antimicrobial prophylaxis for surgery: an advisory statement from the National Surgical Infection Prevention Project. Clin Infect Dis 38:1706–1715

Carrega G, Bartolacci V, Burastero G et al (2008) Etiology of prosthetic joint infections in a tertiary care centre in Italy. Infez Med 16(4):204–208

Carulli C, Villano M, Bucciarelli G et al (2011) Painful knee arthroplasty: definition and overview. Clin Cases Miner Bone Metab 8:23–25

Carulli C, Matassi F, Nistri L et al (2012) Long-term survival of a flat-on-flat total condylar knee arthroplasty fixed with a hybrid cementing technique for tibial components. J Long Term Eff Med Implants 22:305–312

Classen DC, Evans RS, Pestotnik SL et al (1992) The timing of prophylactic administration of antibiotics and the risk of surgical wound infection. N Engl J Med 326:281–286

Corbett KL, Losina E, Nti AA et al (2010) Population-based rates of revision of primary total hip arthroplasty: a systematic review. PLoS One 5:e13520

Crabtree TD, Palletier SJ, Gleason TG et al (1999) Clinical characteristics and antibiotic utilization in surgical patients with Clostridium difficile-associated diarrhea. Am Surg 65:507–511

Cranny G, Elliot R, Weatherly H et al (2008) A systematic review and economic model of switching from non-glycopeptide to glycopeptide antibiotic prophylaxis for surgery. Health Technol Assess 12:1–147

de Beer J, Petruccelli D, Rotstein C et al (2009) Antibiotic prophylaxis for total joint replacement surgery: results of a survey of Canadian orthopaedic surgeons. Can J Surg 52:E229–E234

Engesaeter LB, Lie SA, Espehaug B et al (2003) Antibiotic prophylaxis in total hip arthroplasty: effects of antibiotic prophylaxis seismically and in bone cement on the revision rate of 22170 primary hip replacements followed 0-14 years in the Norwegian Arthroplasty Register. Acta Orthop Scand 74:644–651

Fonseca SN, Kunzle SR, Junqueira MJ et al (2006) Implementing 1-dose antibiotic prophylaxis for prevention of surgical site infection. Arch Surg 141:1109–1113

Fulkerson E, Valle CJ, Wise B et al (2006) Antibiotic susceptibility of bacteria infecting total joint arthroplasty sites. J Bone Joint Surg Am 88:1231–1237

Furuno JP, McGregor JC, Harris AD et al (2006) Identifying groups at high risk for carriage of antibiotic resistant bacteria. Arch Intern Med 166:580–585

Gemmel GC, Edwards DI, Weatherly H, Joint working party of the British Society for Antimicrobial Chemotherapy, Hospital Infection Society and Infection Control Nurses Association et al (2006) Guidelines for the prophylaxis and treatment of methicillin-resistant Staphylococcus aureus (MRSA) infection in UK. J Antimicrob Chemother 57:589–608

Glenny AM, Song F (1999) Antimicrobial prophylaxis in total hip replacement: a systematic review. Health Technol Assess 3:1–57

Goyal N, Miller A, Tripathi M et al (2013) Methicillin-resistant Staphylococcus aureus (MRSA): colonisation and pre-operative screening. Bone Joint J 95B:4–9

Hacek DM, Robb WJ, Paule SM et al (2008) Staphylococcus aureus nasal decolonization in joint replacement surgery reduces infection. Clin Orthop Relat Res 466:1349–1355

Hamilton H, Jamieson J (2008) Deep infection in total hip arthroplasty. Can J Surg 51:111–117

Heath AF (1991) Antimicrobial prophylaxis for arthroplasty and total joint replacement: discussion and review of published clinical trials. Pharmacotherapy 11:157–163

Innocenti M, Carulli C, Matassi F et al (2014) Total knee arthroplasty in patients with hypersensitivity to metals. Int Orthop 38:329–333

Jämsen E, Furnes O, Engesæter LB, Konttinen YT et al (2010) Prevention of deep infection in joint replacement surgery: a review. Acta Orthop 81(6):660–666

Jenkins PJ, Teoh K, Simpson PM et al (2010) Breusch Clostridium difficile in patients undergoing primary hip and knee replacement. J Bone Joint Surg Br 92:994–998

Kalmeijer DM, Coertjens H, van Nieuwland-Bollen PM et al (2002) Surgical site infections in orthopedic surgery: the effect of mupirocin nasal ointment in a double-blind, randomized, placebo-controlled study. Clin Infect Dis 35:353–358

Kock R, Becker K, Cookson B et al (2010) Methicillin-resistant Staphylococcus aureus (MRSA): burden of disease and control challenges in Europe. Euro Surveill 15:19688

Linee Guida ISS (2011) SNLG Antibioticoprofilassi nell'adulto

Matar WY, Jafari MS, Restrepo C et al (2010) Preventing infection in total joint arthroplasty. J Bone Joint Surg Br 92-A(Suppl 2):36–46

Meehan J, Jamali AA, Nguyen H (2009) Prophylactic antibiotics in hip and knee arthroplasty. J Bone Joint Surg Am 91(10):2480–2490
Merollini KMD, Zheng H, Graves N (2013) Most relevant strategies for preventing surgical site infection after total hip arthroplasty: guideline recommendations and expert opinion. Am J Infect Control 41:221–226
Nixon M, Jackson B, Varghese P et al (2006) Methicillin-resistant Staphylococcus aureus in orthopaedic wards: incidence, spread, mortality, cost and control. J Bone Joint Surg Br 88:812–817
Page CP et al (1993) Antimicrobial prophylaxis for surgical wounds. Guidelines for clinical care. Arch Surg 128:79–88
Parvizi J (2013) Prosthetic joint infection: practical management guide. Jaypee Brothers Medical Publishers New Delhi
Parvizi J, Gehrke T (2013) Proceedings of the international consensus meeting on periprosthetic joint infection. Data Trace Publishing Company, Brooklandville
Phillips JE, Crane TP, Noy M et al (2006) The incidence of deep prosthetic infections in a specialist orthopaedic hospital: a 15-year prospective survey. J Bone Joint Surg Br 88:943–948
Pulido L, Ghanem E, Joshi A et al (2008) Periprosthetic joint infection: the incidence, timing, and predisposing factors. Clin Orthop Relat Res 466:1710–1715
Rao N, Cannella B, Crossett LS et al (2008) A preoperative decolonization protocol for staphylococcus aureus prevents orthopaedic infections. Clin Orthop Relat Res 466:1343–1348
Ritter MA (2009) The anatomical graduated component total knee replacement. A long-term evaluation with 20-years survival analysis. J Bone Joint Surg Br 91:45–49
Sewick A, Makani A, Wu C et al (2012) Does dual antibiotic prophylaxis better prevent surgical site infections in total joint arthroplasty? Clin Orthop Relat Res 470:2702–2707
Sharkey PF, Hozack WJ, Rothman RH et al (2002) Why are total knee arthroplasties failing today? Clin Orthop Relat Res 404:7–13
Smith EB, Wynne R, Joshi A et al (2012) Is it time to include vancomycin for routine perioperative antibiotic prophylaxis in total joint arthroplasty patients? J Arthroplasty 27(8 Suppl):55–60
Soriano A et al (2006) Eur J Clin Microbiol Infect Dis 25:35–38
Southorn PA, Plevak DJ, Wright AJ, Wilson WR (1986) Adverse effects of vancomycin administered in the perioperative period. Mayo Clin Proc 61:721–724
Stefánsdóttir A, Johansson Å, Lidgren L et al (2013) Bacterial colonization and resistance patterns in 133 patients undergoing a primary hip- or knee replacement in Southern Sweden. Acta Orthop 84(1):87–91
Tan JA, Naik VN, Lingard L (2006) Exploring obstacles to proper timing of prophylactic antibiotics for surgical site infections. Qual Saf Health Care 1:32–38
Tang WM, Chiu KY, Ng TP et al (2003) Efficacy of a single dose of cefazolin as a prophylactic antibiotic in primary arthroplasty. J Arthroplasty 18:714–718
Toossi N, Adeli B, Timperley AJ et al (2013) Acetabular components in total hip arthroplasty: is there evidence that cementless fixation is better? J Bone Joint Surg Am 95:168–174
Tyllianakis ME, Karageorgos AC, Marangos MN et al (2010) Antibiotic prophylaxis in primary hip and knee arthroplasty: comparison between cefuroxime and two specific antistaphylococcal agents. J Arthroplasty 25(7):1078–1082
Van Kasteren ME et al (2007a) Antibiotic prophylaxis and the risk of surgical site infection following total hip arthroplasty; timely administration is the most important factor. Clin Infect Dis 44:92–97
van Kasteren ME, Mannien J, Ott A et al (2007b) Antibiotic prophylaxis and the risk of surgical site infections following total hip arthroplasty: timely administration is the most important factor. Clin Infect Dis 44:921–927
Vardakas KZ et al (2005) Perioperative anti-infective prophylaxis with teicoplanin compared to cephalosporins in orthopaedic and vascular surgery involving prosthetic material. Clin Microbiol Infect 11: 775–777
Villano M, Carulli C, Puccini S et al (2011) Painful knee arthroplasty: surgical approach. Clinical Cases Miner Bone Metab 8:26–28
Willis-Owen CA, Konyves A, Martin DK (2010) Factors affecting the incidence of infection in hip and knee replacement. An analysis of 5277 cases. J Bone Joint Surg Br 92B:1128–1133
Wymenga A, von Horn J, Theeuwes A et al (1992) Cefuroxime for prevention of post-operative coxitis. One versus three doses tested in a randomized multicenter study of 2651 arthroplasties. Acta Orthop Scand 63:19–24

24 Perspectives: How to Deal with Fever (38 °C) After Arthroplasty: The Infectivologist's Point of View

Tiziana Ascione, Giovanni Balato, and Pasquale Pagliano

Open Questions

- How to differentiate an infectious fever from a noninfectious one during the postoperative period after joint arthroplasty?
- Is there a specific marker demonstrating an early infection in joint reconstruction?
- Should we get culture from wound drainage in a febrile patient who recently underwent arthroplasty surgery?

24.1 Introduction

Infections in the postoperative course after orthopaedic surgery can lead to prolonged hospitalization, increased morbidity and mortality and high costs Blom et al. (2004); Chun et al. (2013); Lora-Tamayo et al. (2013). Postoperative fever in arthroplasty patients is common and may be provoked by many factors including surgical trauma, haematoma in the surgical site and transfusion of blood or blood products Summersell et al. (2003); Tai et al. (2009).

T. Ascione (✉) • P. Pagliano
Department of Infectious Diseases, "D. Cotugno" Hospital, AORN "Dei Colli", Naples, Italy
e-mail: tizianascione@hotmail.com; ppagliano@libero.it

G. Balato
Department of Orthopaedic Surgery, University 'Federico II', Naples, Italy
e-mail: giovannibalato@gmail.com

Early identification of patients with postoperative infections is of great importance in order to establish effective antibiotic therapy Springer and Scuderi (2013). Patients with febrile episodes generally undergo routine laboratory examination including white blood cell count, erythrocyte sedimentation rate (ERS), C-reactive protein (CRP), urine culture, blood culture and chest X-ray to identify the cause of fever Athanassious et al. (2011); Osmon et al. (2013).

Blood markers such as white blood cell count, ERS and CRP employed in daily practice to investigate infective fever are increased for all patients in postoperative surgery and are not helpful in discriminating between early infection and nonspecific inflammatory response due to surgical trauma Shetty and Kasture (2013).

Newer markers such as interleukin-6 have been recently assessed; although these newer markers seem to have better accuracy, their diagnostic utility has not been clearly established. Kinetic properties of such new inflammatory markers are important when their use is assessed in clinical practice as a diagnostic marker for prosthetic joint infection.

Interleukin-6 (IL-6) is produced by stimulated monocytes and macrophages and induces the production of several acute-phase proteins. Its peak is 2 days after uncomplicated arthroplasty and it rapidly returns to a normal value Berbari et al (2012).

CRP is an acute-phase marker that is produced by the liver in response to inflammation. Its levels are elevated to their peak values 2–3 days after

A. Baldini, P. Caldora (eds.), *Perioperative Medical Management for Total Joint Arthroplasty: How to Control Hemostasis, Pain and Infection*, DOI 10.1007/978-3-319-07203-6_24,

surgery and return to normal approximately 3 or 4 weeks after surgery.

Serum procalcitonin is a marker supporting clinical and microbiological findings for more reliable differentiation of infectious from noninfectious causes of fever after orthopaedic surgery Bouaicha et al. (2013). The exact mechanisms underlying procalcitonin induction during or after surgery are unknown. Infection and bacterial endotoxins are strong stimuli for the induction of procalcitonin. The nonspecific induction of procalcitonin production by trauma or tissue injury, however, seems to be lower as compared to a specific induction by bacterial infection. The return of procalcitonin levels to normal within a few days after an uncomplicated postoperative course can be explained by the physiological half-life of procalcitonin of 18–24 h in the absence of further inducing stimuli for procalcitonin production.

Moreover, the diagnostic yield of blood cultures in patient with febrile postoperative arthroplasty is low and seldom contributes to clinical management Anderson and Osland (2009); Sivakumar et al. (2012).

There are currently no evidence-based clinical practice guidelines outlining an approach to the patient with fever following arthroplasty surgery, and fever was found to have low accuracy in the diagnosis of prosthetic joint infection on the basis of current IDSA guidelines.

In an era of escalating health care costs, the development of cost-effective, evidence-based practice algorithm for the evaluation of the febrile patient after arthroplasty is needed to minimize practice variation and limit waste without compromising patient care.

24.2 Analysis of the Literature with Critical Discussion

To evaluate the presence of fever after orthopaedic surgery and the impact of fever on early prosthetic joint infections, we carried out a systematic search of the English language literature using the MEDLINE database with the search strings 'fever AND arthroplasty' and 'diagnostic markers AND arthroplasty' for reports published from January 2000 to March 2014.

On the basis of the findings of the studies retrieved, the value of fever and inflammatory markers during the postoperative period was investigated.

Altogether, fever was reported in 15–37 % of patients undergoing arthroplasty and disappeared about 7 days after surgery regardless of the presence of infection. Fever failed to be a predictive symptom associated to implant infection itself. In the larger study (Ghosh et al. 2006) retrieved, only 3 % of cases reporting fever during the postoperative period were found to have an infection; instead, about 10 % of cases without fever reported a postoperative infection.

Blood cultures had a low sensitivity in febrile patients undergoing arthroplasty. Only 2 out of 141 cultures were positive in 101 patients with fever investigated by Vijaysegaran et al. (2012), and the source of the retrieved microorganism was not found (of note, both cases did not report prosthetic joint infection after a 6-month follow-up period). Similar data are reported by Bindelglass and Pellegrino (2007) investigating 453 cases undergoing arthroplasty. Of five cases with a positive culture retrieved in the study, none reported an infection related to the microorganism cultured and none was found to have a prosthetic joint infection during the follow-up.

Data on procalcitonin value were underreported in studies investigating fever and arthroplasty. However, when we checked the value of this inflammatory marker with the keywords 'diagnostic markers' and 'arthroplasty', we found that when its value was investigated in febrile patients after arthroplasty, there was a significant trend supporting its use in identifying patients with an infection (Hunziker et al. 2010). Unlike CRP and white blood cell count, procalcitonin values were significantly higher in 45 patients with infection compared with 58 uninfected cases on the day of fever onset, day 1 and day 3. Similar data supporting procalcitonin use in association with other biomarkers such as IL-6 and CRP are reported by Glehr et al. (2013) and by Bottner et al. (2007) in smaller studies investigating febrile patients.

The value of IL-6 in patients with prosthetic joint infection was highlighted by the findings of a number of studies, but its value in respect to the

Table 24.1 Main studies investigating the value of fever and biomarkers in patients undergoing arthroplasty

References	No. of cases	Parameters investigation	Positive infection	Follow-up	PJI
Bindelglass and Pellegrino (2007)	453	Blood culture (22 % of cases)	5	6 months	0
Vijaysegaran et al. (2012)	101	Blood culture (141 blood cultures)	2	24 months	0
Ghosh et al. (2006)	170	Fever 62 cases (36 %)	2	19 months	0
		No fever 108 cases	12	19 months	2
Ishii et al. (2013)	400	Fever 149 cases (37 %)	3	4 weeks	1
Czaplicki et al. (2011)	426	Fever 64 cases (15 %)	ND	24 months	2
Ward et al. (2010)	1,100	6 % positive blood	ND	24 month	ND
Hunziker et al. (2010)	103	Procalcitonin	Higher	ND	4
Glehr et al. (2013)	84	Procalcitonin, IL-6, CRP	Higher	ND	ND
Bottner et al. (2007)	31	Procalcitonin, IL-6, CRP	Higher	ND	ND
Randau et al. (2014)	120	Procalcitonin, IL-6 serum IL-6 joint aspirate	Higher	ND	ND

fever itself remained unclear (we have to consider that the relative dosage is not routinely performed in daily practice). In fact Randau et al. (2014) investigated the biomarkers in 120 patients with prosthetic joint infection and found that high serum IL-6 was a valuable and even more accurate marker than either ERS or CRP, but they did not investigate the value of IL-6 in respect to the presence of fever during the perioperative period (Table 24.1).

24.3 New Perspectives

On the basis of the data retrieved by literature search, we construct a diagnostic algorithm useful to examine the patients with postoperative fever after arthroplasty and able to distinguish infectious from noninfectious fever.

We suggest that the presence of fever prompts an accurate clinical examination and laboratory investigation.

In our diagnostic algorithm, continuous fever persisting during the second and third day after arthroplasty can represent indication to dosage of serum procalcitonin and IL-6 (if the dosage is available).

If procalcitonin dosage is elevated, blood culture and other microbiological investigations can be performed on the basis of clinical findings. In fact, the presence of associated symptoms has to guide the choice of subsequent investigation, such as chest X-ray in the presence of pulmonary symptoms or culture of urine in the presence of urinary tract symptoms. Also the surgical site has to be the object of an accurate clinical evaluation for the presence of swelling, warmth and drainage. Culture from an infected surgical site has to be immediately attempted.

Timely administration of adequate antibiotic therapy is an important factor to reduce morbidity and mortality in patients with postoperative infections, and thus a thorough clinical examination and diagnostic algorithm is mandatory.

Antibiotic therapy must be started only in the presence of diagnosis of bacterial infections (Fig. 24.1).

Conclusion

The development of fever during the first few days following arthroplasty is a relatively common finding. However, its relation with perioperative factors remains largely unclear.

Fever in the first few days following surgery is known to be a normal physiological response, and there are no specific tests such as white blood count and CRP that would indicate the presence of infection at this early stage after the operation.

Serum procalcitonin has reliable diagnostic accuracy in predicting underlying infection in patients with a new onset of fever during the early period after orthopaedic surgery. The course of procalcitonin levels is different in a

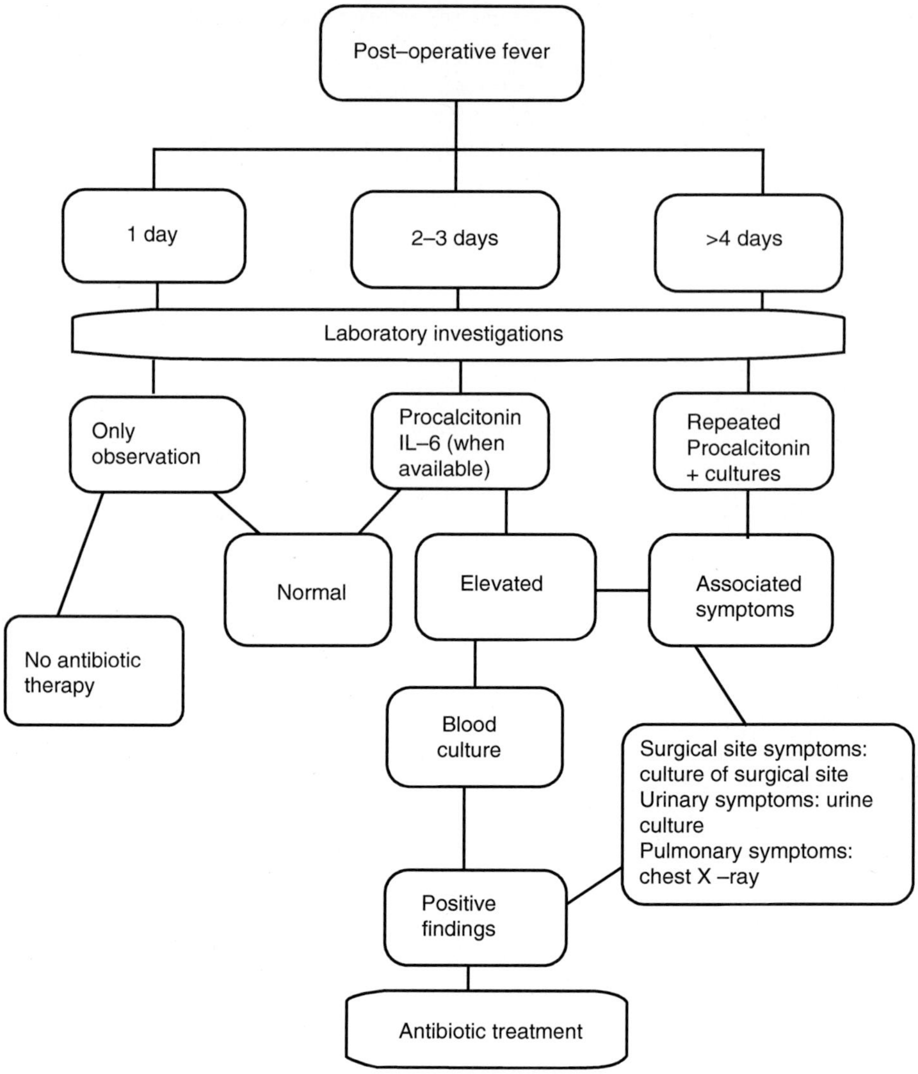

Fig. 24.1 Diagnostic algorithm of patients with fever after arthroplasty

fever of infectious origin compared with fever of noninfectious origin and thus has to be investigated. On the basis of the findings retrieved from the literature, when fever is present, procalcitonin is a reliable marker for infection and more relevant than CRP for the diagnosis of postoperative infection.

IL-6 is considered a valuable early marker of prosthetic joint infection, but its use in diagnosing postoperative infectious fever needs further investigation. Furthermore, its routine use in the clinical practice may be limited in many surgical settings.

Key Points

- With the use of the well-known routine blood, investigations, such as blood cultures, white blood cell count, erythrocyte sedimentation rate and C-reactive protein, it is almost impossible to differentiate an infectious fever from a noninfectious one during the early postoperative period after joint arthroplasty.
- There are currently no evidence-based clinical practice guidelines outlining an

approach to the patient with fever following arthroplasty surgery, and fever was found to have low accuracy in the diagnosis of prosthetic joint infection.

- So far there is no specific marker demonstrating an early infection in joint reconstruction. Serum procalcitonin has shown realable diagnostic accuracy in predicting underlying infection in patients with a new onset of fever during the early period after orthopaedic surgery. Further investigations are needed to demonstrate the usefulness of serum procalcitonin as a diagnostic tool of infection in the early postoperative course.

Adherence to preestablished algorithm in the presence of fever can reduce costs and improve the effectiveness of diagnostic and therapeutic choice.

References

Anderson JT, Osland JD (2009) Blood cultures for evaluation of fever after total joint arthroplasty. Am J Orthop 38:E134–E136

Andres BM, Taub DD, Gurkan I et al (2003) Postoperative fever after total knee arthroplasty: the role of cytokines. Clin Orthop Relat Res 415:221–231

Athanassious C, Samad A, Avery A et al (2011) Evaluation of fever in the immediate postoperative period in patients who underwent total joint arthroplasty. J Arthroplasty 26(8):1404–1408

Berbari E, Mabry T, Tsaras G et al (2012) Inflammatory blood laboratory levels as markers of prosthetic joint infection. J Bone Joint Surg Am 92:2102–2109

Bindelglass DF, Pellegrino J (2007) The role of blood cultures in the acute evaluation of postoperative fever in arthroplasty patients. J Arthroplasty 22:701

Blom AW, Brown J, Taylor AH et al (2004) Infection after total knee arthroplasty. J Bone Joint Surg Br 86:688–691

Bottner F, Wegner A, Winkelmann W et al (2007) Interleukin-6, procalcitonin and TNF-alpha: markers of peri-prosthetic infection following total joint replacement. J Bone Joint Surg Br 89:94–99

Bouaicha S, Blatter S, Moor BK (2013) Early serum procalcitonin level after primary total hip replacement. Mediators Inflamm. Article ID 927636

Chun KC, Kim KM, Chun CH (2013) Infection following total knee arthroplasty. Knee Surg Relat Res 25: 93–99

Czaplicki AP, Borger JE, Politi JR et al (2011) Evaluation of postoperative fever and leukocytosis in patients after total hip and knee arthroplasty. J Arthroplasty 26:1387–1389

Ghosh S, Charity RM, Haidar SG et al (2006) Pyrexia following total knee replacement. Knee 13:324–327

Glehr M, Friesenbichler J, Hofmann G et al (2013) Novel biomarkers to detect infection in revision hip and knee arthroplasties. Clin Orthop Relat Res 471: 2621–2628

Hunziker S, Hugle T, Schuchardt K et al (2010) The Value of serum procalcitonin level for differentiation of infectious from non-infectious causes of fever after orthopaedic surgery. J Bone Joint Surg Am 92:138–148

Ishii Y, Noguchi H, Takeda M et al (2013) Evaluation of fever and its related factors during 4 weeks after primary total hip arthroplasty. Surg Sci 4:1–6

Lora-Tamayo J, Murillo O, Iribarren JA et al (2013) A large multicenter study of methicillin-susceptible and methicillin-resistant Staphylococcus aureus prosthetic joint infections managed with implant retention. Clin Infect Dis 56:182–194

Osmon DR, Berbari EF, Berendt AR et al (2013) Diagnosis and management of prosthetic joint infection: clinical practice guidelines by the infectious diseases society of America. Clin Infect Dis 56: 1–10

Randau TM, Friedrich MJ, Wimmer MD et al (2014) Interleukin-6 in serum and in synovial fluid enhances the differentiation between periprosthetic joint infection and aseptic loosening. PLoS One 9:e89045

Shetty V, Kasture S (2013) Is immediate postoperative fever related to drop in haemoglobin? A comparative study in simultaneous bilateral total knee arthroplasty patients. Eur J Orthop Surg Traumatol 23:345–347

Sivakumar B, Vijaysegaran P, Ottley M et al (2012) Blood cultures for evaluation of early postoperative fever after femoral neck fracture surgery. J Orthop Surg 20:336–340

Springer BD, Scuderi GR (2013) Evaluation and management of the infected total knee arthroplasty. Instr Course Lect 62:349–361

Summersell PC, Turnbull A, Long G et al (2003) Temperature trends in total Hip arthroplasty. A retrospective study. J Arthroplasty 18:426–429

Tai W, Chang C-W, Lin C-J, Lai K-A, Yang C-Y (2009) Elevated temperature trends after total knee arthroplasty. Orthopedics 32:886

Vijaysegaran P, Coulter SA, Coulter C et al (2012) Blood cultures for assessment of postoperative fever in arthroplasty patients. J Arthroplasty 27:375–377

Ward DT, Hansen EN, Takemoto SK et al (2010) Cost and effectiveness of postoperative fever diagnostic evaluation in total joint arthroplasty patients. J Arthroplasty 25:43–48

Perspectives: How to Deal with Fever (38 °C) After Arthroplasty: The Surgeon's Point of View

25

Federica Rosso, Lorenzo Mattei, Matteo Bruzzone, Federico Dettoni, Davide Edoardo Bonasia, and Roberto Rossi

Open Questions

- Is there a relationship between fever and infection in the first postoperative week after joint arthroplasties?
- What are the main causes of fever in the early postoperative period?
- How important is the febrile diagnostic workup?

25.1 Introduction

Fever is a frequent occurrence in the early postoperative period in patients who underwent total hip, knee, or shoulder arthroplasties, but its source and clinical importance is still unclear (Tai et al. 2009). Total joint arthroplasty is one of the most common orthopedic procedures performed in the United States and in Europe, and the orthopedic surgeon should know how to deal with fever and when it is suggestive for infection. The presence of fever in the postoperative period (can) might be correlated with an infection or a serious complication, but in the majority of cases, fever is the result of a noninfectious process (Garibaldi et al. 1985). In literature the incidence of postoperative fever is reported to occur in between 15 and 47 % of cases, with a smaller percentage correlated to infectious processes. For most of the orthopedic surgeons, fever can be overall one of the signs of infection, and it is associated with significant morbidity and mortality (Blom et al. 2004; Lentino 2003). Due to this fear, patients who develop a postoperative pyrexia are often subjected to a routine panel of investigations like chest X-ray (CXR); urinalysis (UA); urine, blood, and wound-swab cultures; serial full blood counts and inflammatory markers; Doppler ultrasound; or venogram to exclude deep vein thrombosis (DVT) to determine the cause of the fever.

F. Rosso • L. Mattei • M. Bruzzone • F. Dettoni •
R. Rossi (✉)
Mauriziano Umberto I Hospital, University of Torino, Torino, Italy
e-mail: federica.rosso@yahoo.it; lorenzo.mattei87@gmail.com; matteo.bruzzone@fastwebnet.it; federicodettoni@tin.it; rossir@fastwebnet.it

D.E. Bonasia
Azienda Ospedaliera Citta` della Salute e della Scienza, Centro Traumatologico Ortopedico Hospital, University of Torino, Torino, Italy
e-mail: davidebonasia@virgilio.it

25.2 Causes of Fever in the Immediate Postoperative

Fever in total knee replacement patients has been correlated to physiological response to surgical trauma; the disturbance of thermoregulation by

A. Baldini, P. Caldora (eds.), *Perioperative Medical Management for Total Joint Arthroplasty: How to Control Hemostasis, Pain and Infection*, DOI 10.1007/978-3-319-07203-6_25,

anesthesia; retained hematoma; the presence of atelectasis, pneumonia, or urinary tract infection; superficial or deep wound infection; deep vein thrombosis; and the response to blood transfusion.

In patients undergoing hip replacement after a proximal femoral fracture, the fever is more frequent and it appears earlier than in patient operated electively. Probably this is due to the fact that the inflammatory response begins at the moment of the trauma, in association with the increased release of inflammatory factors such as interleukin-1β (IL-1β), interleukin-6 (IL-6), and tumor necrosis factor-α (TNF-α). In those patients, fever usually appears at day 0, while it has been demonstrated that in patients operated electively fever usually appears on postoperative day (POD) 2–3 (Petretta et al. 2013). In the last 15 years, extensive data and literature have been produced about the pathophysiology, possible causes, and the role of diagnostic tests in postoperative fever in patients undergoing joint replacement.

25.3 Pathophysiology and Role of Inflammatory Factors

The inflammatory response to total joint arthroplasty surgery could produce a transient release of endogenous factors. IL-1β, IL-6, and TNF-α are involved in the body's inflammatory response to injury, and elective surgery has been shown to cause a temporary elevation in IL-6 serum levels (Frank et al. 2000; Lahat et al. 1992; Miyawaki et al. 1998). This systemic response seems to be even higher in the presence of postoperative fever (Pullicino et al. 1990). One theory for such IL-6 serum elevation is that its production is stimulated by the local inflammatory response at the surgical site. Andres et al. (2003) found elevated levels of IL-1β, IL-6, and TNF-α at the surgical site and elevated IL-6 levels in the serum after total joint arthroplasty. In addition, there were significantly higher levels of drain and serum IL-6 in patients who were febrile than in patients who were afebrile at 24 and 48 h after TKA. A positive correlation was found between serum IL-6, drain IL-6, and serum leukocyte levels, suggesting that TKA is followed by an increased local production of IL-1β, IL-6, and TNF-α at the surgical site that results in the release of IL-6 into the local circulation, leading to leukocytosis and fever.

Other animal studies have shown that subcutaneous injections of pyogenic factors result in a local increase in IL-1 and TNF-α levels, which is followed by a systemic increase in IL-6 and fever (Cooper et al. 1994; Luheshi et al. 1996). In addition, injecting these animals with antibodies against IL-1 or TNF-α resulted in reduction of the febrile response.

25.4 Fever in First 5–7 Postoperative Days

In a retrospective study, Summersell et al. (2003) have analyzed the body temperature before, during, and after surgery in all the patients who underwent a total hip arthroplasty during a period of 2 years. They have recorded a drop in average body temperature of 0.5 °C after surgery, probably as a side effect of anesthetics and low operating room temperature. During POD 1 and 2, the majority of patients experienced an elevation in body temperature above 38 °C. In this casuistry, 62.5 % of patients reached a temperature of >38 °C, the 20 % >38.5 °C, and 3.5 % >39 °C, and no infection was detected in any of these patients.

Ghosh et al. (2006) performed in 2006 a retrospective analysis of the temperature histories of 170 patients who underwent a total knee replacement. Fourteen of these developed a postoperative infection and 2 a prosthetic infection from *S. aureus*. In the 36.5 % of patients, pyrexia was present at some point during the first 5 postoperative days. The highest prevalence was detected during POD 1. They have reported an average temperature (37.5 °C) lower than the one reported from Summersell et al. (2003) (>38 °C). The most interesting conclusion of this study is that they found only 4 patients who developed an infection were febrile in the postoperative period. This may suggest that a lack of fever is a risk for infection, as the patient has not mounted an adequate immune response.

Ishii et al. (2013) found more than half of patients may develop postoperative fever (POF) in the first week, with most developing MT on POD 0 and the latest occurring by POD 3. The four patients who developed fever after POD 7 were associated with urinary tract infection.

Table 25.1 reported most of the literature about development of fever in the postoperative period.

25.5 Characteristic of an Infectious Fever

Most of the authors agree that more than 20 % of patients develop fever after joint replacement, but just in a small percentage of them, this is correlated to an infectious process. There are some fever characteristics that are correlated to a higher probability of joint, pulmonary, or urinary infections. Fever that is not associated with other pulmonary or urinary symptoms or with other joint signs of infection is rarely associated with an infectious process. One of the risk factors for septic fever is the postoperative day in which the patient develops it: it has been demonstrated that fever developing on POD 3–4–5 has a higher risk to be correlated with an infectious problem. Besides, the modality of fever is another crucial point: some authors reported that spiked fever and multiple febrile episodes are highly associated with infection (Czaplicki et al. 2011). Table 25.1 reports the papers we extracted the data from.

25.6 Role of the Workup Tests

The evaluation of fever is often expensive, invasive, and painful and disturbs patient during recovery hours (Cremeans-Smith et al. 2006), having a negative effect on it. To evaluate early postoperative fever, blood and urine cultures, white blood cell counts, chest X -ay (CXR), and urinalysis (UA) are often obtained, although there are no source of infection in the 95 % of febrile episodes. Anyway fever remains the main indication for workup in the postoperative period, both in trauma and in elective patients. In a different study that we reported, the conclusions are the same: sepsis workup is unnecessary if the febrile response progressively decreases.

25.6.1 The Role of CRP and ESR Level as Diagnostic Tool

C-reactive protein (CRP) is a phase protein synthesized by hepatocytes. Usually in healthy people, the plasma level is very low and its increase is not specific for infection.

Orthopedic surgeon sometimes uses the CRP measurement as a diagnostic tool for infection and for monitoring the effect of the treatment. Uncomplicated cardiac surgery, abdominal surgery, and uncomplicated total hip arthroplasty could induce a temporary rise in CRP (Larsson et al. 1992). Larsson et al. (1992) reported a CRP increase in all the patients examined, after an elective orthopedic surgery, and this is probably due to the tissue damage. They observed different peak levels probably correlated to the amount of tissue injured but also to the type of tissue being damaged. They also reported that the operation time, gender, age, drug history, anesthetic, and blood transfusion did not significantly influence CRP response.

Some authors (White et al. 1998) reported that CRP levels begin to increase 6 h after the trauma, with a peak level in 48–72 h, with return to normal level within 3–6 weeks in the absence of complications.

Dupont et al. (2008) reported that CRP level changes in three phases: it firstly increases up to a peak (reached at POD 2–3) of seven to 14 times the normal range. After POD 3 the level falls rapidly and then decreases more slowly until the normalization at three or four postoperative week. A CRP value of 25 mg/l at POD 21 has a 100 % specificity regardless of the location of the infection, but low sensitivity (58.3 %). Gomez-Navalon et al. (2000) reported a sensitivity of 63.3 % and a specificity of 80.1 % for CRP and judged alpha-1 antitrypsin to be more reliable, with a sensitivity of 87.5 % and a specificity of 85.8 % in detecting infections.

Table 25.1 Summary of the articles in the literature about immediate postoperative fever

Author	No of patients	TKA/THA	Mean age (range)	Fever (% patients)	Mean temperature (range)	% of POD fever	Type of workup	% of positive workup	Notes and conclusions
Shetty (2013)	52 patients	Not reported	66.03 (46–83)	25 (48.1 %)	Not reported	Not reported	Not reported	Not reported	Comparison between Hb drop in fever and no fever groups. No differences
Vijaysegaran (2012)	141 blood cultures in 101 patients	58/41 (primary and revisions) +2 SA	Not reported	Only patient with fever	38.5 °C (38°–39.9°)	Not reported	141 blood cultures	2 positive (1.4 %)	Only evaluation of blood cultures. Temperature alone is not an indication to perform blood cultures
Athanassious (2011)	341 patients	195/146	Not reported	31 % TKA, 36 % THA	TKA = 38.3 °C	TKA = 50 % POD 1, 37 % POD 2	In all cases of fever, UA	TKA = 11 positive UA (18.3 %), 0 positive CXR (0 %)	Fever most likely in POD 1–2, a UA and UCS may not be necessary in the immediate postoperative period. A CXR may only be necessary if multiple fever
					THA = 38.3 °C	THA = 58 % POD 1, 33 % POD 2	In second fever, CXR (28 TKA, 18THA)	THA = 7 positive UA (13.4 %), 2 positive CXR (11.1 %)	
Czaplicki (2011)	426 patients	214/212	64.1 (15–94)	TKA = 18 fever (8.4 %), 126 leukocytosis (57.5 %), 13 both (6.1 %)	Not reported	TKA = 9 in POD 2 (50 %)	TKA = 21 additional tests: 8 UA, 6 CXR, 2 blood cultures, 5 other tests	TKA = 6 positive tests (28.6 %), 1 joint infection (0.5 %)	Overall use of testing for fever and leukocytosis without specific physical examination findings is low and should not be performed routinely
				THA = 49 fever (23.1 %), 122 leukocytosis (57.5 %), 22 both (10.4 %)		THA = 25 in POD 1 (51 %)	THA = 39 additional tests: 15 UA, 13 blood cultures, 4 CXR, 7 other tests	THA = 8 positive tests (20.5 %), 1 joint infection (0.5 %)	

Ward (2010)	1,100 patients	562/664 both primary and revisions	55.4 % 51–70 years	161 patients (14.6 %)	Not reported	POD 2–3	69 patients (42.9 %) for a total of 236 diagnostic tests: 71 blood cultures, 59 UA, 49 CXR, 57 other tests	35 positive tests (14.8 %): 23.7 % UA, 5.6 % blood cultures, 2 % CXR	Positive predictor variables are fever after POD 3, multiple days of fever, T max of higher than 39 °C. In the absence of signs and symptoms indicative of pneumonia or septicemia, chest X-Ray and blood cultures are ineffective for fever evaluation
Tai (2009)	186 patients	186 TKA	Not reported	Not reported	37.9 °C	POD 1–2	Not reported	Not reported	Inverse relationship between hemoglobin loss and postoperative temperature
Anderson (2009)	102 sts of blood cultures in 50 patients	39/11 (primary and revisions)	67.3 years	All fever	Not reported	Not reported	All blood cultures	No blood culture is positive	Blood cultures are neither useful nor cost effective in evaluating fever immediately after TJA
Bindelglass (2007)	453 patients	240 TKA, 124 THA, 89 hemiarthroplasty	Not reported	Not reported	Not reported	Not reported	Blood cultures in 40 TKA (16.6 %) and 31 THA (25 %)	2 positive blood cultures (1TKA, 1 THA)	Blood cultures are expensive and do not add relevant information
Ghosh (2006)	170 patients	All TKA	78.5 (47–88)	62/170 (36.5 %)	Not reported	18.2 % in POD1, 16.5 % POD 2	Not reported	4/62 with pyrexia (6.6 %), 14/170 (someone without pyrexia, 8.2 %)	No association between pyrexia and infection, allogenic blood transfusion, hemoglobin loss, use of urinary catheter, rheumatoid arthritis, anesthetic type, and previous pyrexia following TKR. Pyrexia in the first 5 days following TKR is usually a normal physiological response and should not cause undue concern about the presence of infection

(continued)

Table 25.1 (continued)

Author	No of patients	TKA/THA	Mean age (range)	Fever (% patients)	Mean temperature (range)	% of POD fever	Type of workup	% of positive workup	Notes and conclusions
Andres (2003)	20 patients (evaluation of the role of cytokines)	All TKA	68.3 ± 8.6	10 patients with fever compared to 10 without	Not reported	POD 1–2	Blood cultures, UA and urine culture, and a CXR in POD 2 in 10 patients (group fever)	1 positive urine culture	Significantly higher levels of drain and serum IL-6 in patients who were febrile than in patients who were afebrile at 24 and 48 h after TKA
Shaw (1999)	200 patients	100/100 (primary and revisions)	Not reported	38/200 temperature greater than 39 °C (19 %)	Not reported	POD 1	133 urine cultures (66.5 %), 17 CXR (8.5 %), 5 blood cultures (2.5 %)	11 positive urine cultures, no CXR, no blood cultures	A workup for sepsis is not indicate without signs or symptoms
Guinn et al (1999)	118 patients	All TKA (141)	Not reported	80/141 TKA (56.7 %)	Not reported	Not reported	Not reported	Not reported	Fever following TKA was common and was not necessarily a contraindication to discharge
Kennedy (1997)	90 patients	All TKA (92)	Not reported	All T > 37 °C, 17 % > 39 °C	Not reported	Not reported	Not reported	No prosthetic infection	Early postoperative pyrexia after arthroplasty is a normal physiological response, and a significant pyrexia can be predicted by a drop in hematocrit and/or after postoperative transfusion

TKA total knee arthroplasty, *THA* total hip arthroplasty, *SA* shoulder arthroplasty, *POD* postoperative day, *Hb* hemoglobin, *UA* urinalysis, *CXR* chest X-ray

Okafor and Maclellan (1998) also described the trend of CRP. They reported that CRP rises till a mean value of 0.146 g/dl at POD 2 in the normal group versus 0.2 in the infected group. In the infected group, a persistent elevation on day 7 and day 21 was observed. In the same study, the authors have evaluated also the erythrocyte sedimentation rate (ESR); usually the variations were significantly different for day 0 versus POD 2 and day 0 versus POD 7, but not for day 0 versus POD 21. In the infected group, the postoperative values of ESR were significantly different from day 0 value, reflecting the persistent inflammatory state. ESR value depends on multifactorial variable, so the reliability is low and high value has to be interpreted with caution. They concluded that CRP shows less variability between patients and consequently is a better indicator of the acute phase response than ESR, which requires a series of values in order to demonstrate a trend.

25.6.2 The Role of Skin Temperature as Diagnostic Tool

Mehra et al. (2005) demonstrated that there is a significant increase in skin temperature around the operated knee after a TKR. The skin temperature remains significantly elevated at discharge and 6 weeks but returns to normal values by 18 weeks. Elevated skin temperature should not justify starting oral antibiotics. However, a sustained temperature difference and increased CRP, especially around 4–6 postoperative weeks, should alert the surgeon of a possible complication.

25.6.3 The Role of Blood Cultures as Diagnostic Tool

Ward et al. (2010) have performed blood cultures on 35 patients after a total joint arthroplasty. Only 2 out of 35 cultures were positive and both patients had clinical signs of sepsis. They concluded saying positive predictors of sepsis were fever after POD 4, recurrent febrile episode, spikes of temperature >39 °C, and insertion of 2 or more catheter devices. Blood cultures in patients with no sign or symptoms of sepsis were considered ineffective.

Vijaysegaran et al. (2012) have examined 141 blood culture sets drawn from 101 patients. Only 2 were positive and both were identified as contaminants. Similar result was obtained from Anderson and Osland (2009).

Kennedy et al. (1997) did not find any positive cultures on a series of 16 fever patients with a temperature of more than 38 °C. They concluded that there are no correlation between fever and deep infection after arthroplasty.

In an interesting cost-effective evaluation of blood cultures, Sivakumar et al. (2012) have found that the cost of tests is about $3,000 and additional costs are incurred when contaminants were isolated. They concluded that probably blood cultures in patients without other symptoms of sepsis are not cost effective. Also Bindelglass and Pellegrino (2007) have shown similar results. In a study on gynecologic patients, blood cultures were similarly negative in all 77 patients with fever being studied.

25.6.4 The Role of White Cell Counts as Diagnostic Tool

It is well documented in the literature that stress induces demargination of the white blood cell pool, and the operative trauma alone may be the cause of leukocytosis in these patients (Kuhlwein et al. 2001; Landmann et al. 1984; Kumar et al. 2007).

Czaplicki et al. (2011) found that postoperative leukocytosis is much more common than fever in TJA patients (57.5 % versus 15.8 %). They concluded that the overall use of testing for fever and leukocytosis without specific physical examination findings is low and should not be performed routinely because it is not significantly correlating with infections.

25.6.5 The Role of Chest X-Ray (CXR) as Diagnostic Tool

In the evaluation of postoperative chest X-ray in patients with a second postoperative fever, Athanassious et al. (2011) reported only 2 positive tests out of 46 (4 %). Both patients have symptoms of pulmonary impairment. They concluded saying that it could be a useful test in patients developing multiple fever events during the immediate postoperative period, overall if associated with pulmonary symptoms. Also Ward et al. (2010) reported that in febrile patients who underwent a CXR in the absence of other pulmonary symptoms, just 2 % of them had positive results. The authors concluded that CXR in febrile patients without other pulmonary symptoms is unnecessary and not cost effective.

25.6.6 The Role of the Urinalysis (UA) as Diagnostic Tool

Athanassious et al. (2011) support the uselessness of UA in the absence of symptoms such as dysuria or pyuria. Eighteen patients out of 112 have a positive UA, but none of them have positive urine culture that means no urinary tract infections were developed. For Ward et al. (2010), the most common tests performed in patients with fever were urinalyses (24 %, 14/59) and urine cultures (22.5 %, 11/49), followed by blood cultures (7 %, 5/71) and chest radiographs (2 %, 1/49). They reported that just 23.7 % of positive UA were detected, so in the absence of other urinary symptoms, UA is not cost effective.

Petretta et al. (2013) have found 7 on 28 positive UA after the first febrile episode in a trauma population. After the second one, positive urinalyses were 5 on 7 (71 %), but only 2 of them resulted in positive urine cultures and were treated with antibiotics. Both have had symptoms and signs of urinary infection. In all the examined study, patients with positive urine cultures in the preoperative period and with long catheterization time were excluded.

25.6.7 What About Periprosthetic Infection: Role of the Workup

The diagnosis of knee joint infection should meet at least three of the following five criteria: (1) abnormal serology (CRP >1 mg/dl and ESR >30 mm/h), (2) strong clinical and radiological suspicion, (3) positive joint aspiration cultures, (4) evidence of purulence during the revision surgery, and (5) positive intraoperative cultures AAOS (2010). The first step of diagnosis is careful physical examination: reduction in the range of motion (ROM), pain, swelling, erythema, and fever can be correlated to knee prosthesis infection (Chun et al. 2013). Nevertheless, in the early postoperative period, it can be very difficult to distinguish a normal from a pathological symptom. Serology (CRP and ESR) should be the first test to perform, specifically higher for CRP and with equal sensibility. Joint fluid aspiration is an essential test for infection. Synovial fluid white blood cell (WBC) counts greater than 1,700 cells/μL and differential greater than 69 % polymorphonuclear cells should raise a high index of suspicion for infection (Springer and Scuderi 2013). Intraoperative cultures should be done before antibiotics administration. Those cultures must be obtained from different tissues: synovium, synovial fluid, intramedullary tissue, granulation tissue, and bone. Some authors reported that if intraoperative tissue cultures are negative but other clinical examinations suggest infection, the infection treatment should be initiated (Chun et al. 2013).

For early diagnosis, bone scan can be useful; to increase its accuracy, both a Tc-99 and marked WBC scan can be used (Chun et al. 2013). Figure 25.1 shows AAOS algorithm for diagnosis of periprosthetic joint infections of the hip and knee.

25.6.8 Association Between Fever and Hemoglobin Drop

Kennedy et al. (1997) reported an increased risk of febrile-range temperature (>39 °C) with a decrease in hematocrit and the transfusion of blood, but this finding has not been substantiated by other studies of postoperative fever in this population. Shetty and Kasture (2013) and also Andres et al. (2003) did not found any correlation

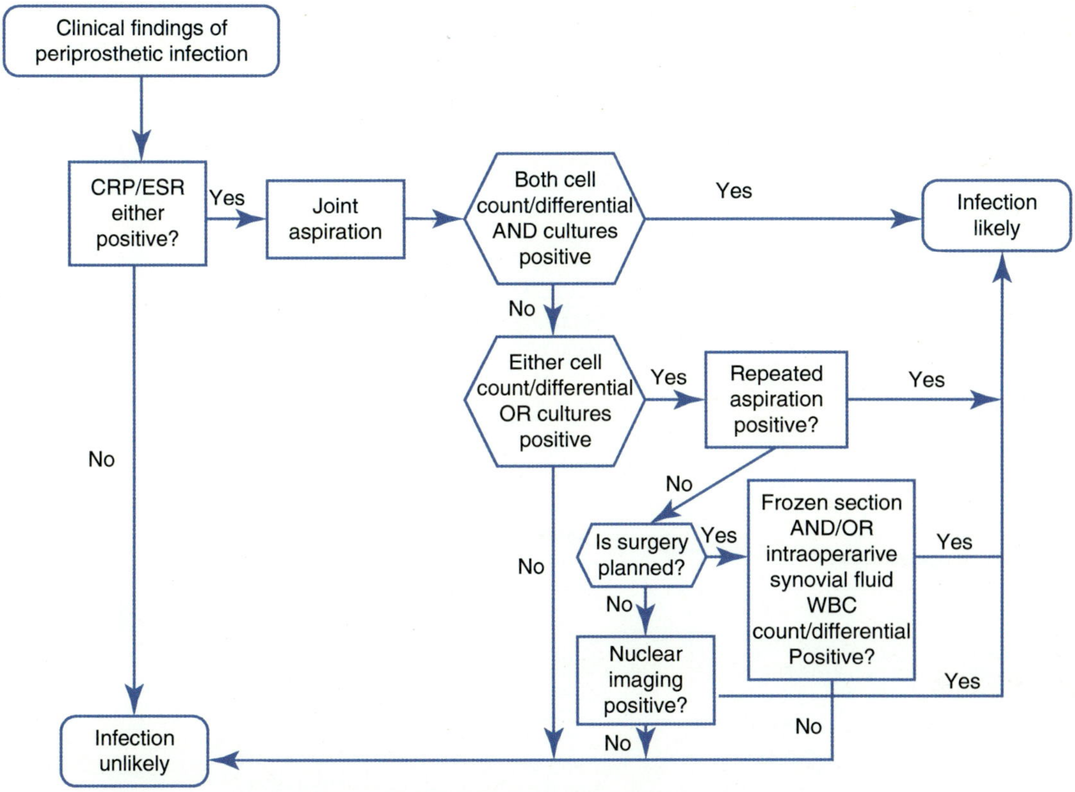

Fig. 25.1 AAOS algorithm for diagnosis of periprosthetic joint infections of the hip and knee

between the development of fever and the hematocrit level or the use of transfusions.

25.6.9 Patient at Risk (Diabetes, HIV, Rheumatoid Arthritis)

In rheumatoid patients, serial measurement of ESR during the same day has revealed a significant diurnal variation, making ESR measurement less accurate as an indicator of postoperative complications in rheumatoid arthritis patients (Larsson et al. 1992). Ghosh et al. (2006) did not find any statistical association between rheumatoid arthritis and development of fever.

There is no other study that shows the trend of fever and the role of diagnostic exam in a high risk population.

25.7 Our Point of View and Diagnostic Algorithm

The lack of correlation between postoperative fever and infection has been reported previously in obstetric/gynecologic (de la Torre et al. 2003), general surgery (Lesperance et al. 2011), and cardio-surgery literature (Frank et al. 2000), and most of the authors consider fever as a physiological response of the organism to the "surgical insult."

Fever alone in the postoperative period is not enough to justify a complete workup made of CXR, UA, and blood and urine cultures. As an initial workup we normally include a full set of vital signs and a focused history and physical examination to assess for focal infections. In the early postoperative period (POD 0–5), we

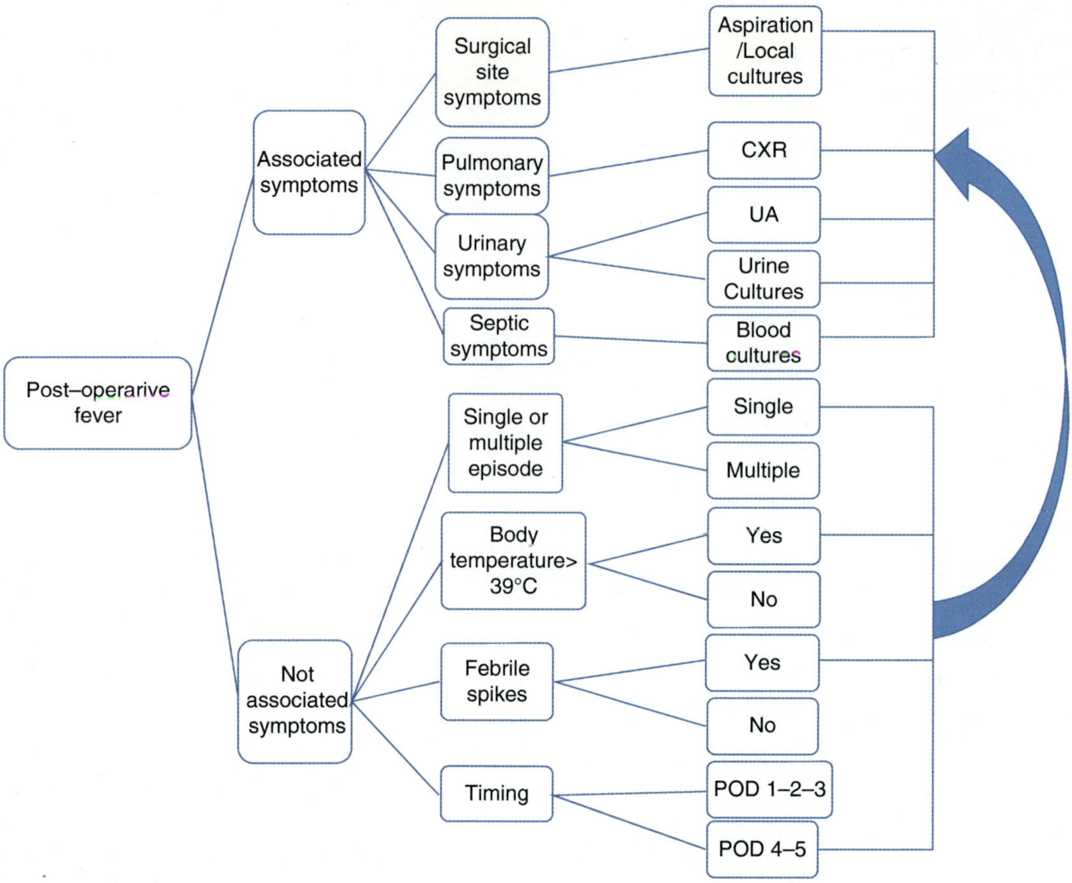

Fig. 25.2 Sample of a diagnostic algorithm for postoperative fever

perform UA in patients with urinary catheters or urinary symptoms, and if positive, we perform urine cultures. In patients with fever and pulmonary symptoms, we perform CXR and sputum cultures. Blood and wound cultures do not seem to play a significant role during this early period, and we normally reserve blood cultures to patients with multiple episode of fever higher than 39 °C, especially if associated with other symptoms of systemic infection, such as tachypnea, tachycardia, or elevated white cell count, overall if it appears after POD 5. Other potential noninfectious etiologies for fever in the postoperative period should also be considered such as atelectasis, deep vein thrombosis, or pulmonary embolus. Again, clinical judgment should be used for investigating these etiologies because routinely ordering tests will result in low yield and unnecessary costs. Figure 25.2 shows our personal diagnostic algorithm in patients with postoperative fever.

Conclusion

Fever in the early postoperative period after a joint replacement is very common, and in few cases, it is associated with an infectious process. The physician should carefully assess the characteristics of the fever, such as the number of episodes, extent, and time trend. As shown in Table 25.1, most of the authors agree that multiple episodes with fever spikes, temperature higher than 39 °C, and development after POD 3 are more likely associated with an infectious process. Before starting with a workup including CXR, UA, and urine and blood cultures, a complete physical and historical examination should be performed to assess other potential sources of infection. In Fig. 25.1 we reported a sample of diagnostic algorithm.

In conclusion the surgeon should be aware that fever is a common postoperative finding, and just in a small percentage of cases, it is associated with an infectious process. A complete workup is unnecessary and not cost effective in the absence of other signs or symptoms of infection. There are some postoperative characteristic of fever that are more suspicious of infection, and the surgeons should know them to avoid useless scaremongering and waste of time, resources, and money.

Key Points

- In literature the incidence of postoperative fever is reported to occur in between 15 and 47 % of cases, with a small percentage correlated to an infectious process.
- In the first postoperative week after total knee and hip replacement, many sources of fever are possible even without prosthesis involvement (surgical site infection). These causes might be the physiological response to surgical trauma, the disturbance of thermoregulation by anesthesia, retained hematoma, pneumonia or urinary tract infection, deep vein thrombosis, and more often the response to blood transfusions. Fever starting on POD 3–4–5 has shown a higher risk of being linked with an infectious status.
- Even though fever remains the main indication for workup in the postoperative period, blood and urine cultures, inflammatory markers, white cell counts, chest X-ray (CXR), and urinalysis (UA), in 95 % of cases, no sources of infection are found. Infection workup is considered unnecessary if the febrile response is progressively decreasing.

References

American Academy of Orthopaedic Surgeons (AAOS) (2010) The diagnosis of periprothetic joint infections of the hip and knee: guideline and evidence report. AAOS, Rosemont

Anderson JT, Osland JD (2009) Blood cultures for evaluation of fever after total joint arthroplasty. Am J Orthop 38:E134–E136

Andres BM, Taub DD, Gurkan I et al (2003) Postoperative fever after total knee arthroplasty: the role of cytokines. Clin Orthop Relat Res 415:221–231. doi:10.1097/01.blo.0000093914.26658.55

Athanassious C, Samad A, Avery A et al (2011) Evaluation of fever in the immediate postoperative period in patients who underwent total joint arthroplasty. J Arthroplasty 26(8):1404–1408

Bindelglass DF, Pellegrino J (2007) The role of blood cultures in the acute evaluation of postoperative fever in arthroplasty patients. J Arthroplasty 22:701

Blom AW, Brown J, Taylor AH et al (2004) Infection after total knee arthroplasty. J Bone Joint Surg Br 86(5):688–691

Chun KC, Kim KM, Chun CH (2013) Infection following total knee arthroplasty. Knee Surg Relat Res 25(3):93–99

Cooper AL, Brouwer S, Turnbull AV et al (1994) Tumor necrosis factor-alpha and fever after peripheral inflammation in the rat. Am J Physiol 267:R1431–R1436

Cremeans-Smith JK, Millington K, Sledjeski E et al (2006) Sleep disruptions mediate the relationship between early postoperative pain and later functioning following total knee replacement surgery. J Behav Med 29:215

Czaplicki AP, Borger JE, Politi JR et al (2011) Evaluation of postoperative fever and leukocytosis in patients after total hip and knee arthroplasty. J Arthroplasty 26(8):1387–1389

de la Torre SH, Mandel L, Goff BA (2003) Evaluation of postoperative fever: usefulness and cost-effectiveness of routine workup. Am J Obstet Gynecol 188:1642

Dupont C, Rodenbach J, Flachaire E (2008) The value of C-reactive protein for postoperative monitoring of lower limb arthroplasty. Ann Readapt Med Phys 51:348–357

Frank SM, Kluger MJ, Kunkel SL (2000) Elevated thermostatic setpoint in postoperative patients. Anesthesiology 93:1426–1431

Garibaldi RA, Brodine S, Matsumiya S et al (1985) Evidence for the non-infectious etiology of early postoperative fever. Infect Control 6:273–277

Ghosh S, Charity RM, Haidar SG et al (2006) Pyrexia following total knee replacement. Knee 13:324–327

Gomez-Navalon LA, Salido Valle JA, Lopez Alonso AL (2000) Alpha-1-antitrypsin in early infections after hip prosthesis surgery. Rev Chir Orthop 86:794–800

Guinn S, Castro FP Jr, Garcia R et al (1999) Fever following total knee arthroplasty. Am J Knee Surg 12(3): 161–164

Ishii Y, Noguchi H, Takeda M et al (2013) Evaluation of fever and its related factors during 4 weeks after primary total hip arthroplasty. Surg Sci 4:1–6. http://dx.doi.org/10.4236/ss.2013.41001

Kennedy JG, Rodgers WB, Zurakowski D et al (1997) Pyrexia after total knee replacement, a cause for concern? Am J Orthop 26(8):549–552, 554

Kuhlwein EC, Irwin MR, Ziegler MG et al (2001) Propranolol affects stress-induced leukocytosis and cellular adhesion molecule expression. Eur J Appl Physiol 86:135

Kumar S, Mehta Y, Vats M et al (2007) An observational study to know the association of leukocytosis and fever with infection in post cardiac surgery patients. Indian Heart J 59:316

Lahat N, Zlotnick AY, Shtiller R et al (1992) Serum levels of IL-1, IL-6 and tumour necrosis factors in patients undergoing coronary artery bypass grafts or cholecystectomy. Clin Exp Immunol 89:255–260

Landmann RM, Müller FB, Perini C et al (1984) Changes of immunoregulatory cells induced by psychological and physical stress: relationship to plasma catecholamines. Clin Exp Immunol 58:127

Larsson S, Thelander U, Friberg S (1992) C-Reactive Protein (PCR) levels after elective orthopedic surgery. Clin Orthop Relat Res 275:237–242

Lentino JR (2003) Prosthetic joint infections: bane of orthopedists, challenge for infectious disease specialists. Clin Infect Dis 36(9):1157–1161

Lesperance R, Lehman R, Lesperance K et al (2011) Early postoperative fever and the "routine" fever work-up: results of a prospective study. J Surg Res 171:245–250. doi:10.1016/j.jss.2010.03.009

Luheshi G, Miller AJ, Brouwer S et al (1996) Interleukin-1 receptor antagonist inhibits endotoxin fever and systemic interleukin-6 induction in the rat. Am J Physiol 270:E91–E95

Mehra A, Langkamer VG, Day A et al (2005) C reactive protein and skin temperature post total knee replacement. Knee 12:297–300

Miyawaki T, Maeda S, Koyama Y et al (1998) Elevation of plasma interleukin-6 level is involved in postoperative fever following major oral and maxillofacial surgery. Oral Surg Oral Med Oral Pathol Oral Radiol Endod 85:146–152

Okafor B, Maclellan G (1998) Postoperative changes of erythrocyte sedimentation rate, plasma viscosity and c-reactive protein levels after hip surgery. Acta Orthop Belg 64(1):52–56

Petretta R, McConkey M, Slobogean GP et al (2013) Incidence, risk factors, and diagnostic evaluation of postoperative fever in an orthopaedic trauma population. J Orthop Trauma 27:558–562

Pullicino EA, Carli F, Poole S et al (1990) The relationship between the circulating concentrations of interleukin 6 (IL-6), tumor necrosis factor (TNF) and the acute phase response to elective surgery and accidental injury. Lymphokine Res 9:231–238

Shaw JA, Chung R (1999) Febrile response after knee and hip arthroplasty. Clin Orthop Relat Res 367: 181–189

Shetty V, Kasture S (2013) Is immediate postoperative fever related to drop in haemoglobin? A comparative study in simultaneous bilateral total knee arthroplasty patients. Eur J Orthop Surg Traumatol 23: 345–347

Sivakumar B, Vijaysegaran P, Ottley M et al (2012) Blood cultures for evaluation of early postoperative fever after femoral neck fracture surgery. J Orthop Surg 20(3):336–340

Springer BD, Scuderi GR (2013) Evaluation and management of the infected total knee arthroplasty. Instr Course Lect 62:349–361

Summersell PC, Turnbull A, Long G et al (2003) Temperature trends in total hip arthroplasty. A retrospective study. J Arthroplasty 18(4):426–429

Tai W, Chang C-W, Lin C-J, Lai K-A, Yang C-Y (2009) Elevated temperature trends after total knee arthoplasty. Orthopedics 32(12):886

Vijaysegaran P, Coulter SA, Coulter C et al (2012) Blood cultures for assessment of postoperative fever in arthroplasty patients. J Arthroplasty 27: 375–377

Ward DT, Hansen EN, Takemoto SK et al (2010) Cost and effectiveness of postoperative fever diagnostic evaluation in total joint arthroplasty patients. J Arthroplasty 25(6 Supp 1):43–48

White J, Kelly M, Dunsmuir R (1998) C-reactive protein level after total hip and total knee replacement. J Bone Joint Surg Br 80B:909–911

Perspectives: Prolonged Wound Drainage (7 Days) After Hip Arthroplasty

26

Lorenzo Castellani and Alberto Farese

Open Questions

- What is considered to be persistent/prolonged wound drainage?
- Can we prevent wound drainage?
- Can we treat it nonsurgically?
- What are the best surgical strategies to address draining?
- Are wound complications more frequent in patients undergoing antithrombotic or anticoagulant therapy?
- Does the routine use of closed suction drainage reduce wound complication and infection rate?
- What are the proper surgical strategies to address persistent (more than 7 days) wound draining?
- Is prolonging antibiotic therapy in persistent wound drainage able to exclude acute deep infection?

L. Castellani (✉)
Reconstructive Articular Surgery Unit, IFCA – Villa Ulivella, Via del Pergolino, 4, Florence 50127, Italy
e-mail: lorenzo.castellani@chirurgiarticolare.it

A. Farese (✉)
Infectious and Tropical Diseases Unit, Azienda Ospedlaiero Universitaria Careggi, Largo Brambilla, 3, Florence 50134, Italy
e-mail: alberto.farese@alice.it

26.1 The Orthopedic Surgeon's Point of View

Lorenzo Castellani

26.1.1 Introduction

Periprosthetic infection remains one of the leading causes of morbidity after total hip and knee arthroplasty. Reported rates of prolonged wound drainage range from 1.3 to 33 %. Persistent wound drainage has been identified as a contributing factor to the development of periprosthetic infection, with infection rates ranging from 1.3 to 50 %. Several studies suggest that with each day of prolonged wound drainage, there is an increased risk of infection. In this chapter, we analyze the literature and we explain our approach for the prevention and control of prolonged wound drainage after hip arthroplasty. We consider persistent wound drainage a continued drainage from the wound that lasts more than 72 h.

26.1.2 EBM Analysis

Several factors contribute in determining a persistent wound drainage; some of them are patient related and can be addressed before surgery; some others depend on surgeons, wound closure

A. Baldini, P. Caldora (eds.), *Perioperative Medical Management for Total Joint Arthroplasty: How to Control Hemostasis, Pain and Infection*, DOI 10.1007/978-3-319-07203-6_26,

and care, and these also can be addressed during surgery and postoperative recovery. We revised the literature considering all factors that can be addressed in order to reduce the incidence of persistent wound drainage.

26.1.3 Patient Status Optimization

26.1.3.1 Malnutrition

Malnutrition is one of the most important factors affecting wound healing. Several published papers highlight the paramount importance of ascertaining nutritional patient status before surgery. Serum transferrin levels have a predictive value in wound healing (Gherini et al. 1993), and serum albumin and total leucocyte count (TLC) correlate with resource consumption, length of stay, and operative time in patients undergoing joint replacement surgery (Lavernia et al. 1999). These parameters may be improved with nutritional supplementation prior to surgery.

26.1.3.2 Diabetes

Diabetes mellitus has the capacity to double the risk of early wound complications after TJA (Galat et al. 2009). Diabetic patients have a significantly higher risk for infection after TJA. Even if diabetes increases the risk of infection, there is no association between controlled and uncontrolled diabetes and the risk of infection using HbA1C as a marker for diabetic control. Based on that evidence there isn't any indication to dose as a predictive factor for infections HbA1C levels before surgery (Iorio et al. 2012; Adams et al. 2013).

26.1.3.3 Anticoagulation

Well-designed studies evaluating the effects of anticoagulation on wound complication and hematoma formation in patients who have undergone reoperation for wound-related problems are lacking. However, one case–control study found that patients with a postoperative INR N 1.5 were more likely to develop hematomas and wound drainage after joint arthroplasty and subsequent infection (Parvizi et al. 2007). Even patients who received low-molecular-weight heparin for prophylaxis had a longer time until the postoperative wound was dry than did those treated with aspirin and mechanical foot compression or those who received Coumadin (warfarin) in another retrospective observational study (Patel et al. 2007).

Although persistent drainage and hematoma formation are recognized to be risk factors for the development of PJI, it is not known if excess anticoagulation is a predisposing factor. Cautious anticoagulation to prevent hematoma formation and/or wound drainage is critical to prevent PJI, and its undesirable consequences and aggressive or excessive anticoagulation must be avoided.

26.1.3.4 Anemia

Both preoperative anemia and allogenic transfusions have been associated with higher rates of PJI (Greenky et al. 2012). A systematic approach to optimizing hemoglobin levels preoperatively that implements oral and possibly intravenous iron, folic acid supplements, and erythropoietin while minimizing blood loss intraoperatively using tranexamic acid, cell salvage, and induced hypotension has been shown to diminish allogenic transfusion requirements (Kotze et al. 2012).

26.1.4 Wound Closure and Medication

A prospective RCT comparing skin adhesives, subcuticular closure, and skin staples for closure of TKA and THA revealed no significant difference in early and late complications, wound cosmetics, or patient satisfaction (Khan et al. 2006). Meticulous closure of deep dead spaces is the main goal during wound closure, regardless of the technique that the surgeon chooses. Barbed bidirectional suture technology has generated interest based on a perception of a more rapid closure and good results reported in the plastic, gynecologic, and general surgery literature as well as more recent reports of use in orthopedic surgery (Eickmann and Quane 2010). Driving much of that interest are the proposed faster closure times, biomechanical strength, cosmetics, and the implications of increased surgical efficiency. Even if preliminary studies based on small samples of orthopedic patients are promising, further investigations are needed in order to evaluate possible drawbacks and cost-effectiveness.

Various wound dressings are used after hip or knee arthroplasty, but the rationale for dressing choice is unclear. The use of occlusive dressing after wound closure has a growing evidence of improving healing and avoiding skin blistering. What's more, occlusive dressing significantly reduces the rate of leakage and number of dressing changes when compared to a traditional adhesive dressing. A comparative evaluation was conducted involving 428 patients undergoing primary elective total hip arthroplasty (THA) or total knee arthroplasty (TKA) in a single hospital (Clarke et al. 2009). Patients received either the traditional postoperative dressing (adhesive dressing with an integral absorbent pad, Mepore) or the new dressing regimen (AQUACEL secured with hydrocolloid dressing, DuoDERM), as well as liquid film-forming acrylate. Patients under the age of 50 and/or with a condition or comorbidity that could compromise wound healing were excluded. A protocol was developed for dressing changes based on the extent of strikethrough. Outcome measures were blister rate, wear time, number of dressing changes, SSI rate, and delayed patient discharge. Patients treated with the new dressing design had a lower blister rate, lower incidence of delayed discharge, longer wear time, fewer dressing changes, and a lower SSI rate. Only four cases of SSIs requiring washout were reported in both groups (one for the new dressing design and three for the traditional dressing), and the rest were successfully treated with antibiotics. To date there have been no revisions for deep infection in either group.

26.1.5 Prolonged Drainage Nonsurgical Treatment

Other interventions, such as antibiotics, are discouraged because they can mask an underlying infection. Currently there is little evidence to support administration of antibiotics to patients with draining wound. Although the rationale for this practice appears logical, in that one is attempting to prevent ingress of infecting organisms through draining wound, the issue of emergence of antibiotic resistance and adverse effects associated with administration of antibiotics cannot be overlooked. In addition administration of an antibiotic is likely to mask the underlying infection or make diagnosis of PJI difficult by influencing the culture results. Negative-pressure wound therapy could be an option for conservative treatment. A Cochrane meta-analysis included trials that compared NPWT with other types of wound dressings or compared one type of NPWT with a different type of NPWT for persistently draining wounds in skin graft patients, orthopedic patients undergoing arthroplasty, and general and trauma surgery. The authors concluded that there is no evidence for the effectiveness of NPWT on the complete healing of wounds expected to heal by primary intention (Webster et al. 2012a, b).

Observation alone is highly discouraged, given the fact that persistent wound drainage is correlated with PJI (Jaberi et al. 2008).

26.1.6 Prolonged Drainage Surgical Treatment

After 5 days of persistent wound drainage, surgical intervention should be carried out to reduce the likelihood of developing a PJI. Saleh et al. (2002) demonstrated that patients who had an average of 5.5 days of drainage were 12.7 times more likely to be infected than those with less wound drainage time. Another study found that each day of prolonged wound drainage increased the risk of wound infection by 42 % following a THA and by 29 % following a TKA (Patel et al. 2007).

Surgery should consist of opening the fascia, performing a thorough irrigation and debridement (I&D) with exchange of modular components, and performing a meticulous fascia and wound reclosure. In case meticulous reconstruction of the fascia and skin is not possible, NPWT might be a viable option, followed by coverage of the wound by a plastic surgeon after cultures and other data exclude early PJI. Deep cultures should be taken at the time of reoperation and antibiotics should be administered according to the sensitivity of the organism. Taking wound swab cultures is misleading because of the high level of contamination from the skin (false positives).

26.1.7 Our Approach

First of all, best practice starts before surgery. We counsel the patient to stop smoking. Patient risk factors like malnutrition, coagulation deficits, anemia, and diabetes are screened out during preoperative evaluation. All these factors can be modified in order to reduce the risk of wound drainage. We routinely evaluate nutritional status, coagulation parameters, blood glucose, and blood cell count at least 1 month before surgery, and we correct abnormal values. We need to recall that, after all, joint arthroplasty is an elective procedure and patients can wait until these issues are addressed.

Intraoperative factors that can assist in wound healing include careful planning of incisions in patients with multiple incisions from previous surgeries. Not only is meticulous handling of soft tissues highly encouraged, but it is equally important to avoid undermining the skin during exposure. During surgery we focus on careful hemostasis and meticulous layer-by-layer suture with resorbable stitches, trying to avoid deep death spaces. We use staples for skin closure. Wound closure, a task often relegated to the most junior of surgeons, is one of the most important aspects of surgery. Proper handling of the tissues and skin during closure and obtaining a watertight, but not strangulated, wound is critical for proper healing.

We use occlusive dressing before we remove sterile draping in the operating room (AQUACEL Hydrofiber Wound Dressing – Convatec, Skillman, NJ 08558, USA). Patients at high risk undergo a lower-intensity joint mobilization program. Dressing is checked daily for wound drainage without removing the patch (Figs. 26.1 and 26.2). If any drainage is suspected, dressing is changed in order to evaluate the amount and quality of fluid coming out from the wound. We do not perform neither wound swab nor antibiotic therapy. We consider to reduce or stop LMWH if hematoma or the need for multiple hemotransfusion is present in combination with wound drainage. If patient is at high risk for wound drainage, when we can't achieve best wound closure at surgery, we apply NPWT in the operating room and we maintain it for the first 4 days. If wound drainage is prolonging more than 5 days postoperatively, surgical wound debridement is performed. Deep cultures are harvested during surgeries. Prosthetic modular components are changed during surgery.

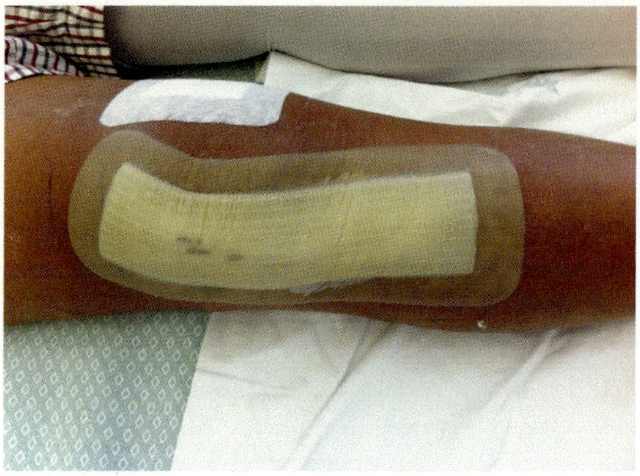

Fig. 26.1 Postoperative occlusive medication with no drainage at day 3 after total knee arthroplasty (AQUACEL Hydrofiber Wound Dressing – Convatec, Skillman, NJ 08558, USA). Absence of wound drainage from the wound is evident

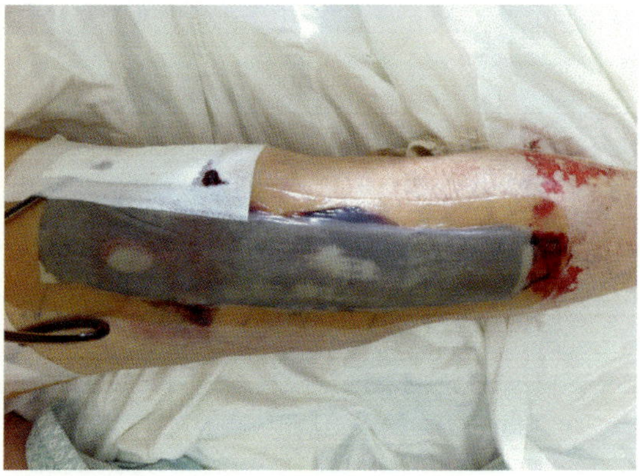

Fig. 26.2 Postoperative occlusive medication with evident drainage at day 1 after revision knee arthroplasty despite the usage of two intra-articular drains

26.1.8 Results

Between January 2013 and March 2014, we performed 271 primary joint replacements, 171 knees and 100 hips.

We have had 13 prolonged (>72 h postoperatively) wound drainage (4.7 %), 8 hips and 5 knees.

8 cases (61.5 %) were associated with superficial hematoma and swelling, and 6 cases (46.1 %) required allogenic transfusions (trigger point Hb <8 g/dl).

Drainage stopped 24 h after LMWH discontinuation or reduction and lower-intensity joint mobilization. None of them developed at date periprosthetic joint infection.

26.1.9 Discussion

In this retrospective review, we found an incidence of prolonged wound drainage apparently higher compared to what you can find in the literature (around 0.5 % in primary; around 10 % in revision – Weiss and Krackow 1993). The first reason is related to what we define "prolonged wound drainage": our numbers are based on drainage that lasts more than 3 days postoperatively. The classical definition of prolonged wound drainage is considered in the literature if drainage persists more than 5 days postoperatively. We didn't have any wound drainage lasting more than 5 days postoperatively. The second point is related to the extensive use of LMWH in our country: we believe that patients receiving excessive anticoagulation during the postoperative period were at high risk of developing wound-related problems. Data from the literature support that theory. Burnett et al. in 2007 showed a high incidence of wound problems related to the use of enoxaparin sodium (Lovenox, enoxaparin sodium; Sanofi-Aventis, Bridgewater, NJ), identifying the use of this drug as predictor of surgical site complications including a prolonged wound drainage over 7 days post-op with an incidence of 5.1 %. This is confirmed by the fact that in our series almost half cases were associated with deep or superficial hematomas and they solved with LMWH discontinuation or reduction. Local guidelines prevent us to reduce patients' coagulation deficits and force us to be meticulous in intraoperative hemostasis. Since we developed a meticulous multimodal approach to prevent blood loss during surgeries, our rate of wound problems reduced consistently even if our standard prophylaxis regimen includes LMWH.

Key Points

- The persistent wound drainage increases the risk of periprosthetic joint infection.
- Meticulous wound closure and control of patient-related risk factors like anemia, malnutrition, anticoagulation, and diabetes can reduce the incidence of persistent wound drainage.
- Strict wound control, adjustments in medical therapy (thromboembolic prophylaxis), and rehab modification should be conducted for drainage that lasts less than 5 days postoperatively.
- Surgical irrigation/debridement and exchange of modularities are suggested in case of drainage lasting more than 5/7 days.

26.2 The Infectivologist's Point of View

Alberto Farese

Definition for persistent wound drainage (PWD) is still controversial: time (48 h to 1 week), site of drainage (wound or site of removed suction drains), type (clear or not, blood or other fluids), amount of secretion, and eventual microbial content of secretion are variously defined in literature (Butt et al. 2011; Dennis 1997; Hansen et al. 2013; Jaberi et al. 2008; Lonner and Lotke 1999; Saleh et al. 2002; Vince et al. 2007). A recent international expert consensus has defined PWD as "continued drainage from the operative incision site for greater than 72 h" with a strong consensus among participants (80 % agree) (Ghanem et al. 2014).

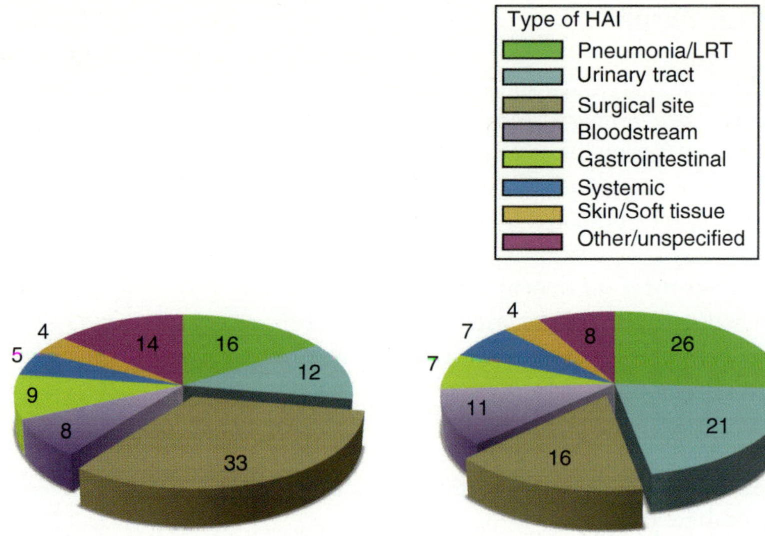

Fig. 26.3 Distribution of HAI types by the presence of HAI on admission: HAI present on admission (*left*); HAI onset during hospitalization (*right*) (Source: European Centre for Disease Prevention and Control (2013))

According to the authors, an area greater than 2×2 cm of drainage covering the medication is also required to fulfill the definition of PWD. However, it is well accepted that PWD after total joint arthroplasty (TJA) is a predictor of a subsequent onset of a TJA infection (Saleh et al. 2002). Patel et al. (2007) estimated that each day of PWD increases the risk of infection by 29 % after total knee arthroplasty and by 42 % after total hip arthroplasty.

Surgical site infections represent a relevant percentage of hospital-acquired infections (HAIs); according to ECDC 2013 point prevalence survey, of a total of 15,000 reported HAIs, the most frequently reported HAI types were respiratory tract infections (23.5 %), followed by surgical site infections (19.6 %). One third of HAIs present at admission were surgical site infections (ECDC 2013, Fig. 26.3). Wound complications after TJA can lead to deep infection with increase of length of hospitalization, need for additional surgery, and adjunctive costs. Any effort to prevent wound complications must be performed in the preoperative period as some risk factors for the development of wound infections or delayed healing (malnutrition, hypokalemia, other infections, decompensated diabetes mellitus, obesity, smoking, renal failure, hypothyroidism, and alcohol abuse) can be corrected. Identification of nasal carriers of methicillin-resistant *Staphylococcus aureus* and decontamination with a short course of mupirocin ointment to the nares may be effective in reducing surgical site infections rates (Rao et al. 2008). Other not preventable factors associated with increased wound complications are prior surgical procedures, immunosuppressive therapy, diverticulosis, rheumatic diseases, and multiple previous incisions. The main topics in the postoperative period are thromboprophylaxis and the use of surgical drains, and both are controversial. Anticoagulation has been associated with increased risk of ecchymosis, hemarthrosis, drainage, and need for transfusion as well as significant bleeding in the gastrointestinal tract and central nervous system (Vince et al. 2007). Parvizi et al. (2007) found that a mean international normalized ratio greater than 1.5 was more prevalent in patients who developed postoperative wound complications and subsequent periprosthetic infection. Finally, patients requiring warfarin seem to have a greater incidence of deep infection, superficial infection, and other wound associated complications (McDougall et al. 2013).

The use of surgical drains for elective TJA is a common practice despite limited evidence to support routine use in noninfected cases; if used, the time of permanence of drains is not well established. Strahovnik et al. (2010) found that the duration of wound drainage did not have any influence on the incidence and duration of prolonged serous drainage; absence of drainage was not associated with PWD, but increased swelling and pain of the thigh were present in these patients. In a perspective randomized trial, Dora et al. (2007) found that to omit closed suction drainage in hip arthroplasty allowed a simpler and faster wound management without any disadvantage. Finally, a recent meta-analysis of randomized controlled trials in hip arthroplasty concludes that there is insufficient evidence to support the routine use of closed suction drainage (Chen et al. 2013). The authors found no statistical difference in wound hematomas, occurrence of postoperative deep vein thrombosis, and postoperative wound infection between groups with and without drainage.

An important issue in PWD is to understand the origin of fluid and if it represents a sign of established deep infection or of a wound closure defect; in case of early postoperative drainage with no evidence of pain, erythema, purulence, or other clinical signs of deep infection, PWD should be managed by wound care for the first 5 days.

Superficial wound cultures are not recommended in this setting: specimens obtained from a wound or a sinus tract often generate polymicrobial results and may misguide diagnosis and treatment. In literature concordance rates between sinus tracts and bone cultures range from 38 to 88 % (Cook and Farrar 1978; Esposito and Gleckman 1977; Mackowiak et al. 1978; Mousa 1997; Patzakis et al. 1994; Perry et al. 1991; Ulug et al. 2009). In a recent study, Tetreault et al. (2013) found 47.3 % of agreement between superficial and deep cultures with bacterial growth in superficial cultures in 80 % of cases without deep infection.

Deep sepsis can be ruled out with a joint aspiration and cell count, differential, and negative culture and sensitivity. There isn't a well-delineated cutoff for the levels of synovial cell count and PMN% in the infected hip arthroplasty (Parvizi et al. 2011). Schinsky et al. (2008), in a chronic setting, propose a threshold of 3,000 cells/μL for leukocytes and 80 % for PMN% for the infected hip arthroplasty. Blood cultures should be obtained if fever is present. Serum tests (erythrocyte sedimentation rate and C-reactive protein) are not useful in this setting as these markers can be elevated up to 60 days in the postoperative period, and they are affected by comedications, comorbidities, age, and sex (Bilgen et al. 2001; Larsson et al. 1992). C-reactive protein seems to be a promising marker of prosthetic joint infection when measured in synovial fluid rather than in serum: in a prospective study by Parvizi et al. (2012), a threshold of 0.06 mg/L for individual ELISA and of 3.7 mg/L for multiplex ELISA provided a sensitivity of 70 and 84 % and a specificity of 100.0 and 97.1 %, respectively. Finally promising methods for diagnosing infection are polymerase chain reaction techniques for detection of microorganisms and analysis of circulating cytokines levels (Bergin et al. 2010; Kobayashi et al. 2008).

Various interventions have been recommended in order to reduce the amount of wound drainage. Negative-pressure wound therapy (NPWT) after total hip arthroplasty was evaluated in a randomized prospective study and compared with standard dressing, and the authors demonstrated a decreased development of postoperative seromas with NPWT (Pachowsky et al. 2012). Hansen et al. (2013) reported cessation of wound drainage after total hip arthroplasty with NPWT in 76 % of cases, while the remaining 24 % required subsequent surgery. However, a previous Cochrane meta-analysis found no evidence for the effectiveness of NPWT in PWD in trauma surgery, arthroplasty, and skin graft patients (Webster et al. 2012a, b).

Antibiotic therapy is not recommended in patients with early PWD for several reasons. First of all, in the absence of signs of deep infection, an antibiotic therapy is unnecessary, and prevention of ingress of germs through draining wound should be warranted by a correct wound care. The emergence of antibiotic resistance actually represents a dramatic challenge in HAIs and any effort should be made in order to prevent this event; to avoid unnecessary and/or inadequate antibiotic prescription is mandatory. In addition antibiotic therapy can cause adverse effects. Finally administration of antibiotics could mask an underlying infection and reduce the sensitivity of microbiological cultures.

Table 26.1 Principal risk factors for multidrug-resistant (MDR) microorganism infection

Cardiovascular diseases
Chronic obstructive pulmonary disease
Chronic renal failure
Diabetes
Hemodialysis
Immunosuppression
Residence in long-term care facilities
Pressure ulcer and previous wound management
Previous antibiotic therapy (last 30 days)
Previous hospitalization (last 90 days)
Previous MDR microorganism colonization

Surgical revision is recommended after 5 days of PWD to reduce the likelihood of a subsequent prosthetic joint infection. During the procedure (exploration, adequate irrigation and debridement, exchange of modular components, and meticulous fascia and layer wound reclose), deep cultures are strongly recommended to drive antibiotic therapy (Ghanem et al. 2014).The number of samples is also important; the isolation of a microorganism from three or more independent samples is highly predictive of infection with a specificity of 99.6 % (Atkins et al. 1998). In case of negative culture (due to low bacterial burden or previous antibiotic therapy) with the presence of clinical signs of infection, an empiric antibiotic therapy covering oxacillin-resistant *Staphylococcus aureus* should be administered until further workup rules out deep infection. In this setting knowledge of local epidemiology and evaluation of patient risk factors for multidrug-resistant microorganism is fundamental to tailor antimicrobial therapy (Table 26.1). In case of positive culture, most common microorganisms and their treatment are summarized in Table 26.2. Staphylococci are the most common agents causing prosthetic joint infection (Kuiper et al. 2013; Saleh et al. 2002). For staphylococcal infections, a pathogen-specific intravenous or highly bioavailable oral antimicrobial therapy (Table 26.2) in combination with rifampin 600 mg orally daily should be administered for 2–6 weeks, followed

Key Points

- Persistent wound drainage can be defined as continued drainage for greater than 72 h.
- Persistent wound drainage is a predictor of subsequent onset of a periprosthetic joint infection.
- In the preoperative period, preventable risk factors for the development of wound infection should be corrected.
- The need for anticoagulant therapy to prevent thromboembolism must be balanced with the risk of subsequent surgical site infection.
- There is insufficient evidence to support the routine use of closed suction drainage.
- In the first 5 days, persistent wound drainage should be managed by wound care.
- Superficial wound cultures are not recommended.
- Synovial fluid white cell count and culture may help to confirm or rule out deep infection.
- Empiric antibiotic therapy is not recommended in persistent wound drainage.
- Irrigation and debridement with modular component change is recommended after 5 days of persistent wound drainage.
- Deep culture is strongly recommended during surgical procedure.
- Gram-positive microorganisms and particularly staphylococci are the most common agents causing prosthetic joint infection.
- Two to 6 weeks of intravenous or highly bioavailable oral antibiotic therapy is needed, followed by oral rifampin plus a companion oral drug.
- C-reactive protein level in the synovial fluid, analysis of circulating cytokines, and polymerase chain reaction techniques for microorganism identification may increase in the future our diagnostic accuracy.

Table 26.2 Treatment of common microorganisms causing prosthetic joint infections Osmon et al. 2013

Microorganism	Preferred treatment	Alternative treatment
Staphylococci, oxacillin susceptible	Oxacillin 2 g IV q4–6 h or ceftriaxone 2 g IV q24 h or cefazolin IV 1–2 g q8 h	Vancomycin 15 mg/kg IV q12 h or teicoplanin 10–12 mg/kg IV q12 h for 3 doses then q24 h or linezolid 600 mg IV/PO q12 h or daptomycin 6 mg/kg IV q24 h
Staphylococci, oxacillin resistant	Vancomycin 15 mg/kg IV q12 h or teicoplanin 10–12 mg/kg IV q12 h for 3 doses then q24 h	Linezolid 600 mg IV/PO q12 h or daptomycin 6 mg/kg IV q24 h
Enterococcus spp., penicillin susceptible	Penicillin G 20–24 million units IV q24 h continuously or in 6 divided doses or ampicillin sodium 12 g IV q24 h continuously or in 6 divided doses ± aminoglycoside	Vancomycin 15 mg/kg IV q12 h or daptomycin 6 mg/kg IV q24 h or linezolid 600 mg PO or IV q12 h or teicoplanin 10–12 mg/kg IV q12 h for 3 doses then q24 h
Enterococcus spp., penicillin resistant	Vancomycin 15 mg/kg IV q12 h or teicoplanin 10–12 mg/kg IV q12 h for 3 doses then q24 h ± aminoglycoside	Linezolid 600 mg PO or IV q12 h or daptomycin 6 mg/kg IV q24 h
Pseudomonas aeruginosa	Cefepime 2 g IV q8 h or meropenem 1 g IV q8 h ± aminoglycoside	Ciprofloxacin 750 mg PO bid or 400 mg IV q8 h or ceftazidime 2 g IV q8 h ± aminoglycoside
Enterobacter spp.	Cefepime 2 g IV q8 h or ertapenem 1 g IV q24 h	Ciprofloxacin 750 mg PO or 400 mg IV q8 h
Enterobacteriaceae	IV *in vitro* β-lactam or carbapenem based on in vitro susceptibilities or ciprofloxacin 750 mg PO bid	
β-hemolytic streptococci	Penicillin G 20–24 million units IV q24 h continuously or in 6 divided doses or ceftriaxone 2 g IV q24 h	Vancomycin 15 mg/kg IV q12 h

Abbreviations: *IV* intravenous, *PO* per oral

by rifampin plus a companion oral drug for a total of 3 months for a total hip arthroplasty infection (Osmon et al. 2013). Rifampin may decrease serum linezolid concentrations in combination therapy (Gebhart et al. 2007; Hoyo et al. 2012).

Best oral companions for rifampin are ciprofloxacin, levofloxacin, cotrimoxazole, and doxycycline. For other microorganisms, a pathogen-specific intravenous or highly bioavailable oral antimicrobial therapy (Table 26.2) should be administered for 4–6 weeks, followed by indefinite chronic oral antimicrobial therapy based on *in vitro* susceptibilities.

References

Adams AL, Paxton EW, Wang JQ et al (2013) Surgical outcomes of total knee replacement according to diabetes status and glycemic control, 2001 to 2009. J Bone Joint Surg Am 95(6):481

Atkins BL, Athanasou N, Deeks JJ et al (1998) Prospective evaluation of criteria for microbiological diagnosis of prosthetic-joint infection at revision arthroplasty. The OSIRIS Collaborative Study Group. J Clin Microbiol 36(10):2932
Bergin PF, Doppelt JD, Hamilton WG et al (2010) Detection of periprosthetic infections with use of ribosomal RNA-based polymerase chain reaction. J Bone Joint Surg Am 92:654–663
Bilgen O, Atici T, Durak K, Karaeminog˘ullari et al (2001) C-reactive protein values and erythrocyte sedimentation rates after total hip and total knee arthroplasty. J Int Med Res 2001;29:7–12
Butt U, Ahmad R, Aspros D et al (2011) Factors affecting wound ooze in total knee replacement. Ann R Coll Surg Engl 93(1):54
Chen ZY, Gao Y, Chen W et al (2014) Is wound drainage necessary in hip arthroplasty? A meta-analysis of randomized controlled trials. Eur J Orthop Surg Traumatol. 24(6):939–46. doi: 10.1007/s00590-013-1284-0
Clarke JV, Deakin AH, Dillon JM et al (2009) A prospective clinical audit of a new dressing design for lower limb arthroplasty wounds. J Wound Care 18(1):5
Cook FV, Farrar WE (1978) Vancomycin revisited. Ann Intern Med 88:813
Dennis DA (1997) Wound complications in total knee arthroplasty. Instr Course Lect 46:165
Dora C, von Campe A, Mengiardi B et al (2007) Simplified wound care and earlier wound recovery without closed suction drainage in elective total hip arthroplasty. A prospective randomized trial in 100 operations. Arch Orthop Trauma Surg 127(10):919–923
Eickmann T, Quane E (2010) Total knee arthroplasty closure with barbed sutures. J Knee Surg 23:163
Esposito AL, Gleckman RA (1977) Vancomycin, a second look. JAMA 238:1756
European Centre for Disease Prevention and Control (2013) Point prevalence survey of healthcare associated infections and antimicrobial use in European acute care hospitals. ECDC, Stockholm
Galat DD, McGovern SC, Larson DR et al (2009) Surgical treatment of early wound complications following primary total knee arthroplasty. J Bone Joint Surg Am 91(1):48
Gebhart BC, Barker BC, Markewitz BA (2007) Decreased serum linezolid levels in a critically ill patient receiving concomitant linezolid and rifampin. Pharmacotherapy 27(3):476–479
Ghanem E, Heppert V, Spangehl M et al (2014) Wound management. J Arthroplasty 29(Suppl 1):84–92
Gherini S, Vaughn BK, Lombardi AV Jr et al (1993) Delayed wound healing and nutritional deficiencies after total hip arthroplasty. Clin Orthop Relat Res 293:188
Greenky M, Gandhi K, Pulido L et al (2012) Preoperative anemia in total joint arthroplasty: is it associated with periprosthetic joint infection? Clin Orthop Relat Res 470(10):2695
Hansen E, Durinka JB, Costanzo JA et al (2013) Negative pressure wound therapy is associated with resolution of incisional drainage in most wounds after hip arthroplasty. Clin Orthop Relat Res 471(10):3230–3236
Hoyo I, Martínez-Pastor J, Garcia-Ramiro S et al (2012) Decreased serum linezolid concentrations in two patients receiving linezolid and rifampicin due to bone infections. Scand J Infect Dis 44(7):548–550
Iorio R, Williams KM, Marcantonio AJ et al (2012) Diabetes mellitus, hemoglobin A1C, and the incidence of total joint arthroplasty infection. J Arthroplasty 27(5):726–9.e1
Jaberi FM, Parvizi J, Haytmanek CT et al (2008) Procrastination of wound drainage and malnutrition affect the outcome of joint arthroplasty. Clin Orthop Relat Res 466(6):1368
Jamsen E, Nevalainen P, Eskelinen A et al (2012) Obesity, diabetes, and preoperative hyperglycemia as predictors of periprosthetic joint infection: a single-center analysis of 7181 primary hip and knee replacements for osteoarthritis. J Bone Joint Surg Am 94(14):e101
Khan RJ, Fick D, Yao F et al (2006) A comparison of three methods of wound closure following arthroplasty: a prospective, randomised, controlled trial. J Bone Joint Surg Br 88(2):238
Kobayashi N, Procop GW, Krebs V et al (2008) Molecular identification of bacteria from aseptically loose implants. Clin Orthop Relat Res 466:1716–1725
Kotze A, Carter LA, Scally AJ (2012) Effect of a patient blood management programme on preoperative anaemia, transfusion rate, and outcome after primary hip or knee arthroplasty: a quality improvement cycle. Br J Anaesth 108(6):943
Kuiper JW, Vos SJ, Saouti R et al (2013) Prosthetic joint-associated infections treated with DAIR (debridement, antibiotics, irrigation, and retention): analysis of risk factors and local antibiotic carriers in 91 patients. Acta Orthop 84(4):380–386
Larsson S, Thelander U, Friberg S (1992) C-reactive protein (CRP) levels after elective orthopedic surgery. Clin Orthop Relat Res 275:237–242
Lavernia CJ, Sierra RJ, Baerga L (1999) Nutritional parameters and short term outcome in arthroplasty. J Am Coll Nutr 18(3):274
Lonner JH, Lotke PA (1999) Aseptic complications after total knee arthroplasty. J Am Acad Orthop Surg 7(5):311
Mackowiak PA, Jones SR, Smith JW (1978) Diagnostic value of sinus-tract cultures in chronic osteomyelitis. JAMA 239:2772
McDougall CJ, Gray HS, Simpson PM et al (2013) Complications related to therapeutic anticoagulation in total hip arthroplasty. J Arthroplasty 28(1):187–192
Mousa HA (1997) Evaluation of sinus tract cultures in chronic bone infection. J Bone Joint Surg Br 79:567
Osmon DR, Berbari EF, Berendt AR et al (2013) Executive summary: diagnosis and management of prosthetic joint infection: clinical practice guidelines by the Infectious Diseases Society of America. Clin Infect Dis 56(1):1–10
Pachowsky M, Gusinde J, Klein A et al (2012) Negative pressure wound therapy to prevent seromas and treat

surgical incisions after total hip arthroplasty. Int Orthop 36(4):719–722

Parvizi J, Ghanem E, Joshi A et al (2007) Does "excessive" anticoagulation predispose to periprosthetic infection? J Arthroplasty 22(6 Suppl 2):24

Parvizi J, Zmistowski B, Berbari EF et al (2011) New definition for prosthetic joint infection. Clin Orthop Relat Res 469:2992–2994

Parvizi J, Jacovides C, Adeli B et al (2012) Mark B. Coventry Award: synovial C-reactive protein: a prospective evaluation of a molecular marker for periprosthetic knee joint infection. Clin Orthop Relat Res 470(1):54–60

Patel VP, Walsh M, Sehgal B et al (2007) Factors associated with prolonged wound drainage after primary total hip and knee arthroplasty. J Bone Joint Surg Am 89(1):33

Patzakis MJ, Wilkins J, Kumar J et al (1994) Comparison of the results of bacterial cultures from multiple sites in chronic osteomyelitis of long bones. A prospective study. J Bone Joint Surg Am 76:664

Perry CR, Pearson RL, Miller GA (1991) Accuracy of cultures of material from swabbing of the superficial aspect of the wound and needle biopsy in the preoperative assessment of osteomyelitis. J Bone Joint Surg Am 73:745

Rao N, Cannella B, Crossett LS et al (2008) A preoperative decolonization protocol for staphylococcus aureus prevents orthopaedic infections. Clin Orthop Relat Res 466(6):1343–1348

Saleh K, Olson M, Resig S et al (2002) Predictors of wound infection in hip and knee joint replacement: results from a 20 year surveillance program. J Orthop Res 20(3):506–515

Schinsky MF, Della Valle CJ, Sporer SM et al (2008) Perioperative testing for joint infection in patients undergoing revision total hip arthroplasty. J Bone Joint Surg Am 90:1869–1875

Strahovnik A, Fokter SK, Kotnik M (2010) Comparison of drainage techniques on prolonged serous drainage after total hip arthroplasty. J Arthroplasty 25(2):244–248

Tetreault MW, Wetters NG, Aggarwal VK et al (2013) Should draining wounds and sinuses associated with hip and knee arthroplasties be cultured? J Arthroplasty 28(8 Suppl):133–136

Ulug M, Ayaz C, Celen MK et al (2009) Are sinus-track cultures reliable for identifying the causative agent in chronic osteomyelitis? Arch Orthop Trauma Surg 129:1565

Vince K, Chivas D, Droll KP (2007) Wound complications after total knee arthroplasty. J Arthroplasty 22(4 Suppl 1):39

Webster J, Scuffham P, Sherriff KL et al (2012a) Negative pressure wound therapy for skin grafts and surgical wounds healing by primary intention. Cochrane Database Syst Rev 4, CD009261 [PUBMED]

Webster J, Scuffham P, Sherriff KL et al (2012b) Negative pressure wound therapy for skin grafts and surgical wounds healing by primary intention. Cochrane Database Syst Rev 18:4

Weiss AP, Krackow KA (1993) Persistent wound drainage after primary total knee arthroplasty. J Arthroplasty 8(3):285–289